D0023492

Handbook of
The Biology of Aging

The Handbooks of Aging
Consisting of Three Volumes

Critical comprehensive reviews of
research knowledge, theories, concepts, and issues

Editor-in-Chief
James E. Birren

Handbook of the Biology of Aging
Edited by Edward J. Masoro and Steven N. Austad

Handbook of the Psychology of Aging
Edited by James E. Birren and K. Warner Schaie

Handbook of Aging and the Social Sciences
Edited by Robert H. Binstock and Linda K. George

Handbook of
The Biology of Aging

Sixth Edition

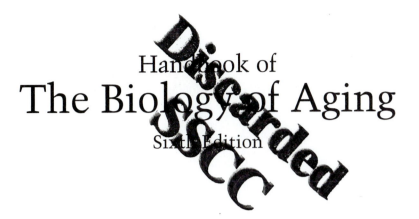

Editors

Edward J. Masoro and Steven N. Austad

AMSTERDAM • BOSTON • HEIDELBERG • LONDON
NEW YORK • OXFORD • PARIS • SAN DIEGO
SAN FRANCISCO • SINGAPORE • SYDNEY • TOKYO

ELSEVIER

Academic Press is an imprint of Elsevier

Academic Press is an imprint of Elsevier
30 Corporate Drive, Suite 400, Burlington, MA 01803, USA
525 B Street, Suite 1900, San Diego, California 92101-4495, USA
84 Theobald's Road, London WC1X 8RR, UK

This book is printed on acid-free paper. ∞

Library of Congress Cataloging-in-Publication Data
Handbook of the biology of aging/editors, E.J. Masoro and S.N. Austad.— 6th ed.
     p. cm. — (The handbooks of aging)
Includes bibliographical references and index.
ISBN 0-12-088387-2 (alk. paper)
1. Aging—Physiological aspects—Handbooks, manuals, etc.   I. Masoro, Edward J.
II. Austad, Steven N., 1946–   III. Series.
QP86.H35 2006
612.6'7—dc22
                                                                2005023985

British Library Cataloguing in Publication Data
A catalogue record for this book is available from the British Library

ISBN 13: 978-0-12-088387-5
ISBN 10: 0-12-088387-2

For all information on all Elsevier Academic Press publications
visit our Web site at www.books.elsevier.com

Printed in the United States of America

05 06 07 08 09 10   9 8 7 6 5 4 3 2 1

Contents

Section II: Non-Mammalian Models

Section III: Mammalian Models

Contributors

Numbers in parentheses indicate the pages on which the authors' contributions begin.

Steven N. Austad (242, 449, 512), University of Texas Health Science Center, Department of Cellular and Structural Biology, Barshop Institute for Longevity and Aging Studies, San Antonio, TX 78245-3207

Nir Barzilai (498), Institute of Aging Research, Division of Endocrinology, Department of Medicine, Albert Einstein College of Medicine, Bronx, NY 10461

Deborah Bell (105), Department of Internal Medicine, University of Kentucky, Lexington, KY 40536-0093

Richard Beyer (295), Department of Environmental Health, University of Washington, Seattle, WA 98105

Richard J. Boys (334), School of Mathematics and Statistics, University of Newcastle, Newcastle Upon Tyne, NEJ7U, UK

Anja K. Brunet-Rossini (243), Department of Biology, Cowley Hall, University of Wisconsin-La Crosse, La Crosse, WI 54601

Joep M. S. Burger (217), Department of Genetics, University of Georgia, Athens, GA 30602-7223

Christy S. Carter (534), Department of Internal Medicine, Section on Geriatrics and Gerontology, Wake Forrest University Health Sciences, Winston-Salem, NC 27147

James W. Curtsinger (267), Department of Ecology, Evolution, and Behavior, University of Minnesota, MN 55108

Lawrence A. Donehower (149), Department of Molecular Virology and Microbiology, Baylor College of Medicine, Houston, TX 77030

Melissa Dumble (149), Department of Molecular Virology and Microbiology, Baylor College of Medicine, Houston, TX 77030

Kenneth M. Fedorka (217), Department of Genetics, University of Georgia, Athens, GA 30602-7223

Thomas Flatt (415), Department of Ecology and Evolutionary Biology, Brown University, Providence, RI 02912

Daniel Ford (400), Molecular and Computational Biology Program, Department of Biological Sciences, University of Southern California, Los Angeles, CA 90089-1340

Catherine Gatza (149), Department of Molecular Virology and Microbiology, Baylor College of Medicine, Houston, TX 77030

Natalia S. Gavrilova (3, 267), Center on Aging, NORC/University of Chicago, Chicago, IL 60637-2745

Leonid A. Gavrilov (3, 267), Center on Aging, NORC/University of Chicago, Chicago, IL 60637-2745

Colin S. Gillespie (334), Institute for Aging and Health, University of Newcastle, Newcastle Upon Tyne, NE46BE UK

Tamara R. Golden (124), Buck Institute for Age Research, Novato, CA 94945

Samuel T. Henderson (360), Institute for Behavioral Genetics, University of Colorado at Boulder, Boulder, CO 80309

George Hinkal (149), Department of Molecular Virology and Microbiology, Baylor College of Medicine, Houston, TX 77030

Konrad T. Howitz (63), BIOMOL Research Laboratories, Inc., Plymouth Meeting, PA 19462

F. Noel Hudson (295), Houston, TX 77040

Felicity Johnson (124), Royston Park SA 5070, Australia

Thomas E. Johnson (360), Institute for Behavioral Genetics, University of Colorado at Boulder, Boulder, CO 80309

Matt Kaeberlein (295), Genome Sciences, University of Washington, Seattle, WA 98195

Thomas B. L. Kirkwood (334), Institute for Aging and Health, University of Newcastle, Newcastle General Hospital, Newcastle Upon Tyne, NE46BE, UK

Jeff W. Leips (181), Department of Biological Sciences, University of Maryland Baltimore County, Baltimore, MD 21250

Nancy Linford (295), Department of Pathology, Box 357705, University of Washington, Seattle, WA 98195-7705

Trudy F. C. Mackay (181), Department of Genetics, North Carolina State University, Raleigh, NC 27695

Edward J. Masoro (43), Department of Physiology at the University of Texas Health Science Center at San Antonio, San Antonio, Texas 78229-3900

Roger J. M. McCarter (470), Department of BioBehavioral Health, Pennsylvania State University, PA 16803

Simon Melov (124), Buck Institute for age Research, Novato, CA 94945

Richard A. Miller (512), University of Michigan, Ann Arbor, MI 48109-0940

Lynette Moore (149), Department of Molecular Virology and Microbiology, Baylor College of Medicine, Houston, TX 77030

Karl Morten (124), Witney, Oxon, OX29 6TD, UK

Radhika Muzumdar (498), Institute of Aging Research, Division of Endocrinology, Department of Medicine, Albert Einstein College of Medicine, Bronx, NY 10461

Elena G. Pasyukova (181), Institute of Molecular Genetics of the Russian, Academy of Sciences, Moscow 123182, Russia

Andrej Podlutsky (449), Geriatric Research, Education and Clinical Center of the South Texas, Veterans Health Care System, San Antonio, TX 78284

David Pritchard (295), Department of Pathology, University of Washington, Seattle, WA 98195

Carole J. Procter (334), Institute for Aging and Health, University of Newcastle, Newcastle Upon Tyne, NE46BE, UK

Daniel E. L. Promislow (217), Department of Genetics, University of Georgia, Athens, GA 30602-7223

Peter S. Rabinovitch (295), Department of Pathology, University of Seattle, WA 98195-7705

Shane L. Rea (360), Institute of Behavioral Genetics, University of Colorado at Boulder, Boulder, CO 80309

Marielisa Rincon (498), Institute for Aging Research and Diabetes Center, Bronx, NY 10461

Natalia V. Roshina (181), Institute of Molecular Genetics of the Russian, Academy of Sciences, Moscow 123182, Russia

Enrique Samper (124), Buck Institute for Age Research, Novato, CA 94945

Daryl P. Shanley (334), Institute for Aging and Health, University of Newcastle, Newcastle General Hospital, Newcastle Upon Tyne, NE46BE, UK

David A. Sinclair (63), Department of Pathology, Boston, MA 02115

William E. Sonntag (534), Department of Physiology and Pharmacology, Wake Forrest University School of Medicine, Winston-Salem, NC 27157-1083

Marc Tatar (415), Division of Biology and Medicine, Department of Ecology and Evolutionary Biology, Brown University, Providence, RI 02916

John Tower (400), Molecular and Computational Biology Program, Department of Biology, University of southern California, Los Angeles, CA 90089-1340

Meng-Ping Tu (415), Department of Genetics and Development, College of Physicians and Surgeons, Columbia University, New York, NY 10032

Gary Van Zant (105), Departments of Internal Medicine and Physiology, University of Kentucky, Markey Cancer Center, Lexington, KY 40536-0093

Darren J. Wilkenson (334), School of Mathematics and Statistics, University of Newcastle, Newcastle Upon Tyne, NEJ7RU, UK

Phyllis M. Wise (570), Department of Physiology and Biophysics, University of Washington, Seattle, WA 98195

Foreword

This volume is one of a series of three handbooks of aging: *Handbook of the Biology of Aging, Handbook of the Psychology of Aging,* and *Handbook of Aging and the Social Sciences. The Handbooks of Aging* series, now in its sixth edition, reflects the exponential growth of research and publications in aging research, as well as the growing interest in the subject of aging. Stimulation of research on aging by government and private foundation sponsorship has been a major contributor to the growth of publications. There has also been an increase in the number of university and college courses related to aging. *The Handbooks of Aging* have helped to organize courses and seminars on aging by providing knowledge bases for instruction and for new steps in research.

The Handbooks are used by academic researchers, graduate students, and professionals, for access and interpretation of contemporary research literature about aging. They serve both as a reference and as organizational tool for integrating a wide body of research that is often cross disciplinary. *The Handbooks* not only provide updates about what is known about the many processes of aging, but also interpretations of findings by well informed and experienced scholars in many disciplines. Aging is a complex process of change involving influences of a biological, behavioral, social, and environmental nature.

Understanding aging is one of the major challenges facing science in the 21st century. Interest in research on aging has become a major focus in science and in the many professions that serve aging populations. Growth of interest in research findings about aging and their interpretation has been accelerated with the growth of populations of older persons in developed and developing countries. As more understanding has been gained about genetic factors that contribute to individual prospects for length of life and life limiting and disabling diseases, researchers have simultaneously become more aware of the environmental factors that modulate the expression of genetic predispositions. These *Handbooks* both reflect and encourage an ecological view of aging, in which aging is seen as a result of diverse forces interacting. These *Handbooks* can help to provide information to guide planning as nations face "age quakes" due to shifts in the size of their populations of young and older persons.

In addition to the rise in research publications about aging, there has been a dramatic change in the availability of scientific literature since the first editions of *The Handbooks of Aging* were published. There are now millions of references available on line. This increases the need for integration of information.

The Handbooks help to encourage integration of information from across disciplines and methods of gathering data about aging.

With so much new information available, one of the editorial policies has been the selection of new chapter authors and subject matter in each successive edition. This allows *The Handbooks* to present new points of view, to keep current, and to explore new topics in which new research has emerged. The sixth edition is thus virtually wholly new, and is not simply an update of previous editions.

I want to thank the editors of the individual volumes for their cooperation, efforts, and wisdom in planning and reviewing the chapters. Without their intense efforts and experience *The Handbooks* would not be possible.

I thank Edward J. Masoro and Steven N. Austad, editors of the *Handbook of the Biology of Aging,* the editors of the *Handbook of Aging and the Social Sciences*, Robert H. Binstock and Linda K. George, and their associate editors, Stephen J. Cutler, Jon Hendricks, and James H. Schulz; and my co-editor of the *Handbook of the Psychology of Aging,* K. Warner Schaie, and the associate editors, Ronald P. Abeles, Margaret Gatz, and Timothy A. Salthouse.

I also want to express my appreciation to Nikki Levy, Publisher at Elsevier, whose experience, long term interest, and cooperation have facilitated the publication of *The Handbooks* through their many editions.

James E. Birren

Preface

The past five years has been a lifetime in aging research. That amount of time has passed since the previous (5th) edition of the *Handbook of the Biology of Aging*. During the year 2000, when the chapters of the previous edition were being written, the research community had at its disposal complete gene sequences of only two multicellular animals (*C. elegans* and *Drosophila melanogaster*). Since then, we have added to that list mice, rats, humans, and a dozen more species, with another 30 species "in process." In the year 2000, we were still coming to terms with claims that a mutation in one gene could extend life and preserve health in a mammal. Now the existence of nine such genes has been documented in mice, and by the time you read this, the total will no doubt have reached double figures. All this is another way of saying that we have a lot of ground to cover in this, the 6th edition of the *Handbook of the Biology of Aging*.

This edition, as previous ones, provides in-depth coverage of the latest and best research as summarized and interpreted by leading investigators in the field. This volume has a particular emphasis on theoretical and technical issues. The first chapter introduces to a wide audience a conceptual approach to aging from the field of engineering, which has considerable relevance for molecular biologists who often think in terms of simple biochemical pathways. That chapter also places a premium on refined demographic analyses of aging, as does a later chapter

recounting how genetics and demography interact in *Drosophila* studies. Other conceptual chapters cover the complex relation between aging and disease, the complexity of the genetic architecture of aging, and the use of computer modeling in the biology of aging. The evolutionary biology of aging crops up in a host of chapters, but specifically in the chapter on senescence in nature and the thoughtful discussion of where future evolutionary studies of aging are likely to go. Readers will also be updated on the theory of hormesis and life extension and how it continues to gain currency in the field. The roles in the aging process of hematopoietic stem cells, mitochondria, and the tumor suppressor gene p53 are also covered, as are issues in the application of the still emerging technology of DNA microarray analysis to aging studies.

Progress in dissecting the genetics and neuroendocrinology of aging in invertebrate models has been so dramatic that five years of progress is difficult to summarize. Yet our authors in Section II, and several in other chapters, perform this job admirably. At the end of that section, there is a chapter that asks what the limits might be to what we can learn about mammalian aging from the study of invertebrates.

The final section is devoted to mammalian aging—either of particular systems such as the muscles or the impact of certain processes such as carbohydrate metabolism or the growth-hormone/IGF-1 system. The mammalian genetics of growth, aging, and their likely relationship also receives a full chapter treatment. The last chapter covers a topic with timely relevance to the modern human condition: female reproductive aging and the complex interplay of brain and ovary that it involves.

We are grateful to the outside reviewers of our chapters: D. J. Anderson, James R. Carey, James R. Cypser, Caleb E. Finch, Kevin Flurkey, Jeff Halter, Eun-Soo Han, Russel Hepple, Peter Hornsby, Pamela L. Larsen, Marc Mangel, James F. Nelson, Linda Partridge, T. T. Samaras, and Heidi Scrable. We are also thankful to our authors, not only for their contributed chapters, but for the alacrity with which they made helpful comments on one another's chapters.

Edward J. Masoro
Steven N. Austad

About the Editors

Edward J. Masoro

Dr. Masoro is Professor Emeritus in the Department of Physiology at the University of Texas Health Science Center at San Antonio (UTHSCSA) where from September of 1973 though May of 1991 he served as Chairman. He was the founding Director of the Aging Research and Education Center of UTHSCSA, which as of 2004 became the Barshop Institute of Longevity and Aging Studies. He now serves as a member of that institute.

Dr. Masoro was the recipient of the 1989 Allied-Signal Achievement Award in Aging Research. In 1990, he received a Geriatric Leadership Academic Award from the National Institute on Aging and the Robert W. Kleemeier Award from the Gerontological Society of America. In 1991, he received a medal of honor from the University of Pisa for Achievements in Gerontology, and in 1993, Dr. Masoro received the Distinguished Service Award from the Association of Chairmen of Departments of Physiology. In addition, he received the 1995 Irving Wright Award of Distinction of the American Federation for Aging Research and the 1995 Glenn Foundation Award. He served as President of the Gerontological Society of America from 1994–1995, as Chairman of the Aging Review Committee of the National Institute on Aging (NIA), and as Chairman of the Board of Scientific Counselors of the NIA.

Dr. Masoro has held faculty positions at Queen's University (Canada), Tufts University School of Medicine, University of Washington, and Medical College of Pennsyvania. Since 1975, Dr. Masoro's research has focused on the influence of food restriction on aging. He has served or is serving in an editorial role for 10 journals and from January 1992 through December 1995, he was the Editor of the *Journal of Gerontology: Biological Sciences*.

Steven N. Austad

Dr. Austad is currently Professor in the Department of Cellular and Structural Biology and the Barshop Institute for Longevity and Aging Studies at the University of Texas Health Science Center at San Antonio. His research centers on the comparative biology of aging and the development of new animal models for aging research.

Dr. Austad was the recipient of the 2003 Robert W. Kleemeier Award from the Gerontological Society of America. He is also a Fellow of the Gerontological Society of America and a past Chair of the Biological Sciences Section of that organization. He received the Phi Kappa Phi/University of Idaho Alumni Assocation's Distinguished Faculty Award, the Fifth Nathan A. Shock Award, and shared the

Geron Corporation-Samuel Goldstein Distinguished Publication Award with former graduate student John. P. Phelan. Previously, he served on the Science Advisory Board of National Public Radio. He is currently an Associate Editor of the *Journals of Gerontology: Biological Sciences* and a Section Editor of *Aging Cell* and *Neurobiology of Aging*. His trade book, *Why We Age* (1997), has been translated into seven languages. He frequently writes and lectures to the general public on topics related to the biology of aging and ethical issues associated with medically extending life.

Section I:

Conceptual and Technical Issues

Chapter 1

Reliability Theory of Aging and Longevity

Leonid A. Gavrilov and Natalia S. Gavrilova

I. Introduction

There is growing interest in scientific explanations of aging and in the search for a general theory that can explain what aging is and why and how it happens.

There is also a need for a general theoretical framework that would allow researchers to handle an enormous amount of diverse observations related to aging phenomena. Empirical observations on aging have become so abundant that a special four-volume encyclopedia, *The Encyclopedia of Aging* (1,591 pages), is now required for even partial coverage of the accumulated facts (Ekerdt, 2002). To transform these numerous and diverse observations into a comprehensive body of knowledge—a general theory of species aging and longevity—is required.

The prevailing research strategy now is to focus on the molecular level in the hopes of understanding the proverbial nuts and bolts of the aging process. In accordance with this approach, many aging theories explain the aging of organ-isms through the aging of organism components. However, this circular reasoning of assuming aging in order to "explain" aging eventually leads to a logical dead end because when moving in succession from the aging of organisms to the aging of organs, tissues, and cells, we eventually come to atoms, which are known not to age. A situation with non-aging components exists not only at the level of atoms, but it may also be observed at higher levels of system organization when its components fail at random with a constant risk of failure independent on age. Even such complex biological structures as cells may sometimes demonstrate a non-aging behavior when their loss follows a simple law of radioactive decay (Burns *et al.*, 2002; Clarke *et al.*, 2000, 2001a,b; Heintz, 2000).

Thus, we come to the following basic question on the origin of aging: How can we explain the aging of a system built of non-aging elements?

This question invites us to start thinking about the possible systemic nature of aging and to wonder whether aging may be a property of the system as a whole. In other words, perhaps we need to broaden our vision and be more concerned with the bigger picture of the aging phenomenon rather than its details.

To illustrate the need for a broad vision, consider the following questions:

- Would it be possible to understand a newspaper article by looking at it through an electronic microscope?
- Would the perception of a picture in an art gallery be deeper and more comprehensive at the shortest possible distance from it?

Evolutionary perspective on aging and longevity is one way to stay focused on the bigger picture (see recent reviews by Charlesworth, 2000; Gavrilova & Gavrilov, 2002; Martin, 2002; Partridge & Gems, 2002). Evolutionary explanations of aging and limited longevity of biological species are based on two major evolutionary theories: the mutation accumulation theory (Charlesworth, 2001; Medawar, 1946) and the antagonistic pleiotropy theory (Williams, 1957). These two theories can be briefly summarized as follows:

1. **Mutation accumulation theory:** From the evolutionary perspective, aging is an inevitable result of the declining force of natural selection with age. For example, a mutant gene that kills young children will be strongly selected against (will not be passed to the next generation), whereas a lethal mutation that affects only people over the age of 80 will experience no selection because people with this mutation will have already passed it on to their offspring by that age. Over successive generations, late-acting deleterious mutations will accumulate, leading to an increase in mortality rates late in life.

2. **Antagonistic pleiotropy theory:** Late-acting deleterious genes may even be favored by selection and be actively accumulated in populations if they have beneficial effects early in life.

Note that these two theories of aging are not mutually exclusive, and both evolutionary mechanisms may operate at the same time. The main difference between the two theories is that in the mutation accumulation theory, genes with negative effects at old age accumulate passively from one generation to the next, whereas in the antagonistic pleiotropy theory, these genes are actively kept in the gene pool by selection (Le Bourg, 2001). The actual relative contribution of each evolutionary mechanism to species aging has not yet been determined, and this scientific problem is the main focus of current research in evolutionary biology.

Evolutionary theories demonstrate that taking a step back from too-close consideration of the details over the "nuts and bolts" of the aging process helps us to gain a broader vision of the aging problem. The remaining question is whether the evolutionary perspective represents the ultimate general theoretical framework for explanations of aging. Or perhaps there may be even more general theories of aging, one step further removed from the particular details?

The main limitation of evolutionary theories of aging is that they are applicable only to systems that reproduce themselves, because these theories are based on the idea of natural selection and the notion of declining force of natural selection with age.

However, aging is a very general phenomenon—it is also observed in technical devices (such as cars), which do not reproduce themselves in a sexual or any other way and which are, therefore, not subject to evolution through natural selection. For this simple reason, the evolutionary explanation of aging based on the idea of declining force of natural selection with age is not applicable to aging technical devices. Thus, there may be a more general explanation of aging, beyond mutation accumulation and antagonistic pleiotropy theories.

The quest for a general explanation of aging (age-related increase in failure rates), applicable both to technical devices and biological systems, invites us to consider the general theory of systems failure known as *reliability theory* (Barlow & Proschan, 1975; Barlow *et al.*, 1965; Gavrilov, 1978; Gavrilov & Gavrilova, 1991, 2001b, 2003b, 2004b,c; Gavrilov *et al.*, 1978).

Reliability theory was historically developed to describe the failure and aging of complex electronic (military) equipment, but the theory itself is a very general theory based on mathematics (probability theory) and a systems approach (Barlow & Proschan, 1975; Barlow *et al.*, 1965). The theory may therefore also be useful in describing and understanding the aging and failure of biological systems. It may be useful in several ways: first, by providing a kind of scientific language (definitions and cross-cutting principles), helping researchers create a logical framework for organizing numerous and diverse observations on aging into a coherent picture. Second, it helps researchers develop an intuition and understanding of the main principles of the aging process through consideration of simple mathematical models, having some features of a real world. Third, reliability theory is useful for generating and testing specific predictions, as well as deeper analyses of already collected data. The purpose of this chapter is to review some applications of reliability theory to the problem of biological aging.

II. General Overview of the Reliability Theory Approach

Reliability theory is a body of ideas, mathematical models, and methods aimed at predicting, estimating, understanding, and optimizing the life span and failure distributions of systems and their components (adapted from Barlow & Proschan, 1975). Reliability theory allows researchers to predict the age-related failure kinetics for a system of given architecture (reliability structure) and given reliability of its components.

A. Definition of Aging and Non-Aging Systems

A reliability-engineering approach to biological aging is appealing because it provides a common scientific language (general framework) for scientists working in different areas of aging research, helping to overcome disruptive specialization and allowing researchers to understand each other.

Specifically, reliability theory helps researchers define more clearly what *is* aging. In reliability theory, *aging* is defined as a phenomenon of *increasing risk of failure* with *the passage of time (age)*. If the risk of failure is not increasing with age (the "old is as good as new" principle), then there is no aging in terms of reliability theory, even if the calendar age of a system is increasing. For example, clocks that count time perfectly are not aging according to reliability theory (although they have a perfect "biomarker" for their continuous age changes—a displayed time and date). Thus, the regular and progressive changes over time *per se* do not constitute aging unless they produce some deleterious outcome (failures). In terms of reliability theory, the *dating problem* of determining the system *age* (time elapsed since system creation) is different from the *performance assessment problem* of a system's *aging* (old becoming not as good as new). Perfect clocks having an ideal marker of their increasing age (time readings) are not aging, but progressively failing clocks are aging (although their "biomarkers" of age at the clock face may stop at a "forever young" date).

Moving to a biological example, we can say that the formation of regular seasonal tree rings tells us everything about tree age but little about tree aging. Moreover, a progressive disruption of the healthy formation of tree rings would indicate tree aging (although this disruption obscures the determination of tree age). In terms of reliability theory, the "biomarkers" of age used in forensics to estimate human ages may have nothing to do with human aging, no matter how accurate these "biomarkers" are in calendar age prediction. For example, an aspartate racemization in the teeth may be ideal for age estimation but not necessarily informative for predicting an increasing risk of death or other types of failure. On the other hand, loss of motor neurons with age would be highly relevant to the problem of human aging, no matter how poorly this loss is correlated with a person's age. These examples illustrate a fundamental difference between *biomarkers of age* (focused on the dating problem of accurate age determination) and *biomarkers of aging* (focused on the performance problem of system deterioration over time).

Thus, reliability theory helps to resolve a confusion that existed in biological aging research when some really important changes related to system deterioration over time were not properly discriminated from other neutral or benign changes closely correlated with calendar age. Reliability theory helps to clarify the difference between age (the passage of time) and aging (deterioration with age)—

concepts that are often confused with each other.[1]

In terms of reliability theory, it is conceivable to imagine at least theoretically that some biological species may not demonstrate aging in certain conditions, although their age is always increasing. "Anti-aging" intervention, according to reliability theory, is not an oxymoron incompatible with the laws of Nature (reversing time), but rather refers to any feasible intervention that delays or prevents "the old becoming not as good as new." Later we will show that non-aging systems are common both in reliability theory and in the real physical world, so becoming old is not synonymous with aging.

B. Notion of System's Failure

The concept of failure is important to the analysis of a system's reliability. In reliability theory, failure is defined as the *event* when a required function is terminated (Rausand & Høyland, 2003). In other words, failure occurs when the system deviates from the optimistically anticipated and

[1]The term *aging* is commonly used by biogerontologists and the public as a synonym to the word *senescence* (progressive deterioration with age). This interpretation of *aging* fits well with the reliability-theory approach, although the term *senescence* itself is not common in reliability theory. The problem with the term *senescence* is that it focuses too narrowly on old ages, when the senescent phenotypes become apparent (e.g., frailty). The term *aging* is more inclusive because it covers any age-related decline in performance, even if its starts early in life (e.g., an increase in human death rates after age 15). See also the second chapter of this book for a critique of other too-broad definitions of aging (Masoro, 2005). It remains to be seen whether the reliability-theory definition of aging will be universally accepted in the future or will be limited to its use in a specialized way as presented in this chapter.

desired behavior (it "fails"). Failures are often classified in two groups:

1. Degradation failures, where the system or component no longer functions properly, and

2. Catastrophic or fatal failures—the end of a system's or a component's life.

Examples of degradation failures in humans would be an onset of different types of health impairments, diseases, or disabilities, whereas catastrophic or fatal failures obviously correspond to death. The notions of aging and failure are related to each other in the following way: when the risk of failure outcomes increases with age ("old is not as good as new"), this is aging by definition. Note that according to reliability theory, aging is not just growing old; instead, aging is a degradation leading to failure (adverse health outcomes)—becoming sick, disabled, frail, and dead. Therefore, from a reliability-theory perspective, the notion of *healthy aging* is an oxymoron, like a healthy dying or a healthy disease. More appropriate terms instead of *healthy aging*, *successful aging*, or *aging well* would be *delayed aging*, *postponed aging*, *slow aging*, *arrested aging*, *negligible aging (senescence)*, or, hopefully, *aging reversal*.

Because the reliability definition of biological aging is linked to health failures (adverse health outcomes, including death), aging without diseases is just as inconceivable as dying without death. Diseases and disabilities are an integral part (outcomes) of the aging process. Not every disease is related to aging, but every progression of disease with age has some relevance to aging: aging is a "maturation" of diseases with age. A more detailed discussion of the relationship between aging and diseases is provided in the second chapter of this book (Masoro, 2005).

Reliability theory also allows us to introduce more "physiological" definitions of failure that are not limited to such failure outcomes as disease, disability, and death but describe a failure in performance tests for speed, strength, endurance, and so on. For example, it is possible to study the age dynamics of failure in sports competitions (marathon records, etc.), thereby making use of rich sports records for the purpose of scientific research on aging. Thus, reliability theory may be useful in studying "physiological" aging too.

Note that a system may have an aging behavior for one particular type of failure, but it may remain as good as new for some other type of failure. Thus, the notion of aging is outcome-specific—it requires specifying a particular type of failure (or group of failures) via which the system deteriorates.

Consequently, legitimate anti-aging interventions may be outcome-specific too, and limited to postponing some specific adverse health outcomes. *Aging* is likely to be a summary term for many different processes leading to various types of degradation failures, and each of these processes deserves to be studied and prevented.[2]

---

[2]One may wonder whether hip replacement surgery would qualify as an "anti-aging intervention" according to its description here. The answer to this question is not as simple as the question itself. It is conceivable that hip replacement therapy may prevent some patients from physical inactivity, stress, depression, loss of appetite, malnutrition, and drug overuse. The result may be that further progression of some diseases and disabilities could indeed slow down compared to patients who did not receive this treatment. In this case we can say that hip replacement therapy helps to oppose aging for some specific types of degradation failures in a particular group of patients (very limited anti-aging effect). It is true, however, that the term *anti-aging intervention* is usually associated with hopes for something far more radical, such as aging reversal in the future, applicable to all older people.

C. Basic Ideas and Formulas of Reliability Theory

Reliability of the system (or its component) refers to its ability to operate properly according to a specified standard (Crowder *et al.*, 1991). Reliability is described by the *reliability function* S(x), which is the probability that a system (or component) will carry out its mission through time x (Rigdon & Basu, 2000). The reliability function (also called the *survival function*) evaluated at time x is just the probability, *P*, that the *failure time X* is beyond time x, $P(X > x)$. Thus, the reliability function is defined as follows:

$$S(x) = \text{P } (X > x) = 1 - \text{P } (X \le x)$$
$$= 1 - F(x)$$

where *F(x)* is a standard *cumulative distribution function* in the probability theory (Feller, 1968). The best illustration for the reliability function *S(x)* is a survival curve describing the proportion of those still alive by time x (the l_x column in life tables).

Failure rate, $\mu(x)$, or instantaneous risk of failure, also called the *hazard rate, h(x)*, or mortality force, is defined as the relative rate for reliability function decline:

$$\mu(x) = -\frac{dS_x}{S_x dx} = -\frac{d \ln S_x}{dx}$$

In those cases when the failure rate is constant (does not increase with age), we have a *non-aging system* (component) that does not deteriorate (does not fail more often) with age:

$$\mu(x) = k = \text{const}$$

The reliability function of non-aging systems (components) is described by the *exponential distribution*:

$$S(x) = S_0 e^{-kx}$$

This *failure law* describes "life span" distribution of atoms of radioactive elements and, therefore, is often called an *exponential decay law*. Interestingly, this failure law is observed in many wild populations with high extrinsic mortality (Finch, 1990; Gavrilov & Gavrilova, 1991). This kind of distribution is observed if failure (death) occurs entirely by chance, and it is also called a "one-hit model" or a "first order kinetics." The non-aging behavior of a system can be detected graphically when the logarithm of the survival function decreases with age in a linear fashion.

Recent studies found that at least some cells in the aging organism might demonstrate a non-aging behavior.[3] Specifically, the rate of neuronal death does not increase with age in a broad spectrum of aging-related neurodegenerative conditions (Heintz, 2000). These include 12 different models of photoreceptor degeneration, "excitotoxic" cell death *in vitro*, loss of cerebellar granule cells in a mouse model, and Parkinson's and Huntington's diseases (Clarke *et al.*, 2000). In this range of diseases, five different neuronal types are affected. In each of these cases, the rate of cell death is best fit by an exponential decay law with constant risk of death independent of age (death by chance only), arguing against models of progressive cell deterioration and aging (Clarke *et al.*, 2000, 2001a). An apparent lack of cell aging is also observed in the case of amyotrophic lateral sclerosis (ALS) (Clarke *et al.*, 2001a), retinitis pigmentosa (Burns *et al.*, 2002; Clarke *et al.*, 2000, 2001a; Massoff *et al.*, 1990), and idiopathic Parkinsonism (Calne, 1994; Clarke *et al.*, 2001b; Schulzer *et al.*, 1994).

---

[3]Non-aging behavior of cells should not be confused with cells' immortality or their ability to self-replicate indefinitely. Instead non-aging behavior means that the risk of cell death (or loss of function) does not depend on cell age.

These observations correspond well with another observation that "an impressive range of cell functions in most organs remain unimpaired throughout the life span" (Finch, 1990, p. 425). These unimpaired functions might reflect the "no-aging" property known as "old as good as new" in survival analysis (Klein & Moerschberger, 1997, p. 38). Thus, we come again to the following fundamental question about the origin of aging: how can we explain the aging of a system built of non-aging elements? This question invites us to think about the possible systemic nature of aging and to wonder whether aging may be a property of the system as a whole. We would again like to emphasize the importance of looking at the bigger picture of the aging phenomenon in addition to its details, and we will suggest a possible answer to the posed question later in this chapter.

If failure rate increases with age, we have an *aging system* (component) that deteriorates (fails more often) with age. There are many failure laws for aging systems, and the most famous one in biology is the *Gompertz law* with exponential increase of the failure rates with age, which is observed for many biological species including humans (Finch, 1990; Gavrilov & Gavrilova, 1991; Gompertz, 1825; Makeham, 1860; Strehler, 1978):

$$\mu(x) = Re^{\alpha x}$$

where x is age, while R and α are positive parameters.

We will show later that there are some exceptions to the Gompertz law and that it is usually applicable within some age windows rather than the entire range of all possible ages.

According to the Gompertz law, the logarithm of failure rates increases linearly with age. This is often used in order to illustrate graphically the validity of the Gompertz law—the data are plotted in the semi-log scale (known as the Gompertz plot) to check whether the logarithm of the failure rate is indeed increasing with age in a linear fashion.

For technical systems, one of the most popular models for the failure rate of aging systems is the Weibull model, the power-function increase in failure rates with age x (Weibull, 1939):

$$\mu(x) = ax^b$$

for $x \geq 0$, where $a, b > 0$

This law was suggested by Swedish engineer and mathematician Waloddi Weibull in 1939 to describe the strength of materials (Weibull, 1939). It is widely used to describe the aging and failure of technical devices (Barlow & Proschan, 1975; Rigdon & Basu, 2000; Weibull, 1951). According to the Weibull law, the logarithm of failure rate increases linearly with the *logarithm* of age, with a slope coefficient equal to parameter b. This is often used in order to illustrate graphically the validity of the Weibull law: the data are plotted in the log-log scale (known as the Weibull plot) to check whether the logarithm of the failure rate is indeed increasing with the *logarithm* of age in a linear fashion.

Both the Gompertz and the Weibull failure laws have their fundamental explanation rooted in reliability theory (Barlow & Proschan, 1975) and are the only two theoretically possible *limiting extreme value distributions* for systems whose life spans are determined by the first failed component (Galambos, 1978; Gumbel, 1958). In other words, as the system becomes more and more complex (contains more vital components, each being critical for survival), its life span distribution may asymptotically approach one of the only two theoretically possible limiting distributions—either Gompertz or Weibull (depending on the early kinetics of failure of system components). The two limit theorems in the statistics of extremes (Galambos, 1978; Gumbel,

1958) make the Gompertz and the Weibull failure laws as fundamental as are some other famous limiting distributions known in regular statistics, such as the normal distribution and the Poisson distribution. It is puzzling, however, why organisms prefer to die according to the Gompertz law, whereas technical devices typically fail according to the Weibull law. One possible explanation of this mystery is suggested later in this chapter.

Because of their fundamental importance for describing mortality kinetics, it may be interesting and useful to compare these two failure laws and their behavior. Figure 1.1A presents the dependence of the logarithm of the failure rate on age (Gompertz plot) for the Gompertz and the Weibull functions. Note that this dependence is strictly linear for the Gompertz function (as expected) and is concave-down for the Weibull function. So the Weibull function looks as if it is *decelerating* with age when compared to the Gompertz function.

Figure 1.1B presents the dependence of the logarithm of the failure rate on the *logarithm* of age (Weibull plot) for the Gompertz and the Weibull functions. Note that this dependence is strictly linear for the Weibull function (as anticipated) and is concave-up for the Gompertz function. So the Gompertz function looks as if it is *accelerating* with the *logarithm* of age when compared to the Weibull function.

This simple graphical method of data analysis is useful in practice because it allows researchers to determine easily whether particular data follow the Gompertz law or the Weibull law (or neither).

Two fundamental differences exist between the Weibull and the Gompertz functions. First, the Weibull function states that the system is immortal at starting age: when age x is equal to zero, the failure rate is equal to zero too, according to the Weibull formula. This means that the system should be initially

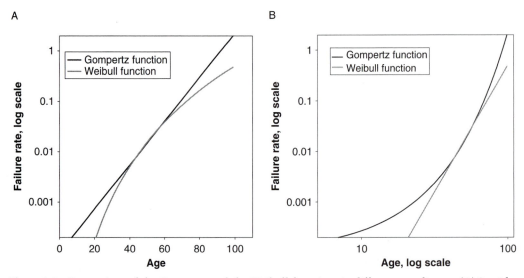

Figure 1.1 Comparison of the Gompertz and the Weibull functions in different coordinates. (A) Semi-log (Gompertz) coordinates. In this case, the Gompertz function produces a straight line, whereas the Weibull function generates a concave-down curve. (B) Log-log (Weibull) coordinates. In this case, the Weibull function produces a straight line, whereas the Gompertz function generates a concave-up curve. By plotting the death rate data in these coordinates, it is possible to determine graphically which particular formula provides the best fit (a better straight line) for the empirical data.

ideal (immortal) in order for the Weibull law to be applicable to it.

On the contrary, the Gompertz function states that the system is already vulnerable to failure at starting age: when age x is equal to zero, the failure rate is already above zero, equal to parameter R in the Gompertz formula. This means that partially damaged systems having some initial damage load are more likely to follow the Gompertz failure law, whereas initially perfect systems are more likely to follow the Weibull law. This profound difference between the two models is often obscured in real life by the period of initially high and then decreasing juvenile mortality that could not be explained by either model.

Second, there is a fundamental difference between the Gompertz and the Weibull functions regarding their response to misspecification of the starting age ("age zero"). This is an important issue because in biology there is an ambiguity regarding the choice of a "true" age, when aging starts. Legally, it is the moment of birth, which serves as a starting moment for age calculation. However, from a biological perspective, there are reasons to consider a starting age as a date either well before the birth date (the moment of conception in genetics, or a critical month of pregnancy in embryology), or long after the birth date (the moment of maturity, when the formation of a body is finally completed).

From a demographic perspective, the starting age at which aging begins is when death rates are the lowest and start to grow—this is about 10 years of age for humans. The uncertainty in starting age has very different implications for data analysis with the Gompertz and the Weibull functions. For the Gompertz function, misspecification of starting age is not as important because the shift in the age scale will still produce the same Gompertz function with the same slope parameter, α. The data generated by the

Gompertz function with different age shifts will all be linear and parallel to each other in the Gompertz plot.

The situation is very different for the Weibull function: it is linear in the Weibull plot for only one particular starting age, and any shifts in starting age produce a different function. Specifically, if a "true" starting age is larger than assumed, the resulting function will be a nonlinear concave-up curve in the Weibull plot, indicating model misspecification and leading to a bias in estimated parameters. Thus, researchers choosing the Weibull function for data analysis first have to resolve an uneasy biological problem: at what age does aging start?

An alternative graceful mathematical solution to this problem would be to move from a standard two-parameter Weibull function to a more general three-parameter Weibull function, which has an additional "location parameter" γ (Clark, 1975):

$$\mu(x) = a(x - \gamma)^b$$

for $x > \gamma$, and $\mu(x)$ is equal to zero otherwise.

Parameters of this formula, including the location parameter γ, could be estimated from the data through standard fitting procedures, thus providing a computational answer to the question "when does aging start?" However, this computational answer might be shocking to researchers unless they are familiar with the concept of initial damage load (Gavrilov & Gavrilova, 1991; 2001b; 2004a), which will be discussed later.

In addition to the Gompertz and the standard two-parameter Weibull laws, a more general failure law was suggested and theoretically justified using the system reliability theory. This law is known as the *binomial failure law* (Gavrilov & Gavrilova, 1991; 2001b), and it represents a special case of the three-parameter

Weibull function with a negative location parameter:

$$\mu(x) = a(x_0 + x)^b$$

The parameter x_0 in this formula is called the *initial virtual age of the system (IVAS)* (Gavrilov & Gavrilova, 1991, 2001b). This parameter has the dimension of time and corresponds to the age by which an initially ideal system would have accumulated as many defects as a real system already has at the starting age (at $x = 0$). In particular, when the system is initially undamaged, the initial virtual age of the system is zero, and the failure rate grows as a power function of age (the Weibull law). However, as the initial damage load increases, the failure kinetics starts to deviate from the Weibull law, and eventually it evolves to the Gompertz failure law at high levels of initial damage load. This is illustrated in Figure 1.2, which represents the Gompertz plot for the data generated by the binomial failure law with different levels of initial damage load (expressed in the units of initial virtual age).

Note that as the initial damage load increases, the failure kinetics evolves from the concave-down curves typical of the Weibull function to an almost linear dependence between the logarithm of failure rate and age (the Gompertz function). Thus, the binomial failure law unifies two different classes of distribution. The biological species dying according to the Gompertz law may have a high initial damage load, presumably because of developmental noise, and a clonal expansion of mutations that occurred in the early development (Gavrilov & Gavrilova, 1991, 2001b, 2003a, 2004a).

The concept of initial virtual age could be practically useful in analysis and interpretation of survival data because it allows us to take into account the initial damage load of the system when observations start. Moreover, this concept allows us to estimate the initial damage load

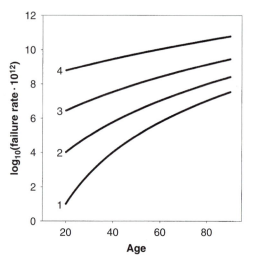

Figure 1.2 Failure kinetics of systems with different levels of initial damage. Dependence 1 is for an initially ideal system (with no damage load). Dependence 2 is for a system with an initial damage load equivalent to damage accumulated by a 20-year-old system. Dependencies 3 and 4 are for systems with an initial damage load equivalent to damage accumulated respectively by a 50-year-old system and a 100-year-old system. Note that high initial damage load transforms the Weibull curve into the Gompertz-like straight line.

1. The Weibull curve for initially ideal systems, $\mu(x) = ax^{10}$, $a = 10^{-24}\ year^{-1}$ Graphs for initially damaged systems:
2. $\mu(x) = a(20 + x)^{10}$
3. $\mu(x) = a(50 + x)^{10}$
4. $\mu(x) = a(100 + x)^{10}$

Adapted from Gavrilov & Gavrilova, 2004c.

from experimental data through fitting procedures.

D. System Reliability and the Concept of Reliability Structure

A branch of reliability theory that studies reliability of an entire system given reliability of its components and its components' arrangement (reliability structure) is called *system reliability theory* (Rausand & Høyland, 2003). System reliability involves the study of the overall performance of systems of interconnected components. The main objective of system reliability is the construction of a model that represents the times-to-failure of the entire system based on the life distributions of the components from which it is composed. Consideration of some basic ideas and models of the system reliability theory is important because living organisms may be represented as structured systems comprised of organs, tissues, and cells.

System reliability theory tells us that how components are arranged strongly affects the reliability of the whole system. The arrangement of components that are important for system reliability is also called *reliability structure* and is graphically represented by a schema of logical connectivity. It is important to understand that the model of logical connectivity focuses only on those components that are relevant for the functioning ability of the system. If the components do not play a direct role in a system's reliability, they usually are not included in the analyzed reliability structure (Rausand & Høyland, 2003). For example, organs of vision are not included in the reliability structure of a living organism if death is the only type of failure to be analyzed (complete failure of vision does not cause an immediate death of the organism). On the other hand, if disability is the type of failure under consideration, then organs of vision should be included in the schema of reliability structure. Therefore, reliability structure does not necessarily reflect a physical structure of the object.

There are two major types of component arrangement (connection) in the system: components connected in series and components connected in parallel (Rausand & Høyland, 2003). Here we consider a simple system of n statistically independent components, where failure of one component does not affect the failure rate of other components of the system.

1. Components Connected in Series

For a system of n independent components connected in series, the system fails if any one of the components fails, much like electrical circuits connected in series.

Thus, the failure of any one component results in the failure of the whole system, such as in Christmas tree lighting chains. Figure 1.3A shows a schema of the logical connectivity of the system in series.

This type of system is also called a *weakest-link system* (Ayyub & McCuen, 2003). In living organisms, many organs and tissues (heart, lung, liver, brain) are vital for the organism's survival, making them a good example of a series-connected component. Thus, the series connection indicates a logical connectivity

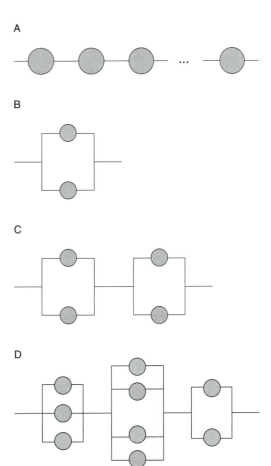

Figure 1.3 Logical schemas of systems with different types of elements connectivity. (A) A system connected in series. (B) A system connected in parallel. (C) A series-parallel system with equal redundancy of system components. (D) A series-parallel system with distributed redundancy.

but not necessarily a physical or an anatomical one. For example, a dominant deleterious mutation leading to a failure of a diploid organism corresponds to a schema of two components (alleles) connected in series (in terms of logical connectivity), although in fact these alleles are physically located at two different homologous chromosomes.

The reliability of a system in series (with independent failure events of the components), S_s, is a product of the reliabilities of its components:

$$S_s = p_1 p_2 \ldots p_n$$

where $p_1 \ldots p_n$ are the reliabilities of the system's components.

This formula explains why complex systems with many critical components are so sensitive to early failures of their components. For example, for a system built of 458 critical components, the initial period of a component's life when its cumulative risk of failure is only 1 percent corresponds to the end of a system's life, when 99 percent of systems have already failed. In other words, by the age when 99 percent of components are still functional ($p = 0.99$), a system built of 458 such critical components has only a 1 percent chance of remaining functional: $P_s = (0.99)^{458} \approx 0.01$. This discrepancy between the lifetimes of systems and the lifetimes of their components is increasing further with growing system complexity (numbers of critical components). Therefore, the early failure kinetics of components is very important in determining the failure kinetics of a complex system for almost its entire life. This helps simplify the analysis of complex system failure by focusing on the early failure kinetics of system components.

The failure rate of a system connected in series is a sum of failure rates of its components (Barlow *et al.*, 1965):

$$\mu_s = \mu_1 + \mu_2 + \cdots + \mu_n$$

If failure rates of all components are equal, the failure rate of the system with n components is $n\mu$. It follows from this formula that if a system's components do not age ($\mu_n = $ const), the entire system connected in series does not age either.

2. Components Connected in Parallel

A parallel system of n independent components fails only when all the components fail (such as in electrical circuits connected in parallel). The logical structure of a parallel system is presented in Figure 1.3B.

An example of a parallel system is a system with components performing an identical function. This function will be destroyed only when *all* the components fail. The number of additional components with the same function in a parallel structure is called a redundancy or a reserve of the system. In living organisms, vital organs and tissues (such as the liver, kidney, or pancreas) consist of many cells performing one and the same specialized function. A recessive deleterious mutation leading to a failure of a diploid organism represents a classic example of two components (alleles) connected in parallel.

For a parallel system with n independent components, the probability of a system's failure, Q, is a product of probabilities of failure for its components, q:

$$Q_s = q_1 q_2 \ldots q_n$$
$$= (1 - p_1)(1 - p_2) \ldots (1 - p_n)$$

Hence, the reliability of a parallel system, S_s, is related to the reliability of its components in the following way:

$$S_s = 1 - Q_s = 1 - (1 - p_1)(1 - p_2) \ldots (1 - p_n)$$

The reliability of a parallel system with components of equal reliability, p, is:

$$S_s = 1 - (1 - p)^n$$

What is important here is the emergence of aging in parallel systems: a parallel system is aging even if it is built of non-aging components with a constant failure rate (see more details in Section IV).

In the real world, most systems are more complex than simply series and parallel structures, but in many cases they can be represented as combinations of these structures.

3. More Complex Types of Reliability Structures

The simplest combination of the two reliability structures is a series-parallel system with equal redundancy, shown in Figure 1.3C.

A general series-parallel system is a system of m subsystems (blocks) connected in series, where each block is a set of n components connected in parallel. It turns out that even if the components themselves are not aging, the system as a whole has an aging behavior—its failure rate grows with age according to the Weibull law and then levels off at advanced ages (Gavrilov & Gavrilova, 1991, 2001b, 2003b). This type of system is important to consider because a living organism can be presented as a system of critical vital organs and tissues connected in series, while each organ consists of specialized cells connected in parallel. The reliability model for this type of system is described in more detail in Section IV.

Another type of reliability structure, a series-parallel system with distributed redundancy, was introduced by Gavrilov and Gavrilova (1991). The series-connected blocks of this system have non-equal redundancy (different numbers of elements connected in parallel), and the elements are distributed between the system's blocks according to some particular distribution law (see Figure 1.3D).

Gavrilov and Gavrilova (1991, 2001b) studied the reliability and failure rate of series-parallel systems with distributed redundancy for two special cases: (1) the redundancy distributed within an organism according to the Poisson law or (2) according to the binomial law. They found that the failure rate of such systems initially grows according to the Gompertz law (in the case of the Poisson distributed redundancy) or binomial failure law (in the case of the binomially distributed redundancy). At advanced ages, the failure rate for both systems asymptotically approaches an upper limit (mortality plateau). Reliability models for these systems are described in Section VI.

Now when the basic concepts of reliability theory are discussed, we may proceed to link them to empirical observations on aging and mortality.

III. Mortality, Failure, and Aging in Biological and Technical Systems

A. Failure Kinetics in Biological and Technical Systems

There is a striking similarity between living organisms and technical devices in the general age pattern of their failures—in both cases, the failure rate usually follows the so-called "bathtub curve" (see Figure 1.4).

The bathtub curve of failure rate is a classic concept presented in many textbooks on reliability theory (Ayyub & McCuen, 2003; Barlow & Proschan, 1975; Rausand & Høyland, 2003). The curve consists of three periods. Initially, the failure rates are high and decrease with age. This period is called the "working-in" period, and the period of "burning-out" of defective components. For example, the risk for a new computer to fail is often higher at the very start, but then those computers that did not fail initially work normally afterwards. The same period exists early in life for most living organisms, including humans, and it is called the *infant mortality period*.

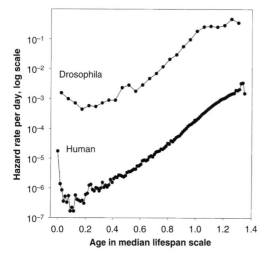

Figure 1.4 "Bathtub" mortality curves for humans and fruit flies. Mortality rates (vertical axis) are calculated in identical units (deaths per day per individual) for both species, whereas the age scale (horizontal axis) is normalized by dividing by the median life span of the species to allow data comparison (a similar approach to age scaling was used by Pearl & Miner, 1935, and Carnes et al., 1998). Mortality for *Drosophila melanogaster* was calculated using data published by Hall (1969). Mortality for humans was calculated using the official Swedish female life table for 1985.

Then follows the second period, called the *normal working period*, corresponding to an age of low and approximately constant failure rates. This period also exists in humans, but unfortunately it is rather short (10 to 15 years) and ends too soon.[4]

Then the third period, the *aging period*, starts, which involves an inexorable rise in the failure rate with age. In most living organisms, including humans, this rise in failure rates follows an explosive exponential trajectory (the Gompertz curve). For humans, the aging period lies approximately within the interval of 20 to 100 years.

Thus, there is a remarkable similarity in the failure patterns of technical and biological systems. This similarity is reinforced further by the fact that at extreme old ages there is a fourth period common to both technical devices and living organisms (Economos, 1979, 1980, 1983, 1985). This period is known in biology as a period of late-life mortality leveling-off (Carey & Liedo, 1995; Clark & Guadalupe, 1995; Economos, 1979; Fukui et al., 1993, 1996; Vaupel et al., 1998), and also as the late-life mortality deceleration law (Fukui et al., 1993, 1996; Khazaeli et al., 1996; Partridge & Mangel, 1999).

Remarkably similar failure patterns of biological and technical systems indicate that there may be some very general principles of system aging and failure (which will be discussed later), despite the obvious differences in specific underlying mechanisms of aging.

B. Mortality Laws in the Biology of Life Span

Attempts to develop a fundamental quantitative theory of aging, mortality, and life span have deep historical roots. In 1825, the British actuary Benjamin Gompertz discovered a law of mortality (Gompertz, 1825) known today as the Gompertz law (Finch, 1990; Gavrilov & Gavrilova, 1991; Olshansky & Carnes, 1997; Strehler, 1978). Specifically, he found that the force of mortality increases in geometrical progression with the age of adult humans. According to the Gompertz law, human mortality rates double about every 8 years of adult age (Finch, 1990; Gavrilov & Gavrilova, 1991; Gompertz, 1825;

---

[4]In countries with low child mortality, this age window with minimal death rates has recently broaden to about 5 to 15 years of age. When the death rates in this age interval are presented in logarithmic scale (sensitive to outliers that are close to zero levels of mortality), this may create an impression of large *relative* differences in death rates. However the death rates are so low in this age group that the absolute differences in death rates are negligible, and it is therefore safe to assume that death rates are "approximately constant."

Makeham, 1860; Strehler, 1978). An exponential (Gompertzian) increase in death rates with age is observed for many biological species including fruit flies (*Drosophila melanogaster*) (Gavrilov & Gavrilova, 1991), nematodes (Brooks *et al.*, 1994; Johnson, 1987, 1990), mosquitoes (Gavrilov, 1980), human lice (*Pediculus humanus*) (Gavrilov & Gavrilova, 1991), flour beetles (*Tribolium confusum*) (Gavrilov & Gavrilova, 1991), mice (Kunstyr & Leuenberger, 1975; Sacher, 1977), rats (Gavrilov & Gavrilova, 1991), dogs (Sacher, 1977), horses (Strehler, 1978), mountain sheep (Gavrilov, 1980), and baboons (Bronikowski *et al.*, 2002).

Gompertz also proposed the first mathematical model to explain the exponential increase in mortality rate with age (Gompertz, 1825). In reality, failure rates of organisms may contain both non-aging and aging terms, as, for example, in the case of the *Gompertz-Makeham law* of mortality (Finch, 1990; Gavrilov & Gavrilova, 1991; Makeham, 1860; Strehler, 1978):

$$\mu(x) = A + Re^{\alpha x}$$

In this formula, the first, age-independent term (Makeham parameter, A) designates the constant, "non-aging" component of the failure rate (presumably due to external causes of death, such as accidents and acute infections), whereas the second, age-dependent term (the Gompertz function, $Re^{\alpha x}$) designates the "aging" component, presumably due to deaths from age-related degenerative diseases such as cancer and heart disease.

The validity of the Gompertz-Makeham law of mortality can be illustrated graphically when the logarithms of death rates without the Makeham parameter $(\mu_x - A)$ are increasing with age in a linear fashion (see Figure 1.6). The log-linear increase in death rates (adjusted for the Makeham term) with age is indeed a very common phenomenon for many

human populations from 35 to 70 years of age (Gavrilov & Gavrilova, 1991).

Note that the slope coefficient α characterizes an "apparent aging rate" (the rapidity of age-deterioration in mortality); if α is equal to zero, there is no apparent aging (death rates do not increase with age).

At advanced ages (after age 80), the "old-age mortality deceleration" takes place: death rates increase with age at a slower pace than expected from the Gompertz-Makeham law. This mortality deceleration eventually produces the "late-life mortality leveling-off" and "late-life mortality plateaus" at extreme old ages (Curtsinger *et al.*, 1992; Economos, 1979, 1983; Gavrilov & Gavrilova, 1991; Greenwood and Irwin, 1939; Vaupel *et al.*, 1998). Actuaries—including Gompertz himself—first noted this phenomenon and proposed a logistic formula for mortality growth with age in order to account for mortality falloff at advanced ages (Beard, 1959, 1971; Perks, 1932). Greenwood and Irwin (1939) provided a detailed description of this phenomenon in humans and even made the first estimates for the asymptotic value of the upper limit to human mortality (see also the chapter by Curtsinger *et al.* in this volume and review by Olshansky, 1998). According to their estimates, the mortality kinetics of long-lived individuals is close to the law of radioactive decay with half-time approximately equal to 1 year.

The same phenomenon of "almost non-aging" survival dynamics at extreme old ages is detected in many other biological species. In some species, the mortality plateau can occupy a sizable part of their life (see Figure 1.5).

Biologists have been well aware of mortality leveling-off since the 1960s. For example, Lindop (1961) and Sacher (1966) discussed mortality deceleration in mice. Strehler and Mildvan (1960) considered mortality deceleration at advanced ages as a prerequisite for all mathematical models

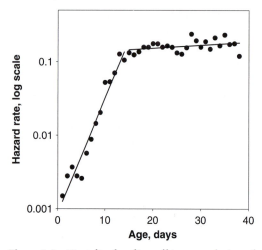

Figure 1.5 Mortality leveling-off in a population of 4,650 male house flies. Hazard rates were computed using the life table of the house fly *Musca domestica*, published by Rockstein & Lieberman (1959).

of aging. Later, Economos published a series of articles claiming a priority in the discovery of a "non-Gompertzian paradigm of mortality" (Economos, 1979, 1980, 1983, 1985). He found that mortality leveling-off is observed in rodents (guinea pigs, rats, and mice) and invertebrates (nematodes, shrimps, bdelloid rotifers, fruit flies, and degenerate medusae *Campanularia Flexuosa*). In the 1990s, the phenomenon of mortality deceleration and leveling-off became widely known after publications demonstrated mortality leveling-off in large samples of *Drosophila melanogaster* (Curtsinger et al., 1992) and medflies (*Ceratitis capitata*) (Carey et al., 1992), including isogenic strains of *Drosophila* (Curtsinger et al., 1992; Fukui et al., 1993, 1996). Mortality plateaus at advanced ages have been observed for some other insects, including the house fly (*Musca vicina*), blowfly (*Calliphora erythrocephala*) (Gavrilov, 1980), fruit flies (*Anastrepha ludens, Anastrepha obliqua, Anastrepha serpentine*), parasitoid wasp (*Diachasmimorpha longiacaudtis*) (Vaupel et al., 1998), and bruchid beetle (*Callosobruchus maculates*) (Tatar et al., 1993). Interestingly, the failure kinetics of

manufactured products (steel samples, industrial relays, and motor heat insulators) also demonstrates the same "non-aging" pattern at the end of their "life span" (Economos, 1979).

The phenomenon of late-life mortality leveling-off presents a theoretical challenge to many models and theories of aging. One interesting corollary from these intriguing observations is that there seems to be no fixed upper limit for individual life span (Gavrilov, 1984; Gavrilov & Gavrilova, 1991; Wilmoth, 1997).[5]

This observation calls for a very general explanation of this apparently paradoxical "no aging at extreme ages" phenomenon, which will be discussed later in this chapter.

Another empirical observation, the *compensation law of mortality*, in its strong form refers to *mortality convergence*, when higher values for the slope parameter α (in the Gompertz function) are compensated by lower values of the intercept parameter *R* in different populations of a given species:

$$\ln(R) = \ln(M) - B\alpha$$

where *B* and *M* are universal species-specific invariants.

Sometimes this relationship is also called the *Strehler-Mildvan correlation* (Strehler, 1978; Strehler & Mildvan, 1960), although that particular correlation was largely an artifact of the opposite biases in parameters estimation caused by not taking into account the age-independent mortality component, the Makeham term *A* (see Gavrilov & Gavrilova, 1991; Golubev, 2004). Parameter *B* is called the species-

---

[5]Note that there is no mathematical limit to life span, even with exponential growth of mortality force (hazard rate). However, this mathematical limit exists if the Gompertz law of exponential growth is applied to probability of death (Gavrilov & Gavrilova, 1991).

specific life span (95 years for humans), and parameter M is called the species-specific mortality rate (0.5 year^{-1} for humans). These parameters are the coordinates for convergence of all the mortality trajectories into one single point (within a given biological species), when extrapolated by the Gompertz function (Gavrilov & Gavrilova, 1979, 1991). This means that high mortality rates in disadvantaged populations (within a given species) are compensated for by a low apparent "aging rate" (longer mortality doubling period). As a result of this compensation, the relative differences in mortality rates tend to decrease with age within a given biological species (see Figure 1.6).

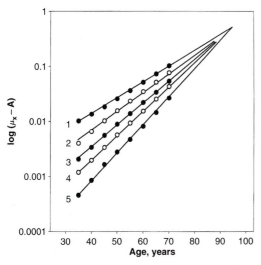

Figure 1.6 Compensation law of mortality. Convergence of mortality rates in different populations at advanced ages. Death rates (with removed age-independent external mortality component, Makeham parameter A) are plotted in a log scale as a function of age in the following countries:

1. India, 1941–1950, males; $A = 0.00676$ year^{-1}
2. Turkey, 1950–1951, males; $A = 0.00472$ year^{-1}
3. Kenya, 1969, males; $A = 0.00590$ year^{-1}
4. England and Wales, 1930–1932, females; $A = 0.00246$ year^{-1}
5. Norway, 1956–1960, females; $A = 0.00048$ year^{-1}

Computed using data from the UN Demographic Yearbook (1967; 1975). Adapted from Gavrilov & Gavrilova, 2003b.

In those cases when the compensation law of mortality is not observed in its strong form, it may still be valid in its weak form—i.e., the relative differences in mortality rates of compared populations tend to decrease with age in many species. Explanation of the compensation law of mortality is a great challenge for many theories of aging and longevity (Gavrilov & Gavrilova, 1991; Strehler, 1978).

There are some exceptions both from the Gompertz law of mortality and the compensation law of mortality that have to be understood and explained. There were reports that in some cases, the organisms die according to the Weibull (power) law (Eakin et al., 1995; Hirsch & Peretz, 1984; Hirsch et al., 1994; Janse et al., 1988; Ricklefs & Scheuerlein, 2002; Vanfleteren et al., 1998). The Weibull law is more commonly applicable to technical devices (Barlow & Proschan, 1975; Rigdon & Basu, 2000; Weibull, 1951), whereas the Gompertz law is more common in biological systems (Finch, 1990; Gavrilov & Gavrilova, 1991; Strehler, 1978). Comparative meta-analysis of 129 life tables for fruit flies as well as 285 life tables for humans demonstrates that the Gompertz law of mortality provides a much better data fit for each of these two biological species compared to the Weibull law (see Gavrilov & Gavrilova, 1991, pp. 55–56, 68–72). Possible explanations for why organisms prefer to die according to the Gompertz law and technical devices typically fail according to the Weibull law are provided elsewhere (Gavrilov & Gavrilova, 1991, 2001b) and will be discussed later in this chapter (see Sections V–VI).

Thus, a comprehensive theory of species aging and longevity should provide answers to the following questions:

1. Why do most biological species deteriorate with age (i.e., die more often as they grow older), whereas some primitive

organisms do not demonstrate such a clear mortality growth with age (Austad, 2001; Finch, 1990; Haranghy & Balázs, 1980; Martinez, 1998)?

2. Specifically, why do mortality rates increase exponentially with age in many adult species (Gompertz law)? How should we handle cases when the Gompertzian mortality law is not applicable?

3. Why does the age-related increase in mortality rates vanish at older ages? Why do mortality rates eventually decelerate compared to predictions of the Gompertz law, demonstrating mortality leveling-off and a late-life mortality plateau?

4. How do we explain the so-called compensation law of mortality (Gavrilov & Gavrilova, 1991)?

Any comprehensive theory of human aging has to explain these last three rules, known collectively as mortality, or failure, laws. And reliability theory, by way of a clutch of equations, covers all of them (Gavrilov & Gavrilova, 1991, 2001b), as will be discussed later.

C. Loss of Redundancy (e.g., Cell Numbers) with Age

Many age changes in living organisms can be explained by cumulative effects of cell loss (either physical or functional) over time. For example, such very common phenomenon as hair graying with age is caused by depletion of hair follicle melanocytes (Commo et al., 2004). Melanocyte density in human epidermis declines gradually with age, at a rate of approximately 0.8 percent per year (Gilchrest et al., 1979). Hair graying is a relatively benign phenomenon, but cell loss can also lead to more serious consequences.

Recent studies suggest that such conditions as atherosclerosis, atherosclerotic inflammation, and consequent thromboembolic complications could be linked

to age-related exhaustion of progenitor cells responsible for arterial repair (Goldschmidt-Clermont, 2003; Libby, 2003; Rauscher et al., 2003). Taking these progenitor cells from young mice and adding them to experimental animals prevents atherosclerosis progression and atherosclerotic inflammation (Goldschmidt-Clermont, 2003; Rauscher et al., 2003).

Age-dependent decline in cardiac function has recently been linked to the failure of cardiac stem cells to replace dying myocytes with new functioning cells (Capogrossi, 2004). Also, it was found that aging-impaired cardiac angiogenic function could be restored by adding endothelial precursor cells derived from young bone marrow (Edelberg et al., 2002).

Chronic renal failure is found to be associated with a decreased number of endothelial progenitor cells (Choi, 2004). People with diminished numbers of nephrons in their kidneys are more likely to suffer from hypertension (Keller et al., 2003), and the number of glomeruli decreases with human age (Nyengaard & Bendtsen, 1992).

Humans generally lose 30 to 40 percent of their skeletal muscle fibers by age 80 (Leeuwenburgh, 2003), which contributes to such adverse health outcomes as sarcopenia and frailty. Loss of striated muscle cells in such places as the rhabdosphincter, from 87.6 percent in a 5-week-old child to only 34.2 percent in a 91-year-old person, has obvious implications for urological failure: incontinence (Strasser et al., 2000).

A progressive loss of dopaminergic neurons in substantia nigra results in Parkinson's disease, loss of GABAergic neurons in striatum produces Huntington's disease, loss of motor neurons is responsible for amyotrophic lateral sclerosis, and loss of neurons in the cortex causes Alzheimer's disease over time (Baizabal et al., 2003). A study of cerebella from normal males age 19 to 84 revealed that the global white matter was reduced by 26 percent with age, and a selective 40 percent loss of both Purkinje and granule cells was observed in the anterior lobe (Andersen *et al.*, 2003).

Furthermore, a 30 percent loss of volume, mostly due to a cortical volume loss, was found in the anterior lobe, which is predominantly involved in motor control (Andersen *et al.*, 2003). Even if the loss of the volume in various brain regions is caused by cell atrophy rather than cell death, it is still indicative for the loss of redundancy (reserve capacity) with age.

Loss of cells with age is not limited to the human species; it is observed in other animals as well. For example, a nematode *C. elegans* demonstrates a gradual, progressive deterioration of muscle, resembling human sarcopenia (Herndon *et al.*, 2002). The authors of this study also found that the behavioral ability of nematode was a better predictor of life expectancy than chronological age.

Interestingly, recent studies have found that caloric restriction can prevent cell loss (Cohen *et al.*, 2004; McKiernan *et al.*, 2004), which may explain why caloric restriction delays the onset of numerous age-associated diseases and can significantly increase life span in mammals (Masoro, 2003). It should be acknowledged, however, that the hypothesis that aging occurs largely because of cell loss remains a subject of debate (Van Zant & Liang, 2003).

In terms of reliability theory, the loss of cells with age is a loss of system redundancy, and therefore this chapter will focus further on the effects of redundancy loss on system aging and failure. Note that the loss of redundancy does not necessarily imply losing cell numbers, because the loss of cell functionality (decrease in proportion of functional cells) could produce the same adverse health outcomes with age.

IV. Explanations of Aging Phenomena Using Reliability Theory

A. Problem of the Origin of Aging

The aging period for most species occupies the greater part of their life span, therefore any model of mortality must explain the existence of this period. It turns out that the phenomena of mortality increase with age and the subsequent mortality leveling-off is theoretically predicted to be an inevitable feature of all reliability models that consider aging as a progressive accumulation of random damage (Gavrilov & Gavrilova, 1991). The detailed mathematical proof of this prediction for some particular models is provided elsewhere (Gavrilov & Gavrilova, 1991, 2001b) and is briefly described in the next sections of this chapter.

The simplest schema, which demonstrates an emergence of aging in a redundant system, is presented in Figure 1.7.

If the destruction of an organism occurs not in one but in two or more sequential random stages, this is sufficient for the phenomenon of aging (mortality increase) to appear and then to vanish at older ages. Each stage of destruction corresponds to one of the organism's vitally important structures being damaged. In the simplest

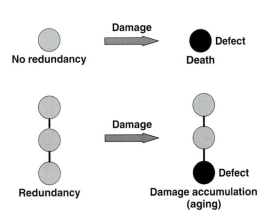

Figure 1.7 Redundancy creates both damage tolerance and damage accumulation (aging).

organisms with unique critical structures, this damage usually leads to death. Therefore, defects in such organisms do not accumulate, and the organisms themselves do not age—they just die when damaged. For example, the inactivation of microbial cells and spores exposed to a hostile environment (such as heat) follows approximately a non-aging mortality kinetics; their semi-logarithmic survival curves are almost linear (Peleg *et al.*, 2003). This observation of non-aging survival dynamics is extensively used in the calculation of the efficacy of sterilization processes in medicine and food preservation (Brock *et al.*, 1994; Davis *et al.*, 1990; Jay, 1996). A similar non-aging pattern of inactivation kinetics is often observed for viruses (Andreadis & Palsson, 1997; Kundi, 1999) and enzymes (Gouda *et al.*, 2003; Kurganov, 2002).

In more complex systems with many vital structures and significant redundancy, every occurrence of damage does not lead to death (unless the environment is particularly hostile). Defects accumulate, therefore, giving rise to the phenomenon of aging (mortality increase). Thus, aging is a direct consequence (tradeoff) of a system's redundancies, which ensure increased reliability and an increased life span of more complex organisms. As defects accumulate, the redundancy in the number of elements finally disappears. As a result of this *redundancy exhaustion*, the organism degenerates into a system with no redundancy (that is, a system with elements connected in series, in which any new defect leads to death). In such a state, no further accumulation of damage can be achieved, and the mortality rate levels off.

The positive effect of a system's redundancy is *damage tolerance*, which decreases the risk of failure (mortality) and increases life span. However, damage tolerance makes it possible for damage to be tolerated and accumulated over time, thus producing the aging phenomenon.

The next section provides a mathematical illustration of these ideas.

B. A Simple Model with Parallel Structure

In this section we show that a system built of non-aging components demonstrates an aging behavior (mortality growth with age) and subsequent mortality leveling-off.

Consider a parallel system built of n non-aging elements with a constant failure rate k and reliability (survival) function e^{-kx} (see also Figure 1.3B). In this case, the reliability function of the entire parallel system is as follows (see also Section II.D):

$$S(x) = 1 - (1 - p)^n = 1 - (1 - e^{-kx})^n$$

This formula corresponds to the simplest case when the failure of elements is statistically independent. More complex models would require specific assumptions or prior knowledge of the exact type of the interdependence in the elements' failure. One of such models known as "the model of the avalanche-like destruction" is described elsewhere (see pp. 246–251 in Gavrilov & Gavrilova, 1991).

Consequently, the failure rate of the entire system, $\mu(x)$, can be written as follows:

$$\mu(x) = -\frac{dS(x)}{S(x)dx} = \frac{nk\,e^{-kx}(1-e^{-kx})^{n-1}}{1 - (1 - e^{-kx})^n}$$

$$\approx nk^n x^{n-1}$$

when $x \ll 1/k$ (early-life period approximation, when $1 - e^{-kx} \approx kx$);

$$\approx k$$

when $x \gg 1/k$ (late-life period approximation, when $1 - e^{-kx} \approx 1$).

Thus, the failure rate of a system initially grows as a power function of age (the Weibull law). Then, the tempo at which the failure rate grows declines, and the failure rate approaches asymptotically an upper limit equal to k. Here we should pay attention to three significant points. First, a system constructed of non-aging elements is now behaving like an aging object; that is, aging is a direct consequence of the redundancy of the system (redundancy in the number of elements). Second, at very high ages, the phenomenon of aging apparently disappears (failure rate levels off) as redundancy in the number of elements vanishes. The failure rate approaches an upper limit, which is totally independent of the initial number of elements but coincides with the rate of their loss (parameter k). Third, the systems with different initial levels of redundancy (parameter n) will have very different failure rates in early life, but these differences will eventually vanish as failure rates approach the upper limit determined by the rate of elements' loss (parameter k). Thus, the compensation law of mortality (in its weak form) is an expected outcome of this illustrative model.

Note also that the identical parallel systems in this example do not die simultaneously when their elements fail by chance. A common view in biology is the idea that all members of a homogeneous population in a hypothetical constant environment should have identical life spans (die simultaneously) so that the survival curve of such a population would look like a rectangle. This idea stems from the basic principles of quantitative genetics, which assume implicitly that every animal of a given genotype has the same genetically determined life span so that all variation of survival time around a genotype mean results from the environmental variance. George Sacher (1977) pointed out that this concept is not applicable to longevity and used an analogy with radioactive decay in his arguments.

Even the simplest parallel system has a specific life span distribution determined entirely by a stochastic nature of the aging process. In order to account for this stochasticity, it was proposed that researchers use a stochastic variance component of life span in addition to genetic and environmental components of phenotypic life span variance (Gavrilov & Gavrilova, 1991). The stochastic nature of a system's destruction also produces heterogeneity in an initially homogeneous population. This kind of induced heterogeneity was observed in isogenic strains of nematodes in which aging resulted in substantial heterogeneity in behavioral capacity among initially homogeneous worms kept in controlled environmental conditions (Herndon et al., 2002).

The graph shown in Figure 1.8 depicts mortality trajectories for five systems with different degrees of redundancy.

System 1 has only one unique element (no redundancy), and it has the highest failure rate, which does not depend on age (no aging). System 2 has two elements connected in parallel (one extra element is redundant), and the failure rate initially increases with age (aging appears). The apparent rate of aging can be characterized by a slope coefficient that is equal to 1. Finally, the failure rate levels off at advanced ages. Systems 3, 4, and 5 have, respectively, three, four, and five elements connected in parallel (two, three, and four extra elements are redundant), and the failure rate initially increases with age at an apparent aging rate (slope coefficient) of 2, 3, and 4, respectively. Finally, the mortality trajectories of each system level off at advanced ages at exactly the same upper limit to the mortality rate.

This computational example illustrates the following general ideas: (1) Aging is a direct consequence of a system's redundancy, and the expression of aging is directly related to the degree of a system's redundancy. Specifically, an apparent

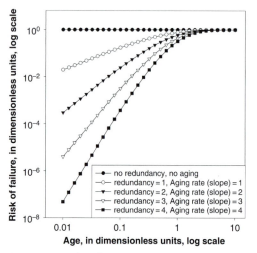

Figure 1.8 Failure kinetics of systems with different levels of redundancy. The dependence of the logarithm of mortality force (failure rate) on the logarithm of age in five systems with different levels of redundancy (computer simulation experiment). Dependence 1 is for the system containing only one unique element (no redundancy). Dependence 2 is for the system containing two elements connected in parallel (degree of redundancy = 1). Dependencies 3, 4, and 5 are for systems containing, respectively, three, four, and five elements connected in parallel (with increasing levels of redundancy). The scales for mortality rates (vertical axis) and for age (horizontal axis) are presented in dimensionless units (μ/k) for mortality rates and kx for age to ensure the generalizability of the results (invariance of graphs on failure rate of the elements in the system, parameter k). Also, the log scale is used to explore the system behavior in a wide range of ages (0.01 to 10 units) and failure rates (0.00000001 to 1.0 units). Adapted from Gavrilov & Gavrilova, 2003b, 2004c.

relative aging rate is equal to the degree of redundancy in parallel systems. (2) All mortality trajectories tend to converge with age so that the compensation law of mortality is observed. (3) All mortality trajectories level off at advanced ages, and a mortality plateau is observed. Thus, the major aging phenomena (aging itself, the compensation law of mortality, late-life mortality deceleration, and late-life mortality plateaus) are already observed in the simplest redundant systems. However, to explain the Gompertz law of

mortality, an additional idea should be taken into account (see the next section).

V. The Idea of High Initial Damage Load: The HIDL Hypothesis

In 1991, Gavrilov and Gavrilova suggested an idea that early development of living organisms produces an exceptionally high load of initial damage, which is comparable with the amount of subsequent aging-related deterioration accumulating during the rest of the entire adult life.

This idea of High Initial Damage Load (the HIDL hypothesis) predicts that even small progress in optimizing the early developmental processes can potentially result in a remarkable prevention of many diseases in later life, postponement of aging-related morbidity and mortality, and significant extension of healthy life span (Gavrilov & Gavrilova, 1991, 2001b, 2003b, 2004a). Thus, the idea of early-life programming of aging and longevity may have important practical implications for developing early-life interventions in promoting health and longevity.

Although this idea may look like a counterintuitive assumption, it fits well with many empirical observations on massive cell losses in early development. For example, the female human fetus at age 4 to 5 months possesses 6 to 7 million eggs (oocytes). By birth, this number drops to 1 to 2 million and declines even further. At the start of puberty in normal girls, there are only 0.3 to 0.5 million eggs—only 4 to 8 percent of initial numbers (Finch & Kirkwood, 2000; Gosden, 1985; Wallace & Kelsey, 2004). It is now well established that the exhaustion of the ovarian follicle numbers over time is responsible for menopause (reproductive aging and failure), and women having higher ovarian reserve have longer reproductive life span (Wallace & Kelsey,

2004). When young ovaries were transplanted to old post-reproductive mice, their reproductive function was restored for a while (Cargill et al., 2003). This example illustrates a general idea that aging occurs largely because of cell loss, which starts early in life.

Massive cell losses in early development create differences between organisms in the numbers of remaining cells, which can be described by the binomial distribution or, at particularly high levels of cell losses, by the Poisson distribution. This, in turn, can produce a quasi-exponential (Gompertzian) pattern of age-specific mortality kinetics with a subsequent mortality deceleration (Gavrilov & Gavrilova, 1991). In some species, including *C. elegans*, the developmental loss of cells seems to be very precise. If adult individuals are identical in the initial numbers of functional cells, one can expect that mortality kinetics in such cases would be closer to the Weibull law rather than the Gompertz law. However, the Gompertz law also can be expected for initially identical organisms if the critical vital organs within a given organism differ by their cell numbers (Gavrilov & Gavrilova, 1991, pp. 252–264; 2001b).

Mathematical proof for this statement was published elsewhere (see Gavrilov & Gavrilova, 1991, pp. 264–272) and will be briefly summarized in Section VI. Here we concentrate on the substantive discussion of the idea of high initial damage load in biological systems.

A. Differences Between Biological and Technical Systems

Biological systems are different from technical devices in at least two aspects. The first fundamental feature of biological systems is that, in contrast to technical (artificial) devices that are constructed out of previously manufactured and tested components, organisms form themselves in ontogenesis through a process of self-assembly out of *de novo* forming and externally untested elements (cells). Moreover, because organisms are formed from a single cell, any defects in early life such as deleterious mutations or deleterious epigenetic modifications (i.e., genomic imprinting) can proliferate by mechanism of clonal expansion, forming large clusters of damaged cells. This proliferation of defects during development of biological systems can make them highly damaged by the time they are formed.

The second property of organisms is the extraordinary degree of miniaturization of their components (the microscopic dimensions of cells as well as the molecular dimensions of information carriers like DNA and RNA), permitting the creation of a huge redundancy in the number of elements. Thus, we can expect that for living organisms, in distinction to many technical (manufactured) devices, the reliability of the system is achieved not by the high initial quality of all the elements but by their huge numbers (redundancy).

The fundamental difference in the manner in which the system is formed (external assembly in the case of technical devices and self-assembly in the case of biological systems) has two important consequences. First, it leads to the macroscopicity of components in technical devices compared to biosystems, since technical devices are assembled "top-down" with the participation of a macroscopic system (man) and must be suitable for this macroscopic system to use (i.e., commensurate with man). Organisms, on the other hand, are assembled "bottom-up" from molecules and cells, resulting in an exceptionally high degree of miniaturization of the component parts. Second, since technical devices are assembled under the control of man, the opportunities to pretest components (external quality control) are incomparably greater than in the self-assembly of biological systems. This inevitably leads to organisms being "littered" with a great number of defective elements. As a result, the reliability of technical devices is assured by the high quality of elements (*fault avoidance*), with a strict limit on their numbers because of size and cost limitations, whereas the reliability of biological systems is assured by an exceptionally high degree of redundancy to overcome the poor quality of some elements (*fault tolerance*).

B. Some Examples Illustrating the HIDL Hypothesis

The idea that living organisms start their lives with a large number of defects is not a new one. Biological justification for this idea was discussed by Dobzhansky, who noted that, from the biological perspective, Hamlet's "thousand natural shocks that flesh is heir to" was an underestimate and that in reality "the shocks are innumerable" (1962, p. 126).

Recent studies have found that troubles in human life start from the very beginning: the cell-cycle checkpoints (which ensure that cells will not divide until DNA damage is repaired and chromosomal segregation is complete) do not operate properly at the early, cleavage stage in human embryos (Handyside & Delhanty, 1997). This produces mosaicism of the preimplantation embryo, where some embryonic cells are genetically abnormal (McLaren, 1998), with potentially devastating consequences in later life.

Most of the DNA damage caused by copy errors during DNA replication also occurs in early life because most cell divisions happen in early development. As a result of extensive DNA damage in early development, many apparently normal tissues of young organisms have a strikingly high load of mutations, including abundant oncogenic mutations and frequent clones of mutated somatic cells (Cha *et al.*, 1994; Deng *et al.*, 1996;

Jonason *et al.*, 1996; Khrapko *et al.*, 2004; Nekhaeva *et al.*, 2002).

Loss of telomeres, eventually leading to such outcomes as genomic instability, cell death (apoptosis), cell senescence, and perhaps to organism's aging (Kim *et al.*, 2002), also begins before birth, and it is directly linked to DNA replication during cell divisions, which are particularly intensive at early stages of growth and development (Collins & Mitchell, 2002; DePinho & Wong, 2003; Forsyth *et al.*, 2002; Kim *et al.*, 2002). In humans, the length of telomeres declines precipitously before the age of 4 (by 25 percent) and then declines further very slowly (Hopkin, 2001).

Another potential source of extensive initial damage is the birth process itself. During birth, the future child is first deprived of oxygen by compression of the umbilical cord (Moffett *et al.*, 1993) and suffers severe hypoxia (often with ischemia and asphyxia). Then, just after birth, a newborn child is exposed to oxidative stress because of acute reoxygenation while starting breathing. It is known that acute reoxygenation after hypoxia may produce an extensive oxidative damage through the same mechanisms that also produce ischemia-reperfusion injury (IRI) and asphyxia-reventilation injury (Martin *et al.*, 2000). Asphyxia is a common occurrence in the perinatal period, and asphyxial brain injury is the most common neurologic abnormality in the neonatal period (Dworkin, 1992) that may manifest in neurologic disorders in later life. The brain damage that occurs after asphyxia may cause long-term neurological consequences in full-term infants (Volpe, 2000) and lead to cerebral palsy, epilepsy, and mental retardation (Hack & Fanaroff, 2000; Hjalmarsson *et al.*, 1988, pp. 28–36). Perhaps the rare geniuses are simply those lucky persons whose early-life brain damage was less extensive than the "normal" level. Thus, using Hamlet's metaphor, we may conclude that humans "suffer the slings and arrows of outrageous fortune" and have "a sea of troubles" from the very beginning of their lives.

It follows from this concept of HIDL that even small progress in optimizing the processes of ontogenesis and increasing the numbers of initially functional elements can potentially result in a remarkable fall in mortality and a significant improvement in life span. This optimistic prediction is supported by experimental evidence (in laboratory mice) of increased offspring life span if future parents are fed antioxidants, which presumably result in protection of parental germ cells against oxidative damage (Harman & Eddy, 1979).

From this point of view, parental characteristics determining the quality of the gametes, and especially maternal characteristics determining the accuracy of the early stages of development, would be expected to have significant influence on the life span of the offspring, which may be in some cases even stronger than the effect of these same properties of the offspring themselves. In other words, the reliability concept leads us to a paradoxical conjecture: sometimes a better predictor of life span may be found not among the characteristics of the organism itself but among the characteristics of its parents.

Gavrilov & Gavrilova (1991) tested this counterintuitive prediction using data on life span and metabolic characteristics of 21 inbred and F_1-hybrid mouse genotypes (several hundred mice) published by

Sacher & Duffy (1979). It was found that the six traits (body weight and resting and average metabolic rates both at young and old ages) of parental genotypes explained 95 percent of variation in mean life span between 16 F_1-hybrid mice genotypes, whereas the same six traits of hybrid mice themselves explained only 25 percent of variation in their mean life span (Gavrilov & Gavrilova, 1991, pp. 175–182). The highest mean life span was observed in the progeny of those parents who had the lowest resting metabolic rate at young age. This observation is consistent with a hypothesis that the differences in progeny life span could be linked to the rates of oxidative DNA damage in parental germ cells. Interestingly, the resting metabolic rate measured in young progeny itself was not predictive for progeny life span (see Table 1.1).

Thus, certain parameters (such as resting metabolic rate at young age) measured in parents could be better predictors of progeny life span compared to the same parameters measured among the progeny itself.

The concept of high initial damage load also predicts that early-life events may affect survival in later adult life through modulating the level of initial damage. This prediction proved to be correct for such early-life indicators as parental age at a person's conception (Gavrilov & Gavrilova, 1997, 2000, 2003a; Gavrilova *et al.*, 2003) and the month of a person's

Table 1.1

Parental Resting Metabolic Rates at Young Age Are Better Predictors of Life Span of Mice Progeny Than the Resting Metabolic Rates (RMR) Measured in Progeny Itself[*]

Variable	Regression Coefficient	Standard Error	t-value	p-value
Maternal RMR	−1054	252	−4.18	0.001
Paternal RMR	−795	254	−3.13	0.009
Progeny RMR	42	205	0.20	0.843

[*]Parameter values for linear regression of progeny life span on parental and progeny resting metabolic rate measured at young age (RMR) for 16 genotypes of F_1-hybrid mice. Computed using data published by Sacher & Duffy (1979).

birth (Doblhammer & Vaupel, 2001; Gavrilov & Gavrilova, 1999, 2003a; Gavrilova *et al.*, 2003). The month of birth may influence a person's life span through early-life exposure to seasonal vitamin deficiencies and seasonal infections during critical periods of child development (Gavrilov & Gavrilova, 2001a). It is known that deficiencies of vitamins B-12, folic acid, B-6, niacin, and vitamins C and E appear to mimic radiation in damaging DNA by causing single- and double-stand breaks, oxidative lesions, or both (Ames, 2004). Vitamin deficiencies had profound seasonality in the past when contemporary adults were born, and these deficiencies may be particularly harmful at the early stages of human development (Gavrilov & Gavrilova, 2001a).

There is mounting evidence now in support of the idea of fetal origins of adult degenerative diseases (Barker, 1998; Kuh & Ben-Shlomo, 1997; Leon *et al.*, 1998; Lucas *et al.*, 1999) and early-life programming of aging and longevity (Gavrilov & Gavrilova, 1991, 2001a, 2003a,b). Women may be particularly sensitive to early-life exposures because they are mosaics of two different cell types (one with active paternal X chromosome and one with active maternal X chromosome), and the pattern of this mosaic is determined early in life. Indeed, this conjecture of stronger female response to early-life exposures is confirmed for such early-life predictors of adult life span as paternal age at a person's conception (Gavrilov & Gavrilova, 1997, 2000, 2003a, 2004a; Gavrilova *et al.*, 2003) and the month of a person's birth (Gavrilov & Gavrilova, 2003a; Gavrilova *et al.*, 2003).

VI. Reliability Models of Aging for Biological Systems

It was demonstrated in Section IV that the aging phenomenon emerges when a system gains some redundancy (reserves).

The failure rate of a simple parallel system built of non-aging elements increases with age, although the initial failure kinetics follows the Weibull law rather then the Gompertz law. This limitation of the model is rooted in the assumption that the system is built of initially ideal structures where all elements are functional from the outset. This standard assumption may be justified for technical devices manufactured from pretested components, but it is not justified for living organisms, presumably replete with defects, for the reasons described earlier. Gavrilov and Gavrilova (1991) proposed a family of reliability models based on the idea of initial damage load, which allows us to explain all three major laws of biological aging and mortality: the Gompertz law, the late-life deceleration law, and the compensation law of mortality (mortality convergence at advanced ages). A brief description of these models is provided below.

A. Highly Redundant System Replete with Defects

The simplest model in this family of reliability models is the model of a series-parallel structure with distributed redundancy *within* the organism (see Gavrilov & Gavrilova, 1991, pp. 252–264; 2001b). If distribution of subsystems within the organism according to initially functional elements can be described by the Poisson law because of high initial damage load, then the failure rate of such series-parallel systems can be approximated initially by the exponential (Gompertz) law with subsequent mortality leveling-off.

According to this model, the compensation law of mortality is inevitable if the "true aging rate" (relative rate of elements' loss) is similar in different populations of a given species (presumably because of homeostasis—stable body temperature, glucose concentration, etc.).

This suggested explanation leads to an interesting testable prediction that for lower organisms with poor homeostasis, there may be deviations from the compensation law of mortality.

B. Partially Damaged Redundant System

The simplest model, which was described earlier, assumed an extremely high level of initial damage load. In a more general model, the distribution of subsystems in the organism according to the number of initially functional elements is described by the binomial rather than Poisson distribution. In this case, the failure rate of a system initially follows the binomial failure law (Gavrilov & Gavrilova, 1991, 2001b).

Thus, if the system is not initially ideal, the failure rate in the initial period of time grows exponentially with age, according to the Gompertz law. A numerical example provided in Figure 1.2 shows that increase in the initial system's damage load (initial virtual age) converts the observed mortality trajectory from the Weibull to the Gompertz one. The model also explains the compensation law of mortality and mortality leveling-off later in life (see Gavrilov & Gavrilova, 1991, 2001b).

Thus, both reliability models described here provide an explanation for a general pattern of aging and mortality in biological species: the exponential growth of failure rate in the initial period, with the subsequent mortality deceleration and leveling-off, as well as the compensation law of mortality.

C. Heterogeneous Population of Redundant Organisms

The models discussed so far examined a situation in which series-connected vital subsystems (blocks) have varying degrees of redundancy *within* each organism, while no additional assumptions were made about possible initial differences between the organisms themselves. In a more general case, the population heterogeneity needs to be taken into account because there is a large variation in the numbers of cells for the organisms of the same species (Finch & Kirkwood, 2000). The model of heterogeneous redundant systems (Gavrilov & Gavrilova, 1991, pp. 264–272) demonstrates that taking into account the heterogeneity of the population also provides an explanation for all the basic laws of mortality. This model assumes that there is a distribution of organisms with regard to their initial redundancy levels (e.g., number of functional cells) within a population under study. If this distribution is close to either the binomial or the Poisson distribution, then a quasi-exponential (Gompertzian) pattern of mortality increase with age is expected initially, with subsequent mortality leveling-off (Gavrilov & Gavrilova, 1991, pp. 264–272).

Figure 1.9 shows computed data for a model in which organisms have a different number of elements (connected in parallel) and are distributed by their redundancy levels according to the Poisson distribution law, with the mean number of elements equal to λ.

Note that the dependence of the logarithm of failure rate on age is almost a linear one, indicating that the initial failure kinetics is indeed close to the Gompertz law. This initial Gompertzian period of failure rate growth can be easily extended for the organism's entire life span in the case of more complex systems with many vital components (built of parallel elements), each being critical for survival (serial connection of a large number of components; see Section II.D).

Figure 1.9 also demonstrates that the populations of organisms with higher mean levels of redundancy (parameter λ) have lower death rates, but these death rates are growing steeper with age (the compensation law of mortality).

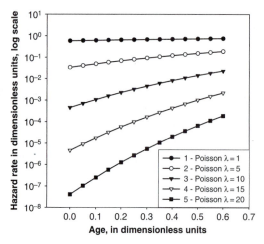

Figure 1.9 Failure kinetics in mixtures of systems with different redundancy levels for the initial age period. The dependence of failure rate as a function of age in mixtures of parallel redundant systems having Poisson distribution by initial numbers of functional elements (mean number of elements, λ = 1, 5, 10, 15, 20). The scales for mortality rates (vertical axis), and for age (horizontal axis) are presented in dimensionless units (μ/k) for mortality rates, and kx for age, to ensure the generalizability of the results (invariance of graphs on failure rate of the elements in the system, parameter k).

D. Accumulation of Defects with Constant Rate of Damage Flow

Another reliability model of aging is obtained after a critical reinterpretation of the assumptions underlying the previously described models. In fact, these models contain an assumption that the death of the organism occurs only when all the elements in a block fail. It is possible that this hypothesis may be justified in a number of cases for some of the organism's subsystems. However, in the majority of cases, the hypothesis seems contentious. For example, it is hard to imagine that a single surviving liver cell (hepatocyte) can assume the functions of an entire destroyed liver. Significantly more realistic is the hypothesis that the system initially contains an enormous number of elements that greatly exceeds the critical number of defects, leading to

the death of the organism. In this case, we arrive at a schema for the accumulation of damage in which the rate of damage flow (equal to the product of the number of elements and their failure rate) turns out to be practically constant in view of the incommensurability of the number of elements and the permitted number of defects (see Gavrilov & Gavrilova, 1991, pp. 272–276).

This model also allows us to take into account the influence of living conditions on the value of the critical number of defects incompatible with the survival of the organism. The key to the solution of this problem is the replacement of the parallel connection hypothesis (assumed in previous models) with the more realistic assumption that there exists a critical number of defects incompatible with the survival of the organism. In this case, it is natural to expect that under harsher conditions, the critical number of defects leading to death might be less than under more comfortable living conditions. In particular, in the wild, when an animal is deprived of care and forced to acquire its own food as well as to defend itself against predators, the first serious damage to the organism can lead to death. It is therefore not surprising that the mortality of many animals (in particular, birds) is practically independent of age in the wild. This follows directly from the single-stage destruction of the organism model. On the other hand, the greater the number of defects the organism can accumulate while remaining alive, the greater its life span will be.

The standard model of defect accumulation with constant rate of damage flow predicts that at the initial moment in time, mortality grows according to a power (Weibull) law of mortality. If we assume that distribution of living organisms according to the number of defects they have is described by the Poisson law, then at the initial moment in time, this model leads to the binomial law of mortality. In this model, the compensation law of mortality can be obtained both as a result of variation in the degree to which the organisms are initially damaged, and of variation in the critical number of defects, dependent on the harshness of living conditions (see Gavrilov & Gavrilova, 1991, pp. 272–276).

Summarizing this brief review of reliability models, note the striking similarity between the conclusions of the considered models. All these models predict a mortality deceleration, no matter what assumptions are made regarding initial population heterogeneity or its complete initial homogeneity. Moreover, these reliability models of aging produce mortality plateaus as inevitable outcomes for any values of considered parameters. The only constraint is that the elementary steps of the multistage destruction process of a system should occur by chance only, independent of age. The models also predict that an initially homogeneous population will become highly heterogeneous for risk of death over time (acquired heterogeneity). The similarity of conclusions obtained from several different models means that it is impossible on the basis of the established mortality phenomena to uncover the correct mechanism behind the age-related destruction of organisms, and further studies are necessary to discriminate between the competing models.

One can of course derive no pleasure from this circumstance, but there are two reasons that give ground for optimism. First, the different models seem to lead to very similar interpretations of certain mortality phenomena. For example, the compensation law of mortality is only possible when the relative rate of redundancy loss is the same in all populations of a given species. This interpretation of the compensation law of mortality is not only a feature of the models described in this chapter but also of other models (Gavrilov, 1978; Gavrilov

et al., 1978; Strehler & Mildvan, 1960). The existence of a multitude of competing models is therefore compatible with the reliable and meaningful interpretation of a number of mortality phenomena because variability of models does not preclude their agreement on a number of issues. Second, if different models lead to the same formulas—for example the binomial law of mortality—this merely makes the problem of interpreting results more complicated for the theoretician, but significantly facilitates the work for the experimenter. Indeed, for the analysis of data, it is preferable to use a formula that is supported not by a single model but by a whole family of models that encompass a wide spectrum of possible situations.

VII. Evolution of Species Reliability

Reliability theory of aging is perfectly compatible with the idea of biological evolution, and it helps to identify key components that may be important for evolution of species reliability and durability (longevity): initial redundancy levels, initial damage load, rate of redundancy loss, and repair potential. Moreover, reliability theory helps evolutionary theories explain how the age of onset of diseases caused by deleterious mutations could be postponed to later ages (as suggested by the mutation accumulation theory of aging)—this could be easily achieved by a simple increase in the initial redundancy levels (e.g., initial cell numbers).

From the reliability perspective, the increase in initial redundancy levels is the simplest way to improve survival at particularly early reproductive ages (with gains fading at older ages). This exactly matches with the higher fitness priority of early reproductive ages emphasized by evolutionary theories. Evolutionary and reliability ideas also help to understand why organisms seem to "choose" a simple but short-term solution to the survival problem through enhancing the systems redundancy, rather than a more permanent but complicated solution based on rigorous repair (with a potential for negligible senescence).

It may be interesting and useful to compare failure rates of different biological species expressed in exactly the same units of risk (risk of death per individual per day). Returning back to the earlier Figure 1.4, we can notice with some surprise that the death rates of young vigorous fruit flies kept in protected laboratory conditions is as high as among very old people! This indicates that fruit flies from the very beginning of their lives have very unreliable design compared to humans. This observation also tells us that young organisms of one biological species may have the same failure risk as old organisms of another species—that is, being old for humans is as good as being young for fruit flies. Note that at extreme old ages, the death rates of fruit flies are well beyond human death rates (see Figure 1.4). In terms of reliability models, this observation suggests that fruit flies are made of less reliable components (presumably cells), which have higher failure rates compared to human cells.

We can ask ourselves a question: is it a general rule that shorter-lived biological species should always have higher death rates within comparable age groups (say, within "young" or "old" age groups)? Traditional evolutionary theories suggest that indeed shorter-lived species should have higher "intrinsic" death rates in protected environments because these rates are shaped in evolution through selection pressure by death rates in the wild (predation, starvation, etc.). In other words, defenseless fruit flies in the wild experience much higher death rates than do humans; therefore a selection pressure

to increase their "intrinsic" reliability was less intensive compared to humans. This traditional evolutionary paradigm also says that birds live longer and have lower "intrinsic" death rates because of adaptation to flight, which improved their survival in the wild and increased a selection pressure to further decrease "intrinsic" death rates (Austad, 2001).

Thus, if a bird (say, a finch) is compared to a similar-sized shorter-lived mammal (say, a rat), the expected picture should be similar to Figure 1.4: a bird should have lower death rates than a rat both in the beginning and in the end of their lives. Interestingly, this prediction of traditional evolutionary paradigm could be confronted with an alternative prediction expected from a reliability paradigm. Reliability paradigm predicts that birds should be very prudent in redundancy of their body structures (because it comes with a heavy cost of additional weight, making flight difficult). Therefore, a flight adaptation should force the birds to evolve in a direction of high reliability of their components (cells) with low levels of redundancy (cell numbers). Thus, reliability paradigm predicts that "intrinsic" death rates of birds in protected environments should be rather high at young ages (because of low redundancy levels), whereas at old ages their death rates might be much lower than in other species (because of higher reliability of their cells). This suggestion of higher reliability of avian cells agrees with the recent findings of increased resistance of these cells to oxidative stress and DNA damage (Holmes & Ottinger, 2003; Ogburn *et al.*, 1998, 2001).

Figure 1.10 presents data on "intrinsic" mortality in Bengalese finches as compared to rats for both species living in protected environments.

Note that the death rates in both species are very close to each other at young ages, but later a *mortality divergence* occurs so that old birds have much lower death rates

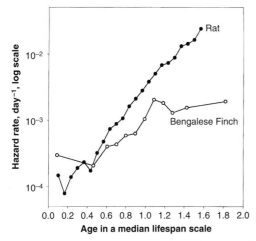

Figure 1.10 Comparative mortality of rats and Bengalese finches expressed in the same units of mortality (per day). Data sources: Bengalese finch, survival data for 39 birds of both sexes in captivity (Eisner, 1967); Rats, survival data for 2,050 female rats kept in a laboratory (Schlettwein-Gsell, 1970).

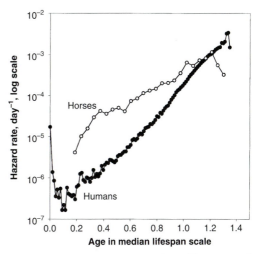

Figure 1.11 Comparative mortality of humans and horses expressed in the same units of mortality (per day). Data sources: Humans, official Swedish female life table for 1985; Horses, survival data for 2,742 thoroughbred mares (Comfort, 1958).

than old rats. These observations match the predictions of a reliability paradigm but not a traditional evolutionary explanation discussed earlier (the initial death rates for birds are much higher than expected from the traditional evolutionary perspective). Thus, a comparison of species death rates may be useful for testing different ideas on evolution of species aging and reliability.

Another interesting observation comes from a comparison of humans with horses (see Figure 1.11). It could be expected that shorter-lived horses should have higher death rates than humans. However, this prediction is only valid for young ages. The data demonstrate that an old horse is not much different from an old man in terms of mortality risk (see Figure 1.11). This example is opposite to observations on finch–rat comparisons and demonstrates a *mortality convergence* between two different biological species (man and horse) at older ages. In terms of reliability models, this observation may indicate that the rates of the late stages of body destruction are

similar in horses and humans, whereas the rates of the early stages of the aging process are vastly different in these two species.

These intriguing findings demonstrate that there are promising opportunities for further comparative studies on the evolution of species reliability and the merging of the reliability and evolutionary theories of aging. This reliability-evolutionary approach could be considered as further development of the earlier comparative studies of species aging and life histories (Austad, 1997, 2001; Gavrilov & Gavrilova, 1991; Holmes *et al.*, 2001; Promislow, 1993, 1994).

Another promising direction for the reliability-evolutionary approach is to study the selection effects for high performance (e.g., the ability to avoid predators). Classic evolutionary theories predict that an exposure to high extrinsic mortality due to predation should produce shorter-lived species (Charlesworth, 2001; Medawar, 1946; Williams, 1957). This prediction could be confronted with the opposite prediction of reliability theory, which says that elimination of weak individuals by predators should increase species life span because of selection for better performance and lower initial damage load. Interestingly, recent studies found an increased life span of guppies evolving in a high predation environment (Reznick *et al.*, 2004) as predicted by the reliability theory of aging.

VIII. Conclusions

Extensive studies of aging have produced many important and diverse findings, which require a general theoretical framework for them to be organized into a comprehensive body of knowledge.

As demonstrated by the success of evolutionary theories of aging, based on a general idea of the declining force of natural selection with age, quite general theoretical considerations can in fact be very useful and practical when applied to aging research (Charlesworth, 2000; Le Bourg, 2001; Martin, 2002; Partridge & Gems, 2002).

In this chapter, we attempted to go one step further in the search for a broader explanation of aging (not limited to biological species only) by applying a general theory of systems failure known as reliability theory. Considerations of this theory lead to the following conclusions:

1. *Redundancy* is a key notion for understanding aging, and the systemic nature of aging in particular. Systems that are redundant in numbers of irreplaceable elements do deteriorate (i.e., age) over time, even if they are built of non-aging elements. The positive effect of system redundancy is *damage tolerance*, which decreases mortality and increases life span. However, damage tolerance makes it possible for damage to be tolerated and accumulated over time, thus producing the aging phenomenon.

2. An apparent aging rate or expression of aging (measured as age differences in failure rates, including death rates) is higher for systems with higher redundancy levels (all other things being equal). This is an important issue because it helps put a correct perspective over fascinating observations of negligible senescence (no apparent aging) observed in the wild and at extreme old ages. Reliability theory explains that some cases of negligible senescence may have a trivial mechanism (lack of redundancies in the system being exposed to a challenging environment) and, therefore, will not help to uncover "the secrets of negligible senescence." The studies of negligible senescence make sense, however, when death rates are also demonstrated to be negligible.

Reliability theory also persuades a re-evaluation of the old belief that aging is somehow related to limited economic or evolutionary investments in systems longevity. The theory provides a completely opposite perspective on this issue—aging is a direct consequence of investments into systems reliability and durability through enhanced redundancy. This is a significant statement because it helps us to understand why the expression of aging (differences in failure rates between younger and older age groups) may be actually more profound in more complex redundant systems (organisms) designed for higher reliability.

3. During the life course, organisms are running out of cells (Gosden, 1985; Herndon *et al.*, 2002), losing reserve capacity (Bortz, 2002; Sehl & Yates, 2001), and this *redundancy depletion* explains the observed "compensation law of mortality" (mortality convergence at older ages) as well as the observed late-life mortality deceleration, leveling-off, and mortality plateaus.

4. Living organisms seem to be formed with a high *load of initial damage*, and

therefore their life span and aging patterns may be sensitive to *early-life conditions* that determine this initial damage load during early development. The idea of early-life programming of aging and longevity may have important practical implications for developing early-life interventions promoting health and longevity.

The theory also suggests that aging research should not be limited to studies of qualitative changes (like age changes in gene expression) because changes in *quantity* (numbers of cells and other functional elements) could be an important driving force in the aging process. In other words, aging may be largely driven by a process of redundancy loss.

The reliability theory predicts that a system may deteriorate with age even if it is built from non-aging elements with constant failure rate. The key issue here is the system's redundancy for irreplaceable elements, which is responsible for the aging phenomenon. In other words, each particular step of system destruction/deterioration may seem to be random (no aging, just occasional failure by chance), but if a system failure requires a sequence of several such steps (not just a single step of destruction), then the system as a whole may have an aging behavior.

Why is this important? Because the significance of beneficial health-promoting interventions is often undermined by claims that these interventions are not proven to delay the process of aging itself, but instead that they simply delay or "cover-up" some particular manifestations of aging.

In contrast to these pessimistic views, the reliability theory says that there may be no specific underlying elementary aging process itself; instead, aging may be largely a property of a redundant system as a whole because it has a network of destruction pathways, each being associated with particular manifestations of aging (types of failure). Therefore, we should not be discouraged by only partial success of each particular intervention, but instead we can appreciate an idea that we do have so many opportunities to oppose aging in numerous different ways.

Thus, the efforts to understand the routes and the early stages of age-related degenerative diseases should not be discarded as irrelevant to understanding "true" biological aging. On the contrary, the attempts to build an intellectual firewall between biogerontological research and clinical medicine are counterproductive. After all, the main reason people are really concerned about aging is because it is related to health deterioration and increased morbidity. The most important pathways of age changes are those that make older people sick and frail (Bortz, 2002).

Reliability theory suggests general answers to both the "why" and the "how" questions about aging. It explains "why" aging occurs by identifying the key determinant of aging behavior: system redundancy in numbers of irreplaceable elements. Reliability theory also explains "how" aging occurs, by focusing on the process of redundancy loss over time as the major mechanism of aging.

Aging is a complex phenomenon (Sehl & Yates, 2001), and a holistic approach using reliability theory may help analyze, understand, and, perhaps, control it. We suggest, therefore, adding reliability theory to the arsenal of methodological approaches applied in aging research.

Acknowledgments

This work was supported in part by grants from the National Institute on Aging.

References

Ames, B. N. (2004). Supplements and tuning up metabolism. *Journal of Nutrition*, 134, 3164S–3168S.

Andersen, B. B., Gundersen, H. J., & Pakkenberg, B. (2003). Aging of the human cerebellum: a stereological study. *Journal of Comparative Neurology, 466,* 356–365.

Andreadis, S., & Palsson, B. O. (1997). Coupled effects of polybrene and calf serum on the efficiency of retroviral transduction and the stability of retroviral vectors. *Human Gene Therapy, 8,* 285–291.

Austad, S. N. (1997). Comparative aging and life histories in mammals. *Experimental Gerontology, 32,* 23–38.

Austad, S. N. (2001). Concepts and theories of aging. In E. J. Masoro & S. N. Austad (Eds.), *Handbook of the biology of aging* (5th ed., pp. 3–22). San Diego, CA: Academic Press.

Ayyub, B. M., & McCuen, R. H. (2003). *Probability, statistics, reliability for engineers and scientists.* Boca Raton, FL: Chapman & Hall/CRC.

Baizabal, J. M., Furlan-Magaril, M., Santa-Olalla, J., & Covarrubias, L. (2003). Neural stem cells in development and regenerative medicine. *Archives of Medical Research, 34,* 572–588.

Barker, D. J. P. (1998). *Mothers, babies, and disease in later life* (2nd ed.). London: Churchill Livingstone.

Barlow, R. E., & Proschan, F. (1975). *Statistical theory of reliability and life testing. Probability models.* New York: Holt, Rinehart and Winston.

Barlow, R. E., Proschan, F., & Hunter, L. C. (1965). *Mathematical theory of reliability.* New York: Wiley.

Beard, R. E. (1959). Note on some mathematical mortality models. In G. E. W. Wolstenholme & M. O'Connor (Eds.), *The lifespan of animals* (pp. 302–311). Boston: Little, Brown.

Beard, R. E. (1971). Some aspects of theories of mortality, cause of death analysis, forecasting and stochastic processes. In W. Brass (Ed.), *Biological aspects of demography* (pp. 57–68). London: Taylor & Francis.

Bortz, W. M. (2002). A conceptual framework of frailty: a review. *Journal of Gerontology: Medical Sciences, 57A,* M283–M288.

Brock, T. D., Madigan, M. T., Martinko, J. M., & Parker, J. (1994). *Biology of microorganisms* (7th ed.), Englewood Cliffs, NJ: Prentice-Hall.

Bronikowski, A. M., Alberts, S. C., Altmann, J., Packer, C., Carey, K. D., & Tatar, M. (2002). The aging baboon: comparative demography in a non-human primate. *Proceedings of the National Academy of Sciences of the USA, 99,* 9591–9595.

Brooks, A., Lithgow, G. J., & Johnson, T. E. (1994). Mortality rates in a genetically heterogeneous population of *Caenorhabditis elegans. Science, 263,* 668–671.

Burns, J., Clarke, G., & Lumsden, C. J. (2002). Photoreceptor death: spatiotemporal patterns arising from one-hit death kinetics and a diffusible cell death factor. *Bulletin of Mathematical Biology, 64,* 1117–1145.

Calne, D. B. (1994). Is idiopathic Parkinsonism the consequence of an event or a process? *Neurology, 44,* 5–10.

Capogrossi, M. C. (2004). Cardiac stem cells fail with aging: a new mechanism for the age-dependent decline in cardiac function. *Circulation Research, 94,* 411–413.

Carey, J. R., & Liedo, P. (1995). Sex-specific life table aging rates in large medfly cohorts. *Experimental Gerontology, 30,* 315–325.

Carey, J. R., Liedo, P., Orozco, D., & Vaupel, J. W. (1992) Slowing of mortality rates at older ages in large medfly cohorts. *Science, 258,* 457–461.

Cargill, Sh. L., Carey, J. R., Muller, H.-G., & Anderson, G. (2003). Age of ovary determines remaining life expectancy in old ovariectomized mice. *Aging Cell, 2,* 185–190.

Carnes, B. A., Olshansky, S. J., & Grahn, D. (1998). An interspecies prediction of the risk of radiation-induced mortality. *Radiation Research, 149,* 487–492.

Cha, R. S., Thilly, W. G., & Zarbl, H. (1994). N-nitroso-N-methylurea-induced rat mammary tumors arise from cells with preexisting oncogenic Hras1 gene mutations. *Proceedings of the National Academy of Sciences of the USA, 91,* 3749–3753.

Charlesworth, B. (2000). Fisher, Medawar, Hamilton and the evolution of aging. *Genetics, 156,* 927–931.

Charlesworth, B. (2001). Patterns of age-specific means and genetic variances of mortality rates predicted by mutation-accumulation theory of aging. *Journal of Theoretical Biology, 210,* 47–65.

Choi, J. H., Kim, K. L., Huh, W., Kim, B., Byun, J., Suh, W., Sung, J., Jeon, E. S., Oh, H. Y., & Kim, D. K. (2004). Decreased number and impaired angiogenic function of endothelial progenitor cells in patients with chronic renal failure. *Arteriosclerosis, Thrombosis, and Vascular Biology*, 24, 1246–1252.

Clark, A. G., & Guadalupe, R. N. (1995). Probing the evolution of senescence in *Drosophila melanogaster* with P-element tagging. *Genetica*, 96, 225–234.

Clark, V. A. (1975). Survival distribution. *Annual Review of Biophysics and Bioengineering*, 4, 431–448.

Clarke, G., Collins, R. A., Leavitt, B. R., Andrews, D. F., Hayden, M. R., Lumsden, C. J., & McInnes, R. R. (2000). A one-hit model of cell death in inherited neuronal degenerations. *Nature*, 406, 195–199.

Clarke, G., Collins, R. A., Leavitt, B. R., Andrews, D. F., Hayden, M. R., Lumsden, C. J., & McInnes, R. R. (2001a). Addendum: a one-hit model of cell death in inherited neuronal degenerations. *Nature*, 409, 542.

Clarke, G., Lumsden, C. J., & McInnes, R. R. (2001b). Inherited neurodegenerative diseases: the one-hit model of neurodegeneration. *Human Molecular Genetics*, 10, 2269–2275.

Cohen, H. Y., Miller, C., Bitterman, K. J., Wall, N. R., Hekking, B., Kessler, B., Howitz, K. T., Gorospe, M., de Cabo, R., & Sinclair, D. A. (2004). Calorie restriction promotes mammalian cell survival by inducing the SIRT1 deacetylase. *Science*, 305, 390–392.

Collins, K., & Mitchell, J. R. (2002). Telomerase in the human organism. *Oncogene*, 21, 564–579.

Comfort, A. (1958). The longevity and mortality of thoroughbred mares. *Journal of Gerontology*, 13, 342–350.

Commo, S., Gaillard, O., & Bernard, B. A. (2004). Human hair greying is linked to a specific depletion of hair follicle melanocytes affecting both the bulb and the outer root sheath. *British Journal of Dermatology*, 150, 435–443.

Crowder, M .J., Kimber, A. C., Smith, R. L., & Sweeting, T. J. (1991). *Statistical analysis of reliability data*. London: Chapman & Hall.

Curtsinger, J. W., Fukui, H., Townsend, D., & Vaupel, J. W. (1992). Demography of genotypes: failure of the limited life-span paradigm in *Drosophila melanogaster*. *Science*, 258, 461–463.

Davis, B. D., Dulbeco, R., Eisen, H. N., & Ginsberg, H. S. (1990). *Microbiology* (4th ed.), Philadelphia: Lippincott.

Deng, G., Lu, Y., Zlotnikov, G., Thor, A. D., & Smith, H. S. (1996). Loss of heterozygosity in normal tissue adjacent to breast carcinomas. *Science*, 274, 2057–2059.

DePinho, R. A., & Wong, K. K. (2003). The age of cancer: telomeres, checkpoints, and longevity. *Journal of Clinical Investigation*, 111, S9–S14.

Doblhammer, G., & Vaupel, J. W. (2001). Lifespan depends on month of birth. *Proceedings of the National Academy of Sciences of the USA*, 98, 2934–2939.

Dobzhansky, T. (1962). *Mankind Evolving. The Evolution of Human Species*. New Haven and London: Yale University Press.

Dworkin, P. H. (1992). *Pediatrics* (2nd ed.), Malvern, PA: Harwal.

Eakin, T., Shouman, R., Qi, Y. L., Liu, G. X., & Witten, M. (1995). Estimating parametric survival model parameters in gerontological aging studies. Methodological problems and insights. *Journal of Gerontology: Biological Sciences*, 50A, B166–B176.

Economos, A. C. (1979). A non-Gompertzian paradigm for mortality kinetics of metazoan animals and failure kinetics of manufactured products. *Age*, 2, 74–76.

Economos, A. C. (1980). Kinetics of metazoan mortality. *Journal of Social and Biological Structures*, 3, 317–329.

Economos, A. C. (1983). Rate of aging, rate of dying and the mechanism of mortality. *Archives of Gerontology and Geriatrics*, 1, 3–27.

Economos, A. C. (1985). Rate of aging, rate of dying and non-Gompertzian mortality—encore . . . *Gerontology*, 31, 106–111.

Edelberg, J. M., Tang, L., Hattori, K., Lyden, D., & Rafii, S. (2002). Young adult bone marrow-derived endothelial precursor cells restore aging-impaired cardiac angiogenic function. *Circulation Research*, 90, E89–E93.

Eisner, E. (1967). Actuarial data for the Bengalese finch (*Lonchura striata*: Fam.Estrildidae) in captivity. *Experimental Gerontology*, 2, 187–189.

Ekerdt, D. J. (Ed.) (2002). *The Macmillan Encyclopedia of Aging*. New York: Macmillan Reference USA.

Feller, W. (1968). *An introduction to probability theory and its applications.* Vol.1, New York: Wiley.

Finch, C. E. (1990). *Longevity, senescence and the genome.* Chicago: University of Chicago Press.

Finch, C. E., & Kirkwood, T. B. L. (2000). *Chance, development, and aging.* New York, Oxford: Oxford University Press.

Forsyth, N. R., Wright, W. E., & Shay, J. W. (2002). Telomerase and differentiation in multicellular organisms: turn it off, turn it on, and turn it off again. *Differentiation*, 69, 188–197.

Fukui, H. H., Ackert, L., & Curtsinger, J. W. (1996). Deceleration of age-specific mortality rates in chromosomal homozygotes and heterozygotes of *Drosophila melanogaster. Experimental Gerontology*, 31, 517–531.

Fukui, H. H., Xiu, L., & Curtsinger, J. W. (1993). Slowing of age-specific mortality rates in *Drosophila melanogaster. Experimental Gerontology*, 28, 585–599.

Galambos, J. (1978). *The asymptotic theory of extreme order statistics.* New York: Wiley.

Gavrilov, L. A. (1978). Mathematical model of aging in animals. *Doklady Akademii Nauk SSSR: Biological Sciences*, 238, 53–55 (English edition).

Gavrilov, L. A. (1980). *Study of life span genetics using the kinetic analysis.* Ph.D. Thesis, Moscow, Russia: Moscow State University.

Gavrilov, L. A. (1984). Does a limit of the life span really exist? *Biofizika*, 29, 908–911.

Gavrilov, L. A., & Gavrilova, N. S. (1979). Determination of species length of life. *Doklady Akademii Nauk SSSR: Biological Sciences*, 246, 905–908 (English edition).

Gavrilov, L. A., & Gavrilova, N. S. (1991). *The biology of life span: a quantitative approach,* New York: Harwood Academic Publisher.

Gavrilov, L. A., & Gavrilova, N. S. (1997). Parental age at conception and offspring longevity. *Reviews in Clinical Gerontology*, 7, 5–12.

Gavrilov, L. A, & Gavrilova, N. S. (1999). Season of birth and human longevity. *Journal of Anti-Aging Medicine*, 2, 365–366.

Gavrilov, L. A., & Gavrilova, N. S. (2000). Human longevity and parental age at conception. In J.-M. Robine, T. B. L. Kirkwood & M. Allard (Eds.). *Sex and longevity: sexuality, gender, reproduction, parenthood* (pp. 7–31). Berlin, Heidelberg: Springer-Verlag.

Gavrilov, L. A., & Gavrilova, N. S. (2001a). Epidemiology of human longevity: the search for appropriate methodology. *Journal of Anti-Aging Medicine*, 4, 13–30.

Gavrilov, L. A., & Gavrilova, N. S. (2001b). The reliability theory of aging and longevity. *Journal of Theoretical Biology*, 213, 527–545.

Gavrilov, L. A., & Gavrilova, N. S. (2003a). Early-life factors modulating lifespan. In S. I. S. Rattan (Ed.), *Modulating aging and longevity* (pp. 27–50). Dordrecht, The Netherlands: Kluwer Academic Publishers.

Gavrilov, L. A., & Gavrilova, N. S. (2003b). The quest for a general theory of aging and longevity. *Science of Aging Knowledge Environment [electronic resource]: SAGE KE*, Vol. 2003 Jul 16, 28, RE5. Available at http://sageke.sciencemag.org.

Gavrilov, L. A., & Gavrilova, N. S. (2004a). Early-life programming of aging and longevity: the idea of high initial damage load (the HIDL hypothesis). *Annals of the New York Academy of Sciences*, 1019, 496–501.

Gavrilov, L. A., & Gavrilova, N. S. (2004b). The reliability-engineering approach to the problem of biological aging. *Annals of the New York Academy of Sciences*, 1019, 509–512.

Gavrilov, L. A., & Gavrilova, N. S. (2004c). Why we fall apart. Engineering's reliability theory explains human aging. *IEEE Spectrum*, 9, 2–7.

Gavrilov, L. A., Gavrilova, N. S., & Iaguzhinskii, L. S. (1978). Basic patterns of aging and death in animals from the standpoint of reliability theory. *Journal of General Biology [Zhurnal Obshchej Biologii]*, 39, 734–742.

Gavrilova, N. S., & Gavrilov, L. A. (2002). Evolution of aging. In D. J. Ekerdt (Ed.), *Encyclopedia of aging* (Vol. 2, pp. 458–467). New York: Macmillan Reference USA.

Gavrilova, N. S., Gavrilov, L. A., Evdokushkina, G. N., Semyonova, V. G. (2003). Early-life predictors of human longevity: analysis of the 19th century birth cohorts. *Annales de Démographie Historique*, 2, 177–198.

Gilchrest, B. A., Blog, F. B., & Szabo, G. (1979). Effects of aging and chronic sun exposure on melanocytes in human skin. *Journal of Investigative Dermatology*, 73, 141–143.

Goldschmidt-Clermont, P. J. (2003). Loss of bone marrow-derived vascular progenitor cells leads to inflammation and atherosclerosis. *American Heart Journal*, 146(4 Suppl), S5–S12.

Golubev, A. (2004). Does Makeham make sense? *Biogerontology*, 5, 159–167.

Gompertz, B. (1825). On the nature of the function expressive of the law of human mortality and on a new mode of determining life contingencies. *Philosophical Transactions of the Royal Society of London*, 115A, 513–585.

Gosden, R. G. (1985). *The biology of menopause: the cause and consequence of ovarian aging.* San Diego: Academic Press.

Gouda, M. D., Singh, S. A., Rao, A. G., Thakur, M. S., & Karanth, N. G. (2003). Thermal inactivation of glucose oxidase: mechanism and stabilization using additives. *Journal of Biological Chemistry*, 278, 24324–24333.

Greenwood, M., & Irwin, J. O. (1939). The biostatistics of senility. *Human Biology*, 11, 1–23.

Gumbel, E. J. (1958). *Statistics of extremes.* New York: Columbia University Press.

Hack, M., & Fanaroff, A. A. (2000). Outcomes of children of extremely low birthweight and gestational age in the 1990s. *Seminars in Neonatology*, 5, 89–106.

Hall, J. C. (1969). Age-dependent enzyme changes in *Drosophila melanogaster*. *Experimental Gerontology*, 4, 207–222.

Handyside, A. H., & Delhanty, J. D. A. (1997). Preimplantation genetic diagnosis: strategies and surprises. *Trends in Genetics*, 13, 270–275.

Haranghy, L., & Balázs, A. (1980). Regeneration and rejuvenation of invertebrates. In N. W. Shock (Ed.), *Perspectives in experimental gerontology* (pp. 224–233). New York: Arno Press.

Harman, D., & Eddy, D. E. (1979). Free radical theory of aging: beneficial effects of adding antioxidants to the maternal mouse diet on life span of offspring: possible explanation of the sex difference in longevity. *Age*, 2, 109–122.

Heintz, N. (2000). One-hit neuronal death. *Nature*, 406, 137–138.

Herndon, L. A., Schmeissner, P. J., Dudaronek, J. M., Brown, P. A., Listner, K. M., Sakano, Y., Paupard, M. C., Hall, D. H., & Driscoll, M. (2002). Stochastic and genetic factors influence tissue-specific decline in ageing *C. elegans. Nature*, 419, 808–814.

Hirsch, A. G., Williams, R. J., & Mehl, P. (1994). Kinetics of medfly mortality. *Experimental Gerontology*, 29, 197–204.

Hirsch, H. R., & Peretz, B. (1984). Survival and aging of a small laboratory population of a marine mollusc, *Aplysia californica*. *Mechanisms of Ageing and Development*, 27, 43–62.

Hjalmarsson, O., Hagberg, B., Hagberg, G., Kubli, F., Patel, N., Schmidt, W., & Linderkamp, O. (Eds.). (1988). *Perinatal events and brain damage in surviving children.* Berlin: Springer-Verlag, pp. 28–36.

Holmes, D. J., & Ottinger, M. A. (2003). Birds as long-lived animal models for the study of aging. *Experimental Gerontology*, 38, 1365–1375.

Holmes, D. J., Fluckiger, R., & Austad, S. N. (2001). Comparative biology of aging in birds: an update. *Experimental Gerontology*, 36, 869–883.

Hopkin, K. (2001). More than a sum our cells. *Science of Aging Knowledge Environment [electronic resource]: SAGE KE*, Vol. 2001 Oct 3, 1, oa4.

Janse, C., Slob, W., Popelier, C. M., & Vogelaar, J.W. (1988). Survival characteristics of the mollusc *Lymnaea stagnalis* under constant culture conditions: effects of aging and disease. *Mechanisms of Ageing and Development*, 42, 263–174.

Jay, J. M. (1996). *Modern food microbiology.* New York: Chapman and Hall.

Johnson, T. E. (1987). Aging can be genetically dissected into component processes using long-lived lines of *Caenorhabditis elegans*. *Proceedings of the National Academy of Sciences of the USA*, 84, 3777–3781.

Johnson, T. E. (1990). Increased life span of age-1 mutants in *Caenorhabditis elegans* and lower Gompertz rate of aging. *Science*, 249, 908–912.

Jonason, A. S., Kunala, S., Price, G. T., Restifo, R. J., Spinelli, H. M., Persing, J. A., Leffell, D. J., Tarone, R. E., & Brash, D. E. (1996). Frequent clones of p53-mutated keratinocytes in normal human skin. *Proceedings of the National Academy of Sciences of the USA*, 93, 14025–14029.

Keller, G., Zimmer, G., Mall, G., Ritz, E., & Amann, K. (2003). Nephron number in patients with primary hypertension. *New England Journal of Medicine*, 348, 101–108.

Khazaeli, A. A., Xiu, L., & Curtsinger, J. W. (1996). Effect of density on age-specific mortality in *Drosophila*: a density supplementation experiment. *Genetica*, 98, 21–31.

Khrapko, K., Ebralidse, K., & Kraytsberg, Y. (2004). Where and when do somatic mtDNA mutations occur? *Annals of the New York Academy of Sciences*, 1019, 240–244.

Kim, Sh. S. H, Kaminker, P., & Campisi, J. (2002). Telomeres, aging and cancer: in search of a happy ending. *Oncogene*, 21, 503–511.

Klein, J. P., & Moeschberger, M. L. (1997). *Survival analysis: techniques for censored and truncated data*. New York: Springer-Verlag.

Kuh, D., & Ben-Shlomo, B. (1997). *A life course approach to chronic disease epidemiology*. Oxford: Oxford University Press.

Kundi, M. (1999). One-hit models for virus inactivation studies. *Antiviral Research*, 41, 145–152.

Kunstyr, I., & Leuenberger, H.-G. W. (1975). Gerontological data of C57BL/6J mice. I. Sex differences in survival curves. *Journal of Gerontology*, 30, 157–162.

Kurganov, B. I. (2002). Kinetics of protein aggregation. Quantitative estimation of the chaperone-like activity in test-systems based on suppression of protein aggregation. *Biochemistry* (Moscow), 67, 409–422.

Le Bourg, É. (2001). A mini-review of the evolutionary theories of aging. Is it the time to accept them? *Demographic Research* [electronic resource], 4, 1–28. Available at http://www.demographic-research.org/volumes/vol4/1/4–1.pdf.

Leeuwenburgh, C. (2003). Role of apoptosis in sarcopenia. *Journal of Gerontology: Biological Sciences*, 58A, B999–B1001.

Leon, D. A., Lithell, H. O., Vågerö, D., Koupilová, I., Mohsen, R., Berglund, L., Lithell, U.-B., & McKeigue, P. M. (1998). Reduced fetal growth rate and increased risk of death from ischaemic heart disease: cohort study of 15,000 Swedish men and women born 1915–29. *British Medical Journal*, 317, 241–245.

Libby, P. (2003). Bone marrow: a fountain of vascular youth? *Circulation*, 108, 378–379.

Lindop, P. J. (1961). Growth rate, lifespan and causes of death in SAS/4 mice. *Gerontologia*, 5, 193–208.

Lucas, A., Fewtrell, M. S., & Cole, T. J. (1999). Fetal origins of adult disease: the hypothesis revisited. *British Medical Journal*, 319, 245–249.

Makeham, W. M. (1860). On the law of mortality and the construction of annuity tables. *Journal of the Institute of Actuaries*, 8, 301–310.

Martin, G. M. (2002). Gene action in the aging brain: an evolutionary biological perspective. *Neurobiology of Aging*, 23, 647–654.

Martin, L. J., Brambrink, A. M., Price, A. C., Kaiser, A., Agnew, D. M., Ichord, R. N., & Traystman, R. J. (2000). Neuronal death in newborn striatum after hypoxia-ischemia is necrosis and evolves with oxidative stress. *Neurobiology of Disease*, 7, 169–191.

Martinez, D. E. (1998). Mortality patterns suggest lack of senescence in hydra. *Experimental Gerontology*, 33, 217–225.

Masoro, E. J. (2003). Subfield history: caloric restriction, slowing aging, and extending life. *Science of aging knowledge environment [electronic resource]: SAGE KE*, Vol. 2003 Feb 26, 8, RE2.

Masoro, E. J. (2005). Are age-associated diseases an integral part of aging? In E. J. Masoro & S. N. Austad (Eds.), *Handbook of the biology of aging* (6th ed.). San Diego, CA: Academic Press.

Massoff, R. W., Dagnelie, G., Benzschawel, T., Palmer, R. W., & Finkelstein, D. (1990). First order dynamics of visual field loss in retinitis pigmentosa. *Clinical Vision Sciences*, 5, 1–26.

McKiernan, S. H., Bua, E., McGorray, J., & Aiken, J. (2004). Early-onset calorie restriction conserves fiber number in aging rat skeletal muscle. *The FASEB Journal*, 18, 580–581.

McLaren, A. (1998). Genetics and human reproduction. *Trends in Genetics*, 14, 427–431.

Medawar, P. B. (1946). Old age and natural death. *Modern Quarterly*, 2, 30–49. [Reprinted in Medawar, P.B. (1958). *The uniqueness of the individual* (pp. 17–43), New York: Basic Books].

Moffett, D. F., Moffett, S. B., & Schauf, C. L. (1993). *Human physiology: foundations and frontiers* (2nd ed.). St. Louis: Mosby.

Nekhaeva, E., Bodyak, N. D., Kraytsberg, Y., McGrath, S. B., Van Orsouw, N. J., Pluzhnikov, A., Wei, J. Y., Vijg, J., & Khrapko, K. (2002). Clonally expanded mtDNA point mutations are abundant in individual cells of human tissues. *Proceedings of the National Academy of Sciences of the USA*, 99, 5521–5526.

Nyengaard, J. R., & Bendtsen, T. F. (1992). Glomerular number and size in relation to age, kidney weight, and body surface in normal man. *Anatomical Record*, 232, 194–201.

Ogburn, C. E., Austad, S. N., Holmes, D. J., Kiklevich, J. V., Gollahon, K., Rabinovitch, P. S., & Martin, G. M. (1998). Cultured renal epithelial cells from birds and mice: enhanced resistance of avian cells to oxidative stress and DNA damage. *Journal of Gerontology: Biological Sciences*, 53A, B287–B292.

Ogburn, C. E., Carlberg, K., Ottinger, M. A., Holmes, D. J., Martin, G. M., & Austad, S. N. (2001). Exceptional cellular resistance to oxidative damage in long-lived birds requires active gene expression. *Journal of Gerontology: Biological Sciences*, 56A, B468–B474.

Olshansky, S. J. (1998). On the biodemography of aging: a review essay. *Population and Development Review*, 24, 381–393.

Olshansky, S. J., & Carnes, B. A. (1997). Ever since Gompertz. *Demography*, 34, 1–15.

Partridge, L., & Gems, D. (2002). The evolution of longevity. *Current Biology*, 12, R544–R546.

Partridge, L., & Mangel, M. (1999). Messages from mortality: the evolution of death rates in the old. *Trends in Ecology and Evolution*, 14, 438–442.

Pearl, R., & Miner, J. R. (1935). Experimental studies on the duration of life. XIY. The comparative mortality of certain lower organisms. *Quarterly Review of Biology*, 10, 60–79.

Peleg, M., Normand, M. D., & Campanella, O. H. (2003). Estimating microbial inactivation parameters from survival curves obtained under varying conditions—the linear case. *Bulletin of Mathematical Biology*, 65, 219–234.

Perks, W. (1932). On some experiments in the graduation of mortality statistics. *Journal of the Institute of Actuaries*, 63, 12–57.

Promislow, D. E. (1993). On size and survival: progress and pitfalls in the allometry of life span. *Journal of Gerontology: Biological Sciences*, 48, B115–B123.

Promislow, D. E. (1994). DNA repair and the evolution of longevity: a critical analysis. *Journal of Theoretical Biology*, 170, 291–300.

Rausand, M., & Høyland, A. (2003). *System reliability theory: models, statistical methods, and applications* (2nd ed.). Hoboken, NJ: Wiley-Interscience.

Rauscher, F. M., Goldschmidt-Clermont, P. J., Davis, B. H., Wang, T., Gregg, D., Ramaswami, P., Pippen, A. M., Annex, B. H., Dong, C., & Taylor, D. A. (2003). Aging, progenitor cell exhaustion, and atherosclerosis. *Circulation*, 108, 457–463.

Reznick, D. N., Bryant, M. J., Roff, D., Ghalambor, C. K., & Ghalambor, D. E. (2004). Effect of extrinsic mortality on the evolution of senescence in guppies. *Nature*, 431, 1095–1099.

Ricklefs, R. E., & Scheuerlein, A. (2002). Biological implications of the Weibull and Gompertz models of aging. *Journal of Gerontology*, 57A, B69–B76.

Rigdon, S. E., & Basu, A. P. (2000). *Statistical methods for the reliability of repairable systems*. New York: Wiley.

Rockstein, M., & Lieberman, H. M. (1959). A life table for the common house fly, *Musca domestica. Gerontologia*, 3: 23–36.

Sacher, G. A. (1966). The Gompertz transformation in the study of the injury-mortality relationship: application to late radiation effects and ageing. In P. J. Lindop & G. A. Sacher (Eds.), *Radiation and ageing* (pp. 411–441). London: Taylor and Francis.

Sacher, G. A. (1977). Life table modification and life prolongation. In C. E. Finch & L. Hayflick (Eds), *Handbook of the biology of aging* (pp. 582–638). New York: Van Nostrand Reinhold.

Sacher, G. A., & Duffy, P. H. (1979). Genetic relation of life span to metabolic rate for inbred mouse strains and their hybrids. *Federation Proceedings*, 38, 184–188.

Schlettwein-Gsell, D. (1970). Survival curves of an old age rat colony. *Gerontologia*, 16, 111–115.

Schulzer, M., Lee, C. S., Mak, E. K., Vingerhoets, F. J. G., & Calne, D. B. (1994). A mathematical model of pathogenesis in idiopathic Parkinsonism. *Brain*, 117, 509–516.

Sehl, M. E., & Yates, F. E. (2001). Kinetics of human aging: I. Rates of senescence between ages 30 and 70 years in healthy people. *Journal of Gerontology: Biological Sciences*, 56A, B198–B208.

Strasser, H., Tiefenthaler, M., Steinlechner, M., Eder, I., Bartsch, G., & Konwalinka, G. (2000). Age dependent apoptosis and loss of rhabdosphincter cells. *Journal of Urology*, 164, 1781–1785.

Strehler, B. L. (1978). *Time, cells, and aging* (2nd ed.). New York and London: Academic Press.

Strehler, B. L., & Mildvan, A. S. (1960). General theory of mortality and aging. *Science*, 132, 14–21.

Tatar, M., Carey, J. R., & Vaupel, J. W. (1993). Long-term cost of reproduction with and without accelerated senescence in *Callosobruchus maculatus*: analysis of age-specific mortality. *Evolution*, 47, 1302–1312.

United Nations (1967). *Demographic Yearbook, 1966*, 18th issue. New York: United Nations.

United Nations (1975). *Demographic Yearbook, 1974*, 26th issue. New York: United Nations.

Vanfleteren, J. R., De Vreese, A., & Braeckman, B. P. (1998). Two-parameter logistic and Weibull equations provide better fits to survival data from isogenic populations of *Caenorhabditis elegans* in axenic culture than does the Gompertz model. *Journal of Gerontology: Biological Sciences*, 53A, B393–B403.

Van Zant, G., & Liang, Y. (2003). The role of stem cells in aging. *Experimental Hematology*, 31, 659–672.

Vaupel, J. W., Carey, J. R., Christensen, K., Johnson, T., Yashin, A. I., Holm, N. V., Iachine, I. A., Kannisto, V., Khazaeli, A. A., Liedo, P., Longo, V. D., Zeng, Y., Manton, K., & Curtsinger, J. W. (1998). Biodemographic trajectories of longevity. *Science*, 280, 855–860.

Volpe, J. (2000). *Neurology of the newborn* (4th ed.). Philadelphia: Saunders.

Wallace, W. H., & Kelsey, T. W. (2004). Ovarian reserve and reproductive age may be determined from measurement of ovarian volume by transvaginal sonography. *Human Reproduction*, 19, 1612–1617.

Weibull, W. A. (1939). A statistical theory of the strength of materials. *Ingeniorsvetenskapsakademiens Handlingar*, 151, 5–45.

Weibull, W. A. (1951). A statistical distribution function of wide applicability. *Journal of Applied Mechanics*, 18, 293–297.

Williams, G. C. (1957). Pleiotropy, natural selection and the evolution of senescence. *Evolution*, 11, 398–411.

Wilmoth, J. R. (1997). In search of limits. In K. W. Wachter & C. E. Finch (Eds.), *Between Zeus and the salmon. The biodemography of longevity* (pp. 38–64). Washington, DC: National Academy Press.

Chapter 2

Are Age-Associated Diseases an Integral Part of Aging?

Edward J. Masoro

I. Introduction

In his essay reviewing the fifth edition of the *Handbook of the Biology of Aging*, Leonard Hayflick (2002) commends the editors for focusing on biogerontology rather than age-associated diseases such as Alzheimer's. Hayflick explains that although he does not view age-associated diseases as an integral part of aging, he does feel that aging provides a substratum for their occurrence. He goes on to say that he places age-associated disease in the province of geriatric medicine rather than biogerontology. A logical extension of this line of thinking would lead one to conclude that although progressive deteriorative physiological changes with age are an integral part of aging, the progression of age-associated pathophysiology is not. Because the validity of such a conclusion seems questionable, I believe that the relationship between aging and age-associated disease warrants further evaluation.

It should be noted that most gerontologists currently share Hayflick's view of aging and disease, although there has long been concern about this relationship. Indeed, in a recent article, Blumenthal (2003) cites 26 papers published since 1880 that address this issue. It appears that Nathan Shock, the towering figure of 20th-century biological gerontology, is responsible for the widely held current view. Shock (1961) posed that the processes of aging and the etiologies of disease are distinct. However, both before and after Shock's pronouncement, contrary views had and have been presented. For example, Perlman (1954) proposed that aging is a disease complex and termed the concept of "normal, healthy senescence" an imaginative figment. Evans (1988) asserted the impossibility of separating disease from aging. And Semsei (2000) suggested that the roots of certain diseases are firmly linked to the aging process itself.

The goal of this chapter is to critically evaluate the relationship between aging and age-associated disease. This evaluation will discuss both how this question has been addressed in the past as well as recent advances in our knowledge of the biology of aging and age-associated diseases. This issue is of interest not only from an academic conceptual perspective, but it also affects the planning, design, and execution of biogerontologic research. Also, as pointed out by Wick and colleagues (2003), the study of age-associated diseases may well be of great value for understanding basic aging processes. However, it is first necessary to review some of the long-held concepts of biological gerontology that have influenced perceptions of the relationship between aging and age-associated diseases.

II. Concepts of Biological Gerontology

There is no better starting point than the definition of aging. A broad, general definition is that aging is what happens to an organism over time (Costa & McCrae, 1995). This definition includes (1) no change with time, (2) beneficial changes with time (such as the maturation of physiological processes during development), and (3) deteriorative changes with time (such as those that occur with advancing adult age). Although this broad definition of the aging of organisms is certainly valid, it is not what is usually meant when biological gerontologists use the term. Nor, for that matter, is it what laypersons mean when discussing the aging of friends and family. Rather, both groups are usually referring solely to those deteriorative changes noted with advancing age, such as diminished physiological capacity or the wrinkling of the skin.

In other words, when biological gerontologists and laypersons use the term *aging*, they are most often referring to senescence. *Senescence* is defined as the progressive deterioration during the adult period of life that underlies an increasing vulnerability to challenges and a decreasing ability of the organism to survive. It is

important to note that organismic senescence (i.e., aging) is a process that starts in early adult life and progresses from that time on. Indeed, athletes in some sports exhibit performance deterioration as early as the last half of the third decade of life; in most sports, deterioration in performance occurs by the middle of the fourth decade. It is also critical not to confuse organismic senescence with cellular senescence, a term for the loss of proliferative ability of cells in culture. In fact, it is the definition of aging as a synonym for organismic senescence that underlies the concept of biological age in contrast to chronological age (Borkan & Norris, 1980) and the search for biomarkers of aging (McClearn, 1997). Thus, aging and senescence will be used as synonyms in this chapter; although not explicitly stated, such is generally the case in other chapters of this book.

Based on this narrow definition of aging, a set of putative fundamental characteristics of aging was developed in the field of biological gerontology during the first half of the 20th century. These, as Strehler (1977) succinctly summarized, include *intrinsicality, universality, progressivity, irreversibility*, and *genetically programmed. Intrinsicality* defines aging as an inherent characteristic of the organism rather than a response to environmental factors. *Universality* confines aging to processes that occur in all members of a species (or all members of a gender of a species; e.g., menopause in the human female). *Progressivity* describes aging as a change that gradually increases in magnitude over time. *Irreversibility* professes that once a change due to aging occurs, it cannot be reversed. *Genetically programmed* originally meant that aging was programmed in the same sense as developmental processes; more recently, it is often modified to mean the influence of genotype on the aging phenotype. It is these putative fundamental characteristics of aging that have, to a great extent, served as the basis for separating biological aging from age-associated disease. Alas, as will become evident in this chapter, it is doubtful that these characteristics have been helpful in clarifying the relationship between aging and age-associated disease.

III. Age-Associated Diseases

The *American Heritage Dictionary* (1996) defines *disease* as "a pathological condition of a part, an organ, or a system of an organism resulting from various causes, such as infection, genetic defect, or environmental stress, and characterized by an identifiable group of signs or symptoms." Although this definition is adequate for the purposes of this chapter, Scully (2004) points out that any definition of disease is problematic because what is called a disease is influenced by both medical advances and by societal culture. Thus, the definition changes with time and differs from place to place.

Although acute infectious diseases occur at all ages, their consequences may be more severe in the elderly because of age-associated deterioration in immune function (Papciak *et al.*, 1996) and in the functioning of most of the other physiological systems (Masoro, 1995). Although genetic diseases are not restricted to the young, they often do occur as congenital diseases or at early postnatal ages (Blumenthal, 1999). Environmental stress can also cause disease at all ages, but because aging decreases the ability to cope with stressors (Shock, 1967), morbidity and mortality are more likely outcomes of stress in the old than in the young. It is reasonable to conclude that the above categories of diseases are not an integral part of aging, even though aging can clearly affect the consequences of such diseases.

However, *age-associated diseases* should not be so readily dismissed as an integral part of aging. Such disease processes cause morbidity and/or mortality primarily at advanced ages and are chronic, or when acute are the result of long-term processes, such as gradual loss of bone and atherogenesis. Brody and Schneider (1986) divided these diseases into two classes: *age-dependent diseases* and *age-related diseases.* They defined *age-dependent diseases* as those in which the pathogenesis appears to involve basic aging processes. Mortality and morbidity caused by these diseases increase exponentially with advancing age. As examples of age-dependent diseases, they listed coronary heart disease, cerebrovascular disease, type II diabetes, osteoporosis, Alzheimer's disease, and Parkinson's disease. They defined *age-related diseases* as those with a temporal relationship to the age of the host but not necessarily related to the aging process. These diseases occur at a specific age, but with a further increase in age they either decline in frequency or increase at a less than exponential rate. Gout, multiple sclerosis, amyotrophic lateral sclerosis (ALS), and many, but certainly not all, cancers are examples of such diseases. The relationship of cancer to aging will be discussed later in this chapter.

Interestingly, in a paper on diseases that cause the death of people 85 years or older, Kohn (1982) divides the diseases into three classes, two of which are similar to the two classes of Brody and Schneider. In Kohn's first class are diseases that are themselves normal aging processes, being progressive and irreversible under usual conditions; examples are atherosclerotic diseases, degenerative joint diseases, and osteoporosis. His second class covers diseases that increase with age but may not be part of the aging process; examples are neoplasia and hypertension. The third class includes diseases with consequences more serious in people of advanced age than in young people; infectious disease is an example. In a paper published some 15 years later, Klima and colleagues (1997) found the causes of death in geriatric patients in Houston, Texas, and Prague, Czech Republic, to be similar to what Kohn reported.

Recently, Horiuchi and colleagues (2003) reported on the causes of death in France from 1979 to 1994 during two periods of life in subjects age 15 to 100-plus years. In one group of subjects age 30 to 54 and a second group of subjects age 65 to 89, the age-specific death rate increased exponentially with increasing age (a measure of population aging). Deaths due to malignant neoplasms, acute myocardial infarctions, hypertensive disease, and liver cirrhosis rose rapidly during the 30- to 54-year age range. During the range of 65 to 89 years, death due to certain infectious diseases, accidents, dementia, heart failure, and cerebrovascular disease rose rapidly. Deaths due to malignant neoplasms and acute myocardial infarction did not rise rapidly in the 65 to 89 age range; thus, the fraction of deaths due to these diseases was less than during the 30 to 54 age range. However, of the people who died between 15 and 100 years old, only 10 percent died between 30 and 54 years and 67 percent died between 65 and 89 years. Thus, the absolute number of deaths due to malignant neoplasms and myocardial infarction was markedly greater in those in the older age range compared to those in the 30- to 54-year age range.

Other investigators have also found that the fraction of deaths due to cancer decreased at advanced ages. Smith (1996) reported that cancer was the cause of 40 percent of deaths that occurred between 50 and 69 years of age but only 4 percent of those that occurred at ages older than 100 years. Miyaishi and colleagues (2000) found that the peak incidence of single cancers occurred between 60 and 64 years of age, and of multiple cancers between 80 and 84 years of age.

It is of interest to note that in humans, the heritability of age-associated diseases is in the same range (<40 percent) as the heritability of life span (Longo & Finch, 2002). However, this claim needs to be tempered because heritability varies among specific age-associated diseases. Nevertheless, this fact and much of the information just presented are compatible with the view that age-associated disease is an integral part of aging. In addition, Urban and colleagues (2002) posed that age-associated autoimmune diseases result from genetic alterations caused by aging processes. And Ames and colleagues (1993) concluded that the oxidant byproducts of normal metabolism cause extensive damage to DNA, proteins, and lipids, thereby contributing to aging and age-associated diseases such as brain dysfunction, cancer, cardiovascular disease, and cataracts. Rattan (1991) proposed that aging and age-associated disease are linked by the failure to maintain the appropriate level and structure of proteins. However, although the views of the Urban and Ames groups and Rattan are provocative, much more work remains to be done to establish their validity.

IV. Primary Aging, Secondary Aging, and "Normal Aging"

The concept of primary and secondary aging was proposed by Busse (1969) to resolve the paradox of viewing intrinsicality as one of the fundamental characteristics of aging, although it was obvious that environmental factors influence both aging and diseases associated with aging. *Primary aging* is defined as the universal changes occurring with age that are not caused by disease or environmental influences. *Secondary aging* is defined as changes involving interactions of primary aging processes with environmental influences and disease processes.

Thus, the concept of primary and secondary aging relegates disease, including age-associated disease, to that of a factor that can influence aging but is not an integral part of the aging process. Because the major thrust of this chapter is to assess whether age-associated diseases are an integral part of aging, further comment on this aspect of the primary and secondary aging concept is more appropriately considered after all other issues have been fully presented. However, placing environmental influences in the category of secondary aging does require comment at this juncture. Although the proximate mechanisms underlying aging are not fully understood, most gerontologists would agree that the long-term accumulation of molecular damage underlies aging, and it is likely that reactive oxygen molecules play an important role in this damage (Barja, 2002). Indeed, many believe that reactive oxygen molecules play a major causative role in aging, but the validity of this view remains to be established. Much of the generation of these reactive oxygen molecules occurs in the mitochondria during the metabolism of fuel, and if these molecules do, indeed, cause aging, it would be classified as primary aging. However, environmental factors (e.g., industrial pollutants), lifestyle (e.g., cigarette smoking), and pharmacological agents also cause the formation of reactive oxygen molecules, and if aging results from reactive oxygen molecules from these sources, it would be classified as secondary aging. Because in both instances aging is proposed to result from the interaction of reactive oxygen molecules with the macromolecules of the organism, it seems illogical to refer to one as primary aging and the other as secondary aging. Indeed, Vieira and colleagues (2000) showed that the effect of genes on the life span of *Drosophila melanogaster* is dependent on environmental factors. For these reasons, it seems highly unlikely that the concept of primary aging and

secondary aging is useful. In fact, it has probably impeded our quest for understanding the biological basis of aging and, even worse, will continue to do so.

An outgrowth of the concept of primary and secondary aging is the concept of *normal aging*, which is defined as senescence in the absence of disease (Shock, 1984). This view was bolstered by the concept of *natural death*, which Fries (1980) defined as death in the absence of disease. Given that with increasing age, most people experience one or more age-associated diseases, "normal aging" and "natural death" must, indeed, be rare occurrences. This is underscored by the report of Hebert (2004) that life expectancy in 2001 in the United Kingdom was 75.7 years for men and 80.4 years for women, and that on average, the projection is that men and women would suffer from poor health during the last 8.7 and 10.1 years of life, respectively. As pointed out by Gessert and colleagues (2002), declaring that someone has "died of old age" does not mean the individual has died without significant pathology.

From 1988 to 1994, the prevalence of diabetes in 60- to 74-year-old American Caucasians was 22.3 percent; it was 29.5 percent in African-Americans of the same age group (Sinclair & Croxon, 2003). The prevalence of osteoarthritis in individuals over 70 years of age is more than 30 percent (Scott, 2003). The prevalence of moderate to severe dementia is estimated at 1 to 2 percent at ages 65 to 70 years, 2 to 5 percent at ages 70 to 75 years, 11 to 20 percent at ages 80 to 85 years, and 39 to 60 percent at ages 90 to 95 years (Elby *et al.*, 1994; Skoog *et al.*, 1996). When dementia is coupled with the many other diseases that become increasingly common with advancing age (coronary heart disease, type II diabetes, congestive heart failure, stroke, osteoporosis, cataracts, Parkinson's disease, many kinds of cancer, and benign prostatic hyperplasia, to name a few), it becomes obvious that aging in the absence of disease is rare, indeed.

In a community-based study of 502 people 90 years of age or older in Stockholm, only 19 percent were found to be free of disease; the remainder had one or more diseases, most of which were age-associated diseases (von Strauss *et al.*, 2000). In a study of 207 Danes who reached their 100th birthday between April 1, 1995, and May 31, 1996, Anderson-Ramberg and colleagues (2001) found that only one was free of age-associated disease, with a mean number of 4.3 such diseases per person. In contrast, based on a study of 424 Americans and Canadians in the age range of 100 to 119 years, Perls' group (Evert *et al.*, 2003) reported that 19 percent were free of disease as compared to the less than 0.5 percent in the Danish study. This apparent discrepancy probably stems from two factors: Perls' group excluded dementia and osteoarthritis in their assessment of age-associated diseases, and they used interviews and questionnaires rather than physical examinations to determine disease status. Subsequently, in reviewing findings from various worldwide centenarian studies, Perls (2004) concluded that the prevalence of dementia is 75 to 85 percent in people age 100 years and older. Moreover, in another paper (Hitt *et al.*, 1999), which emphasizes that centenarians have been healthier than others for most of their lives, Perls' group reported that 37 centenarians with a mean age of 102 suffered from 4.0 diseases or chronic conditions at that age, 3.2 such conditions 5 years earlier, and 2.6 such conditions 10 years earlier. Clearly, even in the healthiest, disease is prevalent at advanced ages.

Investigators have also found a progressive increase with age in the prevalence and severity of age-associated diseases in both rats (Maeda *et al.*, 1985) and mice (Lipman *et al.*, 1999). Although not as exhaustively studied as laboratory rodents, such also appears to be the case for other mammalian species used as animal models in aging research.

Despite the rarity of absence of disease at advanced ages, investigators have used both human subjects and animal models to study "normal aging" by excluding those with discernible disease. In the case of human subjects, the procedure of excluding subjects with discernible diseases, including age-associated diseases, is referred to as "cleaning up" the physiological data (Rowe *et al.*, 1990). Obviously, this procedure limits the study to a small, atypical fraction of the aging population. It also suffers from the fact that advances in medical technology have enhanced detection of diseases previously not discernible. For example, in Lakatta's (1985) studies on the influence of aging on cardiovascular physiology, the thallium-stress test was used to exclude subjects with occult coronary heart disease, a technology not available or not used in earlier studies. Thus, it can be anticipated that advances in medical technology will lead to an ever-decreasing fraction of the elderly in the "normal aging" category.

Finally, the classification of age-associated functional change as either a physiological or pathophysiological process is arbitrary. For example, bone loss occurs with advancing age in almost all, if not all, humans (Kalu, 1995); thus, it is considered an age-associated physiological deterioration. However, when the loss is of sufficient magnitude to have a clinical impact, it is then viewed as a pathophysiological process underlying the age-associated disease osteoporosis. Another example is the age-associated blunting of the baroreflex in healthy humans, which is considered a physiological deterioration (Jones *et al.*, 2003). However, if hypertension results from this physiological deterioration, the individual is said to have a disease (Lakatta & Levy, 2003).

Does the concept of "normal aging" have any value? Potentially, it may be useful as a reductionist tool in aging research. Indeed, reductionism has been a powerful tool in biological science. Unfortunately, this use of "normal aging" is, to a great extent, undermined by the fact that advances in biomedical technology, such as the thallium-stress test discussed above, will result in an ever-changing standard of what is considered "normal aging." Moreover, based on new evidence, what was considered normal may be reclassified as disease. For example, in 1990, a systolic blood pressure of 140 to 160 mmHg was not viewed as hypertension, whereas currently a systolic blood pressure of 140 or above is considered hypertension (Lakatta & Levy, 2003).

V. Evolutionary Theory and Age-Associated Diseases

The currently held concept of the evolution of aging provides strong support for the view that age-associated diseases are an integral part of aging. Specifically, it is believed that aging occurs because the force of natural selection decreases with increasing post-sexual maturational age (Rose, 1991); that is, there is a progressive age-associated post-maturational decrease in the ability of natural selection to eliminate detrimental traits. Lee (2003) points out that this concept should include not only the generation of progeny but, in addition, the intergenerational transfer of food and care, which promotes survival of offspring.

Three genetic mechanisms that affect reproduction and survival have been proposed, and each is compatible with this evolutionary concept. One is termed the *mutation accumulation mechanism* (Medawar, 1952). It proposes that natural selection does not eliminate mutated genes that are expressed throughout life but do not have detrimental effects until late in life; thus, they accumulate in the genome. Specifically, because of predation and other environmental hazards,

most organisms in the wild do not live long enough for these genes to appreciably affect evolutionary fitness. However, in a protected environment where reaching advanced ages becomes the norm, the late-life detrimental effects of these genes result in senescence. There is some empirical evidence in support of this mechanism (Hughes *et al.*, 2002).

Another genetic mechanism, proposed by Williams (1957), is referred to as *antagonistic pleiotropy*. It proposes that those genes that increase evolutionary fitness in early life will be selected for, even if they have catastrophic deleterious effects in late life. Again, the deleterious effects of these genes will be evident only in subjects in protected environments that enable a long life. Although Huntington's disease has been used as a classic example of the mutation accumulation mechanism, there is evidence to indicate that it may instead be an example of the antagonistic pleiotropy mechanism (Frontali *et al.*, 1996).

Kirkwood (1977) proposed a third genetic mechanism, which he terms the *disposable soma theory*. Although this theory does not propose a specific genetic mechanism, it is based on the concept that evolutionary forces tend to form a genome that yields the maximum number of progeny. The premise of this theory is that the fundamental life role of organisms is to utilize free energy in the environment to generate progeny. To do so requires the use of energy for both reproduction and the maintenance of the body (which Kirkwood calls "somatic maintenance"). He proposes that the force of natural selection leads to apportioning the use of energy between reproduction and somatic maintenance so as to maximize evolutionary fitness (i.e., generation of a maximum lifetime yield of viable progeny). As a consequence, less energy is used for somatic maintenance than would be needed for indefinite survival, and this deficit in energy for maintenance is manifested in the deterioration of the organism referred to as aging (the lower the use of energy for somatic maintenance, the greater the rate of aging).

Although Martin (2002) tends to feel that the above three mechanisms have likely played a role in the evolution of aging, he suggests that other genetic mechanisms may also be involved. It is clear that further work is needed to determine the relative importance of each of the proposed mechanisms and of other possible genetic mechanisms as well.

However, Cortopassi (2002) has pointed out that irrespective of specific genetic mechanisms, aging involves a high rate of fixation of alleles that have deleterious effects in the post-reproductive phenotype as compared to the low rate of fixation of such alleles in the pre-reproductive phenotype. Age-associated disease is almost certainly one of the inevitable outcomes of the high rate of fixation of these deleterious alleles. Indeed, Wick and colleagues (2000) subscribe to the view that inherent advantages of biological factors that enhance reproduction in the young adult are paid for by senescent deterioration, including age-associated diseases, in later life. Indeed, Wick and colleagues (2003) have presented evidence that suggests that benign prostate hyperplasia, prostate cancer, atherosclerosis, and Alzheimer's disease are results of antagonistic pleiotropy. They further state that it remains to be shown whether this is also true of other age-associated diseases.

VI. Analysis of Two Major Age-Associated Disease Processes

A consideration of the processes that underlie age-associated diseases provides further insight into their relationship to aging. Atherosclerosis and neoplasia, two major age-associated disease processes, have been chosen for examination.

A. Atherosclerosis

Atherosclerosis is a disorder of the large- and medium-sized arteries that, in humans, underlies most coronary artery disease (myocardial infarction, heart failure) and peripheral vascular disease (aneurysms, gangrene of the extremities) and plays a major role in cerebrovascular disease (Bierman, 1985; Faxon et al., 2004; Scott, 2004). Brody and Schneider (1986) classify both coronary artery disease and cerebrovascular disease in the age-dependent subclass of age-associated diseases. Atherosclerosis is a progressive process that proceeds over several decades but does not usually have clinical consequences until advanced middle age or older (Ross, 1986), when rupture of the advanced atheromatous plaque or thrombosis related to the plaque often causes an acute clinical event (Lusis, 2000). Atherosclerosis occurs in almost all humans (Bierman, 1985); for example, moderate to severe atherosclerosis of the arterial tree was found in all 23 (7 men and 16 women) centenarians. Atherosclerosis is responsible for about 50 percent of all mortality in the United States, Europe, and Japan (Ross, 1993). Although it is almost ubiquitous in humans, atherosclerosis is not commonly seen in rodents or nonhuman primates (Lakatta, 2003). However, the absence of atherosclerosis in these species may be due to diet; for example, atherosclerosis occurs in baboons fed an atherogenic diet (Babiak et al., 1984), a diet similar in composition to that of many humans.

Many of the same factors that underlie the age-associated structural and functional changes in the human cardiovascular system are implicated in the pathogenesis of atherosclerosis (Lakatta, 2003). It appears to start at the intimal surface of the artery, with fatty streaks consisting of lipid-engorged foam cells overlain with intact endothelium; the foam cells are formed by recruitment of monocytes into the subendothelial space, along with the accumulation of modified forms of low-density lipoproteins (Greaves & Gordon, 2001). The lesion slowly progresses in severity, with a continuing recruitment of monocytes and T-lymphocytes plus a migration of smooth muscle cells into the lesion as well as their proliferation. After many decades, the lesion progresses into the fibrous plaque, which also contains smooth muscle cells, activated T-lymphocytes, and monocyte-derived macrophages (Stout, 2003). The chemokine class of cytokines has been postulated to play a role in the migration of monocytes into the developing atherosclerotic lesion (Reape & Groot, 1999); there is evidence that leukotrienes play an important role in the recruitment of T-lymphocytes into the lesion (Jala & Haribabu, 2004).

Witzum (1994) hypothesized that the oxidative modification of low-density lipoproteins is a key event in the pathogenesis of atherosclerosis, and Steinberg (1997) has provided experimental findings in support of this hypothesis. Hypercholesterolemia, hypertension, diabetes, and smoking, the common risk factors for atherosclerosis, are associated with an increased vascular production of reactive oxygen species (Abe & Berk, 1998; Landmesser et al., 2004). Ross (1999) pointed out that atherosclerosis is an inflammatory disease and that oxidized low-density lipoproteins have a role in the arterial inflammatory processes involved in the pathogenesis of these lesions.

Indeed, inflammation appears to play a fundamental role in mediating all stages of atherogenesis, from initiation through progression and, ultimately, thrombotic complications (Libby et al., 2003). An immune and inflammatory response involving endothelial and smooth muscle cells accompanies the accumulation of lipids and fibrous material in atheromatous arteries (Robbie & Libby, 2001). Specifically, pro-inflammatory, oxidized phospholipids generated by the oxidation of low-density lipoprotein phospholipids, particularly those containing arachidonic acid, provoke an immune response (Navab et al., 2004). Bjorkbacka and colleagues (2004) presented evidence that links the pro-inflammatory signaling cascade induced in the arterial wall by elevated plasma lipids to that also used by microbial pathogens. In fact, long-term infections have been viewed as a possible cause of the chronic inflammation that underlies atherogenesis (Becker et al., 2001). Infection and inflammation induce the acute phase response that is characterized by increased levels of certain serum or plasma proteins (e.g., C-reactive protein, amyloid A, and fibrinogen) and the decreased level of others (e.g., albumin, transferrin, and α–fetoprotein). Cytokines from macrophages, monocytes, T-lymphocytes, and endothelial cells mediate the acute phase response; it has been proposed that when inflammation is sustained, the pro-inflammatory cytokines play a pathogenic role in atherogenesis by causing changes in lipoprotein metabolism, which leads to the formation of pro-atherogenic lipoproteins (Khovidhunkit et al., 2004).

The involvement of both oxidative damage and inflammation in the genesis of atherosclerosis indicates that this pathologic process is strongly linked to aging processes. Many biological gerontologists believe that oxidative damage is the major proximate mechanism responsible for senescence (Barja, 2002; Finkel & Holbrook, 2000). Strikingly, de Nigris and colleagues (2003) proposed that oxidation combined with apoptosis, which has also been intimately linked to aging (Zhang & Herman, 2002), promotes the progression of diseased arteries towards atherosclerotic lesions vulnerable to rupture. These are the lesions that give rise to myocardial infarction and ischemic stroke, major age-associated diseases (de Nigris *et al.*, 2003).

Significantly, Krabbe and colleagues (2004) have shown that increased inflammatory activity is also characteristic of aging. Compared to young adults, elderly humans were found to exhibit a two- to four-fold increase in plasma levels of inflammatory mediators such as cytokines (e.g., tumor necrosis factor-alpha and interleukin-6) and in positive acute phase proteins. Indeed, in a cohort of 81-year-old humans, high levels of tumor necrosis factor-alpha in the blood were found to be associated with a high prevalence of atherosclerosis (Bruunsgaard *et al.*, 2000). Krabbe and colleagues (2004) suggest that aging is associated with a dysregulated cytokine response to stimulation and that, in addition to playing this role in atherogenesis, there is also evidence that this dysregulation is involved in other age-associated disorders. In fact, Chung and colleagues (2001) believe that inflammation plays a key role in aging, and they have proposed the "Inflammation Hypothesis of Aging."

Finch and Crimmins (2004) have recently proposed that long-term inflammation underlies many age-associated disorders. Indeed, inflammation has been implicated in many aspects of age-associated deterioration, including age-associated diseases other than those related to atherosclerosis. Chronic low-grade inflammation is associated with age-associated decrease in muscle mass (referred to as *sarcopenia*), which is an important component of frailty in the elderly (Pedersen *et al.*, 2003). Serum markers of inflammation, especially interleukin-6 and C-reactive protein, have been prospectively associated with cognitive decline in the well-functioning elderly (Yaffe *et al.*, 2003) and in age-related macular degeneration (Seddon *et al.*, 2004).

It is particularly striking that inflammatory processes have also been linked to both Alzheimer's disease and vascular dementia (Hofman *et al.*, 1997). Interestingly, in an *in vitro* study, cholesterol ozonolysis products and a related lipid-derived aldehyde were found to modify beta-amyloid so as to dramatically accelerate amyloidgenesis (Zhang *et al.*, 2004); this finding provides a potential chemical link between hypercholesterolemia, oxidative stress, inflammation, atherosclerosis, and sporadic Alzheimer's disease. In fact, many factors contributing to atherogenesis have emerged as potential contributors to Alzheimer's disease (Casserly & Torpol, 2004).

Recently, Rauscher and colleagues (2003) reported still other support for the view that aging underlies atherosclerosis; they found that aging of ApoE$^{-/-}$ mice leads to a failure of bone marrow to produce progenitor cells capable of repairing and rejuvenating arteries. They propose that this age-associated loss of functional endothelial progenitor cells contributes to the development of atherosclerosis. Moreover, Hill and colleagues (2003) observed a strong correlation between the number of circulating endothelial progenitor cells and the Framingham Risk Factor score for coronary artery disease in persons free of clinical disease. Geiger and Van Zant (2002) suggest that a loss in the functional quality of stem cells may play an important role in aging generally, and that research aimed at assessing age-changes in the quality of stem cells in all tissues is needed. However, a cautionary note is in order: it has yet to be clearly established that stem cells undergo senescent deterioration during organismic aging (Park *et al.*, 2004; Van Zant & Liang, 2004).

Although a considerable body of evidence links aging processes and atherogenic processes, a caveat is in order because much of this evidence relates to the role of oxidative damage and inflammation in atherogenesis. As discussed above, many gerontologists do subscribe to the view that oxidative damage and possibly inflammation also play a causal role in aging; however, not all findings support this view. Thus, the recent study by Fontana and colleagues (2004) is of particular significance because it offers a different connection between aging processes and atherosclerosis. They found that severe, self-imposed caloric restriction in humans for a period of 3 to 15 years markedly lowered the risk of developing atherosclerosis. This finding provides yet another link between aging and atherogenesis because caloric restriction markedly retards aging in a spectrum of animal species (Masoro, 2002); for example, in rats, a 40 to 50 percent reduction in food intake increases the mortality rate doubling time from about 100 days to 200 days (Holehan & Merry, 1986). However, this evidence, too, must be viewed with some caution because it has not been established that caloric restriction retards aging in humans.

B. Neoplasia

Although cancer can occur at all ages, the incidence of most types increases with increasing age in humans and animals (Dix, 1989). Although it is true that certain tumors, such as neuroblastoma and Wilms' tumor, occur in childhood, these may well be due to genetic predispositions unrelated to aging. The vast majority of cancers occur at advanced ages, and Brody and Schneider (1986) classify most of them in the *age-related* subclass of age-associated disease because they do not continue to increase exponentially from late middle age on through old-old age. An exception is prostate cancer, which does continue to increase exponentially into old-old age;

thus, prostate cancer is included in the *age-dependent* subclass of age-associated diseases.

Miller (1991) points out that speciation, caloric restriction, and selective breeding, all of which affect the rate of aging, have parallel effects on cancer incidence. On the other hand, DePinho (2000) notes that the increase in tumors in humans between 40 and 80 years of age involves primarily epithelial carcinomas and not mesenchymal and hematopoietic malignancies, and that the opposite is the case for mice between 2 to 4 years (an age range comparable to humans in the 40 to 80 age range). However, this apparent species difference may not be real because it is based primarily on findings with isogenic mouse strains developed for studies on the genetics of lymphoma. In fact, in a recent study with a genetically heterogeneous mouse stock, it was found that at advanced age, fibrosarcoma, mammary adenocarcinoma, and hepatocellular carcinoma were also common and that many other less common cancers also occurred (Lipman *et al.*, 2004).

Indeed, as will be discussed below, there have been many studies opposing and supporting the view that most cancers are an integral part of aging. Donehower and his coworkers (Tyner *et al.*, 2002) presented findings that tend to disassociate cancer and aging. In a p53 mutant mouse with an enhanced p53 activity, they found the expected increase in resistance to cancer and also, surprisingly, shortened longevity and the expression of an age-associated phenotype at a chronological age younger than in the wild type mouse. Donehower (2002) suggests that the pro-aging effects of this mutation may result from a gradual increase in the depletion of stem cell functional capacity due to increased levels of p53 in the mutant mice; he further postulates that this is the "price" of a cancer-free existence during the reproductive phase of adult life. Sharpless and

DePinho (2004) subscribe to this view. Moreover, Maier and colleagues (2004) have confirmed and extended the findings of the Donehower group. They reported that the overexpression of p44 (the short isoform of p53) in mice decreased longevity and caused premature aging and hyperactivation of the IGF-1 signaling axis.

Although at first glance the work of the Donehower group strongly suggests that cancer is not an integral part of aging, there is another possible explanation for their findings. Zhang and Herman (2002) proposed that a defective control of apoptosis is a cause of aging, and Amundson and colleagues (1998) showed that p53 is a positive regulator of apoptosis. Thus, the enhanced p53 activity in the mutant mice of Tyner and colleagues may cause aging by inappropriately enhancing apoptosis, an action that simultaneously protects against the occurrence of cancer.

Several other studies intimately link cancer and aging at both cellular and molecular levels. Cutler and Semsei (1989) were the first to propose that a common mechanism underlies cancer and aging; they suggested that both are initiated and propagated by impaired gene regulation driven by destabilizing processes affecting regulatory elements. In a review article published some 10 years later, DePinho (2000) also linked increased somatic mutations with age as the likely cause of the age-associated increase in cancer. It is striking that somatic mutations have long been considered major factors underlying aging (see review by Vijg & Dolle, 2001). Vijg and Dolle (2002) suggested that an age-associated increase in genome rearrangements leads to cellular senescence or neoplastic transformation or the death of cells. Indeed, Hasty and colleagues (2003) proposed that the age-associated increase in genome instability, driven by oxidative damage, is a primary cause of aging.

Although Liu and colleagues (2003) also pose that both aging and cancer are due to altered genomic function, they believe that an epigenetic mechanism is involved. They point out that both aging and tumorigenesis are characterized by a global hypomethylation of the genomic DNA.

McCullogh and colleagues (1997) found that there was less regression of neoplastically transformed rat liver epithelial cells when the cells were transplanted into the liver of old rats rather than young rats. These investigators suggest that age-associated alterations in tissue microenvironment may permit the development of tumors in late life. Indeed, Bell and Van Zant (2004) proposed that the aging of the stem cell population of the hematopoietic system creates conditions that favor leukemic development, and they suggest that aging of stem cells may similarly promote the occurrence of other types of cancer. Moreover, cancer has been linked to inflammation (Ho et al., 2004; Marx, 2004; Nelson et al., 2004), and Chung and colleagues (2001) have suggested that inflammatory processes play an important role in aging. Indeed, Schwartsburd (2004) recently hypothesized that aging causes chronic inflammation, which plays an important role in the pathogenesis of cancer.

Krtolica and colleagues (2001) proposed that the age-associated increase in cancer is due to a synergism between genetic factors (oncogenic mutations) and epigenetic factors (substances released from the accumulated senescent cells). It has been suggested that the accumulated senescent cells create a microenvironment that favors carcinogenesis (Kim et al., 2002). Although this is an intriguing concept, it must be viewed with caution because neither the prevalence nor the functional significance of senescent cells has been established in the intact organism (Hornsby, 2002).

Very recently, Del Monte and Statuto (2004) proposed that at least some types of cancer (e.g., epidermal cancer) are an integral part of aging. Specifically, they hypothesize that cancers may result from the dysfunction of gap junction intercellular communication because of an age-associated decrease in connexins.

In summary, although there is a substantial body of evidence that shows a close association between aging and cancer, currently available findings do not clearly discriminate among the following three possibilities: (1) many cancers are an integral part of aging; (2) aging provides a favorable environment for the occurrence of cancer; or (3) the occurrence of most cancers requires the passage of time, but in no other way does cancer relate to aging. Ershler and Longo (1997) point out that all three of these possibilities may be involved. Moreover, it is interesting to note that in a review of the issue of aging and cancer, Irminger-Finger (2003) concluded that cancer is very much a part of normal aging. Clearly, this investigator's definition of normal aging differs markedly from that of Shock (1984). Recently, Hasty (2005) and Campisi (2005) have independently presented novel views of the relationship between aging and cancer. Hasty poses that aging acts both to increase life span by preventing cancer in early life and to decrease life span because of functional deterioration in late life. Campisi also proposes that aging protects against the occurrence of cancer in early life, but that the accumulation of senescent cells by late life establishes a cancer-promoting environment. The second component of Campisi's view is not supported by the fact that there is a decreased occurrence of cancer in the 10th and 11th decades of human life.

VII. Summary and Conclusions

The currently available database does not provide a definitive answer to the question of whether age-associated diseases are an integral part of aging. However, the preponderance of evidence indicates it is likely that at least some age-associated diseases, in particular those classified as *age dependent* by Brody and Schneider (1986), are, indeed, an integral part of aging.

In this regard, it is of interest to consider age-associated diseases within the context of the time-honored, fundamental characteristics of aging: intrinsicality, universality, progressivity, irreversibility, and genetically programmed. Aging fits the concept of intrinsicality only in the limited sense that damage to biologically important molecules, such as DNA, proteins, and lipids, is probably the basis of the aging phenotype. Strikingly, it is believed that molecular damage of a similar type underlies age-associated diseases. However, it is important to note that both in what is classically called aging and in age-associated diseases, extrinsic factors often play the major role in causing this intrinsic molecular damage.

As for universality, physiological deteriorations, classically viewed as characterizing the aging phenotype, are not universal, nor are age-associated diseases. For example, deterioration of kidney function has long been considered a hallmark of the human aging phenotype, a view that is based on cross-sectional studies showing a marked decrease in glomerular filtration rate with increasing adult age (Rowe *et al.*, 1976). However, a longitudinal study of 446 participants in the Baltimore Longitudinal Study of Aging revealed marked individual differences in the change with age in glomerular filtration rate, with one-third of participants showing no change (Lindeman *et al.*, 1985). On the other hand, as discussed above, atherosclerosis is almost universal in humans.

Regarding progressivity, most age-associated diseases exhibit an age-associated progression similar to the age-associated physiological deteriorations classically considered components of the aging phenotype.

Strictly speaking, neither the classically recognized components of the aging phenotype nor age-associated diseases exhibit irreversibility. For example, strength exercise programs can result in some increase in muscle mass in the elderly who have experienced a massive age-associated loss in muscle mass (Evans, 1995). Also, treatment with recombinant apoA-I Milano can reverse, to some degree, coronary atherosclerosis in aged people who suffer from acute coronary syndromes (Nissen *et al.*, 2003).

Currently, most biological gerontologists do not believe that aging is programmed in the evolutionary adaptive manner that characterizes development (Rose, 1991). However, the rate of aging is the result of gene-environment interactions (Rowe & Kahn, 1998); this is also true of the occurrence and progression of most age-associated disease processes. In summary, age-associated diseases fit the time-honored, fundamental characteristics of aging at least as well as the classically viewed components of the aging phenotype.

There are many reasons that the concept of "normal aging" (defined as aging in the absence of disease) should be discarded. Aging without the occurrence of age-associated disease is such a rare event that this concept focuses attention on the unique rather than the typical. Of course, some may defend the use of the concept as a reductionist approach to the study of aging, and reductionism has certainly been a powerful tool in biology. However, even in this regard, the concept falls short because, as discussed above, distinguishing between physiological deterioration and pathophysiology is often arbitrary. While the tools for such a determination are improving, the standards used for claiming absence of disease are also changing. Thus, the base to support this kind of reductionist approach to the study of aging is constantly shifting, and that is likely to continue in the foreseeable future.

The most compelling reason to consider age-associated diseases as an integral part of aging comes from our understanding of the evolutionary basis of aging. Specifically, aging is believed to occur because of a progressive age-associated decrease in the force of natural selection; thus, deleterious traits expressed only at advanced ages do not tend to be eliminated by natural selection. Because age-associated diseases do not exhibit deleterious consequences until advanced ages, even if they begin at an early age, current views of the evolutionary basis of aging lead to the conclusion that such diseases are exactly what one would predict to be an integral part of aging.

In conclusion, the question posed in the title of this chapter (Are Age-Associated Diseases an Integral Part of Aging?) has yet to be definitively answered. However, after carefully considering the materials presented in this chapter, I am in total agreement with the following statement made by Robin Holliday (2004) in his debate with Leonard Hayflick: "The distinction between age-related changes that are not pathological and those that are pathological is not at all fundamental." It is my view that rigidly holding to the view that age-associated diseases are not an integral part of aging may have had, and is likely to continue to have, an adverse effect on aging research. It tends to limit the scope of the design of gerontologic studies, and to eliminate the use of experimental models that might well provide unique insights into aging processes.

References

Abe, J., & Berk, B. C. (1998). Reactive oxygen species as mediators of signal transduction and cardiovascular disease. *Trends in Cardiovascular Medicine*, 8, 59–64.

American Heritage Dictionary, 3rd ed. (1996). Boston: Houghton Mifflin.

Ames, B. N., Shigenaga, M. K., & Hagen, T. M. (1993). Oxidants, antioxidants, and the degenerative diseases of aging. *Proceedings of the National Academy of Sciences of the USA*, 90, 7915–7922.

Amundson, S. A., Myers, T. G., & Fornace, A. J. (1998). Roles of p53 in growth arrest and apoptosis: putting on the brakes after genotoxic stress. *Oncogene*, 17, 3287–3299.

Anderson-Ranberg, K., Schroll, M., & Jeune, B (2001). Healthy centenarians do not exist, but autonomous centenarians do: a population-based study of morbidity among Danish centenarians. *Journal of the American Geriatrics Society*, 49, 900–908.

Babiak, J., Gong, E. L., Nichols, A. V., Forte, T. M., Kuehl, T. J., McGill, Jr., H. C. (1984). Characterization of HDL and lipoprotein intermediates to LDL and HDL in the serum of pedigreed baboons fed an atherogenic diet. *Atherosclerosis*, 52, 27–45.

Barja, G. (2002) Endogenous oxidative stress: relationship to aging, longevity, and caloric restriction. *Ageing Research Reviews*, 1, 397–411.

Becker, A. E., de Boer, O. J., & van der Wal, A. C. (2001) The role of inflammation and infection in coronary artery disease. *Annual Review of Medicine*, 52, 289–297.

Bell, D. R., & Van Zant, G. (2004). Stem cells, aging, and cancer. *Oncogene*, 23, 7290–7296.

Bierman, E. L. (1985). Arteriosclerosis and aging. In C. E. Finch & E. L. Schneider (Eds.), *Handbook of the biology of aging* (5th ed., pp. 842–858). New York: Van Nostrand Reinhold.

Bjorkbacka, H., Kunjathoor, V. V., Moore, K. J., Koern, S., Ordija, C. M., Lee, M. A., Means, T., Halmen, K., Luster, A. D., Golenbock, D. T., & Freeman, M. (2004). Reduced atherosclerosis in MyD88-null mice links elevated serum cholesterol to activation of innate immunity signaling pathways. *Nature Medicine*, 10, 416–421.

Blumenthal, H. T. (1999). A view of aging-disease relationship from age 85. *Journal of Gerontology: Biological Sciences*, 54A, B255–B259.

Blumenthal, H. T. (2003). The aging-disease dichotomy: true or false? *Journal of Gerontology*, 58A, 138–145.

Borkan, G. A., & Norris, A. H. (1980). Assessment of biological age using a profile of physical parameters. *Journal of Gerontology*, 35, 177–184.

Brody, J. A., & Schneider, E. L. (1986). Diseases and disorders of aging: a hypothesis. *Journal of Chronic Disease*, 39, 871–876.

Bruunsgaard, H., Skinhoj, P., Pedersen, A. N., Schroll, M., & Pedersen, B. K. (2000). Ageing, tumour necrosis factor-alpha (TNF-α) and atherosclerosis. *Clinical Experimental Immunology*, 121, 255–260.

Busse, E. W. (1969). Theories of aging. In E. W. Busse & E. Pfeiffer (Eds.), *Behavior and adaptation in adult life* (pp. 11–32). Boston: Little Brown.

Campisi, J. (2005). Aging, tumor suppression and cancer: high-wire act! *Mechanisms of Ageing and Development*, 126, 51–58.

Casserly, I., & Torpol, E. (2004). Convergence of atherosclerosis and Alzheimer's disease: inflammation, cholesterol, misfolded proteins. *Lancet*, 363, 1139–1146.

Chung, H. Y., Kim, H. J., & Yu, B. P. (2001). The inflammation hypothesis of aging: molecular modification by caloric restriction. *Annals of the New York Academy of Sciences*, 928, 327–335.

Cortopassi, G. A. (2002). Fixation of deleterious alleles, evolution, and human aging. *Mechanisms of Ageing and Development*, 123, 851–855.

Costa, P. T. Jr., & McCrae, R. R. (1995). Design and analysis of aging studies. In E. J. Masoro (Ed.), *Handbook of physiology* (pp. 25–36). New York: Oxford University Press.

Cutler, R. G., & Semsei, I. (1989). Development, cancer and aging: possible common mechanisms of action and regulation. *Journal of Gerontology: Biological Sciences*, 44, 25–34.

Del Monte, U., & Statuto, M. (2004). Drop of connexins: a possible link between aging and cancer. *Experimental Gerontology*, 39, 273–275.

de Nigris, F., Lerman, A., Ignarro, L. J., Williams-Ignarro, S., Sica, V., Baker, A. H., Lerman, A. O., Geng, Y. J., & Napoli, C. (2003). Oxidative-sensitive mechanisms, vascular apoptosis, and atherosclerosis. *Trends in Molecular Medicine*, 9, 352–359.

DePinho, R. A. (2000). The age of cancer. *Nature*, 408, 248–254.

Dix, D. (1989). The role of aging in cancer incidence: an epidemiological study. *Journal of Gerontology*, 44, (Special Issue) 10–18.

Donehower, L. A. (2002). Does p53 affect organismal aging? *Journal of Cellular Physiology*, 192, 23–33.

Elby, E. M., Parhad, I. M., Hogan, D. B., & Fang, T. S. (1994) Prevalence and types of dementia in the very old: results from the Canadian Study of Health and Aging. *Neurology*, 44, 1593–1600.

Ershler, W. B., & Longo, D. L. (1997). Aging and cancer: issues of basic and clinical science. *Journal of the National Cancer Institute*, 89, 1489–1497.

Evans, J. G. (1988). Aging and disease. In D. Everid & J. Whalen (Eds.), *Research and the aging population* (pp. 38–57). Ciba Foundation Symposium No. 134, Chichester, UK: Wiley.

Evans, W. J. (1995). Effects of exercise on body composition and functional capacity in the elderly. *Journal of Gerontology*, 50A, 147–150.

Evert, J., Lawler, E., Bogan, H., & Perls, T. (2003). Morbidity profiles of centenarians: survivors, delayers, escapers. *Journal of Gerontology: Medical Sciences*, 58A, 232–237.

Faxon, D. P., Fuster, V., Libby, P., Beckman, J. A., Hiatt, W. R., Thompson, R. W., Topper, J. N., Annex, B. H., Rundback, J. A., Fabunmi, R. P., Robertson, R. M., & Loscalzo, J. (2004). Atherosclerotic vascular disease conference group III: pathophysiology. *Circulation*, 109, 2617–2625.

Finch, C. E., & Crimmins, E. M. (2004). Inflammatory exposure and historical changes in human life-spans. *Science*, 305, 1736–1739.

Finkel, T., & Holbrook, N. J. (2000). Oxidants, oxidative stress, and the biology of aging. *Nature*, 408, 239–247.

Fries, J. F. (1980). Aging, natural death, and the compression of morbidity. *New England Journal of Medicine*, 303, 130–135.

Fontana, L., Meyer, T. E., Klein, S., & Holloszy, J. O. (2004). Long-term calorie restriction is highly effective in reducing the risk of atherosclerosis in humans. *Proceedings of the National Academy of Sciences of the USA*, 101, 6659–6663.

Frontali, M., Sabbadini, G., Novelleto, A., Jodice, C., Naso, F., Spadaro, M., Gigcenti, P., Jacopini, A. G., Veneziano, L., Mantuano, E., Malaspina, P., Ulizzi, L., Brice, A., Durr, A., & Terremato, L. (1996). Genetic fitness in Huntington's disease and spinocerebellar ataxia: a population genetics model of CAG repeat expansions. *Annals of Human Genetics*, 60, 423–435.

Geiger, H., & Van Zant, G. (2002). The aging of lympho-hematopoietic stem cells. *Nature Immunology*, 3, 329–333.

Gessert, C. E., Elliott, B. A., & Haller, I. V. (2002). Dying of old age: an examination of death certificates of Minnesota centenarians. *Journal of the American Geriatrics Society*, 50, 1561–1565.

Greaves, D. R., & Gordon, S. (2001). Immunity, atherosclerosis, and cardiovascular disease. *Trends in Immunology*, 22, 180–181.

Hasty, P. (2005). The impact of DNA damage, genetic mutation and cellular responses on cancer prevention, longevity and aging: observations in humans and mice. *Mechanisms of Ageing and Development*, 126, 71–77.

Hasty, P., Campisi, J., Hoeijmakers, J., van Steeg, H., & Vijg, J. (2003). Aging and genome maintenance: lessons from the mouse? *Science*, 299, 1355–1359.

Hayflick, L. (2002). Anarchy in gerontological terminology. *Gerontologist*, 42, 416–421.

Hebert, K. (2004). Life expectancy in Great Britain rises—but later years are still spent in poor health. *British Medical Journal*, 329, 250.

Hill, J. M., Zalos, G., Halcox, J. P. T., Schenke, W. H., Waclawi, W., Quyyumi, A. A., & Finkel, T. C. (2003). Circulating endothelial progenitor cells, vascular function, and cardiovascular risk. *New England Journal of Medicine*, 348, 593–600.

Hitt, R., Young-Xu, Y., Silver, M., & Perls, T. (1999). Centenarians: the older you get, the healthier you have been. *Lancet*, 354, 652.

Ho, E., Boileau, T., & Bray, T. M. (2004). Dietary influence in endocrine-inflammatory interactions in prostate cancer. *Archives of Biochemistry and Biophysics*, 428, 109–117.

Hofman, A., Ott, A., Breteler, M. M., Bots, M. L., Slooter, A. J., van Harskamp, F., van Duijin, C. N., Van Broeckhoven, C., & Grobbee, D. E. (1997) Atherosclerosis, apolipoprotein E, and prevalence of dementia and Alzheimer's disease in the Rotterdam study. *Lancet, 349,* 151–154.

Holehan, A. M., & Merry, B. J. (1986). The experimental manipulation of ageing by diet. *Biological Reviews, 61,* 329–369.

Holliday, R. (2004). The close relationship between biological aging and age-associated pathologies in humans. *Journal of Gerontology: Biological Sciences, 59A,* 543–546.

Horiuchi, S., Finch, C. E., Mesle, F., & Vallin, J. (2003). Differential patterns of age-related mortality increase in middle age and old age. *Journal of Gerontology: Biological Sciences, 58A,* 495–507.

Hornsby, P. J. (2002). Cellular senescence and tissue aging *in vivo. Journal of Gerontology: Biological Sciences, 57A,* B251–B256.

Hughes, K. A., Alipaz, J. A., Drnevitch, J. A., & Reynolds, R. M. (2002). A test of the evolutionary theories of aging. *Proceedings of the National Academy of Sciences of the USA, 99,* 14286–14291.

Irminger-Finger, I. (2003). Geneva Workshop 2002. Cancer, apoptosis, and aging. *Biochimia et Biophysica Acta, 1653,* 41–45.

Jala, V. R., & Haribabu, B. (2004). Leukotrienes and atherosclerosis: new roles for old mediators. *Trends in Immunology, 25,* 315–322.

Jones, P. P., Christou, C., Jordan, J., & Seals, R. (2003). Baroreflex buffering is reduced with age in healthy men. *Circulation, 107,* 1770–1774.

Kalu, D. N. (1995). Bone. In E. J. Masoro (Ed.), *Handbook of physiology* (pp. 395–412). New York: Oxford University Press.

Khovidhunkit, W., Kim. M-S., Memon, R. A., Shivenaga, J. K., Moser, A. H., Feingold, K., & Greenfeld, C. (2004). The pathogenesis of atherosclerosis: effect of infection and inflammation on lipid and lipoprotein metabolism and consequences to the host. *Journal of Lipid Research, 45,* 1169–1196.

Kim, S-h., Kominker, P., & Campisi, J. (2002). Telomeres, aging, and cancer: in search of a happy ending. *Oncogene, 21,* 503–511.

Kirkwood, T. B. L. (1977). Evolution of ageing. *Nature, 270,* 301–304.

Klima, M. P., Povysil, C., & Teasdale, T. A. (1997). Causes of death in geriatric patients: a cross-cultural study. *Journal Gerontology: Medical Sciences, 52A,* M247–M253.

Kohn, R. R. (1982). Cause of death in very old people. *Journal of the American Medical Association, 247,* 2793–2797.

Krabbe, K. S., Pedersen, M., & Bruunsgaard, H. (2004) Inflammatory mediators in the elderly. *Experimental Gerontology, 39,* 687–699.

Krtolica, A., Parrinello, S., Lockett, S., Despres, P-Y, & Campisi, J. (2001). Senescent fibroblasts promote epithelial cell growth and tumorigenesis: a link between cancer and aging. *Proceedings of the National Academy of Sciences of the USA, 98,* 12072–12077.

Lakatta, E. G. (1985). Health, disease, and cardiovascular aging. In Committee on an Aging Society, Institute of Medicine and National Research Council (Ed.), *America's aging-health in an older society* (pp. 73–104). Washington, DC: National Academy Press.

Lakatta, E. G. (2003). Arterial and cardiac aging: major shareholders in cardiovascular disease enterprise: part III: cellular and molecular clues to heart and arterial aging. *Circulation, 107,* 490–497.

Lakatta, E. G., & Levy, D. (2003). Arterial and cardiac aging: major shareholders in cardiovascular disease enterprise: part I: aging arteries: a "set up" for vascular disease. *Circulation, 107,* 139–146.

Landmesser, U., Hornig, B., & Drexler, H. (2004). Endothelial function: a critical determinant in atherosclerosis. *Circulation, 109* [Suppl. II], II-27–II-33.

Lee, R. D. (2003). Rethinking the evolutionary theory of aging. Transfers, not births, shape senescence in social species. *Proceedings of the National Academy of Sciences of the USA, 100,* 9367–9642.

Libby, P., Ridker, P. M., & Maseri, A. (2003). Inflammation and atherosclerosis. *Circulation, 105,* 1135–1143.

Lindeman, R. D., Tobin, J. D., & Shock, N. W. (1985). Longitudinal studies on the rate of decline in renal function with age. *Journal of the American Geriatrics Society, 33,* 278–285.

Lipman, R., Dallal, G. E., & Bronson, R. T. (1999). Lesion biomarkers of aging in B6C3F1 hybrid mice. *Journal of Gerontology: Biological Sciences, 54A,* B466–B477.

Lipman, R., Galecki, A., Burke, D. T., & Miller, R. A. (2004). Genetic loci that influence cause of death in a heterogeneous mouse stock. *Journal of Gerontology: Biological Sciences, 59A,* 977–983.

Liu, L., Wylie, R. C., Andrews, L. G., & Tollefsbol, T. O. (2003). Aging, cancer, and nutrition: the DNA methylation connection. *Mechanisms of Ageing and Development, 124,* 989–998.

Longo, V. D., & Finch, C. E. (2002). Genetics of aging and diseases: from rare mutations and model systems to disease prevention. *Archives of Neurology, 59,* 1706–1708.

Lusis, A. J. (2000). Atherosclerosis. *Nature,* 407, 233–241.

Maeda, H., Gleiser, C. A., Masoro, E. J., Murata, I., McMahan, C., & Yu, B. P. (1985). Nutritional influences of aging of Fischer 344 rats: II. pathology. *Journal of Gerontology, 40,* 671–688.

Maier, B., Gluba, W., Bernier, B., Turner, I., Mohammad, K., Guise, T., Sutherland, A., Thomer, M., & Scrable, H. (2004). Modulation of mammalian life span by the short isoform of p53. *Genes and Development, 18,* 306–319.

Martin, G. M. (2002) The evolutionary substrate of aging. *Archives of Neurology,* 59, 1702–1705.

Marx, J. (2004). Inflammation and cancer: the link grows stronger. *Science, 306,* 966–968.

Masoro, E. J. (Ed.) (1995). *Handbook of physiology,* Section 11, *Aging.* New York: Oxford University Press.

Masoro, E. J. (2002). *Caloric restriction: A key to understanding and modulating aging.* Amsterdam: Elsevier Science.

McClearn, G. E. (1997). Biomarkers of age and aging. *Experimental Gerontology, 32,* 87–94.

McCullough, K. D., Coleman, W. B., Smith, G. J., & Grisham, J. W. (1997).

Age-dependent induction of hepatic tumor regression by the tissue microenvironment after transplantation of neoplastically transformed rat liver epithelial cells into the liver. *Cancer Research,* 57, 1807–1813.

Medawar, P. B. (1952). *An unsolved problem of biology.* Oxford: Oxford University Press.

Miller, R. A. (1991) Gerontology as oncology. *Cancer,* 68, 2496–2501.

Miyaishi, O., Ando, F., Matsuzawa, R., & Isobe, K-I. (2000). Cancer incidence in old age. *Mechanisms of Ageing and Development,* 117, 47–55.

Navab, M., Ananthramaiah, G. M., Reddy, S. T., Van Lenten, B. J., Ansell, B. J., Fonarow, G. C., Vahabzadeh, K., Hama, S., Hough, G., Kamranpour, N., Berliner, J. A., Lusis, A., & Fogelman, A. M (2004). The oxidation hypothesis of atherogenesis: the role of oxidized phospholipids and HDL. *Journal of Lipid Research,* 45, 993–1007.

Nelson, W. G., De Marzo, A. M., DeWeese, T. L., & Isaacs, W. B. (2004). The role of inflammation in the pathogenesis of prostate cancer. *Journal of Urology,* 172, S6–S12.

Nissen, S. E., Tsunoda, T., Turzae, R. M., Schoenhagen, P., Cooper, C. J., Yasin, M., Eaton, G. M., Lauer, M. A., Sheldon, W. S., Grines, C. L., Halpern, S., Crowe, T., Blankenship, J. C., & Kerensky, R. (2003). Effect of recombinant apoA-I Milano on coronary atherosclerosis in patients with acute coronary syndromes. *Journal of the American Medical Association,* 290, 2292–2300.

Papciak, S. M., Song, L., Nagel, J. E., & Adler, W. H. (1996). Immune system. In J. E. Birren (Ed.), *Encyclopedia of gerontology* (Vol. 1, pp. 753–759). San Diego: Academic Press.

Park, I-K., Morrison, S. J., & Clarke, M. I. (2004). *Bmi 1,* stem cells, and senescence. *Journal of Clinical Investigation,* 113, 175–179.

Pedersen, M., Bruunsgaard, H., Weis, N., Hendel, H. W., Andreassen, B. U., Eldrup, E., Dela, F., & Pedersen, B. K. (2003). Circulating levels of TNF-alpha and Il-6-relation to truncal fat mass and muscle mass in healthy elderly individuals and in patients with type-2 diabetes. *Mechanisms of Ageing and Development,* 124, 495–502.

Perlman, R. M. (1954). The aging syndrome. *Journal of the American Geriatrics Society*, 2, 123–129.

Perls, T. (2004). Dementia-free centenarians. *Experimental. Gerontology*, 39, 1587–1593.

Rattan, S. I. S. (1991). Ageing and disease: proteins as the molecular link. *Perspectives in Biology and Medicine*, 34, 526–533.

Rauscher, F., Goldschmidt-Clermont, P., Davis, B. H., Wang, T., Gregg, D., Ramaswami, P., Pippen, A., Annex, B. H., Dong, E., & Taylor, D. A. (2003). Aging, progenitor cell exhaustion, and atherosclerosis. *Circulation*, 108, 457–463.

Reape, T. J., & Groot, P. H. E. (1999). Chemokines and atherosclerosis. *Atherosclerosis*, 147, 213–225.

Robbie, L., & Libby, P. (2001). Inflammation and atherosclerosis. *Annals of the New York Academy of Sciences*, 947, 167–180.

Rose, M. R. (1991). *Evolutionary biology of aging*. New York: Oxford University Press.

Ross, R. (1986). The pathogenesis of atherosclerosis. *New England Journal of Medicine*, 314, 488–500.

Ross, R. (1993). The pathogenesis of atherosclerosis. *Nature*, 801–809.

Ross, R. (1999). Atherosclerosis: an inflammatory disease. *New England Journal of Medicine*, 340, 115–126.

Rowe, J. W., & Kahn, R. W. (1998). *Successful aging*. New York: Pantheon Books.

Rowe, J. W., Andres, R., Tobin, J. D., Norris, A. H., & Shock, N. W. (1976). The effect of age on creatinine clearance in men: a cross-sectional and longitudinal study. *Journal of Gerontology*, 31, 155–163.

Rowe, J. W., Wang, S. Y., & Elahi, D. (1990). Design, conduct, and analysis of human aging research. In E. L Schneider & J. W. Rowe (Eds.), *Handbook of the biology of aging* (3rd ed., pp. 63–71). San Diego: Academic Press.

Schwartsburd, P. M. (2004). Age-promoted creation of a pro-cancer microenvironment: pathogenesis of dyscoordinated feedback control. *Mechanisms of Ageing and Development*, 125, 581–590.

Scott, D. L. (2003). Arthritis in the elderly. In R. Tallis & H. Fillit (Eds.), *Brocklehurst's textbook of geriatric medicine and gerontology* (6th ed., pp. 887–904). London: Churchill Livingstone.

Scott, J. (2004). Pathophysiology and biochemistry of cardiovascular disease. *Current Opinion in Genetics and Development*, 14, 271–279.

Scully, J. L. (2004). What is a disease? *EMBO Report*, 7, 650–653.

Seddon, J. M., Gensler, G., Klein, M. L., & Rifai, N. (2004). Association between C-reactive protein and age-related macular degeneration. *Journal of the American Medical Association*, 291, 704–710.

Semsei, I. (2000). On the nature of aging. *Mechanisms of Ageing and Development*, 117, 93–108.

Sharpless, N. E., & DePinho, R. A. (2004). Telomeres, stem cells, senescence and cancer. *Journal of Clinical Investigation*, 113, 160–168.

Shock, N. W. (1961). Physiological aspects of aging. *Annual Review of Physiology*, 23, 97–122.

Shock, N. W. (1967). Physical activity and the "rate of aging." *Journal of the Canadian Medical Association*, 96, 836–840.

Shock, N. W. (Ed.) (1984). *Normal human aging: the Baltimore longitudinal study of aging* (NIH Publ. 84-2450). Washington, DC: U.S. Government Printing Office.

Sinclair, A. J., & Croxon, S. C. M. (2003). Diabetes mellitus. In R. Tallis & H. Fillit (Eds.), *Brocklehurst's textbook of geriatric medicine and gerontology* (6th ed., pp. 1193–1218). London: Churchill Livingstone.

Skoog, I., Blennow, K., & Marcusson, J. (1996). Dementia. In J. E. Birren (Ed.) *Encyclopedia of gerontology* (Vol. 1, pp. 383–413). San Diego: Academic Press.

Smith, D. W. E. (1996) Cancer mortality at very old ages. *Cancer*, 77, 1367–1372.

Steinberg, D. (1997). Low density lipoprotein oxidation and its pathobiological significance. *Journal of Biological Chemistry*, 272, 20963–20966.

Stout, R. W. (2003). Atherosclerosis and lipid metabolism. In R. Tallis & H. Fillit (Eds.), *Brocklehurst's textbook of geriatric medicine and gerontology* (6th ed., pp. 355–370). London: Churchill Livingstone.

Strehler, B. L. (1977). *Time, cells and aging*. 2nd ed. New York: Academic Press.

Tyner, S. D., Venkatachalam, S., Choi, J., Jones, S., Ghebranious, N., Ingelmann, S., Lu, X., Soron, G, Cooper, B., Brayton, C.,

Park, S. H., Thompson, T., Karsenty, G., Bradley, A., & Donehower, L. (2002). p53 mutant mice that display early aging-associated phenotypes. *Nature*, 415, 45–53.

Urban, L., Bessenyei, B., Marka, M., & Semsei, M. (2002). On the role of aging in the etiology of autoimmunity. *Gerontology*, 179–184.

Van Zant, G., & Liang, Y. (2004). The role of stem cells in aging. *Experimental Hematology*, 31, 659–672.

Viera, C., Pasyukova, E. G., Zeng, Z. B., Hackett, J. B., Lyman, R. F., & Mackay, T. (2000). Genotype-environment interaction for quantitative trait loci affecting life span in *Drosophila melanogaster*. *Genetics*, 154, 213–227.

Vijg, J., & Dolle, M. E. T. (2001). Instability of the nuclear genome and the role of DNA repair. In E. J. Masoro & S. N. Austad (Eds.), *Handbook of the biology of aging* (5th ed., pp. 84–113). San Diego: Academic Press.

Vijg, J., & Dolle, M. E. (2002). Large genome rearrangements as a primary cause of aging. *Mechanisms of Ageing and Development*, 123, 907–915.

Von Straus, E., Fratiglioni, L., Viitanen, M., Forsell, Y., & Winblad, B. (2000). Morbidity and comorbidity in relation to functional status: a community-based study of the oldest old (90+ years). *Journal of the American Geriatrics Society*, 48, 1462–1469.

Wick, G., Berger, P., Jansen-Durr, P., & Grubeck-Loebenstein, B. (2003). A Darwinian-evoltuionary concept of age-related diseases. *Experimental Gerontology*, 38, 13–25.

Wick, G., Jansen-Dürr, Berger, P. Blasko, I., & Grubeck-Loebenstein, B. (2000). Diseases of aging. *Vaccine*, 18, 1567–1583.

Williams, G. C. (1957). Pleiotropy, natural selection, and the evolution of senescence. *Evolution*, 11, 398–411.

Witzum, J. L. (1994). The oxidation hypothesis of atherosclerosis. *Lancet*, 344, 793–795.

Yaffe, K., Lindquist, K., Pennix, B. W., Simonsick, E. M., Pahor, M., Kritchevsky, S., Launer, L., Kuller, L., Rubin, S., & Harris, T. (2003). Inflammatory markers and cognition in well-functioning African American and white elders. *Neurology*, 61, 76–80.

Zhang, Q., Powers, E. T., Nieva, J., Huff, M. E., Dendle, M. A., Bieschke, J., Glabe, C. G., Eschenmoser, A., Wentworth, Jr., P., Lerner, R. A., & Kelly, J. W. (2004) Metabolite-initiated misfolding may trigger Alzheimer's disease. *Proceedings of the National Academy of Sciences of the USA*, 101, 4752–4757.

Zhang, Y., & Herman, B. (2002). Ageing and apoptosis. *Mechanisms of Ageing and Development*, 123, 245–260.

Chapter 3

Dietary Restriction, Hormesis, and Small Molecule Mimetics

David A. Sinclair and Konrad T. Howitz

I. Introduction

This edition of the *Handbook of the Biology of Aging* is being published at an exciting time for aging research. The strict dietary regimen known as caloric restriction (CR) or dietary restriction (DR) is the only way to reliably and dramatically extend life span of mammals without genetic intervention. Animals subjected to DR live longer, not because they spend additional months in a decrepit state, but because they remain more youthful and are somehow protected from the common diseases of aging (Weindruch & Walford, 1988). Since its discovery, it has taken 70 years of intense research, combined with the recent realization that aging is regulated in response to the environment—which some would call a paradigm shift in thinking—to reach a point where many scientists believe we finally understand the principle by which DR works.

One of the main motivations for understanding how DR extends life span, apart from using it as a tool to understand aging, is the hope that with such knowledge we might one day develop molecules that could mimic its health benefits, thus negating the need for us to undergo a similarly strict diet. The ability of DR to extend the maximum life span of mammals is so remarkable that it took numerous studies to reassure the scientific community that DR is a universal effect, not just specific to a particular mouse strain or diet. As a scientific tool, DR meets several important criteria: it is highly effective, the effect is highly reproducible, and the empirical procedure is easily implemented. Besides meeting all these requirements, the great advantage of DR is that it extends the life span of almost every life form it has been tested on, including yeast, worms, flies, spiders, dogs, and fish (Weindruch & Walford, 1988). Although there are exceptional species that do not fit the DR paradigm, namely mayflies and guppies (Carey *et al.*, 2005; Reznick *et al.*, 2004), the broad conservation of the DR effect means that its basic mechanisms are likely to have evolved early in life's history and that we

Handbook of the Biology of Aging, Sixth Edition
Copyright © 2006 by Academic Press. All rights of reproduction in any form reserved.

might tease them out by studying simpler organisms.

Most scientists studying highly complex organisms such as rodents and humans have tended to focus on proximal *causes* of aging. In contrast, researchers studying less complex organisms such as yeast, worms, and flies—which are amenable to unbiased genetic screens for long-lived organisms—have isolated genes that *regulate* the pace of aging. In the past few years, these so-called "longevity genes" have been shown to respond to environmental conditions, such as a lack of food (see Figure 3.1). As we will see in this chapter, the proximal causes of aging and the longevity regulators are both intimately connected to DR and both are essential to understanding what underlies this phenomenon. The effect of DR on the

proximal *causes* of aging and the pathways that *regulate* the pace of aging—the two seemingly separate arenas of aging research—now appear to be manifestations of the same underlying ancient mechanisms that evolved to help organisms survive periods of adversity.

There have been many theories as to how DR works, and many of them have fallen out of favor or have been outright disproved. In this chapter, both the old and new theories of DR will be presented, partly to give a sense of how the field has evolved, but also because it provides a context in which to show how many of these theories can be united under one: the Hormesis Hypothesis of DR (Anderson *et al.*, 2003; Iwasaki *et al.*, 1988; Masoro, 1998; Mattson *et al.*, 2002a; Turturro *et al.*, 2000).

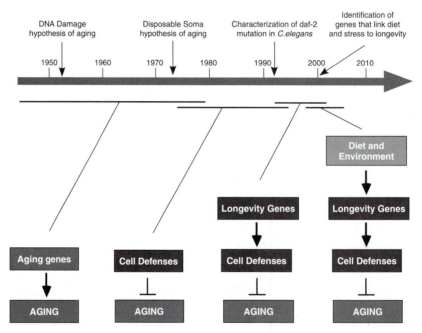

Figure 3.1   Changing views about aging. Before the 1970s, the predominant view was that aging was caused by "death" genes that directed the process, as if it were simply an extension of development. Evolutionary biologists argued that aging is not adaptive for most species, and this idea was laid to rest. During the late 1980s and 1990s, genetic screens in simple organisms such as yeast and worms uncovered single mutations that could dramatically extend life span, seemingly contradicting the complexity of aging. Friedman and Johnson's discovery (1988) of age-1 mutations that extend worm life span was seminal. Around the turn of the 21st century, it became apparent that longevity genes have evolved to protect organisms during times of adversity and that they are activated by low nutrition and other mild biological stress.

This chapter will begin with a summary of the key discoveries in DR research and then will briefly summarize the dramatic physiological effects and health benefits of DR. The central section will summarize the theories about how CR works, dispel some reoccurring myths, and discuss how, with a shift in thinking, many of the current (and valid) theories on DR can be united by the Hormesis Hypothesis. The chapter will conclude by presenting exciting new avenues of research into the development of small molecules that can mimic the beneficial effects of DR, and will attempt to predict where this rapidly moving field might take us in the coming decades.

II. Key Discoveries

A. The DR Paradigm

Throughout human history, numerous societies have touted the health benefits of frugal eating habits, including the Ancient Greeks and Ancient Romans (Dehmelt, 2004). In more recent times, there are also accounts of specific individuals who have fared better on a very lean diet. A fifteenth-century Venetian nobleman named Luigi Cornaro, for example, is famed for his supposed 1,400-calorie diet of meat, bread, and wine, which he maintained from the age of 27 until his death at 103. More recently, Professor Maurice Guéniot, a president of the Paris Medical Academy at the turn of the 20th century, is famed for having lived on a restricted diet and for dying at the age of 102. But of course these are not scientific studies and cannot be treated as more than traditions or anecdotes.

In 1917, Osborne & Mendel (1917) published the first scientific study showing that restricting food extended life, but it had little impact because a publication by Robertson and Gray reported just the opposite (Robertson & Ray, 1920). The first widely recognized study of dietary restriction was conducted between 1934 and 1935, at a time when aging was considered part of an organism's developmental process. To Clive McCay and his colleagues at Cornell University, it seemed reasonable that if the pace of development of an animal were slowed, say by restricting food intake, its life span would correspondingly increase. They tested this idea by substituting 10 to 20 percent of the rats' diet with indigestible cellulose, thus cutting back on their caloric intake (Krystal & Yu, 1994; McCay, 1934). Consistent with predictions, the underfed rats did develop slower and lived substantially longer, although the hypothesis was ultimately proven incorrect.

These first experiments of McCay were not hailed as a breakthrough, partly because they were not performed under strictly controlled conditions on homogeneous groups of animals, and partly because the data conflicted with the current dogma that that poorly fed mice die sooner. But McCay, certain he was right, had already begun another experiment, this time on large cohorts with carefully controlled diets. Over 100 animals were used. He and his colleagues Mary Crowell and Leonard Maynard published a landmark paper titled "The Effect of Retarded Growth Upon the Length of Life Span and Upon the Ultimate Body Size" (McCay et al., 1935). In it they reported:

> the experiment is in its fourth year, but the results are [already] conclusive in showing that the animals that mature slowly have a much greater life span than the rapidly growing ones. . . . This extension of the life span by means of retarded growth indicates that the potential life span for a given species is much longer than has been anticipated. Furthermore, these data suggest that the longer life span of the female may be related to the slower growth rate of the female sex as the animal approaches maturity.

Although their interpretations of the results are now considered incorrect, the results themselves are highly reproducible. They have been validated in dozens of laboratories and with different versions of the diet and using different strains of rats and mice (Krystal & Yu, 1994; Weindruch & Walford, 1988). One recent study went so far as to test three rat and four mouse genotypes each with different life spans and different spectra of disease susceptibility (Turturro et al., 1999). When subjected to DR, all of them lived significantly longer on average and were less prone to age-associated diseases. It is worth noting, however, that the optimal amount of DR is still debated and is likely genotype-specific. Weindruch (1996), for example, severely restricted caloric intake of a strain of mouse by 65 percent (i.e., feeding them 35 percent *ad libitum* amount) and this was their longest-lived group.

To characterize the long-lived animals, Will & McCay (1941) determined their metabolic rate and, to their surprise, found that they had higher cal/kg/h metabolism than the *ad lib* (AL)-fed counterparts. The animals also failed to undergo the usual age-related decline in metabolic rate between 850 to 1,150 days of age (rats typically live ~1,000 days). This DR-dependent increase in metabolic rate has been validated subsequently by multiple rodent studies described below, and for other species such as *Caenorhabditis elegans* and *Drosophila melanogaster* (Braeckman et al., 2002; Hulbert et al., 2004). To this day, the misconception that DR works by slowing metabolic rate persists.

B. Timing of the Diet

Shortly after the work of McCay, a set of researchers began testing the effects of diet composition and implementing DR at different ages and at more moderate levels of restriction. Table 3.1 King & Visscher (1950) reported that 33 percent food restriction was beneficial, whereas 50 percent was too severe. Ross found that a 30 percent reduction in

Table 3.1
The Effect of Different DR Regimes on Rat Mortality Rates

Study	Mortality Rate Doubling Time, MRDT (Years)[a]		
	AL	CR	Ratio CR/AL
Ross, 1959	0.17	0.38	2.23
Berg and Simms, 1960	0.17	0.27	1.59
Ross and Bras, 1973			
10% protein	0.30	0.42	1.40
22% protein	0.28	0.65	2.32
51% protein	0.33	0.57	1.72
Goodrick et al. (1983)			
For 10 months	0.25	0.44	1.76
For 18 months	0.31	0.59	1.90
Yu et al. (1982)	0.30	0.53	1.77
Yu et al. (1985)			
After 6 weeks	0.19	0.27	1.42
6 weeks to 9 months	0.19	0.19	1.00
After 6 months	0.19	0.32	1.63

[a]Post-maturity Mortality Rate Doubling Time (MRDT) is an indicator of the rate of aging of a population. The higher the number, the slower the rate at which mortality increases with age. Adapted from Krystal and Yu, 1994.

caloric intake was close to optimal in rats, with a doubling of life expectancy and an increase in maximum life span of more than 30 percent (Ross, 1972). Carlson and Hoetzel discovered that they could extend the mean and maximum life span of rats about 10 percent by fasting one day out of every four (Carlson & Hoetzel, 1946), but the benefits of restricting food only a few days in a week are highly dependent on the animal's genotype and the age at which the feeding regimen is implemented (Goodrick et al., 1990). Nelson and Halberg (1986) showed that the life span extension is not due to the animals eating only once versus the AL animals who nibble throughout the day.

In 1947, Ball and colleagues (1947) reported that lifelong DR dramatically extends the life span of mice (max life span = 850 days vs. 550 days), whereas DR for the first 240 days had little effect. Switching animals from DR back to a normal AL diet after 8 months gave an intermediate result (max = 600 days). Although it was not appreciated at the time, this paper effectively disproved McCay's hypothesis that DR works by slowing development. There have been numerous studies since, in mice, rats, golden hamsters, worms, flies, and yeast (Krystal & Yu, 1994; Weindruch & Walford, 1988).

Today, it is generally accepted that DR implemented during only the first few months of life of a rodent can have small longevity benefits, but the most efficacious and reliable treatment for extending life span is long-term DR (Weindruch & Walford, 1988). With regards the effect of DR on young animals, it is likely that the diet has lasting effects into adulthood because it permanently alters the endocrinological state of the animal, but this remains to be proven. For flies, there is no lasting effect of DR. In fact, their mortality rate returns to that of well-fed flies within days of being switched to a full diet (Good & Tatar, 2001).

C. Diet Composition

Several laboratories have been instrumental in addressing the question of whether the DR effect is due to the total reduction in food intake or the lack of a specific component. Early on, reduced protein consumption was suspected as the major cause of the effect. Indeed, low-protein diets effectively reduce the incidence of kidney disease and can slightly extend life span (Bras & Ross, 1964; Iwasaki et al., 1988), but total caloric restriction always has a greater effect on life span (Masoro, 1985). Interestingly, Yu and colleagues found that DR animals consume about the same total number of calories during their life span as AL-fed animals (36,000 Kcal), leading to speculation that life span might be related to the total number of calories consumed per rat per lifetime (Yu et al., 1985). Neither the restriction of minerals nor fat affected life span (Iwasaki et al., 1988)

A surprise finding has been that severe restriction of a single amino acid, methionine, is sufficient to extend rat life span (Orentreich et al., 1993; Richie et al., 1994, 2004). The same observations have been made in lower organisms such as yeast, worms, and flies (Bitterman et al., 2003; Braeckman et al., 2001b; Gems et al., 2002; Tatar et al., 2003). For example, yeast life span is extended not only by restricting calories (i.e., glucose) but also by restricting amino acids, nitrogen, or by heat or osmotic stress (Bitterman et al., 2003). Similarly, the life span of flies and worms can be extended not only by restricting their traditional food sources (i.e. yeast and bacteria) but also by mild stresses such as heat shock and overcrowding (Braeckman et al., 2001b; Michalski et al., 2001; Walker et al., 2003). Thus, the important determinant of longevity is not necessarily the restriction of calories, but rather any nutrient deficiency that can invoke a survival response (Braeckman *et al.*, 2001b; Lamming *et al.*, 2004; Turturro *et al.*, 2000). These observations support the Hormesis Hypothesis, which states that DR is a mild stress that provokes a survival response in the organism. This stress response then boosts resistance to biological and chemical insults and counteracts the causes of aging. A more detailed description of this theory is presented in a later section.

In summary, over the past 70 years, the DR paradigm has proven extremely robust. It can be observed for varying extents of restriction, diet composition, time and duration of the treatment, for a variety of different genetic backgrounds and species. It is the robustness and conservation of the DR paradigm that makes it such a powerful tool for the investigation of the mechanisms that cause aging and the pathways that regulate aging in response to environmental conditions.

III. Physiological Effects of DR on Mammals

A large body of literature has been accumulated over the past 70 years on the effects of DR on mammalian physiology. Many of the key findings about the physiological effects of DR are better discussed within the context of specific hypotheses about how DR works (see below). As with previous editions of this book, it is neither possible nor appropriate to present more than a summary of the effects of DR within a chapter of this length. Excellent reviews on the physiological effects of DR have been published elsewhere (Krystal & Yu, 1994; Masoro, 2000; Weindruch & Walford, 1988). Here, our discussion will focus on the effects of DR that are likely to be relevant to understanding the basis of the phenomenon, and on the latest findings at the cellular and molecular levels.

A. Rodents

For both mice and rats, DR is highly effective at slowing age-dependent physiological decline in various tissues and systems, such as muscle (i.e., sarcopenia) and the immune system (Dempsey *et al.*, 1993; McKiernan *et al.*, 2004; Pahlavani, 2004; Spaulding *et al.*, 1997), although there are exceptions (Sun, 2001). DR also delays the occurrence of almost every disease associated with aging, including heart disease, cataracts, diabetes, and neurodegeneration (Weindruch & Walford, 1988). Moreover, DR is the most potent, broadly acting anti-cancer regimen we know of in animal models (Hursting *et al.*, 2003; Raffoul *et al.*, 1999). DR lowers body temperature and increases the physical activity of mice and rats, although neither of these effects is considered a likely cause of increased longevity, with perhaps the exception of its anti-cancer effects (Koizumi *et al.*, 1996; McCarter *et al.*, 1997). Numerous studies have shown that DR animals are more resistant to a variety of toxins and drugs, such as isoproternol, an asthma drug, and ganacyclovir, an antiviral drug (reviewed by Hart *et al.*, 1995). The beneficial action of DR against many of these toxins seems to be two-fold: altered drug metabolism *in vivo*, leading to increased excretion or less conversion of the molecule to its toxic form, and the resistance of individual cells to the toxin or drug.

At the cellular level, DR modulates several fundamental processes that may be intimately involved in aging. For example, DR retards the age-related decline in certain DNA repair capacities (Guo *et al.*, 1998; Lipman *et al.*, 1989; Weraarchakul *et al.*, 1989), although not all types of DNA repair or tissues are affected (Haley-Zitlin & Richardson, 1993; Prapurna & Rao, 1996). The ability of DR to reduce an accumulation of damage to proteins, lipids, and DNA during aging is also well documented in dozens of studies (Dempsey *et al.*, 1993; Moore *et al.*, 1995;

Ward, 1988; Xia *et al.*, 1995). As one example, the rate at which mutations accumulate during aging (or following exposure to DNA-damaging agents such as bleomycin) is markedly lower in DR animals (Aidoo *et al.*, 1999). Hsp70 is a protein-folding chaperone that also blocks apoptosis by binding to Apaf-1 (Ravagnan *et al.*, 2001). The ability of cells to induce hsp70 in response to heat shock remains relatively high in DR animals, seemingly due to the preservation of a transcription factor that binds to the gene's promoter (Heydari *et al.*, 1993; Pahlavani *et al.*, 1995). DR also alters the susceptibility of cells to apoptosis, but in which direction seems to depend on the cell type and the degree of damage inflicted (reviewed in Zhang & Herman, 2002).

Various age-associated changes in hormones, cytokines, and neurotransmitters are attenuated by DR. For example, the decrease in cholinergic and dopaminergic stimulation of inositol phosphate signaling components is reduced (Undie & Friedman, 1993), and the age-dependent decrease in the secretion of growth hormone and IGF-1 is attenuated by DR (D'Costa *et al.*, 1993). Recently, microarray transcriptional profiles of DR animals have identified some of the genes that could underlie the physiological effects of DR. In summary, the genes that are affected by DR indicate increases in gluconeogenesis, the pentose phosphate pathway, and protein turnover (Cao *et al.*, 2001; Prolla, 2002; Sreekumar *et al.*, 2002; Weindruch *et al.*, 2001), with conflicting data on whether genes that regulate apoptosis are decreased (Weindruch *et al.*, 2001) or increased (Cao *et al.*, 2001).

B. Primates

In 1987, the first controlled study of CR in rhesus and squirrel monkeys was initiated at the National Institute on Aging (Ingram *et al.*, 1990). A similar study is also underway at the University of Wisconsin (Kemnitz *et al.*, 1993). To date, the results strongly suggest that the same beneficial effects observed in DR rodents also occur in primates (Edwards *et al.*, 1998; Zainal *et al.*, 2000). The monkeys matured more slowly and achieved shorter stature than controls (Roth *et al.*, 2001). Other notable physiological changes included lower plasma insulin levels; reduced total cholesterol, triglycerides, blood pressure, and arterial stiffness; higher HDL (good cholesterol); and slower decline in circulating levels of a hormonal marker of aging, DHEAS. These biomarkers suggest that DR primates are aging more slowly and will be less likely to incur diseases of aging such as diabetes and cardiovascular disease (Roth *et al.*, 2001). Bone mass is slightly reduced, but in approximate proportion to the smaller body size.

Is there evidence that DR would extend the maximum life span of humans? Short-term markers of DR in rodents appear to occur in people on strict low-calorie diets, and six month pilot-scale trials of DR in humans have been initiated (Roberts *et al.*, 2001). But in the absence of large cohorts of clinically controlled subjects, some researchers have turned to members of the population who have taken it upon themselves to restrict calories, some for as long as a decade. The first of such studies was recently published and, in a sample of 18 individuals who had been on DR for an average of six years, there was good evidence of improved cardiovascular health (Fontana *et al.*, 2004). The DR group also had lower serum levels of various indicators of health such as LDL, triglycerides, fasting glucose, fasting insulin, and C-reactive protein. Blood pressure was lower, and the intima-media of the carotid artery was 40 percent thinner. Members of the Biosphere 2 crew, who were subjected to a low-calorie diet (1,750 to 2,100 kcal/d) for two years, also experienced hematologic, physiologic, hormonal, and biochemical alterations that resembled those of DR rodents and monkeys (Walford *et al.*, 2002). Although these results are encouraging, the longevity benefits and potential health issues arising from long-term DR in humans remain to be established.

IV. Mechanisms of DR

Although there have been many theories on how DR works, we appear to be on the verge of understanding, at least in a general sense, what underlies the phenomenon. Some might argue that there is no reason for such optimism, and that today is no different from yesterday. Clearly, other researchers thought the same thing about their theories, only to be disappointed, so what is so different this time? It is the first time almost all current theories of DR can be integrated

into a single unifying theory. It is also the first theory that can explain most of the observations in the field, many of which were seemingly disconnected. It is as if scientists have been holding the same animal from different ends without realizing it until now. First, we will review how the field of DR restriction evolved; we will then discuss the paradigm shift that led us to where we are today.

A. Early Theories

1. Developmental Delay

Most researchers in the first half of the 20th century believed that aging was part of the developmental process Table 3.2. So, just as there are genes for development, they reasoned there must be genes for aging. This led to the idea that DR worked by slowing development.

Table 3.2
Hypotheses to Explain Life Span Extension by Dietary Restriction

Hypothesis	Evidence For	Evidence Against
Developmental delay	DR slows development; animals with slower development tend to live longer	DR works post-puberty
Decreased metabolic rate	DR lowers body temperature, some evidence for lowering of mutation frequency; good evidence for uncoupling of oxidative phosphorylation, thus reducing ROS	DR does not lower metabolic rate or frequency of certain mutations in mitochondria
Endocrinological changes	DR alters numerous endocrine factors; mice mutant for IGF-1 or growth hormone live longer	Only partial overlap between dwarf and DR mice; IGF-1 mutant mice still respond to DR
Enhanced cell defenses and increased cell survival	Cells from DR and long-lived animals tend to be stress resistant	DR increases rates of cell death in some tissues
Decreased inflammation	Inflammation underlies some diseases of aging and DR reduces the age-associated increase in the inflammatory response	Reports in the literature of the effect of DR on inflammatory responses are inconsistent
Hormesis (i.e., CR) provokes a mild stress response, causing enhanced cell defenses and metabolic changes, coordinated by the endocrine system	CR proven to work via hormesis for budding yeast; long-lived animals have increased stress resistance; fits with evolutionary theories of aging	Hormesis is unproven in mammals

But the hypothesis did not survive long as researchers showed that placing adults on a DR diet also extended life span. Today, the idea that aging is part of a program is no longer considered valid by evolutionary biologists and geneticists alike. Rather, aging is believed to arise due to a lack of selection for health late in life and the inability of organisms to maintain a pristine and immortal soma due to the competing demands of activities such as growth and reproduction (Charlesworth, 2000; Kirkwood & Holliday, 1979; Medawar, 1946).

2. Reduced Metabolic Rate

Existing data on the relationship between metabolic rate (i.e., energy expenditure) and life span are "contradictory and extremely confused" (Speakman et al., 2003). In 1908, German physiologist Max Rubner reported that animals of various sizes utilize a similar number of calories per weight per lifetime (Rubner, 1908), which was the basis for Pearl's Rate of Living Hypothesis (Pearl, 1928). For about 50 years, the theory that life span is proportional to metabolic rate enjoyed center stage. Support for this theory came from indirect evidence and a series of inverse correlations between metabolic rate and life span, and today it is not considered valid. Although there is a rough correlation between metabolic rate and life span, there are many exceptions. For example, a rat and a bat have similar metabolic rates, yet a bat lives around five times longer (Wilkinson & South, 2002). Many researchers also have tended to equate the Rate of Living Hypothesis with the Free-Radical Hypothesis (see Chapter 10), while assuming that reduced metabolic rate means fewer free radicals are generated, when in fact there is currently no scientific merit to the linking of these two theories (Yu, 1993).

The Rate of Living Hypothesis quickly gave rise to the misconception that DR extends life span by lowering metabolic rate. Between 1950 and 1981, four groups showed that reducing the food intake of rats slows metabolic rate per unit body mass (reviewed in Krystal & Yu, 1994). One recent study in primates reported that total daily energy expenditure was lower in the calorie-restricted monkeys than in the AL monkeys, even when corrected for differences in body size using body weight (DeLany et al., 1999). However, numerous other studies, most notably those from Ed Masoro's group, show that DR animals have equal or higher metabolic rates than AL animals, although they do experience an initial drop in metabolic rate in the first six weeks (Duffy et al., 1997; Masoro, 1998; Masoro et al., 1982; McCarter et al., 1985; McCarter & Palmer, 1992; Yu et al., 1985).

In simple eukaryotes and mammals, most studies have failed to find evidence for the Rate of Living Hypothesis. For example, studies by Vanfletteren's group in C. elegans have found no evidence for decreased metabolic rate during CR (Braeckman et al., 2002), and one study reported an increase (Houthoofd et al., 2002). Linda Partridge's group also found no correlation between diet and metabolic rate in D. melanogaster (Braeckman et al., 2002; Hulbert et al., 2004).

A recent study in rodents also found a positive association between metabolic activity and life span (Speakman et al., 2003, 2004). With regards metabolic theories of DR, this finding is consistent with a variation on the theme known as the Uncoupling to Survive Hypothesis, which predicts that increased energy metabolism (therefore greater uncoupling/proton leakage) should be associated with increased longevity (Speakman et al., 2004).

As noted by Masoro (2001), the misconception that DR works by inducing hypometabolism has been perpetuated. This is well illustrated by the following example. Based on a paper by Imai and colleagues in the prestigious journal *Nature*, members of the scientific and lay press published articles suggesting that the yeast Sir2 longevity regulator is activated by reduced metabolic rate, which might free up NAD, a co-substrate of the enzyme. Clearly, claims that increased longevity is caused by reduced metabolic rate should be avoided, no matter how attractive the hypothesis (Masoro, 2001).

3. Laboratory Gluttons

Numerous researchers have speculated that the effect of DR on extending life span might be a laboratory artifact. The argument is the following: DR is a more natural diet for the animal, similar to what it would be in the wild, and that the AL control animals might simply be overfed and more prone to disease (Cutler, 1982; Hayflick, 1994). For this reason, many labs have switched to a controlled diet for the non-restricted animals to ensure that they are not overfeeding. These laboratories report that DR still increases life span to the same extent as an AL diet in these experiments (Pugh *et al.*, 1999).

A fact that supports DR being a *bona fide* natural physiological response is that it improves the health and life span of almost every species it has been tested on. It seems unlikely, but possible, that for all these species—yeast, worms, flies, fish, spiders—it is a case of overfeeding the control organisms. In the wild, yeast and flies often have an abundance of food, far more than is supplied in the lab. Another argument against DR being a laboratory artifact is that animals in their native environment must eat more than DR animals for at least part of their life to be fertile; a lifetime of reduced

energy intake would result in extinction of the species (Austad, 2001). Austad also calculates that the amount of food consumed by a typical laboratory mouse is similar to that in the wild (about 3 kJ/g/day); clearly *ad libitum*-fed mice in the laboratory are not "grossly overfed" (Austad, 2001).

4. Glucocorticoid Cascade

One theory of aging is that steroids that circulate in the blood stream and play a role in the body's stress response, the glucocorticoids, are a cause of aging. Supporting the Glucocorticoid Cascade Hypothesis were several studies that linked chronic stress with accelerated aging. Unfortunately for this model, DR animals have higher, not lower, levels of a key glucocorticoid, corticosterone, and there is no increase in levels of this steroid in older animals as the hypothesis predicted (reviewed in Krystal & Yu, 1994). Although more work is needed in this area, these results present a serious challenge to the glucocorticoid hypothesis.

5. Decreased Fat

Given the negative effects of obesity, it is natural to assume that DR might work by reducing fat stores (Berg & Simms, 1960). Despite early indications that the theory might be correct (Bertrand *et al.*, 1980), over the past 20 years it has been contradicted by numerous studies showing no correlation between body fat and life span (Harrison *et al.*, 1984; Masoro, 1995). A recent study of mice of various genetic backgrounds found no relationship between life span and body mass, fat mass (Speakman *et al.*, 2003). This study did, however, find evidence for higher levels of proton leakage in the mitochondria of longer-lived outbred mouse strains, which supports the Uncoupling to Survive Hypothesis, as described below. In the case of DR rodents, those that maintain a higher level of fat are often longer lived (Masoro, 1995). Another study showed that AL rats kept as lean as CR rats by running on an exercise wheel do not show the same degree of life extension, and there was no increase in maximum longevity in the lean runners compared with controls (Holloszy, 1997).

The Decreased Fat Hypothesis has become popular recently after the demonstration that fat cells secrete factors that can promote aging if present in excess (Barzilai & Gabriely, 2001; Barzilai & Gupta, 1999; Gupta *et al.*, 2000) and the 15 percent increase in life span of mice with a fat-specific knockout of the insulin receptor (FIRKO) (Bluher *et al.*, 2003). While it is possible that fat cells modulate the pace of aging by secreting humoral factors, and more detailed studies of specific fat depots are required, there is currently little evidence that total fat levels play a major role in life span extension by DR.

6. Decreased Inflammation

The Inflammation Hypothesis of Aging, as its name implies, states that the inflammatory process is a major underlying cause of the aging process (Chung *et al.*, 2002). Although the theory is controversial, there is no doubt that inflammation is an important component of many age-associated diseases, including neurodegeneration, heart disease, and vascular dysfunctions of diabetes. Aging is positively correlated with increases in the activity of NF-kB, a ubiquitous pro-inflammatory transcription factor (Chung *et al.*, 2002). Cytokine production is altered in such a way to promote inflammation, such as prostagalandins (PGE$_2$, TXA$_2$, PGH$_2$, and PGG$_2$), MPO, COX-2, iNOS, TNF□, IL-1, IL-6, IFNγ, and TGFβ (Chung *et al.*, 2002; Gen Son *et al.*, 2005). Unfortunately, at least for the cytokines, most age-related changes have only been investigated *in vitro*, and the

results are not always consistent (Chung *et al.*, 2002). Nevertheless, it is well established that DR suppresses inflammation both *in vitro* and *in vivo*. For example, DR suppresses COX-derived ROS generation during aging and blunts the increase in the production of TXA$_2$, PGI$_2$, and PGE$_2$, among others (Cao *et al.*, 2001; Kim *et al.*, 2004). DR is also effective at suppressing inflammation *in vivo*, as recently demonstrated in a rat model of arthritis (Seres *et al.*, 2002). Whether DR extends mammalian life span *primarily* by suppressing inflammation is debatable, but many researchers would agree that it does play some role.

B. Current Theories on DR based on Proximal Causes of Aging

1. Reduced Reactive Oxygen Species (ROS)

The act of living generates reactive oxygen molecules that can damage cellular constituents such as proteins, DNA, and lipids. These molecules are also referred to as free-radicals or reactive oxygen species (ROS). Each human cell receives 10,000 ROS hits per day, which equals 7 trillion insults per second per person. Because our cellular repair systems are not efficient enough to cope with the onslaught, ROS-mediated damage accumulates with time and is considered to be a major cause of aging (Harmon, 1956).

Consistent with the free-radical theory of aging (Harmon, 1956), aged mammals contain high quantities of oxidized lipids and proteins as well as damaged/mutated DNA, particularly the mitochondrial genome (reviewed in Droge, 2003; Dufour & Larsson, 2004). Moreover, mice with an accelerated rate of mutation in mitochondrial DNA exhibit signs of premature aging, such as weight loss, reduced subcutaneous fat, hair loss, osteoporosis, anemia, and reduced fertility (Trifunovic *et al.*, 2004). With regards DR, the diet slows the increase in the rate of lipid peroxidation and the associated loss of fluidity of biological membranes, the accumulation of oxidatively damaged proteins, specifically "carbonylated" proteins, and the increase in oxidative damage to DNA (reviewed in Barja, 2004; Merry, 2002).

Among the many scientists who hypothesize that ROS are a major cause of aging, there is some debate as to whether DR works primarily by decreasing ROS *production* or increasing ROS *defenses* and *repair*. There are data for both these hypotheses, and they are by no means mutually exclusive. Currently, the evidence better supports the lowering of ROS production by DR; the antioxidant defense findings are variable, depending on enzyme(s) and tissues examined. In favor of the first hypothesis, DR has been shown to decrease the production of two key ROS, superoxide radicals and hydrogen peroxide (Sohal et al., 1994b), and to slow the accumulation of ROS-induced damage (Lindsay, 1999; Sohal et al., 1994a; Zainal et al., 2000). The mitochondrial complexes I and III of the electron transport chain are considered to be the major sources of ROS (Barja, 2004; Gredilla et al., 2004; Lopez-Torres et al., 2002). DR also slows the age-dependent increase in iron content of the kidney, thereby reducing ROS damage to that organ (Cook & Yu, 1998). A recent study showed that COX-2-derived ROS production during prostaglandin biosynthesis increases with age in rats, and that this is suppressed by DR (Chung et al., 1999).

There is considerable evidence that ROS *defenses* are also upregulated by DR, but as with most aging theories, the scientific literature on this topic is replete with inconsistencies. The results seem to depend on which enzyme and tissue one looks at (Xia et al., 1995). In support of the ROS repair/defense theory, DR rodents seem to have higher activity of catalase and lower lipid peroxidation than AL controls (Koizumi et al., 1987; Mote et al., 1991), although lower levels of mRNA of other defense genes such as CuZn-superoxide dismutase (SOD), glutathione peroxidase, and epoxide hydrolase, and these do not apparently change with age or diet (Mote et al., 1991). Additional support for the theory comes from a study that reported levels of mRNA and enzymatic activity for SOD, catalase, and glutathione peroxidase remain higher in DR rats versus AL, and that ROS damage is lower (Rao et al., 1990). These findings have been corroborated by subsequent animal studies (Armeni et al., 2003; Xia et al., 1995). Microarray analyses of tissues from DR mice show that mRNA for specific DNA defense enzymes, such as SOD1 and SOD2, are increased relative to *ad lib*-fed mice (Sreekumar et al., 2002; Weindruch et al., 2001). Numerous other studies show that DNA-repair protein levels and activities are higher in DR animals compared to controls (Cabelof et al., 2003; Um et al., 2003).

Although the free-radical theory of DR remains popular, and hundreds of studies have been published on the subject, the experimental evidence so far is not convincing (Lindsay, 1999). Proof that antioxidants are beneficial is mainly limited to the demonstration that they slightly increase average life span in rodents and flies, but there is little evidence to support an increase in maximum life span.

In *Drosophila*, there has been considerable work done in examining this hypothesis, but the data are contradictory. Flies transgenically altered to overexpress human SOD are stress resistant and live up to 40 percent longer (Parkes et al., 1998; Reveillaud et al., 1992; Spencer et al., 2003), but the effect is genotype- and sex-specific (Parkes et al., 1998; Reveillaud et al., 1992; Spencer et al., 2003). Molecules that might soak up ROS, such as melatonin, carnosine, epithalamin (a pineal peptide) and epitalon (a short peptide of Ala-Glu-Asp-Gly), increase average life span of flies up to 16 percent (Izmaylov & Obukhova, 1999; Khavinson et al., 2000; Yuneva et al., 2002). Whether these effects are due to antioxidant properties has not been convincingly demonstrated. Contradicting these studies is the recent demonstration that there is no apparent correlation between ROS production and fly life span, and DR does not reduce ROS production in these animals (Barja, 2004; Merry, 2002; Miwa et al., 2004).

In mammals the situation is no better. A recent study of rat liver and brain reported that DR does not affect the accumulation of a common age-related deletion in mitochondrial DNA (Cassano et al., 2004). There have also been numerous reports that DR has little effect on ROS defense mechanisms and, if anything, DR attenuates the age-dependent increase (Gong et al., 1997; Guo et al., 2001; Luhtala et al., 1994; Rojas et al., 1993; Stuart et al., 2004). This discordance could be due to the fact that many of the studies examined different tissues, or perhaps it is because some measured mRNA levels and others measured protein activity, making direct comparisons between studies difficult. That aside, perhaps the most convincing evidence against the free-radical theory of aging is that mice with an SOD2 deficiency, which have increased oxidative damage, do not show signs of premature aging by a variety of measures (Van Remmen et al., 2003).

2. Alterations in Apoptosis

In response to damage or stress, cells will attempt to repair and defend themselves, but if unsuccessful, they often undergo programmed cell death, or "apoptosis." Aging is generally associated with increased rates of stress-induced apoptosis (Higami & Shimokawa, 2000), and the cumulative effects of cell loss

have been implicated in various diseases, including neurodegeneration, retinal degeneration, cardiovascular disease, and frailty (reviewed in Zhang & Herman, 2002).

The Cell Survival Hypothesis of CR states that the increased life span of mammals is due to an attenuation of cell loss over time, particularly cells that are easily replaced, such as neurons and stem cells (Cohen et al., 2004b). Consistent with this idea, cells cultured from long-lived genetic mutants, such as the p66[sch] knockout mouse and long-lived dwarfs, are typically less prone to stress-induced apoptosis (Migliaccio et al., 1999; Murakami et al., 2003). Numerous studies have examined rates of apoptosis in cells and tissues from DR animals, and the results have been varied. Many studies have reported that DR increases rates of apoptosis (or genes that promote apoptosis), especially rapidly dividing tissues such as skin, pre-neoplastic cells, and the immune system (Cao et al., 2001; Mukherjee et al., 2004; Tsuchiya et al., 2004; Wachsman, 1996). This apparent increase in apoptosis is thought to be a major mechanism by which DR rats maintain healthy cells and are relatively resistant to cancer (James et al., 1998; Zhang & Herman, 2002).

On the other hand, a number of recent studies indicate that DR protects a variety of cell types from apoptosis, including neurons, liver cells, and immune cells (Calingasan & Gibson, 2000; Hiona & Leeuwenburgh, 2004; Monti & Contestabile, 2003; Selman et al., 2003). Recent findings indicate that DR may have a profound effect on brain function and vulnerability to injury and diseases by enhancing neuroprotection and reducing susceptibility to apoptosis. Two studies have reported that neurons of DR animals express high levels of two key apoptosis inhibitors, XIAP and ARC, and are more resistant to stress-induced apoptosis (Hiona & Leeuwenburgh, 2004; Shelke

& Leeuwenburgh, 2003). DR even protects hippocampal neurons from apoptosis due to a presenillin-1 mutation in a mouse model of Alzheimer's disease (Mattson et al., 2002b).

With regards the liver, primary hepatocytes from DR animals are less susceptible to cytotoxins and genotoxins (Shaddock et al., 1995). At the molecular level, expression of p53 and Fas receptor in hepatocytes goes up with aging, but DR suppressed this age-enhanced increase (Ando et al., 2002). The pro-apoptotic gene gadd153/chop is also repressed by DR in liver hepatocytes, causing decreased apoptosis and increased resistance to hydrogen peroxide (Ikeyama et al., 2003). DR has also been reported to suppress apoptosis in aging rat livers, possibly by attenuating the activity of DNase gamma endonuclease (Tanaka et al., 2004). In one notable study, DR fully suppressed TNFalpha-mediated hepatic apoptosis (Hatano et al., 2004).

Lymphocytes in DR mice are much less susceptible to oxidative stress-induced apoptosis due to attenuation of TNF-alpha and Bcl-2 levels (Avula & Fernandes, 2002), and transcripts involved in suppressing apoptosis and promoting cell survival are increased by DR (Weindruch et al., 2001). In a recent study, levels of the SIRT1 (a protein deacetylase homologous to the Sir2 longevity gene in yeast and worms) were shown to be elevated in DR rats, which attenuates cells' susceptibility to apoptosis by sequestering the pro-apoptotic protein Bax away from mitochondria (Cohen et al., 2004b). SIRT1 also deacetylates the FOXO3 transcription factor, tipping the scales even further towards cell protection and survival (Antebi, 2004; Brunet et al., 2004). Sinclair and colleagues propose that SIRT1 protects irreplaceable cells such as neurons and stem cells from death during times of stress, thus maintaining physiological function with age. In summary, it is generally accepted that the rates of apoptosis increase with age and that DR modulates this process, either up or down, depending on the cell type. Whether this contributes to longevity is still hotly debated.

3. Protein Turnover

Several protein modifications accumulate with age, the most widely studied is the carbonyl addition, which results primarily from oxidative damage (Stadtman, 1995). Other modifications include glycation, racemization, isomerization, and deamination. Protein turnover is an efficient way for a cell to maintain functional proteins, and most modified proteins are marked for degradation by cytosolic proteases or the proteosome. There is abundant evidence from biochemical studies and gene expression profiling in C. elegans and mammals that protein turnover rates and overall autophagic processes decline with age and that this decline is attenuated by DR (Del Roso et al., 2003; Lewis et al., 1985; Tavernarakis & Driscoll, 2002). Whether this is a cause or a symptom of aging is not yet clear.

4. Decreased Glucose and Insulin levels

Diabetes mellitus, or type II diabetes, is characterized by a high level of serum glucose, insulin, and the types of cellular alterations seen in the elderly, including glycation and glycooxidation, and the accumulation of advanced glycation end-products (AGE) (see Chapter 19). Furthermore, many organs and tissues of type II diabetic individuals tend to age faster than normal, particularly the cardiovascular system. Thus, one way DR might improve health is by keeping blood glucose and/or insulin levels down (reviewed in Kalant et al., 1988).

Many groups have studied glucose metabolism in DR animals. An important discovery was that DR rats use plasma glucose as fuel at the same rate per unit of metabolic mass as the AL rats while maintaining physiologically significantly lower plasma glucose levels (a 15 mg/dl difference) and markedly lower plasma insulin levels (Masoro *et al.*, 1992). This is due, in large part, to increased glucose uptake in skeletal muscle and fat pads that results from the glucose transporter GLUT-4 localizing to the plasma membrane (Cartee *et al.*, 1994; Dean *et al.*, 1998a; Dean *et al.*, 1998b). The decrease in insulin is attributable to its lower rate of secretion by pancreatic β-cells (Dean *et al.*, 1998b). Although these effects are clearly associated with DR, it remains to be seen whether low glucose and insulin levels are an actual cause of the life span increase. In recent years, many researchers have turned their attention to other endocrine factors, including a related signaling molecule called IGF-1, as described below.

5. IGF-1, Growth Hormone, and Other Endocrinological Changes

It has been known for decades that DR results in changes to hormonal levels, and that some of these changes are associated with increased longevity, but there is now some evidence that these changes actually contribute to the longevity of DR animals. In simple eukaryotes such as worms and flies, disruption of the insulin/IGF-1 signaling pathway increases longevity, and we are now seeing that it is also true for mammals (Tatar *et al.*, 2003). In mice, three transgenic "knocking outs" of endocrine genes have been shown to extend life span, namely the growth hormone (GH) receptor, the insulin receptor (specifically in fat cells), or a heterozygous knockout of the IGF-1 receptor (Bluher *et al.*, 2003; Holzenberger, 2004). Moreover, spontaneous genetic alterations in mice that lead to extensions in

life span are associated with profound alterations in hormonal levels, particularly reductions in IGF-1, namely the Ames dwarf, which are growth hormone–deficient and mutant for *prop-1*, the Snell dwarf, which are mutant for the *pit-1* gene, and little mice, which are mutant in the GH receptor *Ghrhr* gene (Bartke, 2000). For a detailed review, see Chapter 19 by R. Miller and S. Austad in this book.

Whether these dwarf animals are good models for DR is debated (Bluher *et al.*, 2003). Although it is true that IGF-1 and insulin levels are lower in DR animals, Bartke and colleagues reported that the life span of the Ames dwarf, which has already low levels of these factors, can be further increased by CR (Bartke *et al.*, 2001), arguing that they work via different but possibly overlapping mechanisms. This idea is supported by comparing the gene expression profiles of DR versus the GH knockout mouse. Although there was little overlap in gene expression, the effect of CR in GH knockout mice was much lower than wildtype mice (Tsuchiya *et al.*, 2004). Similar conclusions have been reached in the *C. elegans* field, primarily due to the work of Vanfletteren and colleagues. They have provided good evidence that mild DR does not involve altered IGF-1 signaling but that intense DR or starvation does, and together these two "processes" have an additive effect on life span (Houthoofd *et al.*, 2003). In summary, it is clear that the endocrine system is important in determining longevity, and that certain hormones such as IGF-1 seem to play an important role in coordinating a systemic response to CR.

C. The Hormesis Hypothesis and Stress-Responsive Survival Pathways

Over the past five years, a novel hypothesis to explain the effect of DR has gained popularity. It is such a major shift in thinking, and embraces so many of the current theories on DR under one umbrella, that it deserves its own section. A small but rapidly growing number of researchers in the DR field are now major proponents of this new theory known as the Hormesis Hypothesis of DR (Anderson *et al.*, 2003; Iwasaki *et al.*, 1988; Johnson *et al.*, 1996; Masoro, 1998; Mattson *et al.*, 2002a; Turturro *et al.*, 2000). The theory states that the underlying mechanism of DR is the activation of a defense response that evolved to help organisms cope with adverse conditions. These defenses extend life span because they counteract the proximal causes of aging (Masoro & Austad, 1996) (see Figure 3.2). The theory has been recently expanded by Sinclair and Howitz to include the idea that organisms can pick up on chemical cues from other species under stress or DR, either in their food or environment, and use these to activate their own defense pathways in anticipation of adverse conditions to come (Howitz *et al.*, 2003; Lamming *et al.*, 2004). This idea, termed the Xenohormesis Hypothesis, is discussed in more detail in Section V.

1. Hormesis Is an Active Defense Response

In the early 1940s, Southam and Ehrlich (1943) reported that a bark extract known to inhibit fungal growth actually stimulated growth when given at very low concentrations. They coined the term "hormesis" to describe such beneficial actions resulting from the response of an organism to a low-intensity stressor. The word "hormesis" is derived from the Greek word *hormaein*, which means "to excite." The Hormesis Hypothesis of DR proposes that the diet imposes a low-intensity biological stress on the

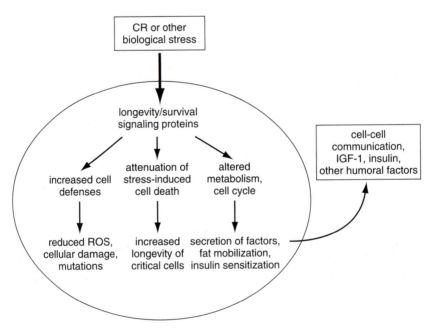

Figure 3.2 The Hormesis Hypothesis of DR. The theory states that DR is a mild stress that provokes a survival response in the organism, which boosts resistance to stress and counteracts the causes of aging. The theory unites previously disparate observations about ROS defenses, apoptosis, metabolic changes, stress resistance, and hormonal changes and is rapidly becoming accepted as the best explanation for the effects of DR.

organism, which elicits a defense response that helps protects it against the causes of aging (Lithgow, 2001; Masoro, 2000; Turturro et al., 1998). It is a major shift in thinking from earlier hypotheses. It suggests that DR is due to an *active* defensive response of the organism as opposed to *passive* mechanisms such as altered mitochondrial metabolism or lower circulating glucose. The genes that seem to control this process are now coming to light, thanks to genetic studies in simple organisms such as worms and flies. The Hormesis Hypothesis makes four key predictions:

1. That DR induces intracellular cell-autonomous signaling pathways that respond to biological stress and low nutrition
2. That the pathways help defend cells (and hence the organism) against the causes of aging
3. That the pathways alter glucose, fat, and protein metabolism to enhance survival during times of adversity
4. That the pathways are under the control of endocrine signaling pathways that ensure that cells in the organism act in a coordinated fashion

Clearly, many of the observations listed under different headings in the previous section are also consistent with the Hormesis Hypothesis. Obvious examples include the DR-associated boost in cell survival and the observed metabolic and endocrine changes. Rather than revisit these observations here, additional evidence for and against the Hormesis Hypothesis will be presented.

2. Genes that Control Survival and Life Span

Prior to 1990, very few researchers suspected the existence of single genes that control aging. This was based in part on the valid assumption that aging was an incredibly complex process that was affected by hundreds, if not thousands, of genes. Then, genetic studies in model organisms in the 1990s began to uncover numerous single gene mutations that extended life span (Friedman & Johnson, 1988; Jazwinski et al., 1993; Kenyon et al., 1993). Today there are dozens of mutations known to extend life span in model organisms (Lee et al., 2003b). It is worth noting that some researchers still do not accept that these genes are particularly relevant to aging research (Hayflick, 1999). This begs the question: what have these researchers overlooked? The major oversight appears to be a failure to realize that organisms possess genetic pathways to promote survival during times of adversity. Long-term activation of these pathways counteracts the causes of aging and hence extends life span (Kenyon, 2001; Sinclair, 2002).

Around the same time as geneticists were formulating these hypotheses to explain the existence of longevity genes, similar ideas about DR were emerging independently. Holliday first proposed that the effect of DR is an evolutionary adaptation that allows organisms to survive periods of low food availability (Holliday, 1989). Masoro and Austad then expanded this idea and provided perhaps the most comprehensive theory on this subject by merging it with the ideas of Kirkwood and the Hormesis concept (Masoro & Austad, 1996). The disposable soma theory of Kirkwood proposes that each organism has limited resources and that these resources can only be allocated to a finite number of cellular activities, the two primary ones being reproduction and somatic maintenance (Kirkwood & Holliday, 1979). During times of perceived adversity such as during DR, organisms divert more of their resources to maintaining their soma until conditions improve. Today there is general consensus among leaders in the DR field that the health benefits of DR derive from an organism's defense response to a perceived threat to its survival.

3. Proof of Hormesis in Budding Yeast

The use of yeast to study longevity mechanisms is now well respected, but when this organism was first proposed as a model for aging in the 1950s and 1960s (Barton, 1950; Johnson, 1966), it was met with considerable skepticism. One reason, no doubt, is that it was difficult to see how a relatively simple unicellular organism could provide information about human aging, which is one of the most complex of biological phenomena, involving trillions of cells in numerous systems and organs. It is becoming clear, however, that all eukaryotes possess surprisingly simple and conserved longevity pathways that govern life span, principally by attenuating the proximal causes of aging in response to adverse conditions (Kenyon, 2001; Sinclair, 2002).

Yeast "replicative" life span is defined as the number of divisions an individual yeast cell undergoes before dying (Bitterman et al., 2003). One attractive feature of S. cerevisiae, as opposed to many other simple eukaryotes, is that the progenitor cell is easily distinguished from its descendants because cell division is asymmetric: a newly formed "daughter" cell is almost always smaller than the "mother" cell that gave rise to it. Yeast mother cells divide about 20 times before dying and undergo characteristic structural and metabolic changes as they age. An alternative measure of yeast aging, "chronological life span," is the length of time a population of yeast cells remains viable in a nondividing state following nutrient deprivation (Longo & Fabrizio, 2002).

Consistent with the Hormesis Hypothesis and findings in other species, longevity of yeast cells and stress

resistance correlate (Fabrizio et al., 2001; Kennedy et al., 1995). Moreover, a variety of low-intensity stresses extend yeast life span, including mild heat, increased salt, low amino acids, or low glucose, the yeast equivalent of CR (Anderson et al., 2003; Bitterman et al., 2003). Remarkably, these life span extensions are facilitated by a single gene, PNC1, which is induced by every treatment known to extend yeast life span (Anderson et al., 2003; Gallo et al., 2004) (see Figure 3.3). By adding more copies of PNC1, researchers were able to mimic the effects of DR and extend life span 60 percent. PNC1

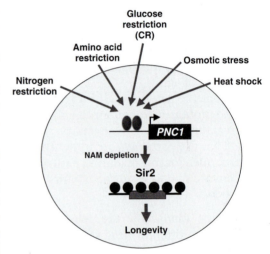

Figure 3.3 *S. cerevisiae* life span extension by DR is due to hormesis. Replicative life span in yeast is extended by caloric restriction (CR) and a variety of mild stresses. The Sir2 enzyme is a nicotinamide (NAM)-sensitive enzyme that extends yeast life span by deacetylating histones and stabilizing repetitive DNA. PNC1 encodes an enzyme that depletes nicotinamide and activates Sir2. PNC1 can be viewed as a "master regulator of aging" that serves as a sensor that translates CR and environmental stress signals into Sir2 activation and longevity (Anderson et al., 2003). By having centralized control of longevity, the system permits new life spans to evolve rapidly in response to a changing environment. The role of NAM and a mammalian equivalent to PNC1, known as PBEF/visfatin/NAMPT, in regulating life span and health in mammals is under investigation by numerous laboratories.

encodes a nicotinamidase that extends yeast life span by depleting the cell of nicotinamide, an inhibitor of the Sir2 longevity enzyme. This system of longevity regulation in yeast explains how multiple, disparate stimuli can lead to the same longevity response and how species may rapidly evolve strategies to suit a changing environment. Whether or not nicotinamide catabolic pathways control Sir2 enzymatic activity in higher organisms is not known.

Interestingly, the *SIR2* gene is conserved in higher eukaryotes, and its ability to extend life span is conserved at least up to worms and flies (Helfand, 2004; Tissenbaum & Guarente, 2001). It is worth noting that there must be alternative pathways for the mediation of life span extension because DR can still extend the life span of certain strains of yeast and worms that lack the Sir2 gene (Kaeberlein *et al.*, 2004; Sinclair & Wood, 2004). A detailed discussion of Sir2 may be found in the section on CR mimetics below.

4. Evidence for Hormesis in Worms and Flies

There is a strong correlation between longevity of various strains of worms and flies and their resistance to various types of stress, including desiccation, heat stress, acetone, ethanol, and paraquat (Arking *et al.*, 1991; da Cunha *et al.*, 1995; Harshman *et al.*, 1999; Houthoofd *et al.*, 2003; Mockett *et al.*, 2001; Wang *et al.*, 2004). Moreover, exposure of organisms to agents or conditions that cause mild biological stress increases life span as well as resistance to other, seemingly unrelated stresses, such as low doses of paraquat, aldehydes, irradiation, heat shock, crowding, and hypergravity (Braeckman *et al.*, 2001b; Hercus *et al.*, 2003; Lints *et al.*, 1993; Minois *et al.*, 1999; Sorensen & Loeschcke, 2001). Arguing that DR is simply another

mild stress, flies and worms subjected to DR are also resistant to a variety of stresses, including heat shock (Tatar *et al.*, 2003). These observations strongly argue that DR does not simply change metabolism or ROS output, as was previously thought, but rather it induces a defense program that provides resistance to a wide array of stresses.

Many of the life span extensions provided by mild stress and crowding have been shown to act through the insulin/IGF-1 pathway, which boosts the activity of a conserved forkhead transcription factor known as daf-16/FOXO. One of the functions of daf-16/FOXO is to increases the transcription of cell defense genes such as SOD2 and HSP70 (Lee *et al.*, 2003a; Murphy *et al.*, 2003). Overexpression of FOXO in the fat body of the fly extends life span via dilp-2, an insulin homolog produced in neurons, indicating that FOXO controls endocrine signaling and that fat is an important tissue for the control of life span (Giannakou *et al.*, 2004; Hwangbo *et al.*, 2004) (see Chapter 10). That said, clearly the insulin/IGF-1 pathway is not the whole story because worm mutants lacking Daf-16 still respond to DR (Braeckman *et al.*, 2001a).

5. Evidence for Hormesis in Mammals

It has been known for a decade that DR boosts serum levels of glucocorticoids, particularly corticosterone, which is a good indicator that the animals are invoking a stress response (Masoro, 2000; Sabatino *et al.*, 1991). As is the case for simple metazoans, DR also increases the resistance of animals to a variety of stresses, including sudden increases in temperature (Heydari *et al.*, 1993) and toxins (Duffy *et al.*, 2001; Masoro, 1998). These observations also extend to the cellular level.

Experiments at the cellular and molecular level strongly support the Hormesis

Hypothesis. The skin cells from long-lived mutant Snell dwarfs are relatively resistance to stress and toxins including UV, light, heat, cadmium, and paraquat (Murakami *et al.*, 2003), and cells cultured in the presence of serum from DR rats are relatively resistant to stresses and pro-apoptotic signals (Cohen *et al.*, 2004b; de Cabo *et al.*, 2003). Subjecting fibroblasts to repeated heat shock also produces similar effects to those seen *in vivo*, including maintenance of the stress protein profile, reduction in the accumulation of damaged proteins, stimulation of proteolysis, and increased resistance to stressors such as ethanol, hydrogen peroxide, and UV (Rattan, 2004).

It has recently been demonstrated that the mammalian homolog of the Sir2 gene that promotes life span in lower organisms, known as SIRT1, is highly induced in the tissues of DR rats (Cohen *et al.*, 2004b). Interestingly, at the cellular level, SIRT1 promotes the resistance of cells to stress-induced death by attenuating p53 and stimulating the Ku70-Bax anti-apoptotic system (Cohen *et al.*, 2004a; Cohen *et al.*, 2004b). SIRT1 also stimulates metabolic changes in cells consistent with DR, including decreases in fatty acid synthesis in adipocytes by deacetylating the nuclear hormone receptor PPARγ (Picard *et al.*, 2004) and increases in glucose production from hepatocytes via PGC-1α and PPARα (Puigserver & Speigelman, 2004). Given that SIRT1 is up-regulated by DR and that the *in vitro* data are consistent with changes seen *in vivo*, it will be interesting to examine whether the overexpression of SIRT1 produces similar effects to DR in transgenic mice.

In summary, although the Hormesis Hypothesis of DR is young and not embraced by the majority of researchers today, it is the best theory we have to explain the multitude of data about DR in mammals and lower organisms. If the theory is right, DR extends life span not simply by *passive* means such as altering glucose metabolism or ROS production, but by triggering an evolutionarily ancient, *active* defense response that allows organisms to survive adversity. The contrast between earlier hypotheses and this one is stark, but only time will tell if the theory will hold up over the coming decades.

V. Small-Molecule CR Mimetics

A. Drug Development Strategies for Mimicking CR

Work on the genetics of aging in yeast, *C. elegans*, *Drosophila*, and rodents suggests that CR might act through conserved signaling pathways to control eukaryotic longevity in response to environmental conditions (Kenyon, 2001). Important elements of a major longevity pathway include insulin/IGF-1 receptor signaling and the FOXO family of transcription factors, whose activity is regulated in part by lysine-acetylation and the action of "sirtuin" NAD^+-dependent deacetylases (see Figure 3.4). The existence of this pathway raises the possibility that small molecule modulators of its constituent proteins could potentially mimic the effects of CR, thereby providing some of its benefits, without the need for actual CR. As an example of this type of CR-mimesis, we will discuss in detail compounds that activate sirtuins.

Other categories of small-molecule CR mimetics include (1) molecules that may mimic CR directly by effects on energy metabolism and (2) molecules identified by their ability to induce gene-expression patterns similar to those induced by CR. Potential CR mimetics that exemplify these approaches are, respectively, 2-deoxyglucose and metformin. These approaches to CR mimetics have been reviewed recently (Ingram *et al.*, 2004) and, because we will not be discussing them further, we refer the reader to that review and some of the recent primary literature on

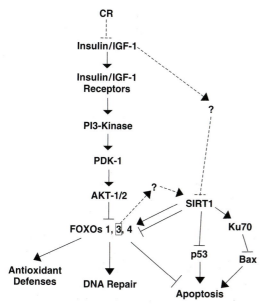

Figure 3.4 Regulatory interactions between SIRT1, the mammalian insulin/IGF-1 signaling pathway, and factors controlling apoptosis. SIRT1 deacetylates the FOXO transcription factors, stimulating transcription of genes involved in antioxidant defense and DNA repair, while repressing transcription of pro-apoptotic genes. SIRT1 exerts additional anti-apoptotic effects by inactivation/destabilization of p53 and by promoting the sequestration of Bax by Ku70. Solid lines indicate that at least one mechanism for the stimulatory or inhibitory effect has been experimentally established (e.g., FOXO3 repression of the expression of BIM, a proapoptotic protein) (Brunet et al., 2004). Dashed lines indicate observed effects for which the mechanism is still unknown. For example, insulin and IGF-1 have been shown in cell culture to reverse the elevation of SIRT1 expression elicited by serum from CR rats (Cohen et al., 2004b).

2-deoxyglucose (Wan et al., 2003; Wan et al., 2004), CR expression profiling (Dhahbi et al., 2004; Weindruch et al., 2001), and metformin (Fulgencio et al., 2001; Spindler et al., 2003).

B. Sirtuin Activating Compounds (STACs)

1. Sirtuins: Conserved Longevity Factors

Yeast Sir2 (Silent information regulator 2) is the founding exemplar of the sirtuins, an apparently ancient group of enzymes which occurs in eukaryotes, the archaea and eubacteria (Laurenson & Rine, 1992; Smith et al., 2000). Originally described as a factor required for maintenance of silencing at telomeres and mating-type loci, Sir2 was subsequently shown to be an enhancer of mother-cell replicative life span in budding yeast (Kaeberlein et al., 1999). The Sir2 enhancement of mother-cell life span has been linked to its stabilization of repetitive DNA, in particular its suppression of the accumulation of extrachromosomal rDNA circles (Kaeberlein et al., 1999; Kobayashi et al., 2004; Sinclair & Guarente, 1997).

The sirtuins represent a distinct class of trichostatin A (TSA)-insensitive protein-lysyl-deacetylases (Class III HDACs) and have been shown to catalyze a reaction that couples lysine deacetylation to the formation of nicotinamide and O-acetyl-ADP-ribose from NAD^+ and the abstracted acetyl group (Imai et al., 2000; Tanner et al., 2000; Tanny & Moazed, 2001). HDACs are named for their role in deacetylation of histone N-terminal tails, an action which typically leads to the formation of condensed chromatin and transcriptional silencing (Strahl & Allis, 2000). However, it is becoming increasingly clear that the effects of HDACs, including those of the sirtuins, are also implemented through deacetylation of transcription factors and other proteins.

There are at least seven human sirtuins, SIRT1–SIRT7 (Frye, 2000). SIRT1, which is located in the nucleus, is the human sirtuin with the greatest homology to Sir2 and has been shown to exert a regulatory effect on multiple transcription factors, including p53 (Langley, 2002; Luo et al., 2001; Vaziri et al., 2001), MyoD (Fulco et al., 2003), FOXO1-3 (Motta et al., 2004; Daitoku et al., 2004), FOXO3 (Brunet et al., 2004; Daitoku et al., 2004; Motta et al., 2004; van der Horst et al., 2004), PPARγ (Picard et al., 2004), and Ku70

(Cohen *et al.*, 2004b). The FOXO effects are perhaps of particular note because they parallel the way in which *C. elegans* DAF16, a FOXO homolog, is required for life span extension by increased Sir2 expression (Tissenbaum & Guarente, 2001). Although there is some disagreement among the FOXO studies—compare FOXO3 effects on p27^{kip1} expression in the study of Motta *et al.* (2004) and that of Brunet *et al.* (2004)—a pattern emerges in which SIRT1 upregulates FOXO-induced transcripts promoting DNA repair (GADD45, Brunet *et al.*, 2004), oxidative stress response (MnSOD, Daitoku *et al.*, 2004; van der Horst *et al.*, 2004), and cell-cycle arrest (p27^{kip1}, Brunet *et al.*, 2004; Daitoku *et al.*, 2004; van der Horst *et al.*, 2004), while repressing pro-apoptotic FOXO-induced transcripts (BIM, Motta *et al.*, 2004; Brunet *et al.*, 2004) (Fas ligand, Brunet *et al.*, 2004).

It has been suggested that SIRT1 promotes cell survival and organismal longevity by delaying apoptosis enough to give antioxidant defenses and repair processes time to succeed (Brunet *et al.*, 2004; Howitz *et al.*, 2003). A variant of this idea, suggested by SIRT1 effects on NF-κB, is that SIRT1 may delay stress-induced p53-dependent apoptosis but may actually make cells more sensitive to apoptosis induced by death receptor ligands such as TNF-α and TRAIL (Yeung *et al.*, 2004).

Sirtuins are inhibited by nicotinamide (NAM), a product of the deacetylation reaction (Bitterman *et al.*, 2002). In yeast, this forms a basis for the regulation of Sir2 activity. Expression of the yeast nicotinamidase, *PNC1*, is upregulated by several longevity-enhancing mild stresses, including calorie restriction suggesting that, at least in yeast, Sir2 stimulation via nicotinamide removal may be the common feature that links several types of hormesis (Anderson *et al.*, 2003). The human functional equivalent of yeast *PNC1* is PBEF/visfatin/NAMPT, which encodes a NAM phosphoribosyl transferase that regulates nicotinamide levels (Fukuhara *et al.*, 2004; Rongvaux *et al.*, 2002). Initial reports indicate that PBEF retains the ability to regulate SIRT1 (Revollo *et al.*, 2004).

Another leading hypothesis on the regulation of Sir2 connects deacetylase activity to energy metabolism by asserting that Sir2 is regulated by the supply of its substrate NAD$^+$ or by the ratio of NAD$^+$ to its reduced form, NADH (Lin *et al.*, 2004). In yeast and *C. elegans*, added copies of sirtuin genes extend life span, and Sir2 activity is boosted by caloric restriction (Anderson *et al.*, 2003; Lin *et al.*, 2000).

Recent work on CR rats has shown that SIRT1 protein levels are elevated in multiple tissues, relative to *ad libitum*-fed controls (Cohen *et al.*, 2004b). Moreover, serum from CR rats elevated SIRT1 expression in cultured human cells, an effect that could be eliminated by the addition IGF-1 and insulin. Of course, this does not negate the possibility that NAD$^+$ and/or nicotinamide levels may also contribute to SIRT1 regulation in mammals. Taken together, the results summarized above suggest that SIRT1 activity plays a central role in the CR-responsive pathway that affects mammalian longevity. SIRT1 expression responds to the known longevity-enhancing stimuli CR and diminished insulin/IGF-1 signaling (Cohen *et al.*, 2004b). On the downstream side, SIRT1 effects on transcription factors and other proteins controlling apoptosis and cell survival, DNA repair, oxidative-stress responses, and lipid metabolism suggest that increased SIRT1 activity may be responsible for eliciting the gene expression changes brought on by CR. SIRT1 effects on mammalian longevity have yet to be directly established. Nevertheless, the demonstration of connections between SIRT1 and insulin/IGF-1 signaling on the one hand and the FOXO transcription factors on the other means that the key elements of the metazoan longevity pathway have been confirmed in mammals.

If SIRT1 is indeed a conduit of CR-derived signals, then interventions that either elevate SIRT1 expression or stimulate SIRT1 activity might mimic CR. Strategies for stimulation of SIRT1 catalytic activity include elevation of the concentration of its substrate, NAD^+, and removal of its reaction product and inhibitor, nicotinamide. Here we will concentrate on the evidence that a number of plant polyphenols can mimic CR via a third mechanism, namely allosteric activation of sirtuins. Plant polyphenols are abundant in various foodstuffs and are themselves produced by plants responding to a variety of environmental stresses. We will end by discussing the idea that polyphenol sirtuin stimulation in plant consumers may represent the species-to-species transfer of a beneficial stress signal, a hypothesis for which we have coined the term *xenohormesis*.

2. Polyphenolic Sirtuin Activators and Their CR-Mimetic Effects

A screen of various small-molecule libraries for modulators of SIRT1 activity identified two compounds, piceatan-nol, a stilbene, and quercetin, a flavone, as stimulators of SIRT1 deacetylase activity (Howitz *et al.*, 2003). Stilbenes and flavones are polyphenols, as are a variety of related plant secondary metabolites such as chalcones, anthocyanidins, and catechins. Screening of additional plant polyphenols identified 15 more SIRT1 activators, the most potent of which was the stilbene resveratrol. Structural features common to these sirtuin-activating compounds (STACs) include two aromatic rings, at least potentially coplanar and *trans* to one another, and hydroxyl functions in one or both of the *meta* positions of one ring and the *para* position of the other (see Figure 3.5).

Kinetic analysis of the resveratrol effect on SIRT1 revealed that it lowered the K_ms for both NAD^+ and the acetylated peptide substrate, while having little or no effect on V_{max} (Howitz *et al.*, 2003). This result suggests that resveratrol is a K-type allosteric effector of SIRT1 (Monod *et al.*, 1965). Qualitatively similar effects on the K_ms of the yeast sirtuin Hst2 can be achieved by deletion of sequences lying N-terminal (NAD^+ and peptide K_ms) and C-terminal (NAD^+ K_m only) to the core catalytic domain (Zhao *et al.*, 2004). On the basis of

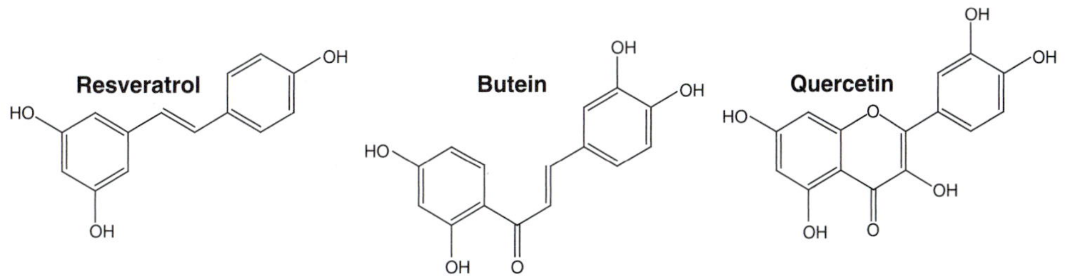

Figure 3.5 Structures of three structurally related polyphenolic sirtuin-activating compounds (STACs): resveratrol (a stilbene in grapes and some Asian herbs), butein (a chalcone in flowers), and quercetin (a flavone in apples and onions). Other STACs include analogs of nicotinamide (NAM) such as isonicotinamide, which activate sirtuins by preventing NAM inhibition. Metabolites of resveratrol, such as sulfated-resveratrol, which can circulate in humans for more than a day, have recently been found to activate sirtuins with the same potency as the native compound. Whether a typical diet can provide sufficient STACs to activate sirtuins in vivo is not yet known, but exogenous addition of resveratrol can extend life span in yeast, worms, and flies—unless they lack the Sir2 gene (Howitz et al., 2003; Wood et al, 2004).

these Hst2 structural and kinetic studies, Zhao and colleagues proposed that a polyphenol-binding-induced reconfiguration of the conserved β1-α2 loop and/or zinc-binding domain could act to enhance sirtuin substrate binding.

Thus far, STACs have been shown to extend life span in *Saccharomyces cerevisiae*, *Drosophila melanogaster*, and *Caenorhabditis elegans* (Howitz *et al.*, 2003; Wood *et al.*, 2004). In each of these model systems, the STACs-induced life span extension required the presence of a functional Sir2/SIRT1 ortholog, and in each case recombinant preparations of these enzymes were activated by STACs *in vitro* (Howitz *et al.*, 2003; Wood *et al.*, 2004). In the two organisms for which this was tested, *Saccharomyces* and *Drosophila*, STACs did not increase the life span extension provided by CR (Howitz *et al.*, 2003; Wood *et al.*, 2004). Clearly this is consistent with the idea that STACs act to extend life span by the same pathway as CR, with direct sirtuin stimulation providing the most straightforward mechanistic explanation.

Resveratrol effects consistent with stimulation of SIRT1 have been observed in several mammalian cell culture systems in which one or more of the relevant SIRT1-targeted acetyl-lysine residues have been identified. Acetylation of lysine 382 increases the activity and stability of p53, and acetyl-lysine-382 is a known target of SIRT1 (Langley, 2002; Luo *et al.*, 2001; Vaziri *et al.*, 2001). Low concentrations of resveratrol (0.5 μM) were shown to diminish the level of UV-induced p53 lysine-382 acetylation in U2OS osteosarcoma cells (Howitz *et al.*, 2003). Parallel experiments with HEK 293 cells showed that this resveratrol-stimulated deacetylation occurred in the presence of transfected wild-type SIRT1, but not in the presence of a dominant-negative, catalytically inactive construct (SIRT1 H363Y) (Howitz *et al.*, 2003).

SIRT1 can reverse the stress-induced acetylation of the DNA repair factor Ku70 at lysines 539 and 542, thereby enhancing Ku70 binding and nuclear sequestration of the pro-apoptotic protein Bax (Cohen *et al.*, 2004b). Resveratrol diminished Bax-induced apoptosis in HEK 293 cells cotransfected with Bax and Ku70, an effect parallel to that obtained by transfection with SIRT1 (Cohen *et al.*, 2004b). Several STACs, including resveratrol, were shown to stimulate sirtuins in HeLa cells (Howitz *et al.*, 2003) and, with the same assay system, resveratrol increased the overall deacetylation rate in a non-small cell lung cancer (NSCLC) line with a high SIRT1 expression level (Yeung *et al.*, 2004). Also in NSCLC cells, SIRT1 downregulates NF-κB-mediated transcription by deacetylation at lysine 310 in the RelA/p65 subunit transactivation domain (Yeung *et al.*, 2004). Resveratrol was shown to decrease the acetylation level of p65 in HEK 293 cells, and the ability of both SIRT1 and resveratrol to repress p65 transactivation in NSCLC cells depended on the presence of lysine 310 (Yeung *et al.*, 2004).

Recently, resveratrol has been shown to enhance SIRT1 action in cellular models of processes of particular relevance to CR effects in mammalian aging: neurodegeneration, fat mobilization, and adipogenesis. Using *in vitro* models of axonal degeneration, Araki and colleagues demonstrated that the mouse *wld^s* mutation delays degeneration by virtue of its overexpression of a fusion protein incorporating the NAD^+-biosynthetic enzyme Nmnat1 (Araki *et al.*, 2004). This delay in degeneration could be mimicked by a 24-hour pretreatment of wild-type neurons with NAD^+, an effect that required SIRT1 expression (Araki *et al.*, 2004). Resveratrol pretreatment afforded protection similar to that obtained with NAD^+, suggesting that both effects were due to stimulation of SIRT1 activity (Araki *et al.*, 2004). Since axonal degeneration is a feature of aging-related neurodegenerative diseases (Raff *et al.*, 2002), these results echo the preventive action of CR on these pathologies.

Sirt1$^{+/-}$ mice display significantly decreased fasting induced mobilization of free fatty acids, an effect that the experiments of Picard and colleagues (2004) have connected to a deficit in SIRT1 repression of the activity of the transcription factor PPARγ in white adipocytes. Resveratrol promoted the mobilization of free fatty acids from primary cultures of rat adipocytes, and the resveratrol-induced fat depletion from 3T3-L1 adipocytes depended on the expression of SIRT1 (Picard *et al.*, 2004). Noting that fat is depleted from white adipose tissue as a consequence of CR, Picard and colleagues suggested that this may be a SIRT1-mediated effect (Picard *et al.*, 2004). Mice that are deficient in PPARγ (PPARγ$^{+/-}$ heterozygotes) have increased insulin sensitivity and experience less aging-related decline in insulin sensitivity than PPARγ$^{+/+}$ mice (Miles *et al.*, 2003). Thus, SIRT1 suppression of PPARγ activity could represent a mechanism that retards the onset of aging-related diseases such as type II diabetes.

C. Is Sirtuin Stimulation by Polyphenols a Case of Xenohormesis?

1. The Roles of Polyphenols in Plant Stress Responses and Stress Signaling

All eukaryotes, including plants, encode sirtuins in their genomes (Frye, 2000; Pandey *et al.*, 2002). The plant polyphe-

nols that activate sirtuins in yeast and animals are produced by plants in response to various types of environmental stress, including drought, nutrient deprivation, and UV-irradiation (Dixon & Paiva, 1995). It therefore seems reasonable to suggest that some plant polyphenols might function as endogenous regulators of plant sirtuins and other stress responses (Howitz *et al.*, 2003). Although plants produce an enormous variety of polyphenols, many of which serve in non-signaling roles (e.g., UV-filters, antioxidants, pigments, antibiotics), it has been argued on evolutionary grounds that the first polyphenols functioned as signaling molecules (Stafford, 1991). Lunularic acid (LA), a stilbenoid, has been proposed to function in "lower" plants (e.g., liverworts) as a stress-response hormone, a role fulfilled by abscisic acid (ABA) in vascular plants (Yoshikawa *et al.*, 2002) (see Figure 3.6). A recent study provided evidence of structural overlap between the stable conformers of ABA and LA and of ABA-like activity by LA in higher plants (Yoshikawa *et al.*, 2002). Noting that synthesis of ABA, unlike that of LA, requires molecular oxygen, Yoshikawa and colleagues propose that LA is the more ancient of the two molecules. In higher plants, there are a few known examples of polyphenols functioning in regulatory roles, for example the flavone-induced pollen germination in petunia (Napoli *et al.*, 1990; Vogt & Taylor, 1995), but in general this is a poorly understood area. The possible existence of endogenous polyphenol regulators of

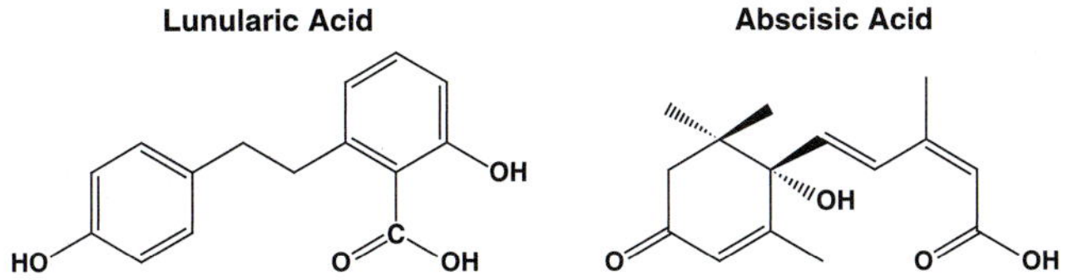

Figure 3.6 Structures of the plant stress hormones, lunularic acid and abscisic acid.

plant sirtuins may provide a fruitful line of inquiry.

2. The Xenohormesis Hypothesis

The question of plant sirtuin regulation aside, why would plant stress molecules, the polyphenol STACs, activate sirtuins from mammals, yeast, nematodes, and insects? One possibility is that the STACs might mimic yet-to-be-discovered endogenous small-molecule regulators in these species. These hypothetical molecules could not be polyphenols, however, because animals lack the enzymes to synthesize them. There are, however, well-known examples of mimicry of chemically unrelated mammalian regulatory molecules by plant secondary metabolites, including the opioids, the cannabinoids, and the weak estrogenic activity of some of the STACs themselves. The notion of mimicry carries with it the implication of survival advantages for the plant. These could range from deterrence of destructive plant consumers to attraction of plant consumers essential for pollination or seed dispersal. However, the fact that plants synthesize and accumulate polyphenol STACs in response to both biotic and abiotic stress suggests to us the possible advantage to plant consuming species of developing or maintaining a capacity to respond to them within the context of their own stress-response pathways.

We propose the term _xenohormesis_ for this concept in order to emphasize that the initial stress and the beneficial response to that stress occur in separate organisms. By serving as early indicators of a deterioration of the food supply and/or the environment in general (e.g., drought), STACs, acting as CR-mimetics, may stimulate plant-consuming organisms to direct resources to cellular and organismal defense and maintenance. The fact, for example, that chronic CR, but not sudden starvation, increases intestinal nutrient transport capacity (Casirola et al., 1996; Ferraris et al., 2001) illustrates how the anticipatory induction of adaptive pathways, by CR-mimetics, could be critical to survival.

Although we have discussed the idea of xenohormesis in the context of sirtuin stimulation, there is no necessity that individual STACs or other plant stress-induced compounds should act only on this target. Rather, the notion is that the overall effect of multiple stress-induced compounds in the diet, perhaps acting on multiple targets and signaling pathways, should strengthen the plant-consuming organism's own stress resistance (Liu, 2003). Indeed, resveratrol effects on numerous targets have been reported (Pervaiz, 2003), including, to name but a few, inhibition of cyclooxygenases (Jang et al., 1997), inhibition of ribonucleotide reductase (Fontecave et al., 1998), and direct chemical scavenging of reactive oxygen species (Frankel et al., 1993). Resveratrol's multiple biological effects—cancer chemoprevention, cardioprotection, and neuroprotection—have been connected, with varying degrees of success, to this plethora of molecular targets (Gescher & Steward, 2003). Due to its capacity to regulate multiple transcription factors, we do feel that polyphenol stimulation of SIRT1 shows great promise as a unifying mechanism behind many of these effects. Xenohormesis, however, as an evolutionary concept, doesn't exclude other possibilities.

The ultimate test of the Xenohormesis Hypothesis is whether it can be shown to actually operate in the realm of nutritional health effects. Epidemiological studies linking consumption of polyphenol-rich foods to the prevention of aging-related diseases (i.e., CR-like health benefits) are consistent with the predictions of STACs-based xenohormesis (Block et al., 1992; Hertog et al., 1993; Keli et al., 1996; Knekt et al., 2002; Sato et al., 2002). However, some studies have raised doubts about whether resveratrol or flavone STACs such as quercetin are sufficiently bioavailable for the effects observed in cell culture to be relevant *in vivo* (Goldberg *et al.*, 2003; Soleas *et al.*, 1997). Plasma concentrations of individual dietary polyphenols rarely rise above the level of 1 to 2 μM, whereas most cell culture effects are observed in the range of 10 to 100 μM (Gescher & Steward, 2003; Goldberg *et al.*, 2003). There are, however, exceptions to this rule (Chang *et al.*, 2000; Basly *et al.*, 2000), and included among these are the sub-micromolar resveratrol effects on SIRT1-dependent p53 deacetylation (Howitz *et al.*, 2003) and Bax-induced apoptosis (Cohen *et al.*, 2004a; Howitz *et al.*, 2003). It also should be noted that because SIRT1 is stimulated by multiple stilbenes, flavones, and chalcones (Howitz *et al.*, 2003), the sum of the plasma concentrations of these effectors may be more relevant than those of individual compounds. One highly valid criticism of mammalian cell culture studies of polyphenol effects is that the vast majority of them have employed the free aglycone forms, rather than the sulfate or glucuronate conjugated metabolites that predominate in the serum *in vivo* (Corder *et al.*, 2003). This concern has recently been somewhat alleviated with respect to resveratrol activation of SIRT1 by the finding that the 3-sulfate and 4'-sulfate forms stimulate SIRT1 *in vitro* to a similar extent as free resveratrol (Calamini *et al.*, 2004). Use of the conjugated forms of resveratrol and other STACs should be given the highest priority in future work on SIRT1 activation and other polyphenol effects.

VI. Conclusions

There have been over a dozen theories to explain the life span–extending effects of DR in mammals and other organisms, but

there is a growing number of scientists who believe we are close to having a grand unifying theory of DR whose basis lies in the idea that DR works by provoking an evolutionarily ancient stress response that keeps organisms alive during adversity. There can be little room for argument that DR meets the narrow, phenomenological definition of hormesis (Masoro, 1998). After all, hormesis, defined simply as an inverted U-shaped dose-response curve, clearly applies to a graph of mortality rate versus dietary restriction, the least being AL and the other extreme being starvation (Turturro *et al.*, 2000).

The broader and more controversial proposition is the one that attributes these hormetic effects to the induction of a single, evolutionarily conserved program, one that activates and coordinates the downstream repair and defense mechanisms that counteract the proximate causes of aging. While the cross-resistances provided by various hormetic stresses are consistent with the existence of such a centralized regulatory mechanism, they don't prove it. However, the Pnc1/Sir2 system, in the case of budding yeast, and the sirtuins together with the insulin/IGF-1/FOXO pathway, in the case of metazoans, appear to have the characteristics one might expect for essential pieces of this regulatory machinery. If this is more than just appearance, biochemical and genetic mapping of the connections between these pathways, upstream hormetic stimuli and downstream gene expression, and anti-aging effects may be key to validating the broader Hormesis Hypothesis of DR.

As noted at the beginning of the chapter, the Hormesis Hypothesis of DR attempts to unite various theories on the proximate causes of aging. In a similar way, the Xenohormesis Hypothesis suggests that many of the health benefits of dietary phytochemicals, particularly those of secondary metabolites produced by plants under stress, may work because they activate an evolutionarily ancient mechanism that allows animals and fungi to pick up on chemical stress signals from plants. As exemplified by the polyphenol STACs, this mechanism is suggested to entail direct stimulation of the hormesis signal transduction machinery, which includes SIRT1 and other proteins that promote health and extend life span. It is important to distinguish this mechanism from actions that directly counteract proximate causes of cellular damage (e.g., chemical antioxidant action) or actions that induce a stress response by actually causing minor damage (conventional hormesis).

While the Hormesis Hypothesis of DR may be young, the Xenohormesis Hypothesis is positively embryonic. The ability to confirm or reject it will depend on identification of the components of hormetic signaling pathways and subsequent assessment of the effects of putative xenohormetic agents on those components. It may also be worthwhile, however, to take the reverse approach to this process and investigate proteins already known to interact with phytochemicals for a possible role in DR physiology. Investigation of the effects of DR on polyphenol-interacting proteins in mammals might provide a line of inquiry into DR signaling that is distinct from, yet complementary to, those currently investigated.

References

Aidoo, A., Desai, V. G., Lyn-Cook, L. E., Chen, J. J., Feuers, R. J., & Casciano, D. A. (1999). Attenuation of bleomycin-induced Hprt mutant frequency in female and male rats by calorie restriction. *Mutation Research*, 430(1), 155–163.

Anderson, R. M., Bitterman, K. J., Wood, J. G., Medvedik, O., & Sinclair, D. A. (2003). Nicotinamide and Pnc1 govern lifespan extension by calorie restriction in S. cerevisiae. *Nature*, 423(6936), 181–185.

Ando, K., Higami, Y., Tsuchiya, T., Kanematsu, T., & Shimokawa, I. (2002). Impact of aging and life-long calorie restriction on expression of apoptosis-related genes in male F344 rat liver. *Microscopy Research and Technique*, 59(4), 293–300.

Antebi, A. (2004). Tipping the balance toward longevity. *Developmental Cell*, 6(3), 315–316.

Araki, T., Sasaki, Y., & Milbrandt, J. (2004). Increased nuclear NAD biosynthesis and SIRT1 activation prevent axonal degeneration. *Science*, 305(5686), 1010–1013.

Arking, R., Buck, S., Berrios, A., Dwyer, S., & Baker, G. T. 3rd (1991). Elevated paraquat resistance can be used as a bioassay for longevity in a genetically based long-lived strain of *Drosophila*. *Developmental Genetics*, 12(5), 362–370.

Armeni, T., Principato, G., Quiles, J. L., Pieri, C., Bompadre, S., & Battino, M. (2003). Mitochondrial dysfunctions during aging: vitamin E deficiency or caloric restriction—two different ways of modulating stress. *Journal of Bioenergetics & Biomembranes*, 35(2), 181–191.

Austad, S. N. (2001). Does caloric restriction in the laboratory simply prevent overfeeding and return house mice to their natural level of food intake? *Science of Aging Knowledge Environment*, 2001(6), pe3.

Avula, C. P., & Fernandes, G. (2002). Inhibition of H2O2-induced apoptosis of lymphocytes by calorie restriction during aging. *Microscopy Research and Technique*, 59(4), 282–292.

Ball, Z. B., Barnes, R. H., & Visscher, M. B. (1947). The effects of dietary caloric restriction on maturity and senescence, with particular reference to fertility and longevity. *American. Journal of Physiology*, 150, 511–520.

Barja, G. (2004). Aging in vertebrates, and the effect of caloric restriction: a mitochondrial free radical production-DNA damage mechanism? *Biological Reviews of the Cambridge Philosophical Society*, 79(2), 235–251.

Bartke, A. (2000). Delayed aging in Ames dwarf mice. Relationships to endocrine function and body size. *Results and Problems in Cell Differentiation*, 29, 181–202.

Bartke, A., Wright, J. C., Mattison, J. A., Ingram, D. K., Miller, R. A., & Roth, G. S. (2001). Extending the lifespan of long-lived mice. *Nature*, 414(6862), 412.

Barton, A. (1950). Some aspects of cell division in *Saccharomyces cerevisiae. Journal of General Microbiology,* 4, 84–86.

Barzilai, N., & Gabriely, I. (2001). The role of fat depletion in the biological benefits of caloric restriction. *Journal of Nutrition,* 131(3), 903S–906S.

Barzilai, N., & Gupta, G. (1999). Revisiting the role of fat mass in the life extension induced by caloric restriction. *Journal of Gerontology Series A Biological Sciences & Medical Sciences,* 54(3), B89–B98.

Basly, J. P., Marre-Fournier, F., Le Bail, J. C., Habrioux, G., Chulia, A. J. (2000). Estrogenic/antiestrogenic and scavenging properties of (E)– and (Z)–resveratrol. *Life Science,* 66(9), 769–77.

Berg, B. N., & Simms, H. S. (1960). Nutrition and longevity in the rat. II. Longevity and onset of disease with different levels of food intake. *Journal of Nutrition,* 71, 255–263.

Bertrand, H. A., Lynd, F. T., Masoro, E. J., & Yu, B. P. (1980). Changes in adipose mass and cellularity through the adult life of rats fed ad libitum or a life-prolonging restricted diet. *Journal of Gerontology,* 35(6), 827–835.

Bitterman, K. J., Anderson, R. M., Cohen, H. Y., Latorre-Esteves, M., & Sinclair, D. A. (2002). Inhibition of silencing and accelerated aging by nicotinamide, a putative negative regulator of yeast sir2 and human SIRT1. *Journal of Biological Chemistry,* 277(47), 45099–45107.

Bitterman, K. J., Medvedik, O., & Sinclair, D. A. (2003). Longevity regulation in *Saccharomyces cerevisiae*: linking metabolism, genome stability, and heterochromatin. *Microbiology and Molecular Biology Reviews,* 67(3), 376–399.

Block, G., Patterson, B., & Subar, A. (1992). Fruit, vegetables, and cancer prevention: a review of the epidemiological evidence. *Nutrition and Cancer,* 18(1), 1–29.

Bluher, M., Kahn, B. B., & Kahn, C. R. (2003). Extended longevity in mice lacking the insulin receptor in adipose tissue. *Science,* 299(5606), 572–574.

Braeckman, B. P., Houthoofd, K., & Vanfleteren, J. R. (2001a). Insulin-like signaling, metabolism, stress resistance and aging in *Caenorhabditis elegans. Mechanisms of Ageing & Development,* 122(7), 673–693.

Braeckman, B. P., Houthoofd, K., & Vanfleteren, J. R. (2001b). Insulin-like signaling, metabolism, stress resistance and aging in *Caenorhabditis elegans. Mechanisms of Ageing & Development,* 122(7), 673–693.

Braeckman, B. P., Houthoofd, K., & Vanfleteren, J. R. (2002). Assessing metabolic activity in aging *Caenorhabditis elegans*: concepts and controversies. *Aging Cell,* 1(2), 82–88; discussion 102–3.

Bras, G., & Ross, M. H. (1964). Kidney disease and nutrition in the rat. *Toxicology & Applied Pharmacology,* 61, 247–262.

Brunet, A., Sweeney, L. B., Sturgill, J. F., Chua, K. F., Greer, P. L., Lin, Y., Tran, H., Ross, S. E., Mostoslavsky, R., Cohen, H. Y., Hu, L. S., Cheng, H. L., Jedrychowski, M. P., Gygi, S. P., Sinclair, D. A., Alt, F. W., & Greenberg, M. E. (2004). Stress-dependent regulation of FOXO transcription factors by the SIRT1 deacetylase. *Science,* 303(5666), 2011–2015.

Cabelof, D. C., Yanamadala, S., Raffoul, J. J., Guo, Z., Soofi, A., & Heydari, A. R. (2003). Caloric restriction promotes genomic stability by induction of base excision repair and reversal of its age-related decline. *DNA Repair (Amsterdam),* 2(3), 295–307.

Calamini, B., Santarsiero, B., Ratia, K., Eggler, A., Malkowski, M., Pezzuto, J. M., & Mesecar, A. (2004). The role of resveratrol and its metabolites in longevity and cancer chemoprevention. *Abstract, 42nd Annual Medicinal Chemistry Meeting in Miniature.*

Calingasan, N. Y., & Gibson, G. E. (2000). Dietary restriction attenuates the neuronal loss, induction of heme oxygenase-1 and blood-brain barrier breakdown induced by impaired oxidative metabolism. *Brain Research,* 885(1), 62–69.

Cao, S. X., Dhahbi, J. M., Mote, P. L., & Spindler, S. R. (2001). Genomic profiling of short- and long-term caloric restriction effects in the liver of aging mice. *Proceedings of the National Academy of Sciences of the USA,* 98(19), 10630–10635.

Carey, J. R., Liedo, P., Muller, H. G., Wang, J. L., Zhang, Y., & Harshman, L. (2005). Stochastic dietary restriction using a Markov-chain feeding protocol elicits complex, life history response in medflies. *Aging Cell,* 4(1), 31–39.

Carlson, A. J., & Hoetzel, F. (1946). Apparent prolongation of the life-span of rats by intermittent fasting. *Journal of Nutrition*, 31, 363–342.

Cartee, G. D., Kietzke, E. W., & Briggs-Tung, C. (1994). Adaptation of muscle glucose transport with caloric restriction in adult, middle-aged, and old rats. *American Journal of Physiology*, 266(5 Pt 2), R1443–R1447.

Casirola, D. M., Rifkin, B., Tsai, W., & Ferraris, R. P. (1996). Adaptations of intestinal nutrient transport to chronic caloric restriction in mice. *American Journal of Physiology*, 271(1 Pt 1), G192–G200.

Cassano, P., Lezza, A. M., Leeuwenburgh, C., Cantatore, P., & Gadaleta, M. N. (2004). Measurement of the 4,834-bp mitochondrial DNA deletion level in aging rat liver and brain subjected or not to caloric restriction diet. *Annals of the New York Academy of Sciences*, 1019, 269–273.

Charlesworth, B. (2000). Fisher, Medawar, Hamilton and the evolution of aging. *Genetics*, 156(3), 927–931.

Chung, H. Y., Kim, H. J., Kim, K. W., Choi, J. S., & Yu, B. P. (2002). Molecular inflammation hypothesis of aging based on the anti-aging mechanism of calorie restriction. *Microscopy Ressearch & Technique*, 59(4), 264–272.

Chung, H. Y., Kim, H. J., Shim, K. H., & Kim, K. W. (1999). Dietary modulation of prostanoid synthesis in the aging process: role of cyclooxygenase-2. *Mechanisms of Ageing & Development*, 111(2–3), 97–106.

Cohen, H. Y., Lavu, S., Bitterman, K. J., Hekking, B., Imahiyerobo, T. A., Miller, C., Frye, R., Ploegh, H., Kessler, B. M., & Sinclair, D. A. (2004a). Acetylation of the C terminus of Ku70 by CBP and PCAF controls Bax-mediated apoptosis. *Molecular Cell*, 13(5), 627–638.

Cohen, H. Y., Miller, C., Bitterman, K. J., Wall, N. R., Hekking, B., Kessler, B., Howitz, K. T., Gorospe, M., de Cabo, R., & Sinclair, D. A. (2004b). Calorie restriction promotes mammalian cell survival by inducing the SIRT1 deacetylase. *Science*, 305(5682), 390–392.

Cook, C. I., & Yu, B. P. (1998). Iron accumulation in aging: modulation by dietary restriction. *Mechanisms of Ageing & Development*, 102(1), 1–13.

Corder, R., Crozier, A., & Kroon, P. A. (2003). Drinking your health? It's too early to say. *Nature*, 426(6963), 119.

Cutler, R. G. (1982). Longevity is determined by specific genes: testing the hypothesis. In R. C. Adelman & G. S. Roth (Eds.), *Testing the theories of aging* (pp. 24–114). Boca Raton, FL: CRC Press.

D'Costa, A. P., Lenham, J. E., Ingram, R. L., & Sonntag, W. E. (1993). Moderate caloric restriction increases type 1 IGF receptors and protein synthesis in aging rats. *Mechanisms of Ageing & Development*, 71(1–2), 59–71.

da Cunha, G. L., da Cruz, I. B., Fiorino, P., & de Oliveira, A. K. (1995). Paraquat resistance and starvation conditions in the selection of longevity extremes in *Drosophila melanogaster* populations previously selected for long and short developmental period. *Developmental Genetics*, 17(4), 352–361.

Daitoku, H., Hatta, M., Matsuzaki, H., Aratani, S., Ohshima, T., Miyagishi, M., Nakajima, T., & Fukamizu, A. (2004). Silent information regulator 2 potentiates Foxo1-mediated transcription through its deacetylase activity. *Proceedings of the National Academy of Sciences of the USA*, 101(27), 10042–10047.

de Cabo, R., Furer-Galban, S., Anson, R. M., Gilman, C., Gorospe, M., & Lane, M. A. (2003). An in vitro model of caloric restriction. *Experimental Gerontology*, 38(6), 631–639.

Dean, D. J., Brozinick, J. T., Jr., Cushman, S. W., & Cartee, G. D. (1998a). Calorie restriction increases cell surface GLUT-4 in insulin-stimulated skeletal muscle. *American Journal of Physiology*, 275(6 Pt 1), E957–E964.

Dean, D. J., Gazdag, A. C., Wetter, T. J., & Cartee, G. D. (1998b). Comparison of the effects of 20 days and 15 months of calorie restriction on male Fischer 344 rats. *Aging (Milano)*, 10(4), 303–307.

Dehmelt, H. (2004). Re-adaptation hypothesis: explaining health benefits of caloric restriction. *Medical Hypotheses*, 62(4), 620–624.

Del Roso, A., Vittorini, S., Cavallini, G., Donati, A., Gori, Z., Masini, M., Pollera, M., & Bergamini, E. (2003). Ageing-related changes in the in vivo function of rat liver macroautophagy and proteolysis. *Experimental Gerontology*, 38(5), 519–527.

DeLany, J. P., Hansen, B. C., Bodkin, N. L., Hannah, J., & Bray, G. A. (1999). Long-term calorie restriction reduces energy expenditure in aging monkeys. *Journals of Gerontology Series A Biological Sciences & Medical Sciences*, 54(1), B5–B11; discussion B12–B13.

Dempsey, J. L., Pfeiffer, M., & Morley, A. A. (1993). Effect of dietary restriction on in vivo somatic mutation in mice. *Mutation Research*, 291(2), 141–145.

Dhahbi, J. M., Kim, H. J., Mote, P. L., Beaver, R. J., & Spindler, S. R. (2004). Temporal linkage between the phenotypic and genomic responses to caloric restriction. *Proceedings of the National Academy of Sciences of the USA*, 101(15), 5524–5529.

Dixon, R. A., & Paiva, N. L. (1995). Stress-induced phenylpropanoid metabolism. *Plant Cell*, 7(7), 1085–1097.

Droge, W. (2003). Oxidative stress and aging. *Advances in Experimental Medicine & Biology*, 543, 191–200.

Duffy, P. H., Leakey, J. E., Pipkin, J. L., Turturro, A., & Hart, R. W. (1997). The physiologic, neurologic, and behavioral effects of caloric restriction related to aging, disease, and environmental factors. *Environmental Research*, 73(1–2), 242–248.

Duffy, P. H., Seng, J. E., Lewis, S. M., Mayhugh, M. A., Aidoo, A., Hattan, D. G., Casciano, D. A., & Feuers, R. J. (2001). The effects of different levels of dietary restriction on aging and survival in the Sprague-Dawley rat: implications for chronic studies. *Aging (Milano)*, 13(4), 263–272.

Dufour, E., & Larsson, N. G. (2004). Understanding aging: revealing order out of chaos. *Biochimica et Biophysica Acta*, 1658(1–2), 122–132.

Edwards, I. J., Rudel, L. L., Terry, J. G., Kemnitz, J. W., Weindruch, R., & Cefalu, W. T. (1998). Caloric restriction in rhesus monkeys reduces low density lipoprotein interaction with arterial proteoglycans. *Journals of Gerontology Series A Biological Sciences & Medical Sciences*, 53(6), B443–B448.

Fabrizio, P., Pozza, F., Pletcher, S. D., Gendron, C. M., & Longo, V. D. (2001). Regulation of longevity and stress resistance by Sch9 in yeast. *Science*, 292(5515), 288–290.

Ferraris, R. P., Cao, Q. X., & Prabhakaram, S. (2001). Chronic but not acute energy restriction increases intestinal nutrient transport in mice. *Journal of Nutrition*, 131(3), 779–786.

Fontana, L., Meyer, T. E., Klein, S., & Holloszy, J. O. (2004). Long-term calorie restriction is highly effective in reducing the risk for atherosclerosis in humans. *Proceedings of the National Academy of Sciences of the USA*, 101(17), 6659–6663.

Fontecave, M., Lepoivre, M., Elleingand, E., Gerez, C., & Guittet, O. (1998). Resveratrol, a remarkable inhibitor of ribonucleotide reductase. *FEBS Letters*, 421(3), 277–279.

Frankel, E. N., Waterhouse, A. L., & Kinsella, J. E. (1993). Inhibition of human LDL oxidation by resveratrol. *Lancet*, 341(8852), 1103–1104.

Friedman, D. B., & Johnson, T. E. (1988). A mutation in the age-1 gene in Caenorhabditis elegans lengthens life and reduces hermaphrodite fertility. *Genetics*, 118(1), 75–86.

Frye, R. A. (2000). Phylogenetic classification of prokaryotic and eukaryotic Sir2-like proteins. *Biochemical & Biophysical Research Communications*, 273(2), 793–798.

Fukuhara, A., Matsuda, M., Nishizawa, M., Segawa, K., Tanaka, M., Kishimoto, K., Matsuki, Y., Murakami, M., Ichisaka, T., Murakami, H., Watanabe, E., Takagi, T., Akiyoshi, M., Ohtsubo, T., Kihara, S., Yamashita, S., Makishima, M., Funahashi, T., Yamanaka, S., Hiramatsu, R., Matsuzawa, Y., & Shimomura, I. (2004). Visfatin: a protein secreted by visceral fat that mimics the effects of insulin. *Science*, 307(5708), 426–430.

Fulco, M., Schiltz, R. L., Iezzi, S., King, M. T., Zhao, P., Kashiwaya, Y., Hoffman, E., Veech, R. L., & Sartorelli, V. (2003). Sir2 regulates skeletal muscle differentiation as a potential sensor of the redox state. *Molecular Cell*, 12(1), 51–62.

Fulgencio, J. P., Kohl, C., Girard, J., & Pegorier, J. P. (2001). Effect of metformin on fatty acid and glucose metabolism in freshly isolated hepatocytes and on specific gene expression in cultured hepatocytes. *Biochemical Pharmacology*, 62(4), 439–446.

Gallo, C. M., Smith, D. L., Jr., & Smith, J. S. (2004). Nicotinamide clearance by Pnc1 directly regulates Sir2-mediated silencing and longevity. *Molecular & Cellular Biology*, 24(3), 1301–1312.

Gems, D., Pletcher, S., & Partridge, L. (2002). Interpreting interactions between treatments that slow aging. *Aging Cell*, 1(1), 1–9.

Gen Son, T., Zou, Y., Pal Yu, B., Lee, J., & Young Chung, H. (2005). Aging effect on myeloperoxidase in rat kidney and its modulation by calorie restriction. *Free Radicals Research*, 39(3), 283–289.

Gescher, A. J., & Steward, W. P. (2003). Relationship between mechanisms, bioavailibility, and preclinical chemopreventive efficacy of resveratrol: a conundrum. *Cancer Epidemiology, Biomarkers & Prevention*, 12(10), 953–957.

Giannakou, M. E., Goss, M., Junger, M. A., Hafen, E., Leevers, S. J., & Partridge, L. (2004). Long-lived *Drosophila* with overexpressed dFOXO in adult fat body. *Science*, 305(5682), 361.

Goldberg, D. M., Yan, J., & Soleas, G. J. (2003). Absorption of three wine-related polyphenols in three different matrices by healthy subjects. *Clinical Biochemistry*, 36(1), 79–87.

Gong, X., Shang, F., Obin, M., Palmer, H., Scrofano, M. M., Jahngen-Hodge, J., Smith, D. E., & Taylor, A. (1997). Antioxidant enzyme activities in lens, liver and kidney of calorie restricted Emory mice. *Mechanisms of Ageing & Development*, 99(3), 181–192.

Good, T. P., & Tatar, M. (2001). Age-specific mortality and reproduction respond to adult dietary restriction in *Drosophila melanogaster*. *Journal of Insect Physiology*, 47(12), 1467–1473.

Goodrick, C. L., Ingram, D. K., Reynolds, M. A., Freeman, J. R., & Cider, N. (1990). Effects of intermittent feeding upon body weight and lifespan in inbred mice: interaction of genotype and age. *Mechanisms of Ageing & Development*, 55(1), 69–87.

Gredilla, R., Phaneuf, S., Selman, C., Kendaiah, S., Leeuwenburgh, C., & Barja, G. (2004). Short-term caloric restriction and sites of oxygen radical generation in kidney and skeletal muscle mitochondria. *Annals of the New York Academy of Sciences*, 1019, 333–342.

Guo, Z., Heydari, A., & Richardson, A. (1998). Nucleotide excision repair of actively transcribed versus nontranscribed DNA in rat hepatocytes: effect of age and dietary restriction. *Experimental Cell Research*, 245(1), 228–238.

Guo, Z. M., Yang, H., Hamilton, M. L., VanRemmen, H., & Richardson, A. (2001). Effects of age and food restriction on oxidative DNA damage and antioxidant enzyme activities in the mouse aorta. *Mechanisms of Ageing & Development*, 122(15), 1771–1786.

Gupta, G., Cases, J. A., She, L., Ma, X. H., Yang, X. M., Hu, M., Wu, J., Rossetti, L., & Barzilai, N. (2000). Ability of insulin to modulate hepatic glucose production in aging rats is impaired by fat accumulation. *American Journal of Physiology*, 278(6), E985–E991.

Haley-Zitlin, V., & Richardson, A. (1993). Effect of dietary restriction on DNA repair and DNA damage. *Mutation Research*, 295(4–6), 237–245.

Harmon, D. (1956). Aging: a theory based on free radical and radiation chemistry. *Journal of Gerontology*, 11, 298.

Harrison, D. E., Archer, J. R., & Astle, C. M. (1984). Effects of food restriction on aging: separation of food intake and adiposity. *Proceedings of the National Academy of Sciences of the USA*, 81(6), 1835–1838.

Harshman, L. G., Moore, K. M., Sty, M. A., & Magwire, M. M. (1999). Stress resistance and longevity in selected lines of *Drosophila melanogaster*. *Neurobiology of Aging*, 20(5), 521–529.

Hart, R. W., Keenan, K., Turturro, A., Abdo, K. M., Leakey, J., & Lyn-Cook, B. (1995). Caloric restriction and toxicity. *Fundamentals of Applied Toxicology*, 25(2), 184–195.

Hatano, E., Tanaka, A., Kanazawa, A., Tsuyuki, S., Tsunekawa, S., Iwata, S., Takahashi, R., Chance, B., & Yamaoka, Y. (2004). Inhibition of tumor necrosis factor-induced apoptosis in transgenic mouse liver expressing creatine kinase. *Liver International*, 24(4), 384–393.

Hayflick, L. (1994). *How and why we age*. New York: Ballantine.

Hayflick, L. (1999). Aging and the genome. *Science*, 283(5410), 2019.

Helfand, S. L. (2004). personal communication, manuscript in press.

Hercus, M. J., Loeschcke, V., & Rattan, S. I. (2003). Lifespan extension of *Drosophila melanogaster* through hormesis by repeated mild heat stress. *Biogerontology*, 4(3), 149–156.

Hertog, M. G., Feskens, E. J., Hollman, P. C., Katan, M. B., & Kromhout, D. (1993). Dietary antioxidant flavonoids and risk of coronary heart disease: the Zutphen Elderly Study. *Lancet*, 342(8878), 1007–1011.

Heydari, A. R., Wu, B., Takahashi, R., Strong, R., & Richardson, A. (1993). Expression of heat shock protein 70 is altered by age and diet at the level of transcription. *Molecular & Cellular Biology*, 13(5), 2909–2018.

Higami, Y., & Shimokawa, I. (2000). Apoptosis in the aging process. *Cell Tissue Research*, 301(1), 125–132.

Hiona, A., & Leeuwenburgh, C. (2004). Effects of age and caloric restriction on brain neuronal cell death/survival. *Annals of the New York Academy of Sciences*, 1019, 96–105.

Holliday, R. (1989). Food, reproduction and longevity: is the extended lifespan of calorie-restricted animals an evolutionary adaptation? *Bioessays*, 10(4), 125–127.

Holloszy, J. O. (1997). Mortality rate and longevity of food-restricted exercising male rats: a reevaluation. *Journal of Applied Physiology*, 82(2), 399–403.

Holzenberger, M. (2004). The GH/IGF-I axis and longevity. *European Journal of Endocrinology*, 151 Supplement 2, S023–S027.

Houthoofd, K., Braeckman, B. P., Johnson, T. E., & Vanfleteren, J. R. (2003). Life extension via dietary restriction is independent of the Ins/IGF-1 signalling pathway in *Caenorhabditis elegans*. *Experimental Gerontology*, 38(9), 947–954.

Houthoofd, K., Braeckman, B. P., Lenaerts, I., Brys, K., De Vreese, A., Van Eygen, S., & Vanfleteren, J. R. (2002). Axenic growth up-regulates mass-specific metabolic rate, stress resistance, and extends life span in *Caenorhabditis elegans*. *Experimental Gerontology*, 37(12), 1371–1378.

Howitz, K. T., Bitterman, K. J., Cohen, H. Y., Lamming, D. W., Lavu, S., Wood, J. G., Zipkin, R. E., Chung, P., Kisielewski, A., Zhang, L. L., Scherer, B., & Sinclair, D. A. (2003). Small molecule activators of sirtuins extend *Saccharomyces cerevisiae* lifespan. *Nature*, 425(6954), 191–196.

Hulbert, A. J., Clancy, D. J., Mair, W., Braeckman, B. P., Gems, D., & Partridge, L. (2004). Metabolic rate is not reduced by dietary-restriction or by lowered insulin/IGF-1 signalling and is not correlated with individual lifespan in *Drosophila melanogaster*. *Experimental Gerontology*, 39(8), 1137–1143.

Hursting, S. D., Lavigne, J. A., Berrigan, D., Perkins, S. N., & Barrett, J. C. (2003). Calorie restriction, aging, and cancer prevention: mechanisms of action and applicability to humans. *Annual Review of Medicine*, 54, 131–152.

Hwangbo, D. S., Gersham, B., Tu, M. P., Palmer, M., & Tatar, M. (2004). *Drosophila* dFOXO controls lifespan and regulates insulin signalling in brain and fat body. *Nature*, 429(6991), 562–566.

Ikeyama, S., Wang, X. T., Li, J., Podlutsky, A., Martindale, J. L., Kokkonen, G., van Huizen, R., Gorospe, M., & Holbrook, N. J. (2003). Expression of the pro-apoptotic gene gadd153/chop is elevated in liver with aging and sensitizes cells to oxidant injury. *Journal of Biological Chemistry*, 278(19), 16726–16731.

Imai, S., Armstrong, C. M., Kaeberlein, M., & Guarente, L. (2000). Transcriptional silencing and longevity protein Sir2 is an NAD- dependent histone deacetylase. *Nature*, 403(6771), 795–800.

Ingram, D. K., Cutler, R. G., Weindruch, R., Renquist, D. M., Knapka, J. J., April, M., Belcher, C. T., Clark, M. A., Hatcherson, C. D., Marriott, B. M., & Roth, G. S. (1990). Dietary restriction and aging: the initiation of a primate study. *Journal of Gerontology*, 45(5), B148–B163.

Ingram, D. K., Anson, R. M., de Cabo, R., Mamczarz, J., Zhu, M., Mattison, J., Lane, M. A., Roth, G. S. (2004). Development of calorie restriction mimetics as a prolongevity strategy. *Annals of the New York Academy of Sciences*, 1019, 412–23.

Iwasaki, K., Gleiser, C. A., Masoro, E. J., McMahan, C. A., Seo, E. J., & Yu, B. P. (1988). The influence of dietary protein source on longevity and age-related disease processes of Fischer rats. *Journal of Gerontology*, 43(1), B5–B12.

Izmaylov, D. M., & Obukhova, L. K. (1999). Geroprotector effectiveness of melatonin: investigation of lifespan of *Drosophila melanogaster. Mechanisms of Ageing & Development*, 106(3), 233–240.

James, S. J., Muskhelishvili, L., Gaylor, D. W., Turturro, A., & Hart, R. (1998). Upregulation of apoptosis with dietary restriction: implications for carcinogenesis and aging. *Environmental Health Perspectives*, 106 Supplement 1, 307–312.

Jang, M., Cai, L., Udeani, G. O., Slowing, K. V., Thomas, C. F., Beecher, C. W., Fong, H. H., Farnsworth, N. R., Kinghorn, A. D., Mehta, R. G., Moon, R. C., & Pezzuto, J. M. (1997). Cancer chemopreventive activity of resveratrol, a natural product derived from grapes. *Science*, 275(5297), 218–220.

Jazwinski, S. M., Chen, J. B., & Sun, J. (1993). A single gene change can extend yeast life span: the role of Ras in cellular senescence. *Advances in Experimental Medicine & Biology*, 330, 45–53.

Johnson, J. R. (1966). Reproductive capacity and mode of death of yeast cells. *Antonie van Leeuwenhoek*, 32, 94–98.

Johnson, T. E., Lithgow, G. J., & Murakami, S. (1996). Hypothesis: interventions that increase the response to stress offer the potential for effective life prolongation and increased health. *Journals of Gerontology Series A Biological Sciences & Medical Sciences*, 51(6), B392–B395.

Kaeberlein, M., Kirkland, K. T., Fields, S., & Kennedy, B. K. (2004). Sir2-Independent Life Span Extension by Calorie Restriction in Yeast. *PLoS Biology*, 2(9), E296.

Kaeberlein, M., McVey, M., & Guarente, L. (1999). The SIR2/3/4 complex and SIR2 alone promote longevity in *Saccharomyces cerevisiae* by two different mechanisms. *Genes & Development*, 13(19), 2570–2580.

Kalant, N., Stewart, J., & Kaplan, R. (1988). Effect of diet restriction on glucose metabolism and insulin responsiveness in aging rats. *Mechanisms of Ageing & Development*, 46(1–3), 89–104.

Keli, S. O., Hertog, M. G., Feskens, E. J., & Kromhout, D. (1996). Dietary flavonoids, antioxidant vitamins, and incidence of stroke: the Zutphen study. *Archives of Internal Medicine*, 156(6), 637–642.

Kemnitz, J. W., Weindruch, R., Roecker, E. B., Crawford, K., Kaufman, P. L., & Ershler, W. B. (1993). Dietary restriction of adult male rhesus monkeys: design, methodology, and preliminary findings from the first year of study. *Journal of Gerontology*, 48(1), B17–B26.

Kennedy, B. K., Austriaco, N. R., Jr., Zhang, J., & Guarente, L. (1995). Mutation in the silencing gene SIR4 can delay aging in *S. cerevisiae*. *Cell*, 80(3), 485–496.

Kenyon, C. (2001). A conserved regulatory mechanism for aging. *Cell*, 105, 165–168.

Kenyon, C., Chang, J., Gensch, E., Rudner, A., & Tabtiang, R. (1993). A *C. elegans* mutant that lives twice as long as wild type. *Nature*, 366(6454), 461–464.

Khavinson, V. K., Izmaylov, D. M., Obukhova, L. K., & Malinin, V. V. (2000). Effect of epitalon on the lifespan increase in *Drosophila melanogaster. Mechanisms of Ageing & Development*, 120(1–3), 141–149.

Kim, J. W., Zou, Y., Yoon, S., Lee, J. H., Kim, Y. K., Yu, B. P., & Chung, H. Y. (2004). Vascular aging: molecular modulation of the prostanoid cascade by calorie restriction. *Journals of Gerontology Series A Biological Sciences & Medical Sciences*, 59(9), B876–B885.

King, J. T., & Visscher, M. B. (1950). Longevity as a function of diet in the C3H mouse. *Faseb Journal*, 9, 70–74.

Kirkwood, T. B., & Holliday, R. (1979). The evolution of ageing and longevity. *Proceedings of the Royal Society of London Series B Biological Sciences*, 205(1161), 531–546.

Knekt, P., Kumpulainen, J., Jarvinen, R., Rissanen, H., Heliovaara, M., Reunanen, A., Hakulinen, T., & Aromaa, A. (2002). Flavonoid intake and risk of chronic diseases. *American Journal of Clinical Nutrition*, 76(3), 560–568.

Kobayashi, T., Horiuchi, T., Tongaonkar, P., Vu, L., & Nomura, M. (2004). SIR2 regulates recombination between different rDNA repeats, but not recombination within individual rRNA genes in yeast. *Cell*, 117(4), 441–453.

Koizumi, A., Wada, Y., Tuskada, M., Kayo, T., Naruse, M., Horiuchi, K., Mogi, T., Yoshioka, M., Sasaki, M., Miyamaura, Y., Abe, T., Ohtomo, K., & Walford, R.L. (1996). A tumor preventive effect of dietary restriction is antagonized by a high housing temperature through deprivation of torpor. *Mechanisms of Ageing & Development*, 92(1), 67–82.

Koizumi, A., Weindruch, R., & Walford, R. L. (1987). Influences of dietary restriction and age on liver enzyme activities and lipid peroxidation in mice. *Journal of Nutrition*, 117(2), 361–367.

Krystal, B. S., & Yu, B. P. (1994). Aging and its modulation by dietary restriction. In B. P. Yu (Ed.), *Modulation of aging processes by dietary restriction* (pp. 1–36). London: CRC Press.

Lamming, D. W., Wood, J. G., & Sinclair, D. A. (2004). Small molecules that regulate lifespan: evidence for xenohormesis. *Molecular Microbiology*, 53(4), 1003–1009.

Langley, E. P. M., Faretta M., Bauer, U.M., Frye, R.A., Minucci, S., Pelicci, P.G., & Kouzarides, T. (2002). Human SIR2 deacetylates p53 and antagonizes PML/p53-induced cellular senescence. *EMBO Journal*, 21(10), 2383–2396.

Laurenson, P., & Rine, J. (1992). Silencers, silencing, and heritable transcriptional states. *Microbiological Reviews*, 56(4), 543–560.

Lee, S. S., Kennedy, S., Tolonen, A. C., & Ruvkun, G. (2003a). DAF-16 target genes that control *C. elegans* life-span and metabolism. *Science*, 300(5619), 644–647.

Lee, S. S., Lee, R. Y., Fraser, A. G., Kamath, R. S., Ahringer, J., & Ruvkun, G. (2003b). A systematic RNAi screen identifies a critical role for mitochondria in *C. elegans* longevity. *Nature Genetics*, 33(1), 40–48.

Lewis, S. E., Goldspink, D. F., Phillips, J. G., Merry, B. J., & Holehan, A. M. (1985). The effects of aging and chronic dietary restriction on whole body growth and protein turnover in the rat. *Experimental Gerontology*, 20(5), 253–263.

Lin, S. J., Defossez, P. A., & Guarente, L. (2000). Requirement of NAD and SIR2 for life-span extension by calorie restriction in *Saccharomyces cerevisiae*. *Science*, 289(5487), 2126–2128.

Lin, S. J., Ford, E., Haigis, M., Liszt, G., & Guarente, L. (2004). Calorie restriction extends yeast life span by lowering the level of NADH. *Genes & Development*, 18(1), 12–16.

Lindsay, D. G. (1999). Diet and ageing: the possible relation to reactive oxygen species. *Journal of Nutrition & Health: Aging*, 3(2), 84–91.

Lints, F. A., Bullens, P., & Le Bourg, E. (1993). Hypergravity and aging in *Drosophila melanogaster*: 7. New longevity data. *Experimental Gerontology*, 28(6), 611–615.

Lipman, J. M., Turturro, A., & Hart, R. W. (1989). The influence of dietary restriction on DNA repair in rodents: a preliminary study. *Mechanisms of Ageing & Development*, 48(2), 135–143.

Lithgow, G. J. (2001). Hormesis: a new hope for ageing studies or a poor second to genetics? *Human Experimental Toxicology*, 20(6), 301–303; discussion 319–320.

Liu, R. H. (2003). Health benefits of fruit and vegetables are from additive and synergistic combinations of phytochemicals. *American Journal of Clinical Nutrition*, 78(3 Suppl), 517S–520S.

Longo, V. D., & Fabrizio, P. (2002). Regulation of longevity and stress resistance: a molecular strategy conserved from yeast to humans? *Cellular & Molecular Life Sciences*, 59(6), 903–908.

Lopez-Torres, M., Gredilla, R., Sanz, A., & Barja, G. (2002). Influence of aging and long-term caloric restriction on oxygen radical generation and oxidative DNA damage in rat liver mitochondria. *Free Radicals in Biology & Medicine*, 32(9), 882–889.

Luhtala, T. A., Roecker, E. B., Pugh, T., Feuers, R. J., & Weindruch, R. (1994). Dietary restriction attenuates age-related increases in rat skeletal muscle antioxidant enzyme activities. *Journal of Gerontology*, 49(5), B231–B238.

Luo, J., Nikolaev, A. Y., Imai, S., Chen, D., Su, F., Shiloh, A., Guarente, L., & Gu, W. (2001). Negative control of p53 by Sir2alpha promotes cell survival under stress. *Cell*, 107(2), 137–148.

Masoro, E. J. (1985). Nutrition and aging: a current assessment. *Journal of Nutrition*, 115(7), 842–848.

Masoro, E. J. (1995). Antiaging action of caloric restriction: endocrine and metabolic aspects. *Obesity Research*, 3 Suppl 2, 241s–247s.

Masoro, E. J. (1998). Influence of caloric intake on aging and on the response to stressors. *Journal of Toxicology & Environmental Health Part B Critical Reviews*, 1(3), 243–257.

Masoro, E. J. (2000). Caloric restriction and aging: an update. *Experimental Gerontology*, 35(3), 299–305.

Masoro, E. J. (2001). Dietary restriction: an experimental approach to the study of the biology of aging. In E. J. Masoro & S. N. Austad (Eds.), *Handbook of the biology of aging* (5th ed., pp. 396–420). New York: Academic Press.

Masoro, E. J., & Austad, S. N. (1996). The evolution of the antiaging action of dietary restriction: a hypothesis. *Journal of Gerontology Series A Biological Sciences & Medical Sciences*, 51(6), B387–B391.

Masoro, E.J., McCarter, R. J., Katz, M. S., & McMahan, C. A. (1992). Dietary restriction alters characteristics of glucose fuel use. *Journal of Gerontology*, 47(6), B202–B208.

Masoro, E. J., Yu, B. P., & Bertrand, H. A. (1982). Action of food restriction in delaying the aging process. *Proceedings of the National Academy of Sciences of the USA*, 79(13), 4239–4241.

Mattson, M. P., Chan, S. L., & Duan, W. (2002a). Modification of brain aging and neurodegenerative disorders by genes, diet, and behavior. *Physiological Reviews*, 82(3), 637–672.

Mattson, M. P., Duan, W., Chan, S. L., Cheng, A., Haughey, N., Gary, D. S., Guo, Z., Lee, J., & Furukawa, K. (2002b). Neuroprotective and neurorestorative signal transduction mechanisms in brain aging: modification by genes, diet and behavior. *Neurobiology of Aging*, 23(5), 695–705.

McCarter, R. J., & Palmer, J. (1992). Energy metabolism and aging: a lifelong study of Fischer 344 rats. *American Journal of Physiology*, 263(3 Pt 1), E448–E452.

McCarter, R., Masoro, E. J., & Yu, B. P. (1985). Does food restriction retard aging by reducing the metabolic rate? *American Journal of Physiology*, 248(4 Pt 1), E488–E490.

McCarter, R. J., Shimokawa, I., Ikeno, Y., Higami, Y., Hubbard, G. B., Yu, B. P., & McMahan, C. A. (1997). Physical activity as a factor in the action of dietary restriction on aging: effects in Fischer 344 rats. *Aging (Milano)*, 9(1–2), 73–9.

McCay, C. M. (1934). Cellulose in the diet of mice and rats. *Journal of Nutrition*, 8, 435–447.

McCay, C. M., Crowell, M. F., & Maynard, L. A. (1935). The effect of retarded growth upon the life-span and upon the ultimate body size. *Journal of Nutrition*, 10, 63.

McKiernan, S. H., Bua, E., McGorray, J., & Aiken, J. (2004). Early-onset calorie restriction conserves fiber number in aging rat skeletal muscle. *Faseb Journal*, 18(3), 580–581.

Medawar, P. B. (1946). Old age and natural death. *Modern Quarterly*, 1, 30–56.

Merry, B. J. (2002). Molecular mechanisms linking calorie restriction and longevity. *International Journal of Biochemistry & Cell Biology*, 34(11), 1340–1354.

Michalski, A. I., Johnson, T. E., Cypser, J. R., & Yashin, A. I. (2001). Heating stress patterns in *Caenorhabditis elegans* longevity and survivorship. *Biogerontology*, 2(1), 35–44.

Migliaccio, E., Giorgio, M., Mele, S., Pelicci, G., Reboldi, P., Pandolfi, P. P., Lanfrancone, L., & Pelicci, P. G. (1999). The p66shc adaptor protein controls oxidative stress response and life span in mammals. *Nature*, 402(6759), 309–313.

Miles, P. D., Barak, Y., Evans, R. M., & Olefsky, J. M. (2003). Effect of heterozygous PPARgamma deficiency and TZD treatment on insulin resistance associated with age and high-fat feeding. *American Journal of Physiology*, 284(3), E618–E626.

Minois, N., Guinaudy, M. J., Payre, F., & Le Bourg, E. (1999). HSP70 induction may explain the long-lasting resistance to heat of *Drosophila melanogaster* having lived in hypergravity. *Mechanisms of Ageing & Development*, 109(1), 65–77.

Miwa, S., Riyahi, K., Partridge, L., & Brand, M. D. (2004). Lack of correlation between mitochondrial reactive oxygen species production and life span in *Drosophila*. *Annals of the New York Academy of Sciences*, 1019, 388–391.

Mockett, R. J., Orr, W. C., Rahmandar, J. J., Sohal, B. H., & Sohal, R. S. (2001).

Antioxidant status and stress resistance in long- and short-lived lines of *Drosophila melanogaster*. *Experimental Gerontology*, 36(3), 441–463.

Monod, J., Wyman, J., & Changeux, J.-P. (1965). On the nature of allosteric transitions. *Journal of Molecular Biology*, 12, 88–118.

Monti, B., & Contestabile, A. (2003). Selective alteration of DNA fragmentation and caspase activity in the spinal cord of aged rats and effect of dietary restriction. *Brain Research*, 992(1), 137–141.

Moore, W. A., Davey, V. A., Weindruch, R., Walford, R., & Ivy, G. O. (1995). The effect of caloric restriction on lipofuscin accumulation in mouse brain with age. *Gerontology*, 41 Suppl 2, 173–185.

Mote, P. L., Grizzle, J. M., Walford, R. L., & Spindler, S. R. (1991). Influence of age and caloric restriction on expression of hepatic genes for xenobiotic and oxygen metabolizing enzymes in the mouse. *Journal of Gerontology*, 46(3), B95–B100.

Motta, M. C., Divecha, N., Lemieux, M., Kamel, C., Chen, D., Gu, W., Bultsma, Y., McBurney, M., & Guarente, L. (2004). Mammalian SIRT1 represses forkhead transcription factors. *Cell*, 116(4), 551–563.

Mukherjee, P., Abate, L. E., & Seyfried, T. N. (2004). Antiangiogenic and proapoptotic effects of dietary restriction on experimental mouse and human brain tumors. *Clinical Cancer Research*, 10(16), 5622–5629.

Murakami, S., Salmon, A., & Miller, R. A. (2003). Multiplex stress resistance in cells from long-lived dwarf mice. *Faseb Journal*, 17(11), 1565–1566.

Murphy, C. T., McCarroll, S. A., Bargmann, C. I., Fraser, A., Kamath, R. S., Ahringer, J., Li, H., & Kenyon, C. (2003). Genes that act downstream of DAF-16 to influence the lifespan of *Caenorhabditis elegans*. *Nature*, 424(6946), 277–283.

Napoli, C., Lemieux, C., & Jorgensen, R. (1990). Introduction of a chimeric chalcone synthase gene into petunia results in reversible co-suppression of homologous genes in trans. *Plant Cell*, 2(4), 279–289.

Nelson, W., & Halberg, F. (1986). Meal-timing, circadian rhythms and life span of mice. *Journal of Nutrition*, 116(11), 2244–2253.

Orentreich, N., Matias, J. R., DeFelice, A., & Zimmerman, J. A. (1993). Low methionine ingestion by rats extends life span. *Journal of Nutrition*, 123(2), 269–274.

Osborne, T. B., & Mendel, L. B. (1917). The effect of retardation of growth upon the breeding period and duration of life of rats. *Science*, 45, 294–295.

Pahlavani, M. A. (2004). Influence of caloric restriction on aging immune system. *Journal of Nutrition, Health & Aging*, 8(1), 38–47.

Pahlavani, M. A., Harris, M. D., Moore, S. A., Weindruch, R., & Richardson, A. (1995). The expression of heat shock protein 70 decreases with age in lymphocytes from rats and rhesus monkeys. *Experimental Cell Research*, 218(1), 310–318.

Pandey, R., Muller, A., Napoli, C. A., Selinger, D. A., Pikaard, C. S., Richards, E. J., Bender, J., Mount, D. W., & Jorgensen, R. A. (2002). Analysis of histone acetyltransferase and histone deacetylase families of Arabidopsis thaliana suggests functional diversification of chromatin modification among multicellular eukaryotes. *Nucleic Acids Research*, 30(23), 5036–5055.

Parkes, T. L., Elia, A. J., Dickinson, D., Hilliker, A. J., Phillips, J. P., & Boulianne, G. L. (1998). Extension of *Drosophila* lifespan by overexpression of human SOD1 in motorneurons. *Nature Genetics*, 19(2), 171–174.

Pearl, R. (1928). *The rate of living*. New York: Alfred Knopf.

Pervaiz, S. (2003). Resveratrol: from grapevines to mammalian biology. *Faseb Journal*, 17(14), 1975–1985.

Picard, F., Kurtev, M., Chung, N., Topark-Ngarm, A., Senawong, T., Machado De Oliveira, R., Leid, M., McBurney, M. W., & Guarente, L. (2004). Sirt1 promotes fat mobilization in white adipocytes by repressing PPAR-gamma. *Nature*, 429(6993), 771–776.

Prapurna, D. R., & Rao, K. S. (1996). Long-term effects of caloric restriction initiated at different ages on DNA polymerases in rat brain. *Mechanisms of Ageing & Development*, 92(2–3), 133–142.

Prolla, T. A. (2002). DNA microarray analysis of the aging brain. *Chemical Senses*, 27(3), 299–306.

Pugh, T. D., Klopp, R. G., & Weindruch, R. (1999). Controlling caloric consumption: protocols for rodents and rhesus monkeys. *Neurobiology of Aging*, 20(2), 157–165.

Puigserver, P., & Speigelman, B. (2004). Personal communication.

Raff, M. C., Whitmore, A. V., & Finn, J. T. (2002). Axonal self-destruction and neurodegeneration. *Science*, 296(5569), 868–871.

Raffoul, J. J., Guo, Z., Soofi, A., & Heydari, A. R. (1999). Caloric restriction and genomic stability. *Journal of Nutrition, Health, & Aging*, 3(2), 102–110.

Rao, G., Xia, E., Nadakavukaren, M. J., & Richardson, A. (1990). Effect of dietary restriction on the age-dependent changes in the expression of antioxidant enzymes in rat liver. *Journal of Nutrition*, 120(6), 602–609.

Rattan, S. I. (2004). Hormetic mechanisms of anti-aging and rejuvenating effects of repeated mild heat stress on human fibroblasts in vitro. *Rejuvenation Research*, 7(1), 40–48.

Ravagnan, L., Gurbuxani, S., Susin, S. A., Maisse, C., Daugas, E., Zamzami, N., Mak, T., Jaattela, M., Penninger, J. M., Garrido, C., & Kroemer, G. (2001). Heat-shock protein 70 antagonizes apoptosis-inducing factor. *Nature Cell Biology*, 3(9), 839–843.

Reveillaud, I., Kongpachith, A., Park, R., & Fleming, J. E. (1992). Stress resistance of *Drosophila* transgenic for bovine CuZn superoxide dismutase. *Free Radical Research Communications*, 17(1), 73–85.

Revollo, J. R., Grimm, A. A., & Imai, S. (2004). The NAD biosynthesis pathway mediated by nicotinamide phosphoribosyltransferase regulates Sir2 activity in mammalian cells. *Journal of Biological Chemistry*, 279(49), 50754–50763.

Reznick, D. N., Bryant, M. J., Roff, D., Ghalambor, C. K., & Ghalambor, D. E. (2004). Effect of extrinsic mortality on the evolution of senescence in guppies. *Nature*, 431(7012), 1095–1099.

Richie, J. P. Jr., Komninou, D., Leutzinger, Y., Kleinman, W., Orentreich, N., Malloy, V., & Zimmerman, J. A. (2004). Tissue glutathione and cysteine levels in methionine-restricted rats. *Nutrition*, 20(9), 800–805.

Richie, J. P. Jr., Leutzinger, Y., Parthasarathy, S., Malloy, V., Orentreich, N., & Zimmerman, J. A. (1994). Methionine restriction increases blood glutathione and longevity in F344 rats. *Faseb Journal*, 8(15), 1302–1307.

Roberts, S. B., Pi-Sunyer, X., Kuller, L., Lane, M. A., Ellison, P., Prior, J. C., & Shapses, S. (2001). Physiologic effects of lowering caloric intake in nonhuman primates and nonobese humans. *Journals of Gerontology Series A Biological Sciences & Medical Sciences*, 56 Spec No 1, 66–75.

Robertson, T. B., & Ray, L. A. (1920). On the growth of relatively long-lived compared with that of relatively short lived animals. *Journal of Biological Chemistry*, 42, 71–107.

Rojas, C., Cadenas, S., Perez-Campo, R., Lopez-Torres, M., Pamplona, R., Prat, J., & Barja, G. (1993). Relationship between lipid peroxidation, fatty acid composition, and ascorbic acid in the liver during carbohydrate and caloric restriction in mice. *Archives of Biochemistry & Biophysics*, 306(1), 59–64.

Rongvaux, A., Shea, R. J., Mulks, M. H., Gigot, D., Urbain, J., Leo, O., & Andris, F. (2002). Pre-B-cell colony-enhancing factor, whose expression is up-regulated in activated lymphocytes, is a nicotinamide phosphoribosyltransferase, a cytosolic enzyme involved in NAD biosynthesis. *European Journal of Immunology*, 32(11), 3225–3234.

Ross, M. H. (1972). Length of life and caloric intake. *American Journal of Clinical Nutrition*, 25(8), 834–838.

Roth, G. S., Ingram, D. K., & Lane, M. A. (2001). Caloric restriction in primates and relevance to humans. *Annals of the New York Academy of Sciences*, 928, 305–315.

Rubner, M. (1908). Das problem der Lebensdauer und seine Beziehungen zum Wachstum under Ehrnarung. *Munich: Oldenburg*, 150–204.

Sabatino, F., Masoro, E. J., McMahan, C. A., & Kuhn, R. W. (1991). Assessment of the role of the glucocorticoid system in aging processes and in the action of food restriction. *Journal of Gerontology*, 46(5), B171–B179.

Sato, M., Maulik, N., & Das, D. K. (2002). Cardioprotection with alcohol: role of both alcohol and polyphenolic antioxidants. *Annals of the New York Academy of Sciences*, 957, 122–135.

Selman, C., Gredilla, R., Phaneuf, S., Kendaiah, S., Barja, G., & Leeuwenburgh, C. (2003). Short-term caloric restriction and regulatory proteins of apoptosis in heart, skeletal muscle and kidney of Fischer 344 rats. *Biogerontology*, 4(3), 141–147.

Seres, J., Stancikova, M., Svik, K., Krsova, D., & Jurcovicova, J. (2002). Effects of chronic food restriction stress and chronic psychological stress on the development of adjuvant arthritis in male long evans rats. *Annals of the New York Academy of Sciences*, 966, 315–319.

Shaddock, J. G., Feuers, R. J., Chou, M. W., Swenson, D. H., & Casciano, D. A. (1995). Genotoxicity of tacrine in primary hepatocytes isolated from B6C3F1 mice and aged ad libitum and calorie restricted Fischer 344 rats. *Mutation Research*, 344(1–2), 79–88.

Shelke, R. R., & Leeuwenburgh, C. (2003). Lifelong caloric restriction increases expression of apoptosis repressor with a caspase recruitment domain (ARC) in the brain. *Faseb Journal*, 17(3), 494–496.

Sinclair, D. A. (2002). Longevity Genes. In R. Abruzzi (Ed.), *The encyclopedia of aging*, Macmillan reference, USA.

Sinclair, D. A., & Guarente, L. (1997). Extrachromosomal rDNA circles—a cause of aging in yeast. *Cell*, 91(7), 1033–1042.

Sinclair, D. A., & Wood, J. G. (2004). Unpublished result.

Smith, J. S., Brachmann, C. B., Celic, I., Kenna, M. A., Muhammad, S., Starai, V. J., Avalos, J. L., Escalante-Semerena, J. C., Grubmeyer, C., Wolberger, C., & Boeke, J. D. (2000). A phylogenetically conserved NAD+-dependent protein deacetylase activity in the Sir2 protein family. *Proceedings of the National Academy of Sciences of the USA*, 97(12), 6658–6663.

Sohal, R. S., Agarwal, S., Candas, M., Forster, M. J., & Lal, H. (1994a). Effect of age and caloric restriction on DNA oxidative damage in different tissues of C57BL/6 mice. *Mechanisms of Ageing & Development*, 76(2–3), 215–224.

Sohal, R. S., Ku, H. H., Agarwal, S., Forster, M. J., & Lal, H. (1994b). Oxidative damage, mitochondrial oxidant generation and antioxidant defenses during aging and in response to food restriction in the mouse. *Mechanisms of Ageing & Development*, 74(1–2), 121–133.

Soleas, G. J., Diamandis, E. P., & Goldberg, D. M. (1997). Resveratrol: a molecule whose time has come? And gone? *Clinical Biochemistry*, 30(2), 91–113.

Sorensen, J. G., & Loeschcke, V. (2001). Larval crowding in *Drosophila melanogaster* induces Hsp70 expression, and leads to increased adult longevity and adult thermal stress resistance. *Journal of Insect Physiology*, 47(11), 1301–1307.

Southam, C. M., & Ehrlich, J. (1943). Effects of extract of western red-cedar heartwood on certain wood decaying fungi in culture. *Phytopathology*, 33, 517–524.

Spaulding, C. C., Walford, R. L., & Effros, R. B. (1997). Calorie restriction inhibits the age-related dysregulation of the cytokines TNF-alpha and IL-6 in C3B10RF1 mice. *Mechanisms of Ageing & Development*, 93(1–3), 87–94.

Speakman, J. R., Talbot, D. A., Selman, C., Snart, S., McLaren, J. S., Redman, P., Krol, E., Jackson, D. M., Johnson, M. S., & Brand, M. D. (2004). Uncoupled and surviving: individual mice with high metabolism have greater mitochondrial uncoupling and live longer. *Aging Cell*, 3(3), 87–95.

Speakman, J. R., van Acker, A., & Harper, E. J. (2003). Age-related changes in the metabolism and body composition of three dog breeds and their relationship to life expectancy. *Aging Cell*, 2(5), 265–275.

Spencer, C. C., Howell, C. E., Wright, A. R., & Promislow, D. E. (2003). Testing an 'aging gene' in long-lived *Drosophila* strains: increased longevity depends on sex and genetic background. *Aging Cell*, 2(2), 123–130.

Spindler, S. R., Dhahbi, J. M., Mote, P. L., Kim, H. J., & Tshuchiya, T. (2003). Rapid identification of candidate CR mimetics using microarrays. *Biogerontology*, 4(Supplement 1), 89.

Sreekumar, R., Unnikrishnan, J., Fu, A., Nygren, J., Short, K. R., Schimke, J., Barazzoni, R., & Nair, K. S. (2002). Effects of caloric restriction on mitochondrial function and gene transcripts in rat muscle. *American Journal of Physiology*, 283(1), E38–E43.

Stadtman, E. R. (1995). Role of oxidized amino acids in protein breakdown and stability. *Methods in Enzymology*, 258, 379–393.

Stafford, H. A. (1991). Flavonoid evolution: an enzymic approach. *Plant Physiology*, 96, 680–685.

Strahl, B. D., & Allis, C. D. (2000). The language of covalent histone modifications. *Nature*, 403(6765), 41–45.

Stuart, J. A., Karahalil, B., Hogue, B. A., Souza-Pinto, N. C., & Bohr, V. A. (2004). Mitochondrial and nuclear DNA base excision repair are affected differently by caloric restriction. *Faseb Journal*, 18(3), 595–597.

Sun, D., Muthukumar, A. R., Lawrence, R. A., & Fernandes, G. (2001). Effects of calorie restriction on polymicrobial peritonitis induced by cecum ligation and puncture in young C57BL/6 mice. *Clinical and Diagnostic Laboratory Immunology*, 8(5), 1003–1011.

Tanaka, K., Higami, Y., Tsuchiya, T., Shiokawa, D., Tanuma, S., Ayabe, H., & Shimokawa, I. (2004). Aging increases DNase gamma, an apoptosis-related endonuclease, in rat liver nuclei: effect of dietary restriction. *Experimental Gerontology*, 39(2), 195–202.

Tanner, K. G., Landry, J., Sternglanz, R., & Denu, J. M. (2000). Silent information regulator 2 family of NAD- dependent histone/protein deacetylases generates a unique product, 1-O-acetyl-ADP-ribose. *Proceedings of the National Academy of Sciences of the USA*, 97(26), 14178–14182.

Tanny, J. C., & Moazed, D. (2001). Coupling of histone deacetylation to NAD breakdown by the yeast silencing protein Sir2: Evidence for acetyl transfer from substrate to an NAD breakdown product. *Proceedings of the National Academy of Sciences of the USA*, 98(2), 415–420.

Tatar, M., Bartke, A., & Antebi, A. (2003). The endocrine regulation of aging by insulin-like signals. *Science*, 299(5611), 1346–1351.

Tavernarakis, N., & Driscoll, M. (2002). Caloric restriction and lifespan: a role for protein turnover? *Mechanisms of Ageing & Development*, 123(2–3), 215–229.

Tissenbaum, H. A., & Guarente, L. (2001). Increased dosage of a sir-2 gene extends lifespan in Caenorhabditis elegans. *Nature*, 410(6825), 227–230.

Trifunovic, A., Wredenberg, A., Falkenberg, M., Spelbrink, J. N., Rovio, A. T., Bruder, C. E., Bohlooly, Y. M., Gidlof, S., Oldfors, A., Wibom, R., Tornell, J., Jacobs, H. T., & Larsson, N. G. (2004). Premature ageing in mice expressing defective mitochondrial DNA polymerase. *Nature*, 429(6990), 417–423.

Tsuchiya, T., Dhahbi, J. M., Cui, X., Mote, P. L., Bartke, A., & Spindler, S. R. (2004). Additive regulation of hepatic gene expression by dwarfism and caloric restriction. *Physiological Genomics*, 17(3), 307–315.

Turturro, A., Hass, B., & Hart, R. W. (1998). Hormesis—implications for risk assessment caloric intake (body weight) as an exemplar. *Human Experimental Toxicology*, 17(8), 454–459.

Turturro, A., Hass, B. S., & Hart, R. W. (2000). Does caloric restriction induce hormesis? *Human Experimental Toxicology*, 19(6), 320–329.

Turturro, A., Witt, W. W., Lewis, S., Hass, B. S., Lipman, R. D., & Hart, R. W. (1999). Growth curves and survival characteristics of the animals used in the Biomarkers of Aging Program. *Journals of Gerontology Series A Biological Sciences & Medical Sciences*, 54(11), B492–B501.

Um, J. H., Kim, S. J., Kim, D. W., Ha, M. Y., Jang, J. H., Chung, B. S., Kang, C. D., & Kim, S. H. (2003). Tissue-specific changes of DNA repair protein Ku and mtHSP70 in aging rats and their retardation by caloric restriction. *Mechanisms of Ageing & Development*, 124(8–9), 967–975.

Undie, A. S., & Friedman, E. (1993). Diet restriction prevents aging-induced deficits in brain phosphoinositide metabolism. *Journal of Gerontology*, 48(2), B62–B67.

van der Horst, A., Tertoolen, L. G., de Vries-Smits, L. M., Frye, R. A., Medema, R. H., & Burgering, B. M. (2004). FOXO4 is acetylated upon peroxide stress and deacetylated by the longevity protein hSir2(SIRT1). *Journal of Biological Chemistry*, 279(28), 28873–28879.

Van Remmen, H., Ikeno, Y., Hamilton, M., Pahlavani, M., Wolf, N., Thorpe, S. R., Alderson, N. L., Baynes, J. W., Epstein, C. J., Huang, T. T., Nelson, J., Strong, R., & Richardson, A. (2003). Life-long reduction in MnSOD activity results in increased DNA damage and higher incidence of cancer but does not accelerate aging. *Physiological Genomics*, 16(1), 29–37.

Vaziri, H., Dessain, S. K., Eaton, E. N., Imai, S. I., Frye, R. A., Pandita, T. K., Guarente, L., & Weinberg, R. A. (2001). hSIR2(SIRT1) Functions as an NAD-Dependent p53 Deacetylase. *Cell*, 107(2), 149–159.

Vogt, T., & Taylor, L. P. (1995). Flavonol 3-O-glycosyltransferases associated with petunia pollen produce gametophyte-specific flavonol diglycosides. *Plant Physiology*, 108(3), 903–911.

Wachsman, J. T. (1996). The beneficial effects of dietary restriction: reduced oxidative damage and enhanced apoptosis. *Mutation Research*, 350(1), 25–34.

Walford, R. L., Mock, D., Verdery, R., & MacCallum, T. (2002). Calorie restriction in biosphere 2: alterations in physiologic, hematologic, hormonal, and biochemical parameters in humans restricted for a 2-year period. *Journals of Gerontology Series A Biological Sciences & Medical Sciences*, 57(6), B211–B224.

Walker, G. A., Thompson, F. J., Brawley, A., Scanlon, T., & Devaney, E. (2003). Heat shock factor functions at the convergence of the stress response and developmental pathways in *Caenorhabditis elegans*. *Faseb Journal*, 17(13), 1960–1962.

Wan, R., Camandola, S., & Mattson, M. P. (2003). Intermittent fasting and dietary supplementation with 2-deoxy-D-glucose improve functional and metabolic cardiovascular risk factors in rats. *Faseb Journal*, 17(9), 1133–1134.

Wan, R., Camandola, S., & Mattson, M. P. (2004). Dietary supplementation with 2-deoxy-D-glucose improves cardiovascular and neuroendocrine stress adaptation in rats. *American Journal of Physiology*, 287(3), H1186–H1193.

Wang, H. D., Kazemi-Esfarjani, P., & Benzer, S. (2004). Multiple-stress analysis for isolation of Drosophila longevity genes. *Proceedings of the National Academy of Sciences of the USA*, 101(34), 12610–12615.

Ward, W. F. (1988). Food restriction enhances the proteolytic capacity of the aging rat liver. *Journal of Gerontology*, 43(5), B121–B124.

Weindruch, R. (1996). The retardation of aging by caloric restriction: studies in rodents and primates. *Toxicologic Pathology*, 24(6), 742–745.

Weindruch, R., & Walford, R. L. (1988). *The retardation of aging and disease by dietary restriction*. Springfield, IL: Charles C. Thomas.

Weindruch, R., Kayo, T., Lee, C. K., & Prolla, T. A. (2001). Microarray profiling of gene expression in aging and its alteration by caloric restriction in mice. *Journal of Nutrition*, 131(3), 918S–923S.

Weraarchakul, N., Strong, R., Wood, W. G., & Richardson, A. (1989). The effect of aging and dietary restriction on DNA repair. *Experimental Cell Research*, 181(1), 197–204.

Wilkinson, G. S., & South, J. M. (2002). Life history, ecology and longevity in bats. *Aging Cell*, 1(2), 124–131.

Will, L. C., & McCay, C. M. (1941). Ageing, basal metabolism, and retarded growth. *Archives of Biochemistry & Biophysics*, 2(481).

Wood, J. G., Rogina, B., Lavu, S., Howitz, K., Helfand, S. L., Tatar, M., & Sinclair, D. (2004). Sirtuin activators mimic caloric restriction and delay ageing in metazoans. *Nature*, 430(7000), 686–689.

Xia, E., Rao, G., Van Remmen, H., Heydari, A. R., & Richardson, A. (1995). Activities of antioxidant enzymes in various tissues of male Fischer 344 rats are altered by food restriction. *Journal of Nutrition*, 125(2), 195–201.

Yeung, F., Hoberg, J. E., Ramsey, C. S., Keller, M. D., Jones, D. R., Frye, R. A., & Mayo, M. W. (2004). Modulation of NF-kappaB-dependent transcription and cell survival by the SIRT1 deacetylase. *Embo Journal*, 23(12), 2369–2380.

Yoshikawa, H., Ichiki, Y., Sakakibara, K. D., Tamura, H., & Suiko, M. (2002). The biological and structural similarity between lunularic acid and abscisic acid. *Bioscience, Biotechnology, & Biochemistry*, 66(4), 840–846.

Yu, B. P. (1993). Need the free radical theory of aging be linked to the metabolic rate theory? *Aging (Milano)*, 5(3), 243–244.

Yu, B. P., Masoro, E. J., & McMahan, C. A. (1985). Nutritional influences on aging of Fischer 344 rats: I. Physical, metabolic, and longevity characteristics. *Journal of Gerontology*, 40(6), 657–670.

Yuneva, A. O., Kramarenko, G. G., Vetreshchak, T. V., Gallant, S., & Boldyrev, A. A. (2002). Effect of carnosine on *Drosophila melanogaster* lifespan.

Bulletin of Experimental Biology & Medicine, 133(6), 559–561.

Zainal, T. A., Oberley, T. D., Allison, D. B., Szweda, L. I., & Weindruch, R. (2000). Caloric restriction of rhesus monkeys lowers oxidative damage in skeletal muscle. *Faseb Journal*, 14(12), 1825–1836.

Zhang, Y., & Herman, B. (2002). Ageing and apoptosis. *Mechanisms of Ageing & Development*, 123(4), 245–260.

Zhao, K., Chai, X., & Marmorstein, R. (2004). Structure and substrate binding properties of cobB, a Sir2 homolog protein deacetylase from Escherichia coli. *Journal of Molecular Biology*, 337(3), 731–741.

Chapter 4

Hematopoietic Stem Cells, Aging, and Cancer

Deborah R. Bell and Gary Van Zant

I. Stem Cells

A. Properties, History, and Significance

Stem cells are the ultimate resource for development, maintenance, regeneration, and repair in an organism. However, a clear distinction must be made between the totipotent potential of embryonic stem cells, which are definitively responsible for an organism's development, and adult somatic stem cells. These adult stem cells, through their abilities of self-renewal and differentiation, help maintain the organism throughout a lifetime of repair and replenishment. These critically important adult stem cells reside in many, if not most, organ systems and are defined by three major characteristics: (1) the lifelong ability to self-renew, (2) extensive proliferation, and (3) differentiation of progeny into multiple lineages (Weissman, 2000a) (see Figure 4.1).

Self-renewal, the quintessential property of a stem cell, enables that cell to make an exact replica of itself during cell division. The resulting daughter cells have precisely the same potential for self-

renewal and multilineage differentiation as the parental cell, thus ensuring a continued supply of stem cells for the life span of the organism (Fuchs & Segre, 2000). From an evolutionary standpoint, the importance of stem cells is demonstrated by comparing the life spans of simple, single-celled organisms and those of higher, more complex animals. For example, in single-celled organisms or very simple multicellular animals, the overall life expectancy of the animal is equal to that of its composite cells. An extreme example of this is the cnidarian *Hydra*, a fresh water polyp that is one of the simplest multicellular animals that still contains differentiated cells types such as epithelial cells, stinging cells, and sensory nerve cells. Amazingly, the *Hydra* can be separated into single cells that reaggregate and reform one or more normal *Hydras* (depending on the size of the initial aggregate) (Muller, 1996). In this regard, most cells of the *Hydra* would be considered stem cells. Furthermore, the *Hydra* would seem immortal because all aged cells in the adult, including nerve cells, are

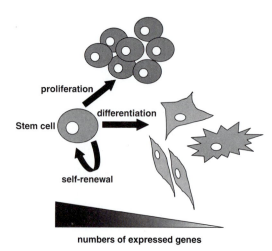

Figure 4.1 Hallmark functions of stem cells.

replaced by a steady supply of stem cells in the animal (Muller, 1996). As animals evolved and became more complex, which coincided with the development of extremely specialized organ systems, the animal's longevity far exceeded that of its individual cells. This process absolutely requires a source of cells to maintain homeostatic balance as the animal faces a lifetime of injury and normal replenishment of worn cells in the various organ systems. This crucial resource is the stem cell pool, and the life spans of these stem cells are either equal to or greater than that of the organism as a whole (Harrison, 1973).

Despite current media coverage and controversies surrounding stem cells and their potential use (i.e., embryonic stem cells in the treatment of injury and disease) (Holden, 2004; Malakoff, 2004; Weissman, 2000b), their existence and clues to their importance were recognized as early as 1945. At this time, a remarkable phenomenon was noted between nonidentical bovine twins. During the rare occurrence when these fraternal twins share a common placenta (and therefore common blood circulation), these animals remain hematopoietic chimeras indefinitely and continue to produce blood cells

from each other during their entire lifetime (Owen, 1945). Presumably, the hematopoietic stem cells (HSCs) shared *in utero* are responsible for this unique chimerism. Experiments in mice in the early 1960s further demonstrated the existence of stem cells in the hematopoietic system. The pioneering work of Till, McCulloch, Becker, and Siminovitch elegantly showed that single cells in the bone marrow of mice could give rise to myeloerythroid colonies in the spleens of irradiated recipients (Till & McCulloch, 1961; Becker et al., 1963). Moreover, when cells from these splenic colonies were transferred to secondary lethally irradiated recipient mice, all blood cell lineages were reconstituted in these animals (Siminovitch et al., 1963). These innovative studies determined that in the bone marrow cells of mice resided cells that (1) could self-renew to be passaged from primary to secondary hosts and (2) could differentiate into multiple lineages, in this case into the various blood cell components, to reconstitute a lethally irradiated animal that was completely dependent on the transplanted cells for survival. These experiments marked the beginning of the stem cell biology field.

Before any discussion about aging in the stem cell compartment, other significant properties of the stem cell must be introduced. Plasticity, one of the most important and perhaps most contentious stem cell properties, refers to flexibility in lineage commitment, thereby allowing a stem cell to cross tissue borders and seed unrelated tissues and organs, even those from different embryonic layers (Blau et al., 2001). For example, two publications have reported the ability of HSCs to convert to hepatocytes (Lagasse et al., 2000) or neurons in the human brain (Mezey et al., 2003). If the concept of plasticity is accurate, then stem cells from a normal, healthy organ could theoretically be used to help regenerate or repair another unrelated tissue

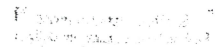

or organ damaged by disease or age. Understandably, this amazing restorative potential has been the driving force behind the flurry of research in stem cell plasticity. More recent evidence has established criteria that would definitively demonstrate plasticity in stem cells; to date, no published reports have fulfilled all such criteria.

To summarize, for a stem cell to be considered "plastic" it would have to satisfy the following conditions: (1) as the cell shifts from one lineage to another, a new lineage-specific *function* should accompany that shift, (2) the genetic profile of the cell should change to fit its new identity, (3) minimal culture or handling of the cell should occur to avoid any extrinsic interference with its developmental program, (4) no cell-cell fusion between the "plastic" cell and a mature cell of the new lineage can occur, and (5) these results must be reproducible (Wagers & Weissman, 2004). Based on these strict criteria, no *bona fide* examples of stem cell plasticity exist; indeed, most reported cases can be explained by cell-cell fusion (Wagers & Weissman, 2004), introduction of heterogenous populations of stem cells into a donor tissue (Orkin & Zon, 2002), or the requirement of induced or natural organ damage or impaired function in the recipient to achieve enhanced performance of the transplanted stem cells in the desired tissue (Grove *et al.*, 2004). However, infusion of donor HSCs may contribute to overall healing and improved outcome in certain cases of organ transplant or disease, albeit via indirect, unidentified mechanisms. Taken together, plasticity of a stem cell, despite hope and initial promise, likely will have little or no bearing on the aging of stem cell populations.

Another fascinating characteristic of stem cells (HSCs in particular) is the wide range of genes they express. Counterintuitive to the prevailing belief of stem cells as "resting" and waiting to become activated as necessary in response to some cellular signal, purified HSCs express a vast array of genes as compared to committed progenitor cells (Terskikh *et al.*, 2003) (see Figure 4.1). Of the differentially expressed genes examined, nearly half were seen in the stem cell population, with relatively few genes expressed by more committed progenitors. In contrast, a limited but distinct set of lineage-specific genes was upregulated in the progenitor cells. These data suggest that stem cells are quite active transcriptionally, allowing them to constantly assess their environment and respond quickly to the needs of or changes experienced by the organism. Active transcriptional status usually means an open chromatin configuration, which could account for DNA damage or liabilities over time, especially over the stem cell's (and the organism's) long lifetime. In this regard, active and robust gene expression in a stem cell could be important during aging.

Finally, an additional characteristic of stem cells that potentially could be affected by advancing age is their proliferative capacity. In much the same way that stem cells traditionally were considered "inactive" in terms of gene expression (which we now know to be untrue), they were further thought to be sedentary as far as cell cycle progression is concerned. Again, the stem cell (in particular the HSC) has proven to be much more dynamic than once believed. These cells are far from quiescent; on the contrary, the most primitive stem cells actively cycle. Each day between 8 and 10 percent of these primitive stem cells progress through the cell cycle, and all cells in the HSC pool undergo cell division every one to three months, depending on the mouse strain studied (Bradford *et al.*, 1997; Cheshier *et al.*, 1999). Not only does this implicate the stem cell as an active entity, it introduces additional mechanisms for DNA damage (mismatches, open chromatin structure) that could accumulate during the lifetime of the cell. Cell proliferation, therefore, is another factor to be considered during the aging of a stem cell.

B. Hematopoietic Stem Cells

Many of the preceding descriptions about stem cell biology and characteristics cite the hematopoietic system as an example. HSCs are likely the most highly studied stem cells to date because of their early discovery (Till, 1961), their isolation from both mice and humans (Baum *et al.*, 1992; Spangrude *et al.*, 1988), and their clinical applications, such as the critical components in bone marrow transplantation (Reya *et al.*, 2001). Because of the extensive literature dedicated to the HSC, this stem cell population will be the focus of this chapter.

The HSC displays all the hallmarks of a stem cell, including the capacity to self-renew and differentiate into all necessary blood cell lineages. This is clearly demonstrated in the ability of a single transplanted stem cell to reconstitute and rescue a lethally irradiated recipient mouse. Classic limiting dilution assays by Smith and colleagues show that single HSCs do indeed generate multilineage clones capable of long-term self-renewal (Smith *et al.*, 1991). HSCs differentiate in a hierarchical manner, with the most primitive stem cells, or long-term HSCs, retaining the ability to self-renew indefinitely (see Figure 4.2). These, in turn, give rise to short-term HSCs that self renew in approximately eight weeks and multipotent progenitors that can self-renew in less than two weeks. At this point, lineage-restricted progenitors emerge, which ultimately give rise to all of the differentiated cells of the hematopoietic system (Reya *et al.*, 2001). As seen in Figure 4.2, as differentiation increases, the ability to self renew decreases.

II. Stem Cell Aging

Stem cells are uniquely sensitive to damage accumulation from both intrinsic and extrinsic sources because they are

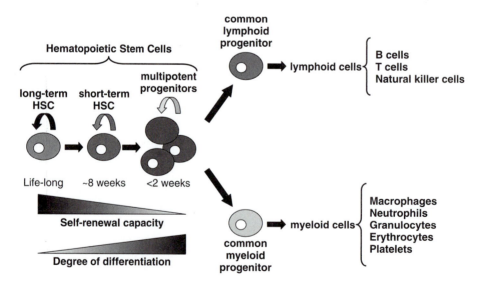

*adapted from Reya, Morrison, Clarke, and Weissman, 2001

Figure 4.2 Self-renewal and differentiation in the stem cell hierarchy.

long-lived. One of the main perpetrators of damage is reactive oxygen species (ROS) that are generated by normal cellular metabolism. Long-term exposure to ROS is detrimental to many macromolecules, including proteins, lipids, and nucleic acids. Whereas damage to any of these molecules may affect cellular function, harm to the nucleic acids and proteins that constitutes chromatin in stem cells is particularly deleterious because it can be passed on to progeny (Harman, 1981; Johnson *et al.*, 1999). Another source of damage to stem cells is associated with their lifetime of cell division. As mentioned in the previous section, stem cells are not quiescent, and enter the cell cycle on a regular basis. Repeated rounds of DNA replication can result in the incorporation of numerous copy errors into the genome. Under normal circumstances, the cell has sophisticated proofreading and editing enzymes to correct these potentially hazardous mistakes. However, over a lifetime of use, the function of these enzymes may decline due to ROS exposure, for example (Johnson *et al.*, 1999), and lead to mutation. Whereas mutation in a single long-lived differentiated cell may have

serious consequences for that individual cell, mutation in a stem cell could have potentially disastrous effects because this genome will be perpetuated as the progeny of that stem cell differentiates.

Although stem cells from other tissues have been identified (i.e., in the central nervous system, liver, and skin), much less is known about them, and virtually no data concerning their properties during aging have been published. The study of stem cell aging in systems other than the hematopoietic is in its infancy. Likewise, data will be presented describing the functional consequences of aging on HSCs. Factors such as replicative stress and editing errors that occur in all cells, including the long-lived stem cell, are important in limiting organismal longevity and hence contribute to the decline of the individual with age.

A. Stem Cell Aging Theories

Various hypotheses have been put forth to explain stem cell usage as an organism ages. The first was proposed nearly 40 years ago and is referred to as the *clonal succession theory* (see Figure 4.3a). This theory suggests that the stem cell

A. Clonal succession theory: total # of stem cells decreases over time

B. "Equal contribution" theory: total # of stem cells remains constant over time

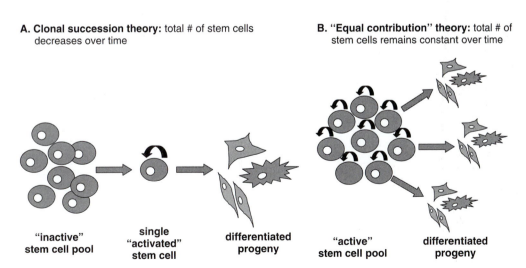

"inactive" stem cell pool   single "activated" stem cell   differentiated progeny   "active" stem cell pool   differentiated progeny

Figure 4.3 Theories of stem cell usage.

pool as a whole is maintained in a quiescent state, held in check until needed by the organism. When required, one or at most only a few stem cells become active and leave the pool to proliferate and supply the necessary differentiated cells to the organism (Kay, 1965). According to the tenets of this theory, the activated clone would never rejoin the primitive pool of resting stem cells; therefore, over time, the supply of stem cells would diminish, and aging would proceed. Injury or disease could accelerate this stem cell diminution and thereby contribute to aging. To counteract this loss of critical stem cells with time, one could postulate that a sufficiently large pool of stem cells would be present at birth to meet the needs of the organism during periods of crisis or a lifetime of wear and tear, or both. In this regard, a mouse with an average life span of approximately 2 years would require far fewer stem cells than humans with their life expectancies of nearly 80 years. However, one study unexpectedly showed that HSC numbers are relatively conserved in mammals (Abkowitz et al., 2002). That is, the total number of HSCs in the bone marrow of mice, cats, and humans was similar and not commensurate with either the size or the potential life span of the organism. These data argue against a model of sequential activation and subsequent depletion of a non-renewable stem cell population.

An alternative theory that takes into account the compelling data that demonstrate that HSCs actively cycle and are not quiescent (Bradford et al., 1997; Cheshier et al., 1999) can be termed the "equal contribution" model. In this case, all members of the primitive stem cell pool are active and in a homeostatic balance of self-renewal, proliferation, or differentiation (see Figure 4.3b). This theory suggests that the total number of stem cells does not decrease during the lifetime of the animal due to the self-renewal properties of the stem cells. Therefore, depletion of stem cell numbers does not occur and hence does not drive aging. This model agrees with data from mouse chimera experiments that show equal contribution by most (perhaps all) HSCs to blood formation simultaneously (Harrison et al., 1987).

In view of this model, advancing age poses a special problem with regard to stem cells: does the ability to self-renew prevent aging of this critical cell population? Certain limited evidence exists that seems to argue against stem cell aging. For example, experiments analyzing stem cell properties in a large animal model (the dog) show little age-related differences in the HSC populations in young versus old bone marrow (Zaucha et al., 2001). Additionally, although not directly related to the self-renewal properties of stem cells, is the observation that many common diseases responsible for death in mammals, including humans, are not diseases of stem cell origin, such as heart disease or renal failure (Van Zant & Liang, 2003). However, greater evidence is mounting in favor of age-related changes that affect stem cell properties, especially in the hematopoietic system.

B. Mouse Aging Data

1. Intrinsic Factors

Because of the similarities in the blood-forming processes between mice and humans and the availability of numerous inbred laboratory mouse strains, much of the data on stem cells and aging generated to date has been in the mouse. Several general characteristics have been determined with regard to stem cell aging. To begin, in the murine hematopoietic system, HSCs are not immortal and can only be serially passaged to recipient mice for five generations at most (Ogden & Mickliem, 1976; Siminovitch et al., 1964). Subsequent transplants and manipulations do not fully reconstitute and rescue lethally irradiated recipient mice and suggest that repeated rounds of self-renewal and lineage replenishment exert a lasting effect on the stem cells. Although these serial transplantations may not precisely recapitulate the natural aging process and may further be magnified by differentiation of the transplanted stem cells as well, similar mechanisms are involved and hence can provide clues as to what is happening as the mouse ages. Another stem cell characteristic affected by advancing age is the ability to "home." Stem cells must be able to find their way from one site in the bone marrow, enter and travel through the bloodstream, and finally recognize other positions in the bone marrow where they are needed. The same is true of transplanted stem cells: they must be able to locate appropriate locations in the bone marrow to lodge from the bloodstream following transplantation (Cao et al., 2004). This process of traveling to and recognizing the correct spot to reside by a stem cell is called *homing*, and diminished homing efficiency of HSCs in mice is observed with regard to age. Indeed, old stem cells have a significantly reduced ability to home to the proper location as compared to young stem cells following transplantation (Morrison et al., 1996). Finally, other observations between young and old mice have shown that changes occur in the developmental potential in aged stem cells of hematopoietic origin. Specifically, as murine bone marrow is serially transplanted (as mentioned before, this is a process likened, but not identical, to aging), or when bone marrow from aged donors is used in transplantation experiments, stem cells lose their ability to differentiate into the lymphoid lineage. Hence, hematopoietic maturation is skewed toward myeloid precursors and away from the B and T cell lineages (Spangrude et al., 1995; Sudo et al., 2000). All of these data indicate that despite their ability to continually self-renew, stem

cells are not immune to the inevitable passage of time.

In addition to these studies that directly examine the effects of aging on stem cells, many investigators have exploited the intrinsic differences among inbred mouse strains to look at age-related alterations in HSCs. One of the best examples of these experiments involves analyses of allophenic mice, which provide hints about naturally occurring differences in hematopoietic cells and their life spans between two inbred strains of mice. These innovative experiments involve creating chimeric animals by aggregating cells from two different strains of mice (in this case, the commonly used C57BL/6 [B6] and DBA/2 [D2] mice) at the embryonic stage. The resulting animals are composed of cells from both B6 and D2 mice. Amazingly, stem cells derived from the D2 mice, which are short-lived (by 34 percent) compared to B6 mice, stopped contributing to hematopoiesis at a time corresponding to their normal life span. After this time, all hematopoietic cells in the allophenic mice came from the longer-lived B6 mice (Van Zant et al., 1990). This convincingly demonstrates that HSCs do indeed age and that there are functional consequences of this aging. Adding to this data are observations from other investigators who use inbred strains of laboratory mice to show wide variations in HSC characteristics and natural life span (Van Zant et al., 1983). Specifically, many researchers have used recombinant mouse strains to identify quantitative trait loci (QTLs) responsible for the complex traits (including aging) exhibited by different mouse strains (Abiola et al., 2003). For example, studies from this laboratory have shown that old mice (24 months old) have greater numbers of primitive HSCs compared to young mice (6 weeks old), but the total number of HSCs per animal is strain-dependent. Five commonly used mouse strains were assayed in these experiments (C3H/He, CBA/J, DBA/2, BALB/c, and C57BL/6). A decrease in stem cell cycling activity in older mice of each strain tested was demonstrated, and this decrease had a statistically significant negative correlation with the maximal expected life span of that particular strain. However, the degree of proliferative decrease was also strain-dependent (de Haan et al., 1997). These results were further investigated in light of extrinsic (such as growth factor) controls on HSC proliferation and pool size. In this study, the effects of stimulation by the growth factor flk-2/flt-3 ligand (FL), which has been proposed to be important in maintaining HSC numbers and regulating their proliferation, were assessed in the stem cell compartment of the same five mouse strains analyzed previously. Interestingly, following incubation with FL, a correlation was noted among the following characteristics: life span of the various mouse strains, HSC proliferation, and HSC pool size. Specifically, FL only elicited a stimulatory effect on stem cell cycling in strains of mice with a naturally larger pool of stem cells, such as the D2 mice, which are also relatively short-lived. Using the power of recombinant inbred mice and QTL mapping, a putative region on mouse chromosome 18 was identified as responsible for this trait. In addition, this region of mouse chromosome 18 shows synteny with human chromosome 5q, deletions of which are important in hematologic cancers (de Haan & Van Zant, 1997). Further analysis of HSC cell turnover and cycling in recombinant inbred mice had a dramatic association with mean life span in mice, and two additional QTLs on mouse chromosomes 7 and 11 were identified as possible loci for the genes responsible for these traits (de Haan & Van Zant, 1999a). Detailed experiments entirely focused on the informative recombinant inbred mice generated by crossing the B6 and D2

lines (called BXD strains) identified other QTLs important in HSC biology and aging. Analysis of all 35 BXD strains of mice available to determine QTLs responsible for the changes in stem cell numbers as mice age from 2 to 20 months identified several potential contributing loci, including those found on chromosomes 2, 14, and X (de Haan & Van Zant, 1999b). When thinking about how vital and complex stem cell regulation and maintenance is, it is not surprising that several chromosomal locations could be responsible for this regulation. Using newer and more reliable database resources with higher resolution, the potential locus on mouse chromosome 2 can be considered a bona fide "aging locus" because in B6 mice this site appears to be responsible for the increased numbers of HSCs noted in old B6 mice (Geiger et al., 2001). Senescence, or the limitation of proliferative capacity due to exhaustive rounds of cellular cycling, is also genetically regulated and age-related in HSCs (Chen et al., 2000), as evidenced by both competitive repopulation and serial transplantation studies in mice in vivo. To be precise, B6 mice (longer-lived) have a delayed onset of senescence compared to D2 mice (shorter-lived). Decreased repopulating ability with increasing HSC age in D2 mice suggests that these cells do senesce; however, HSCs from old B6 mice repopulate recipients better than do those from young B6 mice, an odd contradiction. This could be explained if B6 stem cells simply have a higher proliferative limit than D2 stem cells. If this is true, then only repeated serial transplantations requiring extensive proliferation would uncover functional deterioration (i.e., loss of repopulating ability) over time in B6 stem cells (Chen et al., 2000). As stated earlier in this section, this is indeed the case: serial transplantation recovery by HSCs is affected with increasing age. Initial experiments indicate that a potential locus on mouse chromosome 12 may be responsible for the senescent phenotype. In all of these reports, no specific candidate genes have been identified in the putative QTLs shown to be responsible for the suggested traits. Analysis of candidate genes in these loci is an area of active research by many investigators.

2. Extrinsic Factors

While most data published on the aging of HSCs focus on intrinsic factors, such as genetic components specific to each cell, an important related topic concerns certain extrinsic factors, such as the cellular microenvironment, and how this crucial milieu of cells, cytokines, and soluble growth factors change and affect HSCs with advancing age. The supporting stromal cells of the microenvironment help to maintain HSCs by supporting their localization, survival, or self-renewal, or any combination thereof. This concept of an HSC niche was first proposed many years ago (Schofield, 1978) and has since been expanded and intensely studied to provide a more complete understanding of stem cells to enhance their manipulation and applications in treating disease.

The bone-forming cells of the bone marrow, or osteoblasts, now appear to be critically important factors in the stem cell niche (Zhu & Emerson, 2004). Experiments examining hematopoietic recovery in mice following treatment with 5-fluorouracil have shown in vivo that stimulated HSCs are found in direct proximity to osteoblasts (Heissig et al., 2002). However, an unsettling contradiction was noted with regard to the numbers of osteoblasts present in the bone marrow and the numbers of HSCs: osteoblasts vastly outnumber the HSCs (Taichman et al., 1996). This raises the question of how do HSCs "choose" with which osteoblast to associate. Are certain osteoblasts somehow different and specialized to function

as a stem cell niche? Or, is it more likely that other cells in the bone marrow, such as the mesenchymal cells (i.e., endothelial cells), also are part of the HSC niche and their association with osteoblasts truly defines the niche? Data supporting this model were shown by analyzing the expression of certain HSC-specific recognition molecules (i.e., c-Kit ligand) on the surface of osteoblasts; no such expression was detected, thereby suggesting that other accessory cells that do express such necessary factors must be associated with the osteoblasts to allow HSCs to home to their proper niche (Taichman et al., 1996). These data lead to an important point regarding aging: both the endothelial cells of the bone marrow and the primitive HSCs develop from a common hematopoietic precursor, the hemangioblast (Zhu & Emerson, 2004). It is therefore highly likely that these accessory cells of the stroma also will show similar age-related changes that will influence the biology and chemistry of the microenvironment (Wineman et al., 1996). Finally, to further address the role of the aged environment and its potential impact on HSC function in mice, bone marrow transplantation studies were performed in young and old recipients. Regardless of the age of the bone marrow donor, an increased autoimmune response in the old recipients was detected compared to the young (Doria et al., 1997). This supports the notion of age-related impairment of the stroma that, in turn, causes improper functioning of the immune system. Thus, the microenvironment of the aging HSC is another important factor to consider during the process of cancer development, which will be discussed in Section III.

C. Human Aging Data

While data from mouse models of stem cell aging are considerably more thorough, reports demonstrating similar age-related functional decline in human

HSCs are compelling. First, studies analyzing the lengths of telomeres (which are specialized structures on the ends of chromosomes) in both human somatic cells and HSCs have shown progressive telomere shortening after cellular proliferation, which leads to termination of cell division or replicative senescence. Accumulation of senescent cells with repeated cellular cycling, as occurs over time with progressing age, is theorized to contribute to tissue deterioration (Baird & Kipling, 2004). Unlike human somatic cells, which express no (or very low levels of) telomerase (the enzyme responsible for maintaining telomere length), human HSCs do express detectable levels of telomerase. Despite this fact, HSCs also display shortening of telomeres with age (Allsopp & Weissman, 2002). A recent interesting observation in cultured human cells also lends further evidence to the importance of age-related telomere shortening in somatic and presumably HSCs. As mentioned earlier in this discussion, oxidative stress contributes to cellular aging. It is known that oxidative stress can also increase the rate of telomere shortening (Kawanishi & Oikawa, 2004). Thus, oxidative stress can directly affect chromosomes and lead to cellular senescence and aging in many human cells, including HSCs. Next, studies using primitive hematopoietic cells obtained from human umbilical cord blood and bone marrow from both adults and the elderly show a steady decline in cell function that begins after birth and progresses throughout life. Specifically, increases in progenitor cell numbers with advancing age were demonstrated in the samples tested, which correlates with data obtained in mice; however, there was a concomitant decrease in proliferative capacity in those same progenitor cells. Samples from children with bone marrow failure and a propensity to develop leukemia also showed comparable proliferative deficiencies, as did the samples from the elderly, indicating a potential link between hematopoietic deficiencies or aging, or both, with cancer (Marley et al., 1999). Also, as seen in murine HSCs, differentiation potential is affected in stem cells from the elderly. Primitive human CD34 + cells have a diminished capacity to generate T cells when examined in vitro (Offner et al., 1999). This last example of reduced T and B cell number and activity with advancing age is related to the well-documented decrease in immune system function in older individuals (Globerson & Effros, 2000; Miller, 2000; Miller et al., 1997), and this could clearly affect an organism's ability to achieve long life. Impaired T cell monitoring and destruction of cancerous cells is highly affected in the elderly (Aspinall, 2000). Therefore, this could represent a direct link between dysfunctional stem cell differentiation, loss of immune prowess, and increased cancer development due to advancing age.

D. Health Impact of Aging Hematopoietic Stem Cells

As humans age, small, seemingly innocuous changes in hematopoiesis occur, which include anemia, diminished immune responses (discussed above), and an overall decrease in bone marrow cellularity (Lipschitz et al., 1981). Although these may be tolerated sufficiently in otherwise healthy individuals, times of hematopoietic stress (such as that following myeloablative chemotherapeutic treatment or infection) exacerbate these subtle changes. Not only is response to such stress slowed in the elderly, but complete recovery is unusual even after significant periods of time, resulting in anemias or other hematopoietic deficiencies (Botnick et al., 1982; Kim et al., 2003; Marley et al., 1999). With regard to hematopoietic changes in the elderly, anemia is common, and nearly one-third of the cases seen are unexplained (Guralnik *et al.*, 2004). As the mean age of the population increases, so does the percentage of accompanying anemias (Cesari *et al.*, 2004; Penninx *et al.*, 2003). In fact, by age 85, the prevalence of anemia is greater than 20 percent (Guralnik *et al.*, 2004). As mentioned earlier, this usually does not present complications in a healthy patient, and most elderly anemic patients go untreated; however, even mildly anemic patients can have unfavorable outcomes following heart complications such as myocardial infarction. The decline in hemoglobin in older individuals is not sufficient to explain the extent of anemia observed. Dysregulated red blood formation in the bone marrow is a plausible culprit of this anemia. Ultimately, the HSC is responsible for erythropoiesis, and because other developmental abnormalities are seen in aging stem cells (such as reduced T and B cell production), it is possible the aging HSC also fails to produce the number of red blood cells necessary to prevent anemia. This anemia could therefore reflect an underlying weak myelodysplasia; indeed, evidence suggests that myelodysplastic syndromes are stem cell disorders (Liesveld *et al.*, 2004). Age-associated changes in function and accumulation of damage, particularly in chromatin, in HSCs may account for the dramatic increase in cancer seen after the age of 65.

III. Stem Cells and Cancer

Progressing age is the most significant risk factor in cancer development; indeed, between the ages of 40 to 80 years, there is an exponential increase in cancer incidence rates, after which the incidence of cancer levels off (DePinho, 2000). Ultimately, the overall risk of developing an invasive cancer in one's lifetime is 1 in 3 for women and 1 in 2 for men (ACS, 2000). These statistics not only apply to the solid tumors that commonly are cited today, such as pancre-

atic, lung, prostate, and colon cancer, but also to cancers of the hematopoietic system, namely leukemias. For example, acute myeloid leukemia (AML), for which the majority of data is available, is more than three times as likely to occur in someone age 65 versus an individual who is 35 years old (NCI, 2000). Furthermore, the median age at diagnosis of patients with AML is 65 years (Lowenberg *et al.*, 1999). Clearly, this is a disease that predominates in older persons. In addition to the prevalence of AML in older individuals is their poor response to treatment. Following standard chemotherapy treatment, an initial remission is seen in 65 to 75 percent of younger AML patients (<60 years old). Unfortunately, the same standard treatment protocols in older AML patients (>60 years) result in a much lower remission rate (30 to 50 percent) and a death rate that is twice as high (20 percent) as that observed in young persons with AML (Baudard *et al.*, 1994; Bishop *et al.*, 1996; Estey *et al.*, 1995; Leith *et al.*, 1997; Mayer *et al.*, 1994; Rowe *et al.*, 1995; Schiller & Lee, 1997; Stone *et al.*, 1995; Taylor *et al.*, 1995). A sustainable remission is achieved in only 10 to 20 percent of elderly AML patients overall (Goldstone *et al.*, 2001). As an increasing proportion of our population gets older due to modern medical advances, health challenges of the elderly will become even more critical to science and medicine. The statistics cited above demonstrate that AML will be an important concern in an ever-growing segment of the population.

A. Stem Cell Origin of Leukemia

Cancers of the hematopoietic system, or leukemias, originate from and are sustained by cancer stem cells. Leukemias provide the most convincing data that normal stem cells can become cancer stem cells through the acquisition of mutations, and it is this leukemic stem cell (LSC) that is responsible for the disease (Reya et al., 2001). Studies of human AML have begun to define the genetic alterations and chromosome translocations associated with the various subtypes of the disease (Dash & Gilliland, 2001). AML is a heterogeneous disease clinically and includes many subtypes (M0–M7) as defined by the French-American-British (FAB) classification system (Mirro, 1992). Despite this heterogeneity, the leukemias are quite similar at the level of the stem cell and share many of the same immunophenotypic markers as normal HSCs (Bonnet & Dick, 1997; Lapidot et al., 1994). With the advent of improved methods of detection and isolation of stem cells (such as fluorescence activated cell sorting), it is now possible to analyze the functional and molecular characteristics of both normal HSCs and LSCs. Recent reports formally have described the existence of leukemic stem cells in AML and strongly suggest that these LSCs give rise to the disease (Jordan, 2002). Specifically, when CD34 + /CD38-cells, previously defined as containing the stem cell population of normal bone marrow, were isolated from the bone marrow of patients with AML and transplanted into the non-obese diabetic/severe combined immunodeficient (NOD/SCID) mouse, leukemic disease was evident and transferable (Bonnet & Dick, 1997). This indicates that, just like the normal HSC, the leukemic stem cell also displays the cell surface marker phenotype of CD34 + /CD38-. Other evidence supporting the stem cell origin of AML comes from studies on the various subtypes of the disease. As mentioned previously, AML subtype classification is based on the morphologies and genetic abnormalities of the leukemic cells (FAB subtypes) (Brendel & Neubauer, 2000). Interestingly, the AML subtypes M0, M1, M2, M4, and M5 all contain LSCs with similar immunophenotypes, even though each of these subtypes of leukemia displays a different clinical disease (Guzman & Jordan, 2004). While the phenotypically identical LSCs (CD34 + /CD38-) from each of the AML subtypes when transplanted into NOD/SCID mice contained the leukemia-initiating cells, the resulting disease was similar to that observed in the donor patient (Wang et al., 1998). These results indicate that the initial transformed cell was a primitive stem cell that took the wrong developmental pathway, presumably depending on the mutation that occurred. All of these data point to a transformed stem cell source of leukemia.

B. The Two-Hit Model

An important corollary to this discussion of a stem cell origin of AML is the theory that cancer, in general, results from a series of genetic changes that, over time, confer unique properties to a cell that lead to a progression from normalcy to malignancy (Hanahan & Weinberg, 2000). These genetic alterations include, but are not limited to, independence in growth signaling, escape from apoptosis, and endless ability to replicate. Likewise, AML progression is theorized to result from a stepwise accumulation of genetic mutations. This buildup of mutations takes place over the life span of an individual, which is why AML is more than three times as likely to occur in someone aged 65 years versus an individual who is 35 years old (NCI, 2000). The mutation buildup generally results from two sources: (1) replicative stress and (2) exposure to damaging extrinsic factors. Repeated rounds of cell division, as occurs in a long-lived stem cell, provide ample opportunity for mistakes such as DNA mismatches and other editing errors to be incorporated into the genome. These types of errors can be directly responsible for alterations in gene regulation or function, or both. Additionally, exposure to repeated extrinsic insults, such as ROS, can lead to mutation accumulation in crucial cells like HSCs. As mentioned earlier, this will obviously have serious consequences in a long-lived, terminally differentiated cell, but it will likely have a dire outcome in a stem cell responsible for life-long tissue repair and replenishment. In summary, given that the origin of AML is an HSC that has undergone oncogenic mutations, it is reasonable to propose that an *aging* stem cell is a likely target for this leukemic transformation.

Acute myeloid leukemias are composed of leukemic cells that not only have proliferation or survival advantages, or both, over other cells of the hematopoietic system, but also have diminished, poor differentiation compared to normal cells (Deguchi & Gilliland, 2002). The current "two-hit" model of AML cites mutation in a cellular kinase that results in a constant growth-promoting signal, and mutation in a hematopoietic transcription factor that leads to disrupted developmental potential as the important elements driving leukemogenesis (Dash & Gilliland, 2001; Deguchi & Gilliland, 2002). Clinically, support for the acquisition of cooperating mutations in the development of AML is well documented. In nearly all cases of chronic myeloid leukemia (CML), a translocation exists that constitutively activates a tyrosine kinase. Common translocations associated with CML include BCR/ABL, TEL/ABL, TEL/PDGFβR, and TEL/JAK2 (Deguchi & Gilliland, 2002). Expression of these constitutively active kinases results in increased proliferation or survival of affected cells without a block in cellular differentiation. It is the subsequent gain of mutations involving transcription factors that provides the differentiation block and causes the onset of acute disease. Examples of CML progression to AML (or CML blast crisis) provide supporting evidence for this hypothesis. Cases of CML patients with BCR/ABL-positive disease progressing to acute leukemia with ensuing acquisition of either the Nup98/HoxA9 or AML1/ETO translocations are documented (Golub et al., 1994; Yamamoto et al., 2000). These data point to the need for multiple cooperating mutations during leukemogenesis.

Given the differences in life span between mice (3 years) and humans (~80 years), it is logical that development of a "second hit" would occur more quickly in the mouse. In fact, most processes occur faster in mice compared to humans (i.e., metabolism, reproduction, etc.). Additionally, the most common cancers that affect elderly mice and humans are not the same and therefore are likely to develop and progress in different ways. Specifically, old mice tend to develop sarcomas and lymphomas, whereas elderly humans more commonly develop epithelial cancers such as breast and colon cancers (DePinho, 2000). Considering all the variance between mouse and human physiology, it is not surprising that development of mutations necessary to transform cells occur at different rates.

C. Age as the "Second Hit" in Cancer

The work summarized in this section corresponds strongly with a model of multistep leukemogenesis, in which the main culprits of disease consist of an altered transcription factor that causes a differentiation block, and of an activated kinase that can provide limitless growth and survival signals. The combination of these events is critical to disease development. But, as evidenced by the increase in leukemia incidence with advancing age, these detrimental mutations obviously take place over a long period of time. Aging, therefore, must also be a key player in this scenario. Because stem cells are known to be the source of AML and the effects of aging on the stem cell population, we favor a model of AML in which aging may be considered a secondary age-related event in leukemogenesis (see Figure 4.4). However, the models in Figure 4.4 (A and B) are not necessarily mutually exclusive. For the sake of simplicity, models A and B were shown as separate events. But secondary mutations (A) that help drive leukemogenesis may be direct results of the age-related changes brought about by increasing age (B). Effects on DNA repair mechanisms and repeated exposure to environmental insults, both internal and external, may cause enough genomic instability to permit the formation and escape from detection of the translocations and point mutations/duplications commonly seen in human AMLs. In this regard, aging would provide and promote conditions permissive to leukemic transformation. Aging stem cells also display decreased developmental potential, which could be similar to the effects of a mutated transcription factor and skew the differentiation of progeny. Furthermore, decreased monitoring by the immune system, another issue in older individuals, may allow disease to progress more efficiently and aggressively. Finally, the increased cellular senescence seen with advancing age in mice could directly contribute to leukemic progression. Krtolica *et al.* (2001) showed that senescent fibroblasts can permit epithelial cells to become malignant. Given that HSCs and the surrounding stromal cells do age, senescence and cancer development may be inevitable outcomes of this process. Therefore, age may be just as important a factor in AML development as the altered genes themselves.

A. Current "Two–Hit" theory of leukemogenesis

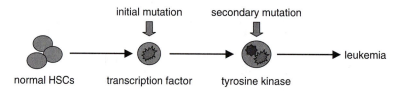

B. Age as a secondary event in the development of leukemia

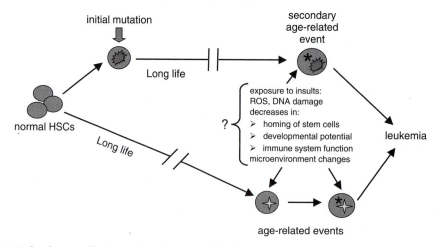

Figure 4.4 Role of stem cell aging in development of leukemia.

IV. Conclusions

The study of stem cells, with their promise of curing injury and disease, has led to discoveries that necessitate monitoring and caution as well as those that inspire excitement and hope. The evidence presented here not only should entice further research into the incredible potential of stem cells but should also cause reflection about the inevitabilities of being such a long-lived cell. The natural course of aging and its undeniable association with cancer is not lost in a stem cell despite its amazing ability to self-renew and restore (some) tissues in times of need. The identification of malignant stem cells in cancers other than the hematopoietic system, such as the breast and brain, provides increasing evidence consistent with a general model of stem cell origin of disease. To the extent that at least some, and perhaps most, malignancies are stem cell-derived, cancer may provide some of the strongest evidence yet supporting the concept of stem cell aging.

References

Abiola, O., Angel, J. M., Avner, P., Bachmanov, A. A., Belknap, J. K., Bennett, B., Blankenhorn, E. P., Blizard, D. A., Bolivar, V., Brockmann, G. A., Buck, K. J., Bureau, J. F., Casley, W. L., Chesler, E. J., Cheverud, J. M., Churchill, G. A., Cook, M., Crabbe, J. C., Crusio, W. E., Darvasi, A., de Haan, G., Dermant, P., Doerge, R. W., Elliot, R. W., Farber, C. R., Flaherty, L., Flint, J., Gershenfeld, H., Gibson, J. P., Gu, J., Gu. W., Himmelbauer, H., Hitzemann, R., Hsu, H. C., Hunter, K., Iraqi, F. F., Jansen, R. C., Johnson, T. E., Jones, B. C., Kempermann, G., Lammert, F., Lu, L., Manly, K. F., Matthews, D. B., Medrano, J. F., Mehrabian, M., Mittlemann, G., Mock, B. A., Mogil, J. S., Montagutelli, X., Morahan, G., Mountz, J. D., Nagase, H., Nowakowski, R. S., O'Hara, B. F., Osadchuk, A. V., Paigen, B., Palmer, A. A., Peirce, J. L., Pomp, D., Rosemann, M., Rosen, G. D., Schalkwyk, L. C., Seltzer, Z., Settle, S., Shimomura, K., Shou, S., Sikela, J. M., Siracusa, L. D., Spearow, J. L., Teuscher, C., Threadgill, D. W., Toth, L. A., Toye, A. A., Vadasz, C., Van Zant, G., Wakeland, E., Williams, R. W., Zhang, H. G., & Zou, F. (2003). The nature and identification of quantitative trait loci: a community's view. *Nature reviews. Genetics,* 4, 911–916.

Abkowitz, J. L., Catlin, S. N., McCallie, M. T., & Guttorp, P. (2002). Evidence that the number of hematopoietic stem cells per animal is conserved in mammals. *Blood,* 100, 2665–2667.

ACS. (2000). Cancer facts and figures. *Annual Report of the American Cancer Society,* 1–7.

Allsopp, R. C., & Weissman, I. L. (2002). Replicative senescence of hematopoietic stem cells during serial transplantation: does telomere shortening play a role? *Oncogene,* 21, 3270–3273.

Aspinall, R. (2000). Longevity and the immune response. *Biogerontology,* 1, 273–278.

Baird, D. M., & Kipling, D. (2004). The extent and significance of telomere loss with age. *Annals of the New York Academy of Sciences,* 1019, 265–268.

Baudard, M., Marie, J. P., Cadiou, M.,Viguie, F., &, Zittoun, R. (1994). Acute myelogenous leukemia in the elderly: retrospective study of 235 consecutive patients. *British Journal of Haematology,* 86, 82–91.

Baum, C. M., Weissman, I. L., Tsukamoto, A. S., Buckle, A. M., & Peault, B. (1992). Isolation of a candidate human hematopoietic stem-cell population. *Proceedings of the National Academy of Sciences of the USA,* 89, 2804–2808.

Becker, A. J., McCulloch, E. A., & Till, J. E. (1963). Cytological demonstration of the clonal nature of spleen colonies derived from transplanted mouse marrow cells. *Nature,* 197, 452–454.

Bishop, J. F., Matthews, J. P., Young, G. A., Szer, J., Gillett, A., Joshua, D., Bradstock, K., Enno, A., Wolf, M. M., Fox, R., Cobcroft, R., Herrmann, R., Van Der Weyden, M., Lowenthal, R. M., Page, F., Garson, O. M., & Juneja, S. (1996). A randomized study of high-dose cytarabine in induction in acute myeloid leukemia. *Blood,* 87, 1710–1717.

Blau, H. M., Brazelton, T. R., & Weimann, J. M. (2001). The evolving concept of a stem cell: entity or function? *Cell*, 105, 829–841.

Bonnet, D., & Dick, J. E. (1997). Human acute myeloid leukemia is organized as a hierarchy that originates from a primitive hematopoietic cell. *Nature Medicine*, 3, 730–737.

Botnick, L. E., Hannon, E. C., Obbagy, J., & Hellman, S. (1982). The variation of hematopoietic stem cell self-renewal capacity as a function of age: further evidence for heterogenicity of the stem cell compartment. *Blood*, 60, 268–271.

Bradford, G. B., Williams, B., Rossi, R., & Bertoncello, I. (1997). Quiescence, cycling, and turnover in the primitive hematopoietic stem cell compartment. *Experimental Hematology*, 25, 445–453.

Brendel, C., & Neubauer, A. (2000). Characteristics and analysis of normal and leukemic stem cells: current concepts and future directions. *Leukemia*, 14, 1711–1717.

Cao, Y. A., Wagers, A. J., Beilhack, A., Dusich, J., Bachmann, M. H., Negrin, R. S., Weissman, I. L., & Contag, C. H. (2004). Shifting foci of hematopoiesis during reconstitution from single stem cells. *Proceedings of the National Academy of Sciences of the USA*, 101, 221–226.

Cesari, M., Penninx, B. W., Lauretani, F., Russo, C. R., Carter, C., Bandinelli, S., Atkinson, H., Onder, G., Pahor, M., & Ferrucci, L. (2004). Hemoglobin levels and skeletal muscle: results from the InCHIANTI study. *Journals of Gerontology. Series A. Biological Sciences and Medical Sciences*, 59, M249–M254.

Chen, J., Astle, C. M., & Harrison, D. E. (2000). Genetic regulation of primitive hematopoietic stem cell senescence. *Experimental Hematology*, 28, 442–450.

Cheshier, S. H., Morrison, S. J., Liao, X., & Weissman, I. L. (1999). In vivo proliferation and cell cycle kinetics of long-term self-renewing hematopoietic stem cells. *Proceedings of the National Academy of Sciences of the USA*, 96, 3120–3125.

Dash, A., & Gilliland, D. G. (2001). Molecular genetics of acute myeloid leukaemia. *Best Practice & Research. Clinical Haematology*, 14, 49–64.

de Haan, G., & Van Zant, G. (1997). Intrinsic and extrinsic control of hemopoietic stem cell numbers: mapping of a stem cell gene. *Journal of Experimental Medicine*, 186, 529–536.

de Haan, G., & Van Zant, G. (1999a). Dynamic changes in mouse hematopoietic stem cell numbers during aging. *Blood*, 93, 3294–3301.

de Haan, G., & Van Zant, G. (1999b). Genetic analysis of hemopoietic cell cycling in mice suggests its involvement in organismal life span. *FASEB Journal*, 13, 707–713.

de Haan, G., Nijhof, W., & Van Zant, G. (1997). Mouse strain-dependent changes in frequency and proliferation of hematopoietic stem cells during aging: correlation between lifespan and cycling activity. *Blood*, 89, 1543–1550.

Deguchi, K., & Gilliland, D. G. (2002). Cooperativity between mutations in tyrosine kinases and in hematopoietic transcription factors in AML. *Leukemia*, 16, 740–744.

DePinho, R. (2000). The age of cancer. *Nature*, 408, 248–254.

Doria, G., Mancini, C., Utsuyama, M., Frasca, D., & Hirokawa, K. (1997). Aging of the recipients but not of the bone marrow donors enhances autoimmunity in syngeneic radiation chimeras. *Mechanisms of Ageing and Development*, 95, 131–142.

Estey, E. H., Kantarjian, H., Keating, M. J. (1995). Therapy for acute myeloid leukemia. In R. Hoffman, Z. E. Ben, S. Shattel, B. Furce, & M. Cohen (Eds.), *Hematology, basic principles and practice* (2nd ed., Chapter 65). New York: Churchill Livingstone.

Fuchs, E., & Segre, J. A. (2000). Stem cells: a new lease on life. *Cell*, 100, 143–155.

Geiger, H., True, J. M., de Haan, G., & Van Zant, G. (2001). Age- and stage-specific regulation patterns in the hematopoietic stem cell hierarchy. *Blood*, 98(10), 2966–2972.

Globerson, A., & Effros, R. B. (2000). Ageing of lymphocytes and lymphocytes in the aged. *Immunology Today*, 21, 515–521.

Goldstone, A. H., Burnett, A. K., Wheatley, K., Smith A. G., Hutchinson, R. M., & Clark, R. E. (2001). Attempts to improve treatment outcomes in acute myeloid leukemia (AML) in older patients: the results of the United Kingdom Medical Research Council AML 11 trial. *Blood*, 98, 1302–1311.

Golub, T. R., Barker, G. F., Lovett, M., & Gilliland, D. G. (1994). Fusion of PDGF receptor beta to a novel ets-like gene, tel, in chronic myelomonocytic leukemia with t(5;12) chromosomal translocation. *Cell,* 77, 307–316.

Grove, J. E., Bruscia, E., & Krause, D. S. (2004). Plasticity of bone marrow-derived stem cells. *Stem Cells,* 22, 487–500.

Guralnik, J. M., Eisenstaedt, R. S., Ferrucci, L., Klein, H. G., & Woodman, R. C. (2004). Prevalence of anemia in persons 65 years and older in the United States: evidence for a high rate of unexplained anemia. *Blood,* 104, 2263–2268.

Guzman, M. L., & Jordan, C. T. (2004). Considerations for targeting malignant stem cells in leukemia. *Cancer Control,* 11, 97–104.

Hanahan, D., & Weinberg, R. A. (2000). The hallmarks of cancer. *Cell,* 100, 57–70.

Harman, D. (1981). The aging process. *Proceedings of the National Academy of Sciences of the USA,* 78, 7124–7128.

Harrison, D. E. (1973). Normal production of erythrocytes by mouse marrow continuous for 73 months. *Proceedings of the National Academy of Sciences of the USA* 70, 3184–3188.

Harrison, D. E., Lerner, C., Hoppe, P. C., Carlson, G. A., & Alling, D. (1987). Large numbers of primitive stem cells are active simultaneously in aggregated embryo chimeric mice. *Blood,* 69, 773–777.

Heissig, B., Hattori, K., Dias, S., Friedrich, M., Ferris, B., Hackett, N. R., Crystal, R. G., Besmer, P., Lyden, D., Moore, M. A., Werb, Z., & Rafii, S. (2002). Recruitment of stem and progenitor cells from the bone marrow niche requires MMP-9 mediated release of kit-ligand. *Cell,* 109, 625–637.

Holden, C. (2004). Stem cell research. Advocates keep pot boiling as Bush plans new centers. *Science,* 305, 461.

Johnson, F. B., Sinclair, D. A., & Guarente, L. (1999). Molecular biology of aging. *Cell,* 96, 291–302.

Jordan, C. T. (2002). Unique molecular and cellular features of acute myelogenous leukemia stem cells. *Leukemia,* 16, 559–562.

Kawanishi, S., & Oikawa, S. (2004). Mechanism of telomere shortening by oxidative stress. *Annals of the New York Academy of the Sciences,* 1019, 278–284.

Kay, H. E. (1965). How many cell-generations? *Lancet,* 15, 418–419.

Kim, M., Moon, H. B., & Spangrude, G. J. (2003). Major age-related changes of mouse hematopoietic stem/progenitor cells. *Annals of the New York Academy of Sciences,* 996, 195–208.

Krtolica, A., Parrinello, S., Lockett, S., Desprez, P-Y., & Campisi, J. (2001). Senescent fibroblasts promote epithelial cell growth and tumorigenesis: A ling between cancer and aging. *Proceedings of the National Academy of Sciences of the USA,* 98, 12072–12077.

Lagasse, E., Connors, H., Al-Dhalmy, M., Reitsma, M., Dohse, M., Osborne, L., Wang, X., Finegold, M., Weissman, I. L., & Grompe, M. (2000). Purified hematopoietic stem cells can differentiate into hepatocytes *in vivo. Nature Medicine,* 6, 1229–1234.

Lapidot, T., Sirard, C., Vormoor, J., Murdoch, B., Hoang, T., Caceres-Cortes, J., Minden, M., Paterson, B., Caligiuri, M. A., & Dick, J. E. (1994). A cell initiating human acute myeloid leukaemia after transplantation into SCID mice. *Nature,* 367, 645–648.

Leith, C. P., Kopecky, K. J., Godwin, J., McConnell, T., Slovak, M. L., Chen, I. M., Head, D. R., Appelbaum, F. R., & Willman, C. L. (1997). Acute myeloid leukemia in the elderly: assessment of multi-drug resistance (MDR1) and cytogenetics distinguishes biologic subgroups with remarkably distinct responses to standard chemotherapy. A Southwest Oncology Group Study. *Blood,* 89, 3323–3329.

Liesveld, J. L., Jordan, C. T., & Phillips, G. L. (2004). The hematopoietic stem cell in myelodysplasia. *Stem Cells,* 22, 590–599.

Lipschitz, D. A., Mitchell, C. O., & Thompson, C. (1981). The anemia of senescence. *American Journal of Hematology,* 11, 47–54.

Lowenberg, B., Downing, J. R., & Burnett, A. (1999). Acute myeloid leukemia. *New England Journal of Medicine* 341, 1051–1062.

Malakoff, D. (2004). Election 2004. The calculus of making stem cells a campaign issue. *Science,* 305, 760.

Marley, S. B., Lewis, J. L., Davidson, R. J., Roberts, I. A., Dokal, I., Goldman, J. M., & Gordon, M. Y. (1999). Evidence for a continuous decline in haemopoietic cell function from birth: application to evaluating bone marrow failure in children. *British Journal of Haematology*, 106, 162–166.

Mayer, R. J., Davis, R. B., Schiffer, C. A., Berg, D. T., Powell, B. L., Schulman, P., Omura, G. A., Moore, J. O., Mclntyre, O. R., & Frei, E., 3rd (1994). Intensive postremission chemotherapy in adults with acute myeloid leukemia. *New England Journal of Medicine*, 331, 896–903.

Mezey, E., Key, S., Vogelsang, G., Szalayova, I., Lange, G. D., & Crain, B. (2003). Transplanted bone marrow generates new neurons in human brains. *Proceedings of the National Academy of Sciences of the USA*, 100, 1364–1369.

Miller, R. A. (2000). Effect of aging on T lymphocyte activation. *Vaccine*, 18, 1654–1660.

Miller, R. A., Chrisp, C., & Galecki, A. (1997). CD4 memory T cell levels predict life span in genetically heterogenous mice. *FASEB Journal*, 11, 775–783.

Mirro, J. Jr. (1992). Pathology and immunology of acute leukemia. *Leukemia*, 6 Suppl 4, 13–15.

Morrison, S. J., Wandycz, A. M., Akashi, K., Globerson, A., & Weissman, I. L. (1996). The aging of hematopoietic stem cells. *Nature Medicine*, 2, 1011–1016.

Muller, W. A. (1996). Pattern formation in the immortal Hydra. *Trends in Genetics*, 12, 91–96.

NCI. (2000). *SEER Cancer Statistics Review 1975–2000*.

Offner, F., Kerre, T., DeSmedt, M., & Plum, J. (1999). Bone marrow CD34+ cells generate fewer T cells in vitro with increasing age and following chemotherapy. *British Journal of Haematology*, 104, 801–808.

Ogden, D. A., & Mickliem, H. S. (1976). The fate of serially transplanted bone marrow cell populations from young and old donors. *Transplantation*, 22, 287–293.

Orkin, S. H., & Zon, L. I. (2002). Hematopoiesis and stem cells: plasticity versus developmental heterogeneity. *Nature Immunology*, 3, 323–328.

Owen, R. (1945). Immunogenetic consequences of vascular anastomoses between bovine twins. *Science*, 102, 400.

Penninx, B. W., Guralnik, J. M., Onder, G., Ferrucci, L., Wallace, R. B., & Pahor, M. (2003). Anemia and decline in physical performance among older persons. *American Journal of Medicine*, 115, 104–110.

Reya, T., Morrison, S. J., Clarke, M. F., & Weissman, I. L. (2001). Stem cells, cancer, and cancer stem cells. *Nature*, 414, 105–111.

Rowe, J. M., Anderson, J. W., Mazza, J. J., Bennett, J. M., Paietta, E., Hayes, F. A., Oette, D., Cassileth, P. A., Stadtmauer, E. A., & Wiernik, P. H. (1995). A randomized placebo-controlled phase III study of granulocyte-macrophage colony-stimulating factor in adult patients (>55–70 years of age) with acute myelogenous leukemia: A study of the Eastern Cooperative Oncology Group (E1490). *Blood*, 86, 457–462.

Schiller, G., & Lee, M. (1997). Long-term outcome of high-dose cytarabine-based consolidation chemotherapy for older patients with acute myelogenous leukemia. *Leukemia & Lymphoma*, 25, 111–119.

Schofield, R. (1978). The relationship between the spleen colony-forming cell and the haemopoietic stem cell. *Blood Cells*, 4, 7–25.

Siminovitch, L., McCulloch, E. A., & Till, J. E. (1963). The distribution of colony-forming cells among spleen colonies. *Journal of Cellular Physiology*, 62, 327–336.

Siminovitch, L., Till, J. E., & McCulloch, E. A. (1964). Decline in colony-forming ability of marrow cells subjected to serial transplantation into irradiated mice. *Journal of Cellular Physiology*, 64, 23–31.

Smith, L. G., Weissman, I. L., & Heimfeld, S. (1991). Clonal analysis of hematopoietic stem-cell differentiation in vivo. *Proceedings of the National Academy of Sciences of the USA*, 88, 2788–2792.

Spangrude, G. J., Brooks, D. M., & Tumas, D. B. (1995). Long-term repopulation of irradiated mice with limiting numbers of purified hematopoietic stem cells: in vivo expansion of stem cell phenotype but not function. *Blood*, 85, 1006–1016.

Spangrude, G. J., Heimfeld, S., & Weissman, I. L. (1988). Purification and characterization of mouse hematopoietic stem cells. *Science, 241,* 58–62.

Stone, R. M., Berg, D. T., George, S. L., Dodge, R. K., Paciucci, P. A., Schulman, P., Lee, E. J., Moore, J. O., Powell, B. L., & Schiffer, C. A. (1995). Granulocyte-macrophage colony-stimulating factor after initial chemotherapy for elderly patients with primary acute myelogenous leukemia. *New England Journal of Medicine, 332,* 1671–1677.

Sudo, K., Ema, H., Morita, Y., & Nakauchi, H. (2000). Age-associated characteristics of murine hematopoietic stem cells. *Journal of Experimental Medicine, 192,* 1273–1280.

Taichman, R. S., Reilly, M. J., & Emerson, S. G. (1996). Human osteoblasts support human hematopoietic progenitor cells in vitro bone marrow cultures. *Blood, 87,* 518–524.

Taylor, P. R., Reid, M. M., Stark, A. N., Brown, N., Hamilton, P. J., & Proctor, S. J. (1995). De novo acute myeloid leukemia in patients over 55-years-old: a population based study of incidence, treatment and outcome. *Leukemia, 9,* 231–237.

Terskikh, A. V., Miyamoto, T., Chang, C., Diatchenko, L., & Weissman, I. L. (2003). Gene expression analysis of purified hematopoietic stem cells and committed progenitors. *Blood, 102,* 94–101.

Till, J. E., & McCulloch, E. A. (1961). A direct measurement of the radiation sensitivity of normal mouse bone marrow cells. *Radiation Research, 14,* 1419–1430.

Van Zant, G., & Liang, Y. (2003). The role of stem cells in aging. *Experimental Hematolology, 31,* 659–672.

Van Zant, G., Eldridge, P. W., Behringer, R. R., & Dewey, M. J. (1983). Genetic control of hematopoietic kinetics revealed by analyses of allophenic mice and stem cell suicide. *Cell, 35,* 639–645.

Van Zant, G., Holland, B. P., Eldridge, P. W., & Chen, J. J. (1990). Genotype-restricted growth and aging patterns in hematopoietic stem cell populations of allophenic mice. *Journal of Experimental Medicine, 171,* 1547–1565.

Wagers, A. J., & Weissman, I. L. (2004). Plasticity of adult stem cells. *Cell, 116,* 639–648.

Wang, J. C. Y., Lapidot, T., Cashman, J. D., Doedens, M., Addy, L., Sutherland, D. R., Nayar, R., Laraya, P., Minden, M., Keating, A., Eaves, A. C., Eaves, C. J., & Dick, J. E. (1998). High level engraftment of NOD/SCID mice by primitive normal and leukemic hematopoietic cells from patients with chronic myeloid leukemia in chronic phase. *Blood, 91,* 2406–2414.

Weissman, I. L. (2000a). Stem cells: units of development, units of regeneration, and units in evolution. *Cell, 100,* 157–168.

Weissman, I. L. (2000b). Translating stem and progenitor cell biology to the clinic: barriers and opportunities. *Science, 287,* 1442–1446.

Wineman, J., Moore, K., Lemischka, I., & Muller-Sieburg, C. (1996). Functional heterogeneity of the hematopoietic microenvironment: rare stromal elements maintain long-term repopulating stem cells. *Blood, 87,* 4082–4090.

Yamamoto, K., Nakamura, Y., Saito, K., & Furusawa, S. (2000). Expression of the NUP98/HOXA9 fusion transcript in the blast crisis of Philadelphia chromosome-positive chronic myelogenous leukaemia with t(7;11)(p15;p15). *British Journal of Haematology, 109,* 423–426.

Zaucha, J. M., Yu, C., Mathioudakis, G., Seidel, K., Georges, G., Sale, G., Little, M. T., Torok-Storb, B., & Storb, R. (2001). Hematopoietic responses to stress conditions in young dogs compared with elderly dogs. *Blood, 98,* 322–327.

Zhu, J., & Emerson, S. G. (2004). A new bone to pick: osteoblasts and the haematopoietic stem-cell niche. *Bioessays, 26,* 595–599.

Chapter 5

Mitochondria: A Critical Role in Aging

Tamara R. Golden, Karl Morten, Felicity Johnson, Enrique Samper,
and Simon Melov

The mitochondrial theory of aging was proposed by Harman over 30 years ago (Harman, 1972), and though the past three decades have seen a plethora of correlative data in support of this theory, only recently has the hypothesis been tested directly. An outgrowth of the free-radical theory of aging (Harman, 1956), the mitochondrial theory of aging proposes that mitochondria are the source of the majority of reactive oxygen species (ROS) produced by the cell and that important targets of these mitochondrially generated ROS are mitochondrial components, including the mtDNA. According to the theory, age-related cumulative damage to the mtDNA causes a concomitant decrease in mitochondrial function and perhaps a further increase in the mitochondrial production of damaging free-radicals, leading to a "vicious cycle" of escalating ROS production and mtDNA damage. The reduced mitochondrial bioenergetic capability, as well as the increasing oxidative damage to cellular components, is hypothesized to contribute to the pathophysiology of aging.

I. The Mitochondrion

The mitochondrion is an essential organelle, playing a central role in much of metabolism. The site of oxidative phosphorylation, mitochondria provide the majority of energy, in the form of ATP, that fuels cellular processes. Electrons derived from the oxidation of dietary carbohydrate, fat, and protein are fed into the electron transport chain (ETC), localized in the inner mitochondrial membrane. The electrons are passed through the four ETC complexes before terminally combining with molecular oxygen to form water. In the process, an electrochemical gradient is formed across the inner mitochondrial membrane that drives the synthesis of ATP.

It has been estimated that as much as 0.4 to 4 percent of respired oxygen is converted to the radical superoxide in the course of normal oxidative metabolism (Boveris, 1984; Hansford et al., 1997). This superoxide is formed at sites in complexes I and III of the ETC (Boveris et al., 1976; Takeshige & Minakami, 1979; Turrens &

Boveris, 1980). In isolated brain mitochondria, the main site of mitochondrial radical production has been reported to be at complex I, on the matrix side of the inner mitochondrial membrane (Kudin *et al.*, 2004). However, debate surrounds the relative importance of each site *in vivo* and whether radicals are generated at high enough levels to cause damage to cellular components, including the mtDNA (Chen *et al.*, 2003; Liu *et al.*, 2002a; St-Pierre *et al.*, 2002).

Mammalian mtDNA is a circular genome of approximately 16,500 bp, encoding 13 polypeptides of the respiratory chain, two ribosomal RNAs and 22 tRNAs. In addition to the transcribed region, mtDNA also contains a non-coding D-loop region believed to be involved in mtDNA maintenance, replication, and transcription (Bogenhagen & Clayton, 2003; Gillum & Clayton, 1978; Holt & Jacobs, 2003). The remainder of the proteins required for mitochondrial function are encoded by nuclear genes. Mammalian cell culture models and studies in *S. cerevisiae* indicate that mtDNA molecules exist in nucleoids, discrete structures containing 2 to 10 mtDNA molecules combined with protein factors involved in replication and transcription (Iborra *et al.*, 2004; Legros *et al.*, 2004; Miyakawa *et al.*, 1987). The mitochondrial nucleoids appear to be directly tethered to the inner mitochondrial membrane and closely associated with the mitochondrial protein import machinery (Iborra *et al.*, 2004; Legros *et al.*, 2004). Attachment of mtDNA to the inner mitochondria membrane is proposed to facilitate respiratory chain assembly but also places mtDNA in close proximity to the major cellular site of ROS production, the ETC.

With hundreds of mitochondria per cell, and tens of mtDNA molecules per mitochondrion, an average cell may contain over a thousand copies of mtDNA. The mtDNA is inherited maternally, and numerous variants exist in the human population, but usually a single mtDNA variant populates an egg, resulting in a homoplasmic individual. Alternatively, more than one variant may be passed to the offspring, resulting in heteroplasmy, in which a single cell contains multiple different mtDNA sequences. Heteroplasmy can also develop as a result of the accumulation of somatic mutations to the mtDNA during the lifetime of the individual. In this case, the mutations are stochastic, with different unique mutations accumulating to different frequencies in each cell. The fraction of mitochondrial genomes that need to be mutated (the "mutational load" of a cell) *in vivo* before mitochondrial or cellular functions are affected remains unknown, although studies of mitochondrial disease have indicated that for dramatic phenotypes such as clinically significant myopathies, the majority of mtDNA needs to be mutant.

II. Evidence for Increased Oxidative Damage to Mitochondrial Components with Age

A. Mitochondrial DNA Mutations and Aging

The age-related increases in the levels of both oxidative damage and mutational load of mtDNA predicted by the mitochondrial theory of aging have been described in multiple species and organ systems. However, whether this damage affects mitochondrial function or significantly modulates the physiology of aging has remained controversial (Jacobs, 2003a,b; Pak *et al.*, 2003a,b).

Age-related duplications and concatenations of mtDNA were first described using electron microscopy (Piko & Matsumoto, 1977; Piko *et al.*, 1978). With the advent of PCR, age-related increases in large scale deletions of the mtDNA have been described in *C. elegans* (Melov *et al.*,

1994; Melov *et al.*, 1995a), *Drosophila melanogaster* (Yui *et al.*, 2003), mouse (Tanhauser & Laipis, 1995), rat (Filburn *et al.*, 1996), monkey (Lee *et al.*, 1993), and human (Cortopassi & Arnheim, 1990; Melov *et al.*, 1995b; Melov *et al.*, 1999a). New technologies have also shown that point mutations in the control region of human mtDNA increase with age (Michikawa *et al.*, 1999). However, determining the total mutational load of the mtDNA in any one tissue or cell remains a difficult proposition because age-related somatic mutations are stochastic, resulting in heteroplasmy. Generally, studies have focused on quantifying a specific deletion (e.g., the so-called "common deletion" in human mtDNA) or detecting point mutations through sequencing of a small segment of the mitochondrial genome. Neither of these approaches provides a comprehensive picture of the potential total mutational load in a cell or tissue.

Studies that have quantified specific mutations have found that the observed prevalence of any one mutation in aged tissue has been low, generally below 1 percent in homogenized tissue samples, though one report found the common deletion reached more than 10 percent in the putamen (Corral-Debrinski *et al.*, 1992). This is far below the level of mutational load known to be associated with pathology in mitochondrial diseases, in which a mutant form of mtDNA may be inherited from the mother (Holt *et al.*, 1988; Wallace, 1994). For example, characteristic mtDNA deletions are present at levels between 45 and 75 percent in affected tissues of patients with the mitochondrial disease Kearne Sayre Syndrome (KSS) (Zeviani *et al.*, 1988). In addition, cell culture studies in which mtDNA from one cell is introduced into a cell line depleted of its own mtDNA (ρ^0 cells), generating "cybrid" cells, indicate that a significant majority of the mitochondrial genomes (60 to 90 percent) must be mutant for a disease-related mutation to cause a phenotype (Hayashi *et al.*,

1991; King *et al.*, 1992; Trounce *et al.*, 1994). Therefore, it has remained unclear whether the age-related increases in mitochondrial mutations that have been detected can play a role in phenotypes associated with aging.

Two hypotheses have been formulated as to how age-related mtDNA mutations may be deleterious. The first is based on the observation that a single mutation can be found at very high levels within an individual cardiomyocyte (Khrapko *et al.*, 1999) or muscle fiber (Schwarze *et al.*, 1995; Wanagat *et al.*, 2001) and that these mutations co-localize with regions of impaired mitochondrial function (Fayet *et al.*, 2002; Wanagat *et al.*, 2002). This has lead to the hypothesis that discrete mutations may, through clonal expansion, reach a prevalence within a single cell at which they are capable of affecting the function of that cell. In this model, each cell would have its own unique mutation, making any one mutation difficult to detect when a homogenized tissue or population of cells is studied. Alternatively, it has been hypothesized that multiple, random mtDNA mutations may be present in an individual cell, and though each is in low amount, enough mutations accumulate such that a substantial fraction of the mtDNA in the cell is damaged, with significant phenotypes arising as a result.

Recent work in support of the first hypothesis includes studies of adult stem cells. Stem cells at the base of colonic crypts were discovered to accumulate deleterious mtDNA mutations at a relatively high frequency of 5×10^{-5} mutations per genome (Taylor *et al.*, 2003). In several cases, the mtDNA mutations reached levels of prevalence in the crypt cells at which they could be expected to affect tissue function. The authors attributed an age-related decline in cytochrome oxidase activity (complex IV of the ETC) in colonic crypts to this expansion of stem cell mtDNA mutations.

The second hypothesis, that an increase in random mtDNA mutations can influence aging, is supported by work demonstrating that a high load of point mutations accumulates in agedhuman brain, such that as many as three mutations per mitochondrial genome are present in aged individuals (Simon *et al.*, 2004). In addition, this hypothesis was directly tested by a recent study that demonstrated the importance of mtDNA maintenance (Trifunovic *et al.*, 2004). In this study, the endogenous mouse mitochondrial DNA polymerase (PolgA) was replaced with an enzyme with reduced exonuclease activity, resulting in impaired proofreading during DNA replication. The load of point mutations per mtDNA molecule increased approximately threefold, although no single mutation or "hot spot" for mutations was observed. In addition, the total amount of mtDNA decreased by 30 percent, although mitochondrial transcript levels remained unchanged. The increase in mutational load resulted in reduced life span, and the development of some age-related pathologies, including loss of bone density, weight loss, cardiomyopathy, anemia, and reduced fertility. This mouse model demonstrates that it is possible for an increase in random mtDNA mutations to affect tissue function and supports the hypothesis that the age-related increase in mutational load described in many systems could potentially contribute to some of the phenotypes associated with aging.

Because maternally transmitted mtDNA mutations are more likely to be homoplasmic, they are much easier to associate with a disease or aging than the random somatic mtDNA mutations generated as a result of oxidative damage. In combination with certain nuclear backgrounds or environmental factors, specific mtDNA variants may affect respiratory chain function and aging (Chinnery *et al.*, 1999; Niemi *et al.*, 2003). The mtDNA D-loop variant has been best characterized in relation to age-related conditions. In this variant, cytosine replaces thymidine at position 16,189,

resulting in a very long polycytosine tract in the D-loop region of the mtDNA. It is believed that this results in mitochondrial DNA polymerase slippage during replication, resulting in a heteroplasmic length variation of the tract (Marchington *et al.*, 1997). It has been proposed that subsequent instability in the D-loop region, which plays a role in mtDNA replication and transcription, could result in reduced mtDNA copy number over time (Poulton *et al.*, 1998). The 16,189 variant has been shown to have a positive association with type II diabetes, dilated cardiomyopathy, low body fat at birth, iron loading associations in haemachromatosis, and stroke (Casteels *et al.*, 1999; Kim *et al.*, 2002; Liou *et al.*, 2004; Livesey *et al.*, 2004; Poulton *et al.*, 2002), although this has not been confirmed in other studies (Gibson *et al.*, 2004; Gill-Randall *et al.*, 2001).

A recent study identified a novel mitochondrial mutation that can be a risk factor in a set of the most common age-related diseases. Wilson and colleagues identified an mtDNA mutation that predisposed a family to hypomagnesemia, hypertension, and hypercholesterolemia, all risk factors for cardiovascular disease (Wilson *et al.*, 2004). Interestingly, the mutation did not increase incidence of type II diabetes or insulin resistance, phenotypes frequently observed with mitochondrial DNA mutations (discussed below). How the mutation, which impairs the ability of tRNA^{Ile} to bind to the ribosome, causes the phenotypes measured is unknown, but the study supports the hypothesis that mtDNA mutations can contribute to age-related phenotypes.

B. Oxidative Damage to Mitochondrial Proteins and Membranes and Aging

Numerous studies have been aimed at detecting age-related increases in oxidative damage to protein or lipid components of the mitochondrion (Berlett & Stadtman, 1997; Linton *et al.*, 2001). Aging has been

---

associated with both an increase in oxidative damage to proteins and a decrease in protein turnover and repair (Stadtman, 2004). The age-related increase in protein modifications includes cross-linkages, fragmentation, carbonylation, glycation, and advanced glycation endproduct (AGE) formation (Berlett & Stadtman, 1997). Recent evidence indicates that in blood lymphocytes, some proteins are selectively modified with age (Poggioli *et al.*, 2004), indicating that there may be a nonrandom pattern of protein damage associated with aging. Oxidative damage to proteins may lead to dysfunction and/or aggregation of the damaged proteins, which can result in their being targeted for removal and degradation (Cuervo & Dice, 1998; Levine, 2002).

Numerous lines of evidence support mitochondria as the primary source of ROS (Chance *et al.*, 1979; Li *et al.*, 1995). Hence, mitochondrial proteins, including the complexes of the ETC and members of other metabolic pathways, are likely to be particularly susceptible to modifications as a result of oxidative damage. Certain cellular components are known to be sensitive to oxidative stress. Specifically, proteins containing iron-sulfur clusters (Fe-S proteins) are highly sensitive to superoxide. This is exemplified in the *sod2* nullizygous mouse model, which lacks the mitochondrial form of superoxide dismutase (SOD2)(Li *et al.*, 1995). Activities of two Fe-S containing enzymes, aconitase and succinate dehydrogenase (SDH, complex II of the ETC), are severely decreased in multiple tissues in this model (Hinerfeld *et al.*, 2004; Li *et al.*, 1995; Melov *et al.*, 1998; Melov *et al.*, 1999b), and protein levels of SDH have been demonstrated to be depressed in mitochondria isolated from the cerebral cortex of these mice (Hinerfeld *et al.*, 2004). Superoxide is proposed to oxidize 4Fe-4S clusters, resulting in the release of free iron (Flint *et al.*, 1993). In the case of the SOD2 null mouse, it is

hypothesized that elevated levels of superoxide disrupt a structurally important Fe-S cluster of SDH, resulting in reduced levels of assembled complex in the mitochondria (Hinerfeld *et al.*, 2004).

Aconitase has been specifically examined as a target of oxidative damage with respect to aging. In the house fly (Yan *et al.*, 1997), oxidation to mitochondrial aconitase was found to increase with age, and a corresponding age-related decrease in aconitase activity was described. The adenine nucleotide translocase has also been identified as a mitochondrial protein that increasingly is oxidatively damaged with age in flies (Yan & Sohal, 1998). In other studies via proteomic profiling, heart mitochondrial protein was compared in young and old rats (Kanski *et al.*, 2004), resulting in the identification of oxidative modifications to 48 proteins with age. Among the group were many metabolic enzymes, including succinate dehydrogenase and aconitase (Kanski *et al.*, 2004). In addition, numerous oxidatively modified proteins have been identified in bovine heart sub-mitochondrial particles, the majority localized in the mitochondrial matrix (Choksi *et al.*, 2004).

Once damaged, mitochondrial proteins are removed and recycled either via autophagy, where the entire organelle is degraded by lysosomal enzymes, or via the mitochondrion's own internal protein turnover mechanisms. Studies indicate that protein turnover declines with age, although surprisingly little is known about the mechanisms of mitochondrial protein degradation. Recent studies define the AAA proteases, which are ATP-dependent, membrane-bound, and responsible for membrane protein turnover in mitochondria, chloroplasts, and eubacteria (Korbel *et al.*, 2004). Mitochondrial forms of this protease from *S. cerevisiae* appear to play a direct role in dismantling the proteins embedded in the mitochondrial membrane (Korbel *et al.*, 2004). In aged mice, it was found that as levels of a mitochondrial protease (Lon protease) decreased with age, levels of oxidatively modified proteins, specifically aconitase, increased with age (Bota *et al.*, 2002).

Membrane lipids are also major targets of cellular damage induced by oxygen radicals. In the mitochondria, this problem is particularly acute because of the close proximity of mitochondrial membranes to the sites of ROS production. Although the mechanism of superoxide-induced lipid peroxidation is not fully understood, it is proposed to occur via the reaction of superoxide with nitric oxide, producing the potent oxidant peroxynitrite (Rubbo *et al.*, 1994). Nitric oxide can freely diffuse across membranes and is produced in a variety of mammalian cells, including endothelium, neuronal cells, smooth muscle cells, macrophages, platelets, and fibroblasts.

Polyunsaturated fatty acids of membrane lipids are susceptible to peroxidation by ROS (Esterbauer *et al.*, 1991). The lipid peroxides (lipid-OOH) formed can decompose in the presence of transition metals such as iron to give alkoxy (lipid-O) radicals. These lipid radicals may alter membrane fluidity and subsequently affect the activity of membrane-bound proteins and membrane permeability, ultimately leading to cell degeneration (Gutteridge *et al.*, 1979; Halliwell & Gutteridge, 1984). Studies have shown that lipid peroxidation levels are increased in patients with neurodegenerative diseases such as Alzheimer's disease, where lipoprotein oxidation is increased in the cerebrospinal fluid of patients compared to age-matched controls (Sayre *et al.*, 1997). Lipid peroxidation also results in the fragmentation of polyunsaturated fatty acids, giving rise to aldehydes, alkenals, and hydroxyalkenals such as malonaldehyde and 4-hydroxynonenal (HNE) (Esterbauer *et al.*, 1991), which have been implicated in the damage of protein and DNA.

The HNE lipid peroxidation product is particularly reactive, with levels increased in hypertrophic and ischemic/reperfusion damaged hearts (Eaton *et al.*, 1999). Recent evidence indicates that the formation of HNE-protein adducts is a key event in many free-radical-related effects in the heart and other tissues (Poli & Schaur, 2000), and that aging increases the susceptibility to these modifications (Lucas & Szweda, 1998). The mitochondrial proteins pyruvate dehydrogenase E2 subunit and NADP+-isocitrate dehydrogenase appear particularly sensitive to HNE attack and inactivation (Benderdour *et al.*, 2003; Millar & Leaver, 2000). Interestingly, several recent reports suggest that the superoxide-generated lipid peroxidation product HNE has a direct signaling role in reducing further superoxide production by activating the mitochondrial uncoupling protein UCP2 and ANT (Brand *et al.*, 2004). It has been proposed that the regulation of respiratory chain activity by superoxide and lipid peroxidation could be important in cells exposed to a fluctuating mixture of glucose and fatty acids and may coordinate the response to a variable nutrient supply (Brand *et al.*, 2004).

According to the mitochondrial theory of aging, the accumulation of damage to mitochondrial components, including mtDNA, protein, and lipid, should affect mitochondrial function. However, to date, convincing evidence for an age-related decline in mitochondrial function or bioenergetic capacity has been lacking, primarily due to the lack of application of appropriate tools for measuring mitochondrial function with age coupled with an expertise in biogerontology.

III. Mitochondrial Dysfunction and Aging

A. Mitochondria Function and Longevity

Several studies suggest that mitochondrial structure and function decline with age in human and animal tissue samples (Bowling *et al.*, 1993; Gabbita *et al.*, 1997;

Ojaimi *et al.*, 1999; Sugiyama *et al.*, 1993; Takasawa *et al.*, 1993), cultured human fibroblasts (Greco *et al.*, 2003), and in human skeletal muscle *in vivo* (Wilson *et al.*, 2004). In contrast, other studies have found no decrease in mitochondrial function with age (Barrientos *et al.*, 1996; Sharman & Bondy, 2001; Takai *et al.*, 1995; Zucchini *et al.*, 1995). Frequently, studies that do describe an age-related effect find that the mitochondrial complexes affected, and the degree of change in activity, are tissue-specific. Generally, it appears that complex I of the ETC is most likely to decrease with age, and post-mitotic tissues such as heart and brain are more likely to be affected than mitotic tissues such as liver (Bowling *et al.*, 1993; Sugiyama *et al.*, 1993; Takasawa *et al.*, 1993).

Additional evidence of mitochondrial dysfunction accompanying aging of post-mitotic cells is the appearance of enlarged mitochondria, showing partial loss of cristae, swelling, and mtDNA damage (Beregi *et al.*, 1988; Coleman *et al.*, 1987; Terman *et al.*, 2004). These bioenergetically impaired and enlarged organelles have been termed *giant mitochondria* and appear to coexist with their smaller counterparts in a heterogeneous pool. Autophagocytosis has been determined to be important to the development of this mixed population of mitochondria (Terman *et al.*, 2003). By studying cultured cardiomyocytes, with and without an inhibitor of autophagy, it was concluded that the appearance of giant mitochondria with age was due to selective recycling. Smaller mitochondria displayed a faster turnover, accumulating more rapidly but also returning to pretreatment levels once the inhibitor was removed. In contrast, the accumulation of giant mitochondria was less rapid but irreversible, indicating evasion of autophagy could play a critical role in the mitochondrial population of an aging cell.

In cell culture experiments, several attributes of mitochondrial function were found to decline with age in fibroblasts from 53 human donors ranging in age from 1 to 103 years old (Greco *et al.*, 2003). Specifically, mitochondrial protein synthesis rates, control of complex I over respiration rates, control of mitochondrial membrane potential over respiration rates, coupling efficiency of ATP synthesis to oxygen consumption (P:O ratio), and the control of ADP over respiration rates (RCR) were found to decrease significantly with age. In addition, the authors observed a trend toward a decrease in mtDNA content and toward a decrease in respiration rates with age. Unfortunately, when cell cultures are used—even low-passage cultures such as in this study—it is difficult to rule out an effect of donor age on the adaptation of the fibroblasts to culture that might contribute to the effects measured.

Similarly, studies of isolated mitochondria prepared from tissue biopsies are complicated by the potential that mitochondria from older individuals might be more fragile or otherwise differently affected by preparation methods, thereby affecting the experimental outcome. Therefore, *in vivo* studies are especially relevant to understanding whether mitochondrial function truly changes with age. Recently, a 40 percent decrease in oxidative phosphorylation capacity of skeletal muscle was reported between young (18- to 39-year-old) and older (61- to 84-year-old) individuals measured *in vivo* (Petersen *et al.*, 2003). Unlike Greco *et al*, these authors propose that the age-related decline they observed is due to a loss of mitochondrial number or function rather than a decrease in coupling. There is a great need for more *in vivo* studies of this type to better understand the dynamics of mitochondrial function with age.

One approach that may help answer whether it is the coupling of mitochondrial bioenergetic functions or the activities of rate-limiting mitochondrial enzymes that are declining with age may be use of

Metabolic Control Analysis (MCA). MCA can be applied to determine the capacity of the mitochondrion to regulate metabolism via different enzyme components in the key pathways. This approach considers that at any one time, a pathway shares the control of the pathway's flux or "flow-through" among the components of that pathway. Using inhibitors of each individual step of the pathway, the relative control of each step over the entire pathway (the flux control coefficient for that step) is experimentally determined. These empirical measurements can form the basis of mathematical models, allowing one to predict the response of the pathway to a perturbation. MCA reveals the degree of plasticity a particular pathway has at any one time but does not tell us definitively what is happening *in vivo*. And to the extent that measurements are made on isolated enzymes or mitochondria, MCA is subject to the same concerns discussed above regarding the preparation of intact mitochondria from aged tissues. Likewise, it does not tell us what occurs in the long term, but instead gives a window into one time point in the dynamic process of aging.

MCA has been increasingly used to describe mitochondrial function in a variety of biological contexts. MCA has described the suprastructure of the ETC (Bianchi *et al.*, 2004), demonstrating that complexes I and III are associated with each other. This work led the field into new paradigms, where ETC complexes in selective "supercomplexes" act as single enzymes with respect to Coenzyme Q. Whether the supercomplexes are always in association or selectively associate at different stages of cell development remains to be determined. MCA has also been applied to describing the relationship between the TCA cycle, oxidative phosphorylation, and mitochondrial Ca^{2+} dynamics in heart mitochondria (Cortassa *et al.*, 2003) and between ATP production, heme biosynthesis, and phos-

pholipid synthesis (Vo *et al.*, 2004) in human cardiac mitochondria. In the latter case, computation of a subset of the optimal flux distributions for each of the pathways examined showed high correlations, indicating that the *in silico* modeling results were more likely to be of physiological significance (Vo *et al.*, 2004). MCA has been applied to aging in rat liver mitochondria, where it revealed an age-related decrease in respiration and the control of respiration under conditions of maximum respiration (Darnold *et al.*, 1990). These studies reveal the power of metabolic control analysis in exploring the daunting complexity of mitochondrial biochemistry and bioenergetics as they relate to disease and aging.

Although control coefficients have long been used to describe the weight of one enzyme in a pathway on the flux of that pathway, thresholds and their associated hypotheses are relatively new. The threshold of an ETC complex describes the amount of its contribution that may be inhibited before the total electron flux is affected. This concept has been applied to understanding the mutational load required for biochemical defects in mitochondrial diseases (Davey & Clark, 1996; Mazat *et al.*, 2001; Rossignol *et al.*, 1999). The flux through the ETC is relevant to the aging process because it is related to the rate of production of ROS. Small reductions in metabolic flux through the ETC occur at the cost of increased upstream substrate levels (Mazat *et al.*, 2001). This increased concentration of reduced upstream substrates allows a larger generation of ROS. This idea is supported by the observation that mice with a greater proton leak live longer (Speakman *et al.*, 2004). The impaired mitochondrial ETC activities reported in the work discussed above may result in increased ROS production, which would be expected to damage mitochondrial components, and may even damage the nuclear DNA, as discussed below.

B. Mitochondrial Dysfunction and Genetic Instability in Aging

It has been speculated that the mitochondrial genome can sustain more DNA damage than the nuclear genome without critical loss of function because there are thousands of mitochondrial genomes per cell (Lieber & Karanjawala, 2004) and because wobble in the genetic code of the mtDNA allows for more mutation in protein coding regions without concomitant changes in amino acid sequence. Recently it has been shown that mice deficient in Rnaseh1, a critical factor for mitochondrial DNA replication, show an embryonic lethal phenotype at days 8.5 to 10.5 of embryonic development (E8.5–E10.5), highlighting the essential role of mitochondrial DNA during development (Cerritelli *et al.*, 2003). The Rnaseh1 null embryos have only 1 percent of the normal levels of mitochondrial DNA by E8.5 and undetectable levels of cytochrome oxidase (COX-1) activity, indicating a severe mitochondrial dysfunction. This mitochondrial dysfunction leads to massive apoptosis at day 9.5 of embryonic development. Of note, mice deficient in mitochondrial transcription factor A (mtTFA−/−) show similar developmental abnormalities and apoptosis in embryos and in the hearts of conditional knock-out mtTFA−/− animals (Larsson *et al.*, 1998).

Initial evidence that mitochondrial dysfunction can lead to nuclear damage comes from studies in which Paraquat, a superoxide generator and mitochondrial toxin, induced chromosomal instability in Chinese hamster fibroblasts (Nicotera *et al.*, 1985). Additional recent studies have shown that primary mouse zygotes treated with the protonophore FCCP undergo mitochondrial membrane depolarization, increased ROS production, reduced viability, and induced chromosomal transloca-

tions and end-to-end fusions (Liu *et al.*, 2002b). The onset of genomic instability in the FCCP-treated mouse zygotes was ameliorated by the antioxidant NAC, a thiol-reducing antioxidant, verifying that the induced ROS are responsible for this insult. The relationship between mitochondrial dysfunction and nuclear DNA damage was strengthened by a recent study showing that primary $sod2^{-/-}$ mouse embryonic fibroblasts display increased levels of superoxide, leading directly or indirectly to nuclear gene destabilization, including very high levels of non-reciprocal translocations as well as chromosomal breaks and fragments and end-to-end fusions (Samper *et al.*, 2003). This highlights the importance of mitochondrial function in the absence of chemical inhibitors for the maintenance of genomic integrity. Therefore, there is increasing evidence that mitochondrial dysfunction and ROS production can lead to nuclear genomic instability in a variety of cases, thereby establishing a novel link between mitochondria and genomic stability in cancer and aging.

Evidence for the relationship between genomic instability and aging is increasing steadily. To date, all "premature aging" syndromes in humans, including Down syndrome (Maluf & Erdtmann, 2001; Scarfi *et al.*, 1990; Shubber *et al.*, 1991), dyskeratosis congenita (Marciniak *et al.*, 2000; Vulliamy *et al.*, 2001), HS progeria (De Sandre-Giovannoli *et al.*, 2003; Eriksson *et al.*, 2003), Werner syndrome (Epstein, 1985), and ataxia telangiectasia (Barlow *et al.*, 1996) show increased levels of genomic instability or have defects in nuclear architecture. These "premature aging" syndromes recapitulate several, though not all, aspects of normal aging (for an excellent discussion of the merits and drawbacks of "accelerated aging" models and paradigms, see Hasty *et al.*, 2003; Hasty and Vijg, 2004a,b; Miller, 2004a,b). The premature aging phenotypes associated with these diseases can be recapitulated in mice deficient for DNA repair, such as mice deficient in ATM (Wong *et al.*, 2003), Ku86−/− (Vogel *et al.*, 1999), WRN−/− (Chang *et al.*, 2004), telomerase (Herrera *et al.*, 1999; Rudolph *et al.*, 1999; Samper *et al.*, 2001), and XPD (de Boer *et al.*, 2002), among others. In the case of mice deficient for telomerase, ATM, and WRN, a "premature aging" phenotype is displayed when the substantial telomere reserve of laboratory *Mus musculus* is eroded by progressive generations in the absence of telomerase. In addition to deficiency in DNA repair or transcription, defects in DNA segregation can lead to profound premature aging. The hypomorphic mutation of BubR1, a spindle assembly checkpoint protein, again shows progressive levels of aneuploidy with age and a whole array of "premature aging" phenotypes *in vivo* (Baker *et al.*, 2004).

C. Mitochondrial Dysfunction and DNA Instability in Cancer

Cancer is predominantly a disease of old age, as its incidence increases exponentially with age. It was recognized by Warburg more than 50 years ago that the metabolism of cancer cells appears to shift toward glycolysis instead of oxidative phosphorylation for ATP production, indicating that there may be a connection between mitochondrial function and cancer (Warburg, 1956). One of the most accepted hallmarks of cancer cells is aneuploidy, an imbalance in DNA copy number of either whole or partial chromosomes (Lengauer *et al.*, 1998). This DNA imbalance can arise via many different paths, from defects in DNA repair, DNA segregation, cell cycle proteins, increased mitogenic signaling, and possibly mitochondrial dysfunction. Conceptually, mitochondrial dysfunction can precipitate the onset of nuclear genomic instability by a variety of mechanisms. For example, mitochondrial dysfunction can lead to the increased production of ROS, direct oxida-

tion/ breakage of DNA, increased mitogenic signaling, reduction in DNA repair, or increased oxidation of zinc finger-containing proteins such as Sp-1 or P53 (Hainaut & Mann, 2001; Hussain *et al.*, 2003; Vafa *et al.*, 2002; Woo & Poon, 2004). At a more molecular level, it has been shown that increased ROS drive the Ras mitogenic signaling cascades and result in chromosomal aneuploidy (Arnold *et al.*, 2001; Irani *et al.*, 1997; Lee *et al.*, 1999; Woo & Poon, 2004).

When investigators began searching for mechanistic links between mitochondrial dysfunction and colorectal carcinogenesis, they discovered that up to 70 percent of human colorectal tumors show mutations in the mitochondrial DNA (Polyak *et al.*, 1998). Further support for a role of mitochondrial dysfunction in cancer comes from a variety of studies that have shown that mutations in the nuclear genes SDHB, SDHC, and SDHD, which encode subunits of the mitochondrial complex II (Succinate dehydrogenase), predispose patients to paragangliomas (head and neck tumors of the parasympathetic ganglia) and pheochromocytoma (catecholamine-producing tumors of the adrenal ganglia)(Astuti *et al.*, 2001; Baysal *et al.*, 2000; Gimm *et al.*, 2000; Niemann & Muller, 2000). Additional evidence that mitochondrial function is important in transformation comes from studies that show that mutations in fumarate hydratase, an enzyme of the TCA cycle, are associated with human neoplasias (Lehtonen *et al.*, 2004; Tomlinson *et al.*, 2002). The fumarate hydratase gene is a tumor-suppressor protein that, when mutated, predisposes patients to uterine fibroids and leiomyomata (benign smooth muscle tumors) together with an associated predisposition to type II renal cell carcinoma. In the case of germline mutations of fumarate hydratase, patients usually survive a few months, with a maximal life span of approximately 30 years (Tomlinson *et al.*, 2002).

Additional evidence comes from studies of the Superoxide dismutase 2 (*sod2*) gene, the main defense against ROS in the mitochondria. The *sod2* gene is thought to be a novel tumor suppressor (Kinnula & Crapo, 2004). Certain polymorphisms in the *sod2* gene have been found to correlate with higher incidence of breast cancer (Mitrunen *et al.*, 2001). Importantly, the *sod2* locus at 6q25 in human cells is frequently deleted in a number of lymphomas and other tumors. The exact role of SOD2 as a tumor suppressor is still being elucidated. Two possibilities are that increased steady-state levels of superoxide may lead to increased mutagenesis of tumor suppressor genes, increased proliferation, or decreased DNA repair. Alternatively, *sod2* mutations may induce tumorigenesis by inactivating mitochondrial complex II (SDH) (see above).

Direct support for the role of SOD2 as a novel tumor suppressor comes from recent studies of the laboratory of Dr. Arlan Richardson that have indicated that mice hemizygous for *sod2* have a 61 percent incidence of lymphoma at 24 to 28 months of age versus an incidence of 22 percent in the wild-type mice (Van Remmen *et al.*, 2003). It is noteworthy that the increased lymphomagenesis has been attributed to an increase in the stages of initiation and/or promotion rather than to an increase in aggressiveness as measured by PCNA positivity and pathological grade staging.

It was recently argued that mice hemizygous for *sod2* constitute a test of the free-radical theory of aging (Van Remmen *et al.*, 2003). Because the mice exhibit increased levels of oxidative damage due to the lack of one copy of *sod2*, they were hypothesized to have a shortened life span, but they did not. This result is interesting, especially in light of the increased cancer incidence, but a great deal of caution should be used when interpreting negative results, particularly in the context of genetic models. For example, it was estab-

lished in the early 1990s that mutations in the amyloid precursor protein (APP) could cause a familial form of Alzheimer's disease (AD). Consequently, many groups undertook the construction of transgenic mice that overexpressed the mutant form of APP in the hopes of faithfully recapitulating key features of the neuropathology of AD. It was learned that choice of genetic background was a critical feature for creation of a mouse model of AD. Early mouse models of the transgenic overexpression of mutant APP (in FVB/N mice) did not recapitulate any aspects of the neuropathology of AD but did cause an early death (Hsiao *et al.*, 1995). Some of these authors went on to develop different mouse models, experimenting with the APP gene on different genetic backgrounds, and in 1996 they published what was hailed as the first broadly successful animal model of AD (Hsiao *et al.*, 1996). The take-home message is that genetic background, choice of promoter, tissue specificity, and compensatory processes within the animal as a result of expression or lack of expression of a gene all can confound the interpretation of the result. With respect to *sod2*, it is interesting to contrast the lack of an effect on life span in the heterozygous mouse with the increase in life span observed when *sod2* is overexpressed in *Drosophila* (Sun *et al.*, 2002). Perhaps endogenous levels of superoxide-related damage are limiting under laboratory conditions for *Drosophila* but are not for mice on a C57BL/6 genetic background under the environmental conditions used in this study (Van Remmen *et al.*, 2003).

IV. Mitochondrial Dysfunction and Age-Associated Disease

A. Mitochondrial Dysfunction in Alzheimer's and Parkinson's Diseases

In addition to the potential association between mitochondrial function and cancer discussed above, age-related neurodegenerative disorders, including Alzheimer's and Parkinson's diseases, as well as the age-related metabolic disorder type II diabetes, have long been associated with mitochondrial dysfunction (Bonilla *et al.*, 1999; Duara *et al.*, 1986; Maassen *et al.*, 2004; Metter *et al.*, 1990; Ristow, 2004; Sims *et al.*, 1980). Evidence of damage to mitochondria, as well as evidence of decreased mitochondrial function, has been associated with each of these age-associated diseases.

Respiratory chain dysfunction has been transmitted to cybrid cells by introducing mtDNA from cells of Alzheimer's and Parkinson's patients (Khan *et al.*, 2000; Trimmer *et al.*, 2004; Veech *et al.*, 2000), despite the fact that no obvious mutations were detected in the mtDNA. It has been argued that mtDNA from these patients may contain multiple stochastic mtDNA mutations, the levels of which are too low to detect via standard approaches. In other studies, numerous known deleterious mtDNA mutations were identified in brains of Alzheimer's patients (Coskun *et al.*, 2004).

Histochemical evidence suggests that mitochondrial function is impaired in the brains of patients with Alzheimer's disease (AD) (Hirai *et al.*, 2001). Also, in the early stages of Alzheimer's disease, there is reduced brain glucose utilization (Chandrasekaran *et al.*, 1996; Rapoport *et al.*, 1996), yet it is difficult to determine the role of mitochondrial dysfunction in Alzheimer's disease. There is much evidence of oxidative damage in AD brains; however, chronic inflammation is associated with AD and can be a source of ROS, and recent studies indicate that the amyloid plaques associated with the disease are themselves a source of ROS (Bush *et al.*, 1999; McLellan *et al.*, 2003). In addition, beta-amyloid, widely believed to be to be a key factor in the disease, can directly inhibit mitochondrial enzymes (Casley *et al.*, 2002). Hence, though reduced mitochondrial function may be

associated with the disease, it is not possible to assign cause and effect.

A role for mitochondrial function is easier to support in Parkinson's disease (PD). As with AD, familial cases of PD have been highly informative in identifying candidate proteins and pathways that may be involved in the more abundant sporadic PD. Genetic studies have identified mutations in proteins associated with the formation of Lewy bodies (alpha-synuclein), protein degradation (ubiquitin carboxy-terminal hydrolase-1 and parkin), and in the cell's oxidative stress response (DJ-1) (Bonifati *et al.*, 2003; Kitada *et al.*, 1998; Leroy *et al.*, 1998; Singleton *et al.*, 2003). A series of common themes are emerging from these studies that implicate the mitochondrion as the central player in PD. Overexpression of alpha-synuclein and inactivation of parkin both result in mitochondrial dysfunction (Beal, 2004; Palacino *et al.*, 2004). Inhibition of mitochondrial complex I leads to the increased production and aggregation of alpha synuclein and impairs the ubiquitin-proteosome system (Shamoto-Nagai *et al.*, 2003; Sherer *et al.*, 2002). The normal form of DJ-1 protects against oxidative stress, whereas the mutant form associated with familial PD does not. The recent discovery of mutations in PINK-1, a putative mitochondrial protein kinase, which directly cause PD adds even more weight to the hypothesis that mitochondria play a pivotal role in the development of PD (Valente *et al.*, 2004).

Parkinson's disease is associated with a profound and selective loss of dopaminergic neurons in the nigrostriatal pathway of the brain (Graybiel *et al.*, 1990). Postmortem studies have consistently implicated oxidative damage in PD pathogenesis (Jenner, 2003). Dopamine metabolism and/or mitochondrial dysfunction are the leading candidates for the source of damaging radicals (Beal, 2003; Fiskum *et al.*, 2003). One of the earliest observations linking mitochondrial dysfunction to the development of Parkinson's disease came from the accidental exposure of a group of intravenous drug users to the compound 1-methyl-4-phenyl-1,2,5,6-tetrahydropyridine (MPTP) (Langston *et al.*, 1983). Exposure to the complex I inhibitor MPTP resulted in an acute and permanent form of Parkinson's disease. Epidemiological studies also suggest that environmental agents, including pesticides, might be important factors in PD pathogenesis (Di Monte *et al.*, 2002). When administered to rats, the pesticide rotenone (a mitochondrial complex I inhibitor) caused a Parkinson's-like pathology (Betarbet *et al.*, 2000).

B. Age-Related Mitochondrial Dysfunction and Type II Diabetes

Type II diabetes is now well established as a polygenic disease linked to numerous polymorphisms, none of which individually appears capable of causing the disease (Gloyn, 2003). The primary cause of type II diabetes is unknown; whether the development of insulin resistance or failure of pancreatic β-cells to produce insulin is the primary cause is an area of intense debate (for reviews see Ashcroft & Rorsman, 2004; Saltiel & Kahn, 2001). Mitochondrial dysfunction has long been known to cause diabetes, as pathogenic mtDNA mutations are associated with mitochondrial encephalopathy lactic acidosis and stroke-like episodes (MELAS) and Kearne Sayre Syndrome, causing diabetes as part of these multisystem disorders (Maassen *et al.*, 2004). Although the mtDNA 3,243 bp tRNA leucine mutation causes the severe MELAS syndrome when found at high levels, at low levels the mutation can cause diabetes with no other tissue involvement (Guillausseau *et al.*, 2001; Maassen, 2002; Suzuki, 2004). A recent report examining levels of the mtDNA 3243 tRNA leucine mutation in a diabetic patient showed that levels of the mutation did not rise above 30 percent in the pancreatic islets and indi-

vidual β-cells, while much higher levels (>60 percent) were found in muscle and brain with no obvious pathology (Lynn *et al.*, 2003). This suggests that β-cells may be especially sensitive to mitochondrial dysfunction.

There is a growing body of evidence implicating mitochondrial dysfunction as a key risk factor in the development of both insulin resistance and β-cell failure in type II diabetes. Two recent gene-expression studies on muscle from type II diabetics showed a coordinate reduction of genes involved in oxidative phosphorylation (Mootha *et al.*, 2003; Patti *et al.*, 2003). This is consistent with an earlier finding that decreased whole-body aerobic capacity is decreased in type II diabetics and their first-degree relatives (Nyholm *et al.*, 1996; Schneider *et al.*, 1984).

One of the characteristics of human type II diabetes is the link between obesity and the development of the disease. The accumulation of triglycerides in the muscle of diabetics has led to the proposition that reduced glucose uptake, in conjunction with increased fatty acid oxidation, results in increased mitochondrial ROS production. This is supported by a recent report that showed that heart and skeletal muscle mitochondria, although producing very little superoxide or hydrogen peroxide when respiring on complex I or II substrates, produced large amounts of superoxide from complex I when respiring on the fatty acid palmityl carnitine (St-Pierre *et al.*, 2002). In addition, fatty acids are particularly prone to oxidative damage, forming cytotoxic lipid peroxides that can further damage DNA and proteins as discussed above. One study suggests that increasing the load of fatty acids on the mitochondrial membrane will lead to the entrance of neutral fatty acids into the mitochondrial matrix where they are prone to oxidation (Ho *et al.*, 2002). Consistent with this idea is the finding that skeletal muscle of obese insulin-resistant subjects contained a higher amount of intramyocellular lipids, and, more importantly, these lipids showed a higher degree of peroxidation (Russell *et al.*, 2003). In the short term, increased levels of mitochondrial radicals produced as a result of increased fatty acid oxidation could affect the control of insulin signaling pathways, resulting in insulin resistance. In the long term, a buildup of reactive oxidized mitochondrial lipids would damage mitochondrial proteins and impair mitochondrial function.

V. Conclusions

In conclusion, it is clear that mitochondrial components, including the mitochondrial genome, as well as the membranes and proteins central to mitochondrial function accumulate damage with age. However, whether this damage is responsible for some aspects of aging or is merely associated with aging and age-related disease remains an open question. Evidence continues to accumulate demonstrating that interfering with mitochondrial function and mitochondrial production of reactive oxygen species can influence life span (Lee *et al.*, 2003; Melov *et al.*, 2000; Sun *et al.*, 2002). Despite the continued debate as to which aspects of mitochondrial biology are important to aging and age-related disease, it is clear that mitochondria play a critical role in aging.

References

Arnold, R. S., Shi, J., Murad, E., Whalen, A. M., Sun, C. Q., Polavarapu, R., Parthasarathy, S., Petros, J. A., & Lambeth, J. D. (2001). Hydrogen peroxide mediates the cell growth and transformation caused by the mitogenic oxidase Nox1. *Proceedings of the National Academy of Sciences of the USA*, 98, 5550–5555.

Ashcroft, F., & Rorsman, P. (2004). Type 2 diabetes mellitus: not quite exciting enough? *Human Molecular Genetics*, 13 Spec No 1, R21–R31.

Astuti, D., Latif, F., Dallol, A., Dahia, P. L., Douglas, F., George, E., Skoldberg, F., Husebye, E. S., Eng, C., & Maher, E. R. (2001). Gene mutations in the succinate dehydrogenase subunit SDHB cause susceptibility to familial pheochromocytoma and to familial paraganglioma. *American Journal of Human Genetics*, 69, 49–54.

Baker, D. J., Jeganathan, K. B., Cameron, J. D., Thompson, M., Juneja, S., Kopecka, A., Kumar, R., Jenkins, R. B., de Groen, P. C., Roche, P., & van Deursen, J. M. (2004). BubR1 insufficiency causes early onset of aging-associated phenotypes and infertility in mice. *Nature Genetics*, 36, 744–749.

Barlow, C., Hirotsune, S., Paylor, R., Liyanage, M., Eckhaus, M., Collins, F., Shiloh, Y., Crawley, J. N., Ried, T., Tagle, D., & Wynshaw-Boris, A. (1996). Atm-deficient mice: a paradigm of ataxia telangiectasia. *Cell*, 86, 159–171.

Barrientos, A., Casademont, J., Rotig, A., Miro, O., Urbano-Marquez, A., Rustin, P., & Cardellach, F. (1996). Absence of relationship between the level of electron transport chain activities and aging in human skeletal muscle. *Biochemical and Biophysical Research Communications*, 229, 536–539.

Baysal, B. E., Ferrell, R. E., Willett-Brozick, J. E., Lawrence, E. C., Myssiorek, D., Bosch, A., van der Mey, A., Taschner, P. E., Rubinstein, W. S., Myers, E. N., Richard, C. W. 3rd, Cornelisse, C. J., Devilee, P., & Devlin, B. (2000). Mutations in SDHD, a mitochondrial complex II gene, in hereditary paraganglioma. *Science*, 287, 848–851.

Beal, M. F. (2003). Mitochondria, oxidative damage, and inflammation in Parkinson's disease. *Annals of the New York Academy of Sciences*, 991, 120–131.

Beal, M. F. (2004). Commentary on "Alpha-synuclein and mitochondria: a tangled skein." *Experimental Neurology*, 186, 109–111.

Benderdour, M., Charron, G., DeBlois, D., Comte, B., & Des Rosiers, C. (2003). Cardiac mitochondrial NADP+-isocitrate dehydrogenase is inactivated through 4-hydroxynonenal adduct formation: an event that precedes hypertrophy development. *Journal of Biological Chemistry, 278,* 45154–45159.

Beregi, E., Regius, O., Huttl, T., & Gobl, Z. (1988). Age-related changes in the skeletal muscle cells. *Zeitschrift fur Gerontologie,* 21, 83–86.

Berlett, B. S., & Stadtman, E. R. (1997). Protein oxidation in aging, disease, and oxidative stress. *Journal of Biological Chemistry,* 272, 20313–20316.

Betarbet, R., Sherer, T. B., MacKenzie, G., Garcia-Osuna, M., Panov, A. V., & Greenamyre, J. T. (2000). Chronic systemic pesticide exposure reproduces features of Parkinson's disease. *Nature Neuroscience,* 3, 1301–1306.

Bianchi, C., Genova, M. L., Parenti Castelli, G., & Lenaz, G. (2004). The mitochondrial respiratory chain is partially organized in a supercomplex assembly: kinetic evidence using flux control analysis. *Journal of Biological Chemistry,* 279, 36562–36569.

Bogenhagen, D. F., & Clayton, D. A. (2003). The mitochondrial DNA replication bubble has not burst. *Trends in Biochemical Sciences,* 28, 357–360.

Bonifati, V., Rizzu, P., van Baren, M. J., Schaap, O., Breedveld, G. J., Krieger, E., Dekker, M. C., Squitieri, F., Ibanez, P., Joosse, M., van Dongen, J. W., Vanacore, N., van Swieten, J. C., Brice, A., Meco, G., van Duijn, C. M., Oostra, B. A., & Heutink, P. (2003). Mutations in the DJ-1 gene associated with autosomal recessive early-onset Parkinsonism. *Science,* 299, 256–259.

Bonilla, E., Tanji, K., Hirano, M., Vu, T. H., DiMauro, S., & Schon, E. A. (1999). Mitochondrial involvement in Alzheimer's disease. *Biochimica et Biophysica Acta,* 1410, 171–182.

Bota, D. A., Van Remmen, H., & Davies, K. J. (2002). Modulation of Lon protease activity and aconitase turnover during aging and oxidative stress. *FEBS Letters,* 532, 103–106.

Boveris, A. (1984). Determination of the production of superoxide radicals and hydrogen peroxide in mitochondria. *Methods in Enzymology,* 105, 429–435.

Boveris, A., Cadenas, E., & Stoppani, A. O. (1976). Role of ubiquinone in the mitochondrial generation of hydrogen

peroxide. *Biochemical Journal,* 156, 435–444.

Bowling, A. C., Mutisya, E. M., Walker, L. C., Price, D. L., Cork, L. C., & Beal, M. F. (1993). Age-dependent impairment of mitochondrial function in primate brain. *Journal of Neurochemistry,* 60, 1964–1967.

Brand, M. D., Affourtit, C., Esteves, T. C., Green, K., Lambert, A. J., Miwa, S., Pakay, J. L., & Parker, N. (2004). Mitochondrial superoxide: production, biological effects, and activation of uncoupling proteins. *Free Radical Biology and Medicine,* 37, 755–767.

Bush, A. I., Huang, X., & Fairlie, D. P. (1999). The possible origin of free radicals from amyloid beta peptides in Alzheimer's disease. *Neurobiology of Aging,* 20, 335–337; discussion 339–342.

Casley, C. S., Canevari, L., Land, J. M., Clark, J. B., & Sharpe, M. A. (2002). Beta-amyloid inhibits integrated mitochondrial respiration and key enzyme activities. *Journal of Neurochemistry,* 80, 91–100.

Casteels, K., Ong, K., Phillips, D., Bendall, H., & Pembrey, M. (1999). Mitochondrial 16189 variant, thinness at birth, and type-2 diabetes. ALSPAC study team. Avon Longitudinal Study of Pregnancy and Childhood. *Lancet,* 353, 1499–1500.

Cerritelli, S. M., Frolova, E. G., Feng, C., Grinberg, A., Love, P. E., & Crouch, R. J. (2003). Failure to produce mitochondrial DNA results in embryonic lethality in Rnaseh1 null mice. *Molecular Cell,* 11, 807–815.

Chance, B., Sies, H., & Boveris, A. (1979). Hydroperoxide metabolism in mammalian organs. *Physiological Reviews,* 59, 527–605.

Chandrasekaran, K., Hatanpaa, K., Brady, D. R., & Rapoport, S. I. (1996). Evidence for physiological down-regulation of brain oxidative phosphorylation in Alzheimer's disease. *Experimental Neurology,* 142, 80–88.

Chang, S., Multani, A. S., Cabrera, N. G., Naylor, M. L., Laud, P., Lombard, D., Pathak, S., Guarente, L., & DePinho, R. A. (2004). Essential role of limiting telomeres in the pathogenesis of Werner syndrome. *Nature Genetics,* 000, 000–000.

Chen, Q., Vazquez, E. J., Moghaddas, S., Hoppel, C. L., & Lesnefsky, E. J. (2003).

Production of reactive oxygen species by mitochondria: central role of complex III. *Journal of Biological Chemistry*, 278, 36027–36031.

Chinnery, P. F., Howell, N., Andrews, R. M., & Turnbull, D. M. (1999). Mitochondrial DNA analysis: polymorphisms and pathogenicity. *Journal of Medical Genetics*, 36, 505–510.

Choksi, K. B., Boylston, W. H., Rabek, J. P., Widger, W. R., & Papaconstantinou, J. (2004). Oxidatively damaged proteins of heart mitochondrial electron transport complexes. *Biochimica et Biophysica Acta*, 1688, 95–101.

Coleman, R., Silbermann, M., Gershon, D., & Reznick, A. Z. (1987). Giant mitochondria in the myocardium of aging and endurance-trained mice. *Gerontology*, 33, 34–39.

Corral-Debrinski, M., Horton, T., Lott, M. T., Shoffner, J. M., Beal, M. F., & Wallace, D. C. (1992). Mitochondrial DNA deletions in human brain: regional variability and increase with advanced age. *Nature Genetics*, 2, 324–329.

Cortassa, S., Aon, M. A., Marban, E., Winslow, R. L., & O'Rourke, B. (2003). An integrated model of cardiac mitochondrial energy metabolism and calcium dynamics. *Biophysical Journal*, 84, 2734–2755.

Cortopassi, G. A., & Arnheim, N. (1990). Detection of a specific mitochondrial DNA deletion in tissues of older humans. *Nucleic Acids Research*, 18, 6927–6933.

Coskun, P. E., Beal, M. F., & Wallace, D. C. (2004). Alzheimer's brains harbor somatic mtDNA control-region mutations that suppress mitochondrial transcription and replication. *Proceedings of the National Academy of Sciences of the USA*, 101, 10726–10731.

Cuervo, A. M., & Dice, J. F. (1998). How do intracellular proteolytic systems change with age? *Frontiers in Bioscience*, 3, D25–43.

Darnold, J. R., Vorbeck, M. L., & Martin, A. P. (1990). Effect of aging on the oxidative phosphorylation pathway. *Mechanisms of Ageing and Development*, 53, 157–167.

Davey, G. P., & Clark, J. B. (1996). Threshold effects and control of oxidative phosphorylation in nonsynaptic rat brain mitochondria. *Journal of Neurochemistry*, 66, 1617–1624.

de Boer, J., Andressoo, J. O., de Wit, J., Huijmans, J., Beems, R. B., van Steeg, H., Weeda, G., van der Horst, G. T., van Leeuwen, W., Themmen, A. P., Meradji, M., & Hoeijmakers, J. H. (2002). Premature aging in mice deficient in DNA repair and transcription. *Science*, 296, 1276–1279.

De Sandre-Giovannoli, A., Bernard, R., Cau, P., Navarro, C., Amiel, J., Boccaccio, I., Lyonnet, S., Stewart, C. L., Munnich, A., Le Merrer, M., & Levy, N. (2003). Lamin A truncation in Hutchinson-Gilford progeria. *Science*, 300, 2055.

Di Monte, D. A., Lavasani, M., & Manning-Bog, A. B. (2002). Environmental factors in Parkinson's disease. *Neurotoxicology*, 23, 487–502.

Duara, R., Grady, C., Haxby, J., Sundaram, M., Cutler, N. R., Heston, L., Moore, A., Schlageter, N., Larson, S., & Rapoport, S. I. (1986). Positron emission tomography in Alzheimer's disease. *Neurology*, 36, 879–887.

Eaton, P., Li, J. M., Hearse, D. J., & Shattock, M. J. (1999). Formation of 4-hydroxy-2-nonenal-modified proteins in ischemic rat heart. *American Journal of Physiology*, 276, H935–H943.

Epstein, C. J. (1985). Werner's syndrome and aging: a reappraisal. *Advances in Experimental Medicine and Biology*, 190, 219–228.

Eriksson, M., Brown, W. T., Gordon, L. B., Glynn, M. W., Singer, J., Scott, L., Erdos, M. R., Robbins, C. M., Moses, T. Y., Berglund, P., Dutra, A., Pak, E., Durkin, S., Csoka, A. B., Boehnke, M., Glover, T. W., & Collins, F. S. (2003). Recurrent de novo point mutations in lamin A cause Hutchinson-Gilford progeria syndrome. *Nature*, 423, 293–298.

Esterbauer, H., Schaur, R. J., & Zollner, H. (1991). Chemistry and biochemistry of 4-hydroxynonenal, malonaldehyde and related aldehydes. *Free Radical Biology and Medicine*, 11, 81–128.

Fayet, G., Jansson, M., Sternberg, D., Moslemi, A. R., Blondy, P., Lombes, A., Fardeau, M., & Oldfors, A. (2002). Ageing muscle: clonal expansions of mitochondrial DNA point mutations and deletions cause focal impairment of mitochondrial function. *Neuromuscular Disorders*, 12, 484–493.

Filburn, C. R., Edris, W., Tamatani, M.,
Hogue, B., Kudryashova, I., & Hansford, R. G.
(1996). Mitochondrial electron transport
chain activities and DNA deletions in regions
of the rat brain. *Mechanisms of Ageing and
Development*, 87, 35–46.

Fiskum, G., Starkov, A., Polster, B. M., &
Chinopoulos, C. (2003). Mitochondrial
mechanisms of neural cell death and
neuroprotective interventions in
Parkinson's disease. *Annals of the New
York Academy of Sciences*, 991, 111–119.

Flint, D. H., Tuminello, J. F., & Emptage, M. H.
(1993). The inactivation of Fe-S cluster
containing hydro-lyases by superoxide.
Journal of Biological Chemistry, 268,
22369–22376.

Gabbita, S. P., Butterfield, D. A., Hensley, K.,
Shaw, W., & Carney, J. M. (1997). Aging and
caloric restriction affect mitochondrial
respiration and lipid membrane status: an
electron paramagnetic resonance
investigation. *Free Radical Biology and
Medicine*, 23, 191–201.

Gibson, A. M., Edwardson, J. A., Turnbull, D.
M., McKeith, I. G., Morris, C. M., &
Chinnery, P. F. (2004). No evidence of an
association between the T16189C mtDNA
variant and late onset dementia. *Journal of
Medical Genetics*, 41, e7.

Gill-Randall, R., Sherratt, E. J., Thomas, A. W.,
Gagg, J. W., Lee, A., & Alcolado, J. C. (2001).
Analysis of a polycytosine tract and
heteroplasmic length variation in the
mitochondrial DNA D-loop of patients with
diabetes, MELAS syndrome and race-
matched controls. *Diabetic Medicine*, 18,
413–416.

Gillum, A. M., & Clayton, D. A. (1978).
Displacement-loop replication initiation
sequence in animal mitochondrial DNA
exists as a family of discrete lengths.
*Proceedings of the National Academy of
Sciences of the USA*, 75, 677–681.

Gimm, O., Armanios, M., Dziema, H.,
Neumann, H. P., & Eng, C. (2000). Somatic
and occult germ-line mutations in SDHD, a
mitochondrial complex II gene, in
nonfamilial pheochromocytoma. *Cancer
Research*, 60, 6822–6825.

Gloyn, A. L. (2003). The search for type 2
diabetes genes. *Ageing Research Reviews*,
2, 111–127.

Graybiel, A. M., Hirsch, E. C., & Agid, Y.
(1990). The nigrostriatal system in
Parkinson's disease. *Advances in
Neurology*, 53, 17–29.

Greco, M., Villani, G., Mazzucchelli, F.,
Bresolin, N., Papa, S., & Attardi, G. (2003).
Marked aging-related decline in efficiency
of oxidative phosphorylation in human
skin fibroblasts. *FASEB Journal*, 17,
1706–1708.

Guillausseau, P. J., Massin, P., Dubois-
LaForgue, D., Timsit, J., Virally, M., Gin, H.,
Bertin, E., Blickle, J. F., Bouhanick, B.,
Cahen, J., Caillat-Zucman, S., Charpentier, G.,
Chedin, P., Derrien, C., Ducluzeau, P. H.,
Grimaldi, A., Guerci, B., Kaloustian, E.,
Murat, A., Olivier, F., Paques, M., Paquis-
Flucklinger, V., Porokhov, B., Samuel-
Lajeunesse, J., & Vialettes, B. (2001).
Maternally inherited diabetes and deafness:
a multicenter study. *Annals of Internal
Medicine*, 134, 721–728.

Gutteridge, J. M., Richmond, R., & Halliwell, B.
(1979). Inhibition of the iron-catalysed
formation of hydroxyl radicals from
superoxide and of lipid peroxidation by
desferrioxamine. *Biochemical Journal*, 184,
469–472.

Hainaut, P., & Mann, K. (2001). Zinc binding
and redox control of p53 structure and
function. *Antioxidants and Redox
Signaling*, 3, 611–623.

Halliwell, B., & Gutteridge, J. M. (1984). Free
radicals, lipid peroxidation, and cell
damage. *Lancet*, 2, 1095.

Hansford, R. G., Hogue, B. A., & Mildaziene, V.
(1997). Dependence of H2O2 formation by
rat heart mitochondria on substrate
availability and donor age. *Journal of
Bioenergetics and Biomembranes*, 29, 89–95.

Harman, D. (1956). Aging: a theory based on
free radical and radiation chemistry.
Journal of Gerontology, 11, 298–300.

Harman, D. (1972). The biologic clock: the
mitochondria? *Journal of the American
Geriatrics Society*, 20, 145–147.

Hasty, P., & Vijg, J. (2004a). Accelerating
aging by mouse reverse genetics: a rational
approach to understanding longevity. *Aging
Cell*, 3, 55–65.

Hasty, P., & Vijg, J. (2004b). Rebuttal to
Miller: 'Accelerated aging: a primrose path
to insight?' *Aging Cell*, 3, 67–69.

Hasty, P., Campisi, J., Hoeijmakers, J., van Steeg, H., & Vijg, J. (2003). Aging and genome maintenance: lessons from the mouse? *Science, 299,* 1355–1359.

Hayashi, J., Ohta, S., Kikuchi, A., Takemitsu, M., Goto, Y., & Nonaka, I. (1991). Introduction of disease-related mitochondrial DNA deletions into HeLa cells lacking mitochondrial DNA results in mitochondrial dysfunction. *Proceedings of the National Academy of Sciences of the USA, 88,* 10614–10618.

Herrera, E., Samper, E., Martin-Caballero, J., Flores, J. M., Lee, H. W., & Blasco, M. A. (1999). Disease states associated with telomerase deficiency appear earlier in mice with short telomeres. *EMBO Journal, 18,* 2950–2960.

Hinerfeld, D., Traini, M. D., Weinberger, R. P., Cochran, B., Doctrow, S. R., Harry, J., & Melov, S. (2004). Endogenous mitochondrial oxidative stress: neurodegeneration, proteomic analysis, specific respiratory chain defects, and efficacious antioxidant therapy in superoxide dismutase 2 null mice. *Journal of Neurochemistry, 88,* 657–667.

Hirai, K., Aliev, G., Nunomura, A., Fujioka, H., Russell, R. L., Atwood, C. S., Johnson, A. B., Kress, Y., Vinters, H. V., Tabaton, M., Shimohama, S., Cash, A. D., Siedlak, S. L., Harris, P. L., Jones, P. K., Petersen, R. B., Perry, G., & Smith, M. A. (2001). Mitochondrial abnormalities in Alzheimer's disease. *Journal of Neuroscience, 21,* 3017–3023.

Ho, J. K., Duclos, R. I., Jr., & Hamilton, J. A. (2002). Interactions of acyl carnitines with model membranes: a (13)C-NMR study. *Journal of Lipid Research, 43,* 1429–1439.

Holt, I. J., & Jacobs, H. T. (2003). Response: the mitochondrial DNA replication bubble has not burst. *Trends in Biochemical Sciences, 28,* 355–356.

Holt, I. J., Harding, A. E., & Morgan-Hughes, J. A. (1988). Deletions of muscle mitochondrial DNA in patients with mitochondrial myopathies. *Nature, 331,* 717–719.

Hsiao, K. K., Borchelt, D. R., Olson, K., Johanrisdottir, R., Kitt, C., Yunis, W., Xu, S., Eckman, C., Younkin, S., Price, D., Iadecola, C., Clark, H. B., Carlson, G. (1995). Age-related CNS disorder and early death in transgenic FVB/N mice overexpressing Alzheimer amyloid precursor proteins. *Neuron, 15,* 1203–1218.

Hsiao, K., Chapman, P., Nilsen, S., Eckmnan, C., Harigaya, Y., Younkin, S., Yang, F., Cole, G. (1996). Correlative memory deficits, A beta elevation, and amyloid plaques in transgenic mice. *Science, 274,* 99–102.

Hussain, S. P., Hofseth, L. J., & Harris, C. C. (2003). Radical causes of cancer. *Nature Reviews. Cancer, 3,* 276–285.

Iborra, F. J., Kimura, H., & Cook, P. R. (2004). The functional organization of mitochondrial genomes in human cells. *BMC Biology, 2,* 9.

Irani, K., Xia, Y., Zweier, J. L., Sollott, S. J., Der, C. J., Fearon, E. R., Sundaresan, M., Finkel, T., & Goldschmidt-Clermont, P. J. (1997). Mitogenic signaling mediated by oxidants in Ras-transformed fibroblasts. *Science, 275,* 1649–1652.

Jacobs, H. T. (2003a). Rebuttal to Pak et al.: new data, chestnuts. *Aging Cell, 2,* 19–20.

Jacobs, H. T. (2003b). The mitochondrial theory of aging: dead or alive? *Aging Cell, 2,* 11–17.

Jenner, P. (2003). Oxidative stress in Parkinson's disease. *Annals of Neurology, 53* Suppl 3, S26–S36; discussion S36–S28.

Kanski, J., Behring, A., Pelling, J., & Schoneich, C. (2004). Proteomic identification of 3-nitrotyrosine-containing rat cardiac proteins: effect of biological aging. *American Journal of Physiology. Heart and Circulatory Physiology, 000,* 000–000.

Khan, S. M., Cassarino, D. S., Abramova, N. N., Keeney, P. M., Borland, M. K., Trimmer, P. A., Krebs, C. T., Bennett, J. C., Parks, J. K., Swerdlow, R. H., Parker, W. D. Jr., & Bennett, J. P. Jr. (2000). Alzheimer's disease cybrids replicate beta-amyloid abnormalities through cell death pathways. *Annals of Neurology, 48,* 148–155.

Khrapko, K., Bodyak, N., Thilly, W. G., van Orsouw, N. J., Zhang, X., Coller, H. A., Perls, T. T., Upton, M., Vijg, J., & Wei, J. Y. (1999). Cell-by-cell scanning of whole mitochondrial genomes in aged human heart reveals a significant fraction of myocytes with clonally expanded deletions [In Process Citation]. *Nucleic Acids Research, 27,* 2434–2441.

Kim, J. H., Park, K. S., Cho, Y. M., Kang, B. S., Kim, S. K., Jeon, H. J., Kim, S. Y., &

Lee, H. K. (2002). The prevalence of the mitochondrial DNA 16189 variant in non-diabetic Korean adults and its association with higher fasting glucose and body mass index. *Diabetic Medicine,* 19, 681–684.

King, M. P., Koga, Y., Davidson, M., & Schon, E. A. (1992). Defects in mitochondrial protein synthesis and respiratory chain activity segregate with the tRNA(Leu(UUR)) mutation associated with mitochondrial myopathy, encephalopathy, lactic acidosis, and strokelike episodes. *Molecular and Cellular Biology,* 12, 480–490.

Kinnula, V. L., & Crapo, J. D. (2004). Superoxide dismutases in malignant cells and human tumors. *Free Radical Biology and Medicine,* 36, 718–744.

Kitada, T., Asakawa, S., Hattori, N., Matsumine, H., Yamamura, Y., Minoshima, S., Yokochi, M., Mizuno, Y., & Shimizu, N. (1998). Mutations in the parkin gene cause autosomal recessive juvenile parkinsonism. *Nature,* 392, 605–608.

Korbel, D., Wurth, S., Kaser, M., & Langer, T. (2004). Membrane protein turnover by the m-AAA protease in mitochondria depends on the transmembrane domains of its subunits. *EMBO Reports,* 5, 698–703.

Kudin, A. P., Bimpong-Buta, N. Y., Vielhaber, S., Elger, C. E., & Kunz, W. S. (2004). Characterization of superoxide-producing sites in isolated brain mitochondria. *Journal of Biological Chemistry,* 279, 4127–4135.

Langston, J. W., Ballard, P., Tetrud, J. W., & Irwin, I. (1983). Chronic Parkinsonism in humans due to a product of meperidine-analog synthesis. *Science,* 219, 979–980.

Larsson, N. G., Wang, J., Wilhelmsson, H., Oldfors, A., Rustin, P., Lewandoski, M., Barsh, G. S., & Clayton, D. A. (1998). Mitochondrial transcription factor A is necessary for mtDNA maintenance and embryogenesis in mice. *Nature Genetics,* 18, 231–236.

Lee, A. C., Fenster, B. E., Ito, H., Takeda, K., Bae, N. S., Hirai, T., Yu, Z. X., Ferrans, V. J., Howard, B. H., & Finkel, T. (1999). Ras proteins induce senescence by altering the intracellular levels of reactive oxygen species. *Journal of Biological Chemistry,* 274, 7936–7940.

Lee, C. M., Chung, S. S., Kaczkowski, J. M., Weindruch, R., & Aiken, J. M. (1993). Multiple mitochondrial DNA deletions associated with age in skeletal muscle of rhesus monkeys. *Journal of Gerontology,* 48, B201–B205.

Lee, S. S., Lee, R. Y., Fraser, A. G., Kamath, R. S., Ahringer, J., & Ruvkun, G. (2003). A systematic RNAi screen identifies a critical role for mitochondria in *C. elegans* longevity. *Nature Genetics,* 33, 40–48.

Legros, F., Malka, F., Frachon, P., Lombes, A., & Rojo, M. (2004). Organization and dynamics of human mitochondrial DNA. *Journal of Cell Science,* 117, 2653–2662.

Lehtonen, R., Kiuru, M., Vanharanta, S., Sjoberg, J., Aaltonen, L. M., Aittomaki, K., Arola, J., Butzow, R., Eng, C., Husgafvel-Pursiainen, K., Isola, J., Jarvinen, H., Koivisto, P., Mecklin, J. P., Peltomaki, P., Salovaara, R., Wasenius, V. M., Karhu, A., Launonen, V., Nupponen, N. N., & Aaltonen, L. A. (2004). Biallelic inactivation of fumarate hydratase (FH) occurs in nonsyndromic uterine leiomyomas but is rare in other tumors. *American Journal of Pathology,* 164, 17–22.

Lengauer, C., Kinzler, K. W., & Vogelstein, B. (1998). Genetic instabilities in human cancers. *Nature,* 396, 643–649.

Leroy, E., Boyer, R., Auburger, G., Leube, B., Ulm, G., Mezey, E., Harta, G., Brownstein, M. J., Jonnalagada, S., Chernova, T., Dehejia, A., Lavedan, C., Gasser, T., Steinbach, P. J., Wilkinson, K. D., & Polymeropoulos, M. H. (1998). The ubiquitin pathway in Parkinson's disease. *Nature,* 395, 451–452.

Levine, R. L. (2002). Carbonyl modified proteins in cellular regulation, aging, and disease. *Free Radical Biology and Medicine,* 32, 790–796.

Li, Y., Huang, T. T., Carlson, E. J., Melov, S., Ursell, P. C., Olson, J. L., Noble, L. J., Yoshimura, M. P., Berger, C., Chan, P. H., & et al. (1995). Dilated cardiomyopathy and neonatal lethality in mutant mice lacking manganese superoxide dismutase. *Nature Genetics,* 11, 376–381.

Lieber, M. R., & Karanjawala, Z. E. (2004). Ageing, repetitive genomes and DNA damage. *Nature Reviews. Molecular Cell Biology,* 5, 69–75.

Linton, S., Davies, M. J., & Dean, R. T. (2001). Protein oxidation and ageing. *Experimental Gerontology*, 36, 1503–1518.

Liou, C. W., Lin, T. K., Huang, F. M., Chen, T. L., Lee, C. F., Chuang, Y. C., Tan, T. Y., Chang, K. C., & Wei, Y. H. (2004). Association of the mitochondrial DNA 16189 T to C variant with lacunar cerebral infarction: evidence from a hospital-based case-control study. *Annals of the New York Academy of Sciences*, 1011, 317–324.

Liu, Y., Fiskum, G., & Schubert, D. (2002a). Generation of reactive oxygen species by the mitochondrial electron transport chain. *Journal of Neurochemistry*, 80, 780–787.

Liu, L., Trimarchi, J. R., Smith, P. J., & Keefe, D. L. (2002b). Mitochondrial dysfunction leads to telomere attrition and genomic instability. *Aging Cell*, 1, 40–46.

Livesey, K. J., Wimhurst, V. L., Carter, K., Worwood, M., Cadet, E., Rochette, J., Roberts, A. G., Pointon, J. J., Merryweather-Clarke, A. T., Bassett, M. L., Jouanolle, A. M., Mosser, A., David, V., Poulton, J., & Robson, K. J. (2004). The 16189 variant of mitochondrial DNA occurs more frequently in C282Y homozygotes with haemochromatosis than those without iron loading. *Journal of Medical Genetics*, 41, 6–10.

Lucas, D. T., & Szweda, L. I. (1998). Cardiac reperfusion injury: aging, lipid peroxidation, and mitochondrial dysfunction. *Proceedings of the National Academy of Sciences of the USA*, 95, 510–514.

Lynn, S., Borthwick, G. M., Charnley, R. M., Walker, M., & Turnbull, D. M. (2003). Heteroplasmic ratio of the A3243G mitochondrial DNA mutation in single pancreatic beta cells. *Diabetologia*, 46, 296–299.

Maassen, J. A. (2002). Mitochondrial diabetes: pathophysiology, clinical presentation, and genetic analysis. *American Journal of Medical Genetics*, 115, 66–70.

Maassen, J. A., LM, T. H., Van Essen, E., Heine, R. J., Nijpels, G., Jahangir Tafrechi, R. S., Raap, A. K., Janssen, G. M., & Lemkes, H. H. (2004). Mitochondrial diabetes: molecular mechanisms and clinical presentation. *Diabetes*, 53 Suppl 1, S103–S109.

Maluf, S. W., & Erdtmann, B. (2001). Genomic instability in Down syndrome and Fanconi anemia assessed by micronucleus analysis and single-cell gel electrophoresis. *Cancer Genetics and Cytogenetics*, 124, 71–75.

Marchington, D. R., Hartshorne, G. M., Barlow, D., & Poulton, J. (1997). Homopolymeric tract heteroplasmy in mtDNA from tissues and single oocytes: support for a genetic bottleneck. *American Journal of Human Genetics*, 60, 408–416.

Marciniak, R. A., Johnson, F. B., & Guarente, L. (2000). Dyskeratosis congenita, telomeres and human ageing. *Trends in Genetics*, 16, 193–195.

Mazat, J. P., Rossignol, R., Malgat, M., Rocher, C., Faustin, B., & Letellier, T. (2001). What do mitochondrial diseases teach us about normal mitochondrial functions . . . that we already knew: threshold expression of mitochondrial defects. *Biochimica et Biophysica Acta*, 1504, 20–30.

McLellan, M. E., Kajdasz, S. T., Hyman, B. T., & Bacskai, B. J. (2003). *In vivo* imaging of reactive oxygen species specifically associated with thioflavine S-positive amyloid plaques by multiphoton microscopy. *Journal of Neuroscience*, 23, 2212–2217.

Melov, S., Hertz, G. Z., Stormo, G. D., & Johnson, T. E. (1994). Detection of deletions in the mitochondrial genome of *Caenorhabditis elegans*. *Nucleic Acids Research*, 22, 1075–1078.

Melov, S., Lithgow, G. J., Fischer, D. R., Tedesco, P. M., & Johnson, T. E. (1995a). Increased frequency of deletions in the mitochondrial genome with age of *Caenorhabditis elegans*. *Nucleic Acids Research*, 23, 1419–1425.

Melov, S., Shoffner, J. M., Kaufman, A., & Wallace, D. C. (1995b). Marked increase in the number and variety of mitochondrial DNA rearrangements in aging human skeletal muscle. *Nucleic Acids Research*, 23, 4122–4126

Melov, S., Schneider, J. A., Day, B. J., Hinerfeld, D., Coskun, P., Mirra, S. S., Crapo, J. D., & Wallace, D. C. (1998). A novel neurological phenotype in mice lacking mitochondrial manganese superoxide dismutase. *Nature Genetics*, 18, 159–163.

Melov, S., Coskun, P., Patel, M., Tuinstra, R., Cottrell, B., Jun, A. S., Zastawny, T. H.,

Dizdaroglu, M., Goodman, S. I., Huang, T. T., Miziorko, H., Epstein, C. J., & Wallace, D. C. (1999a). Mitochondrial disease in superoxide dismutase 2 mutant mice. *Proceedings of the National Academy of Sciences of the USA*, 96, 846–851.

Melov, S., Schneider, J. A., Coskun, P. E., Bennett, D. A., & Wallace, D. C. (1999b). Mitochondrial DNA rearrangements in aging human brain and in situ PCR of mtDNA. *Neurobiology of Aging*, 20, 565–571.

Melov, S., Ravenscroft, J., Malik, S., Gill, M. S., Walker, D. W., Clayton, P. E., Wallace, D. C., Malfroy, B., Doctrow, S. R., & Lithgow, G. J. (2000). Extension of life-span with superoxide dismutase/catalase mimetics. *Science*, 289, 1567–1569.

Metter, E. J., Kuhl, D. E., & Riege, W. H. (1990). Brain glucose metabolism in Parkinson's disease. *Advances in Neurology*, 53, 135–139.

Michikawa, Y., Mazzucchelli, F., Bresolin, N., Scarlato, G., & Attardi, G. (1999). Aging-dependent large accumulation of point mutations in the human mtDNA control region for replication [see comments]. *Science*, 286, 774–779.

Millar, A. H., & Leaver, C. J. (2000). The cytotoxic lipid peroxidation product, 4-hydroxy-2-nonenal, specifically inhibits decarboxylating dehydrogenases in the matrix of plant mitochondria. *FEBS Letters*, 481, 117–121.

Miller, R. A. (2004a). 'Accelerated aging': a primrose path to insight? *Aging Cell*, 3, 47–51.

Miller, R. A. (2004b). Rebuttal to Hasty and Vijg: 'Accelerating aging by mouse reverse genetics: a rational approach to understanding longevity'. *Aging Cell*, 3, 53–54.

Mitrunen, K., Sillanpaa, P., Kataja, V., Eskelinen, M., Kosma, V. M., Benhamou, S., Uusitupa, M., & Hirvonen, A. (2001). Association between manganese superoxide dismutase (MnSOD) gene polymorphism and breast cancer risk. *Carcinogenesis*, 22, 827–829.

Miyakawa, I., Sando, N., Kawano, S., Nakamura, S., & Kuroiwa, T. (1987). Isolation of morphologically intact mitochondrial nucleoids from the yeast, Saccharomyces cerevisiae. *Journal of Cell Science*, 88 (Pt 4), 431–439.

Mootha, V. K., Lindgren, C. M., Eriksson, K. F., Subramanian, A., Sihag, S., Lehar, J., Puigserver, P., Carlsson, E., Ridderstrale, M., Laurila, E., Houstis, N., Daly, M. J., Patterson, N., Mesirov, J. P., Golub, T. R., Tamayo, P., Spiegelman, B., Lander, E. S., Hirschhorn, J. N., Altshuler, D., & Groop, L. C. (2003). PGC-1alpha-responsive genes involved in oxidative phosphorylation are coordinately downregulated in human diabetes. *Nature Genetics*, 34, 267–273.

Nicotera, T. M., Block, A. W., Gibas, Z., & Sandberg, A. A. (1985). Induction of superoxide dismutase, chromosomal aberrations and sister-chromatid exchanges by paraquat in Chinese hamster fibroblasts. *Mutation Research*, 151, 263–268.

Niemann, S., & Muller, U. (2000). Mutations in SDHC cause autosomal dominant paraganglioma, type 3. *Nature Genetics*, 26, 268–270.

Niemi, A. K., Hervonen, A., Hurme, M., Karhunen, P. J., Jylha, M., & Majamaa, K. (2003). Mitochondrial DNA polymorphisms associated with longevity in a Finnish population. *Human Genetics*, 112, 29–33.

Nyholm, B., Mengel, A., Nielsen, S., Skjaerbaek, C., Moller, N., Alberti, K. G., & Schmitz, O. (1996). Insulin resistance in relatives of NIDDM patients: the role of physical fitness and muscle metabolism. *Diabetologia*, 39, 813–822.

Ojaimi, J., Masters, C. L., Opeskin, K., McKelvie, P., & Byrne, E. (1999). Mitochondrial respiratory chain activity in the human brain as a function of age. *Mechanisms of Ageing and Development*, 111, 39–47.

Pak, J. W., Herbst, A., Bua, E., Gokey, N., McKenzie, D., & Aiken, J. M. (2003a). Mitochondrial DNA mutations as a fundamental mechanism in physiological declines associated with aging. *Aging Cell*, 2, 1–7.

Pak, J. W., Herbst, A., Bua, E., Gokey, N., McKenzie, D., & Aiken, J. M. (2003b). Rebuttal to Jacobs: the mitochondrial theory of aging: alive and well. *Aging Cell*, 2, 9–10.

Palacino, J. J., Sagi, D., Goldberg, M. S., Krauss, S., Motz, C., Wacker, M., Klose, J.,

& Shen, J. (2004). Mitochondrial dysfunction and oxidative damage in parkin-deficient mice. *Journal of Biological Chemistry*, 279, 18614–18622.

Patti, M. E., Butte, A. J., Crunkhorn, S., Cusi, K., Berria, R., Kashyap, S., Miyazaki, Y., Kohane, I., Costello, M., Saccone, R., Landaker, E. J., Goldfine, A. B., Mun, E., DeFronzo, R., Finlayson, J., Kahn, C. R., & Mandarino, L. J. (2003). Coordinated reduction of genes of oxidative metabolism in humans with insulin resistance and diabetes: Potential role of PGC1 and NRF1. *Proceedings of the National Academy of Sciences of the USA*, 100, 8466–8471.

Petersen, K. F., Befroy, D., Dufour, S., Dziura, J., Ariyan, C., Rothman, D. L., DiPietro, L., Cline, G. W., & Shulman, G. I. (2003). Mitochondrial dysfunction in the elderly: possible role in insulin resistance. *Science*, 300, 1140–1142.

Piko, L., & Matsumoto, L. (1977). Complex forms and replicative intermediates of mitochondrial DNA in tissues from adult and senescent mice. *Nucleic Acids Research*, 4, 1301–1314.

Piko, L., Meyer, R., Eipe, J., & Costea, N. (1978). Structural and replicative forms of mitochondrial DNA from human leukocytes in relation to age. *Mechanisms of Ageing and Development*, 7, 351–365.

Poggioli, S., Mary, J., Bakala, H., & Friguet, B. (2004). Evidence of preferential protein targets for age-related modifications in peripheral blood lymphocytes. *Annals of the New York Academy of Sciences*, 1019, 211–214.

Poli, G., & Schaur, R. J. (2000). 4-Hydroxy-nonenal in the pathomechanisms of oxidative stress. *IUBMB Life*, 50, 315–321.

Polyak, K., Li, Y., Zhu, H., Lengauer, C., Willson, J. K., Markowitz, S. D., Trush, M. A., Kinzler, K. W., & Vogelstein, B. (1998). Somatic mutations of the mitochondrial genome in human colorectal tumours. *Nature Genetics*, 20, 291–293.

Poulton, J., Brown, M. S., Cooper, A., Marchington, D. R., & Phillips, D. I. (1998). A common mitochondrial DNA variant is associated with insulin resistance in adult life. *Diabetologia*, 41, 54–58.

Poulton, J., Luan, J., Macaulay, V., Hennings, S., Mitchell, J., & Wareham, N. J. (2002).

Type 2 diabetes is associated with a common mitochondrial variant: evidence from a population-based case-control study. *Human Molecular Genetics*, 11, 1581–1583.

Rapoport, S. I., Hatanpaa, K., Brady, D. R., & Chandrasekaran, K. (1996). Brain energy metabolism, cognitive function and down-regulated oxidative phosphorylation in Alzheimer disease. *Neurodegeneration*, 5, 473–476.

Ristow, M. (2004). Neurodegenerative disorders associated with diabetes mellitus. *Journal of Molecular Medicine*, 82, 510–529.

Rossignol, R., Malgat, M., Mazat, J. P., & Letellier, T. (1999). Threshold effect and tissue specificity. Implication for mitochondrial cytopathies. *Journal of Biological Chemistry*, 274, 33426–33432.

Rubbo, H., Radi, R., Trujillo, M., Telleri, R., Kalyanaraman, B., Barnes, S., Kirk, M., & Freeman, B. A. (1994). Nitric oxide regulation of superoxide and peroxynitrite-dependent lipid peroxidation. Formation of novel nitrogen-containing oxidized lipid derivatives. *Journal of Biological Chemistry*, 269, 26066–26075.

Rudolph, K. L., Chang, S., Lee, H. W., Blasco, M., Gottlieb, G. J., Greider, C., & DePinho, R. A. (1999). Longevity, stress response, and cancer in aging telomerase-deficient mice. *Cell*, 96, 701–712.

Russell, A. P., Gastaldi, G., Bobbioni-Harsch, E., Arboit, P., Gobelet, C., Deriaz, O., Golay, A., Witztum, J. L., & Giacobino, J. P. (2003). Lipid peroxidation in skeletal muscle of obese as compared to endurance-trained humans: a case of good vs. bad lipids? *FEBS Letters*, 551, 104–106.

Saltiel, A. R., & Kahn, C. R. (2001). Insulin signalling and the regulation of glucose and lipid metabolism. *Nature*, 414, 799–806.

Samper, E., Flores, J. M., & Blasco, M. A. (2001). Restoration of telomerase activity rescues chromosomal instability and premature aging in Terc−/− mice with short telomeres. *EMBO Reports*, 2, 800–807.

Samper, E., Nicholls, D. G., & Melov, S. (2003). Mitochondrial oxidative stress causes chromosomal instability of mouse embryonic fibroblasts. *Aging Cell*, 2, 277–285.

Sayre, L. M., Zelasko, D. A., Harris, P. L., Perry, G., Salomon, R. G., & Smith, M. A. (1997). 4-Hydroxynonenal-derived advanced lipid peroxidation end products are increased in Alzheimer's disease. *Journal of Neurochemistry*, 68, 2092–2097.

Scarfi, M. R., Cossarizza, A., Monti, D., Bersani, F., Zannotti, M., Lioi, M. B., & Franceschi, C. (1990). Age-related increase of mitomycin C-induced micronuclei in lymphocytes from Down's syndrome subjects. *Mutation Research*, 237, 247–252.

Schneider, S. H., Amorosa, L. F., Khachadurian, A. K., & Ruderman, N. B. (1984). Studies on the mechanism of improved glucose control during regular exercise in type 2 (non-insulin-dependent) diabetes. *Diabetologia*, 26, 355–360.

Schwarze, S. R., Lee, C. M., Chung, S. S., Roecker, E. B., Weindruch, R., & Aiken, J. M. (1995). High levels of mitochondrial DNA deletions in skeletal muscle of old rhesus monkeys. *Mechanisms of Ageing and Development*, 83, 91–101.

Shamoto-Nagai, M., Maruyama, W., Kato, Y., Isobe, K., Tanaka, M., Naoi, M., & Osawa, T. (2003). An inhibitor of mitochondrial complex I, rotenone, inactivates proteasome by oxidative modification and induces aggregation of oxidized proteins in SH-SY5Y cells. *Journal of Neuroscience Research*, 74, 589–597.

Sharman, E. H., & Bondy, S. C. (2001). Effects of age and dietary antioxidants on cerebral electron transport chain activity. *Neurobiology of Aging*, 22, 629–634.

Sherer, T. B., Betarbet, R., Stout, A. K., Lund, S., Baptista, M., Panov, A. V., Cookson, M. R., & Greenamyre, J. T. (2002). An in vitro model of Parkinson's disease: linking mitochondrial impairment to altered alpha-synuclein metabolism and oxidative damage. *Journal of Neuroscience*, 22, 7006–7015.

Shubber, E. K., Hamami, H. A., Allak, B. M., & Khaleel, A. H. (1991). Sister-chromatid exchanges in lymphocytes from infants with Down's syndrome. *Mutation Research*, 248, 61–72.

Simon, D. K., Lin, M. T., Zheng, L., Liu, G. J., Ahn, C. H., Kim, L. M., Mauck, W. M., Twu, F., Beal, M. F., & Johns, D. R. (2004). Somatic mitochondrial DNA mutations in cortex and substantia nigra in aging and Parkinson's disease. *Neurobiology of Aging*, 25, 71–81.

Sims, N. R., Bowen, D. M., Smith, C. C., Flack, R. H., Davison, A. N., Snowden, J. S., & Neary, D. (1980). Glucose metabolism and acetylcholine synthesis in relation to neuronal activity in Alzheimer's disease. *Lancet*, 1, 333–336.

Singleton, A. B., Farrer, M., Johnson, J., Singleton, A., Hague, S., Kachergus, J., Hulihan, M., Peuralinna, T., Dutra, A., Nussbaum, R., Lincoln, S., Crawley, A., Hanson, M., Maraganore, D., Adler, C., Cookson, M. R., Muenter, M., Baptista, M., Miller, D., Blancato, J., Hardy, J., & Gwinn-Hardy, K. (2003). alpha-Synuclein locus triplication causes Parkinson's disease. *Science*, 302, 841.

Speakman, J. R., Talbot, D. A., Selman, C., Snart, S., McLaren, J. S., Redman, P., Krol, E., Jackson, D. M., Johnson, M. S., & Brand, M. D. (2004) Uncoupled and surviving: individual mice with high metabolism have greater mitochondrial uncoupling and live longer. *Aging Cell*, 3, 87–95.

St-Pierre, J., Buckingham, J. A., Roebuck, S. J., & Brand, M. D. (2002). Topology of superoxide production from different sites in the mitochondrial electron transport chain. *Journal of Biological Chemistry*, 277, 44784–44790.

Stadtman, E. R. (2004). Role of oxidant species in aging. *Current Medicinal Chemistry*, 11, 1105–1112.

Sugiyama, S., Takasawa, M., Hayakawa, M., & Ozawa, T. (1993). Changes in skeletal muscle, heart and liver mitochondrial electron transport activities in rats and dogs of various ages. *Biochemistry and Molecular Biology International*, 30, 937–944.

Sun, J., Folk, D., Bradley, T. J., & Tower, J. (2002). Induced overexpression of mitochondrial Mn-superoxide dismutase extends the life span of adult Drosophila melanogaster. *Genetics*, 161, 661–672.

Suzuki, S. (2004). Diabetes mellitus with mitochondrial gene mutations in Japan. *Annals of the New York Academy of Sciences*, 1011, 185–192.

Takai, D., Inoue, K., Shisa, H., Kagawa, Y., & Hayashi, J. (1995). Age-associated changes of mitochondrial translation and respiratory function in mouse brain. *Biochemical and Biophysical Research Communications, 217,* 668–674.

Takasawa, M., Hayakawa, M., Sugiyama, S., Hattori, K., Ito, T., & Ozawa, T. (1993). Age-associated damage in mitochondrial function in rat hearts. *Experimental Gerontology, 28,* 269–280.

Takeshige, K., & Minakami, S. (1979). NADH- and NADPH-dependent formation of superoxide anions by bovine heart submitochondrial particles and NADH-ubiquinone reductase preparation. *Biochemical Journal, 180,* 129–135.

Tanhauser, S. M., & Laipis, P. J. (1995). Multiple deletions are detectable in mitochondrial DNA of aging mice. *Journal of Biological Chemistry, 270,* 24769–24775.

Taylor, R. W., Barron, M. J., Borthwick, G. M., Gospel, A., Chinnery, P. F., Samuels, D. C., Taylor, G. A., Plusa, S. M., Needham, S. J., Greaves, L. C., Kirkwood, T. B., & Turnbull, D. M. (2003). Mitochondrial DNA mutations in human colonic crypt stem cells. *Journal of Clinical Investigation, 112,* 1351–1360.

Terman, A., Dalen, H., Eaton, J. W., Neuzil, J., & Brunk, U. T. (2003). Mitochondrial recycling and aging of cardiac myocytes: the role of autophagocytosis. *Experimental Gerontology, 38,* 863–876.

Terman, A., Dalen, H., Eaton, J. W., Neuzil, J., & Brunk, U. T. (2004). Aging of cardiac myocytes in culture: oxidative stress, lipofuscin accumulation, and mitochondrial turnover. *Annals of the New York Academy of Sciences, 1019,* 70–77.

Tomlinson, I. P., Alam, N. A., Rowan, A. J., Barclay, E., Jaeger, E. E., Kelsell, D., Leigh, I., Gorman, P., Lamlum, H., Rahman, S., Roylance, R. R., Olpin, S., Bevan, S., Barker, K., Hearle, N., Houlston, R. S., Kiuru, M., Lehtonen, R., Karhu, A., Vilkki, S., Laiho, P., Eklund, C., Vierimaa, O., Aittomaki, K., Hietala, M., Sistonen, P., Paetau, A., Salovaara, R., Herva, R., Launonen, V., & Aaltonen, L. A. (2002). Germline mutations in FH predispose to dominantly inherited uterine fibroids, skin leiomyomata and papillary renal cell cancer. *Nature Genetics, 30,* 406–410.

Trifunovic, A., Wredenberg, A., Falkenberg, M., Spelbrink, J. N., Rovio, A. T., Bruder, C. E., Bohlooly, Y. M., Gidlof, S., Oldfors, A., Wibom, R., Tornell, J., Jacobs, H. T., & Larsson, N. G. (2004). Premature ageing in mice expressing defective mitochondrial DNA polymerase. *Nature, 429,* 417–423.

Trimmer, P. A., Borland, M. K., Keeney, P. M., Bennett, J. P., Jr., & Parker, W. D., Jr. (2004). Parkinson's disease transgenic mitochondrial cybrids generate Lewy inclusion bodies. *Journal of Neurochemistry, 88,* 800–812.

Trounce, I., Neill, S., & Wallace, D. C. (1994). Cytoplasmic transfer of the mtDNA nt 8993 T—>G (ATP6) point mutation associated with Leigh syndrome into mtDNA-less cells demonstrates cosegregation with a decrease in state III respiration and ADP/O ratio. *Proceedings of the National Academy of Sciences of the USA, 91,* 8334–8338.

Turrens, J. F., & Boveris, A. (1980). Generation of superoxide anion by the NADH dehydrogenase of bovine heart mitochondria. *Biochemical Journal, 191,* 421–427.

Vafa, O., Wade, M., Kern, S., Beeche, M., Pandita, T. K., Hampton, G. M., & Wahl, G. M. (2002). c-Myc can induce DNA damage, increase reactive oxygen species, and mitigate p53 function: a mechanism for oncogene-induced genetic instability. *Molecular Cell, 9,* 1031–1044.

Valente, E. M., Abou-Sleiman, P. M., Caputo, V., Muqit, M. M., Harvey, K., Gispert, S., Ali, Z., Del Turco, D., Bentivoglio, A. R., Healy, D. G., Albanese, A., Nussbaum, R., Gonzalez-Maldonado, R., Deller, T., Salvi, S., Cortelli, P., Gilks, W. P., Latchman, D. S., Harvey, R. J., Dallapiccola, B., Auburger, G., & Wood, N. W. (2004). Hereditary early-onset Parkinson's disease caused by mutations in PINK1. *Science, 304,* 1158–1160.

Van Remmen, H., Ikeno, Y., Hamilton, M., Pahlavani, M., Wolf, N., Thorpe, S. R., Alderson, N. L., Baynes, J. W., Epstein, C. J., Huang, T. T., Nelson, J., Strong, R., & Richardson, A. (2003). Life-long reduction in MnSOD activity results in increased DNA damage and higher incidence of cancer but does not accelerate aging. *Physiological Genomics, 16,* 29–37.

Veech, G. A., Dennis, J., Keeney, P. M., Fall, C. P., Swerdlow, R. H., Parker, W. D., Jr., &

Bennett, J. P., Jr. (2000). Disrupted mitochondrial electron transport function increases expression of anti-apoptotic bcl-2 and bcl-X(L) proteins in SH-SY5Y neuroblastoma and in Parkinson disease cybrid cells through oxidative stress. *Journal of Neuroscience Research*, 61, 693–700.

Vo, T. D., Greenberg, H. J., & Palsson, B. O. (2004). Reconstruction and functional characterization of the human mitochondrial metabolic network based on proteomic and biochemical data. *Journal of Biological Chemistry*, 279, 39532–39540.

Vogel, H., Lim, D. S., Karsenty, G., Finegold, M., & Hasty, P. (1999). Deletion of Ku86 causes early onset of senescence in mice. *Proceedings of the National Academy of Sciences of the USA*, 96, 10770–10775.

Vulliamy, T. J., Knight, S. W., Mason, P. J., & Dokal, I. (2001). Very short telomeres in the peripheral blood of patients with X-linked and autosomal dyskeratosis congenita. *Blood Cells, Molecules, and Diseases*, 27, 353–357.

Wallace, D. C. (1994). Mitochondrial DNA mutations in diseases of energy metabolism. *Journal of Bioenergetics and Biomembranes*, 26, 241–250.

Wanagat, J., Cao, Z., Pathare, P., & Aiken, J. M. (2001). Mitochondrial DNA deletion mutations colocalize with segmental electron transport system abnormalities, muscle fiber atrophy, fiber splitting, and oxidative damage in sarcopenia. *FASEB Journal*, 15, 322–332.

Wanagat, J., Wolff, M. R., & Aiken, J. M. (2002). Age-associated changes in function, structure and mitochondrial genetic and enzymatic abnormalities in the Fischer 344 × Brown Norway F(1) hybrid rat heart. *Journal of Molecular and Cellular Cardiology*, 34, 17–28.

Warburg, O. (1956). On the origin of cancer cells. *Science*, 123, 309–314.

Wilson, F. H., Hariri, A., Farhi, A., Zhao, H., Petersen, K. F., Toka, H. R., Nelson-Williams, C., Raja, K. M., Kashgarian, M., Shulman, G. I., Scheinman, S. J., & Lifton, R. P. (2004). A Cluster of Metabolic Defects Caused by Mutation in a Mitochondrial tRNA. *Science*, 000, 000–000.

Wong, K. K., Maser, R. S., Bachoo, R. M., Menon, J., Carrasco, D. R., Gu, Y., Alt, F. W., & DePinho, R. A. (2003). Telomere dysfunction and Atm deficiency compromises organ homeostasis and accelerates ageing. *Nature*, 421, 643–648.

Woo, R. A., & Poon, R. Y. (2004). Activated oncogenes promote and cooperate with chromosomal instability for neoplastic transformation. *Genes and Development*, 18, 1317–1330.

Yan, L. J., & Sohal, R. S. (1998). Mitochondrial adenine nucleotide translocase is modified oxidatively during aging. *Proceedings of the National Academy of Sciences of the USA*, 95, 12896–12901.

Yan, L. J., Levine, R. L., & Sohal, R. S. (1997). Oxidative damage during aging targets mitochondrial aconitase. *Proceedings of the National Academy of Sciences of the USA*, 94, 11168–11172.

Yui, R., Ohno, Y., & Matsuura, E. T. (2003). Accumulation of deleted mitochondrial DNA in aging Drosophila melanogaster. *Genes and Genetic Systems*, 78, 245–251.

Zeviani, M., Moraes, C. T., DiMauro, S., Nakase, H., Bonilla, E., Schon, E. A., & Rowland, L. P. (1988). Deletions of mitochondrial DNA in Kearns-Sayre Syndrome. *Neurology*, 38, 1339–1346.

Zucchini, C., Pugnaloni, A., Pallotti, F., Solmi, R., Crimi, M., Castaldini, C., Biagini, G., & Lenaz, G. (1995). Human skeletal muscle mitochondria in aging: lack of detectable morphological and enzymic defects. *Biochemistry and Molecular Biology International*, 37, 607–616.

Chapter 6

p53 and Mouse Aging Models

Catherine Gatza, George Hinkal, Lynette Moore, Melissa Dumble, and
Lawrence A. Donehower

I. Introduction to p53

Since the original identification of p53 in 1979 (Lane & Crawford, 1979; Linzer & Levine, 1979), much attention has been focused on this important protein and its links to cancer. A decade after its discovery, it was found to be a prototypical tumor suppressor protein (Levine *et al.*, 2004). At least half of all human cancers exhibit mutations in the p53 gene, and it has been estimated that 80 percent of human cancers have a functional defect in p53 signaling (Levine, 1997; Lozano & Elledge, 2000). Mice deficient in p53 are profoundly susceptible to early tumors (Donehower *et al.*, 1992). Although the role of p53 in suppressing tumorigenesis is now well established, recent mouse model and human studies suggest a link between p53 and organismal aging (Donehower, 2002; Maier *et al.*, 2004; Tyner *et al.*, 2002; Van Heemst *et al.*, 2005). This chapter will discuss various mouse models of aging, with a particular emphasis on the potential role of p53 in regulating cellular senescence and organismal aging.

A primary function of p53 is to protect the normal dividing cell from stress-induced damage. In an unstressed cell, p53 exists at low basal levels in the cytoplasm; it is activated by a number of cellular insults, including DNA damage, hypoxia, and aberrant growth signaling (Giaccia & Kastan, 1998; Levine, 1997; Ljungman, 2000; Vousden, 2002). Activation results in a stabilization of protein levels and the translocation of p53 to the nucleus, where it functions as a transcription factor to regulate target genes via a conserved p53 consensus sequence (Ashcroft & Vousden, 1999). The cellular outcome of p53 activation depends on many variables, but generally results in the onset of either cell cycle arrest or apoptosis (Oren, 2003; Vousden & Lu, 2002) (see Figure 6.1).

Post-translational modifications play an important role in activating p53 (Bode & Dong, 2004). There are many sites of phosphorylation and acetylation on p53 (Appella & Anderson, 2001; Bode & Dong, 2004; Brooks & Gu, 2003; Xu, 2003). Many of these phosphorylations can occur

Handbook of the Biology of Aging, Sixth Edition

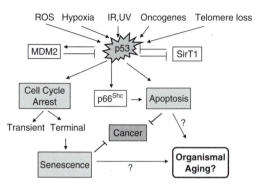

Figure 6.1 Activation of p53 signaling suppresses cancer and may influence organismal aging. Activation of p53 upon cellular stress results in translocation to the nucleus and transcription of target genes that affect anti-proliferative outcomes. These can include apoptosis or cell cycle arrest. In some cases, cell cycle arrest induced by p53 can be permanent in nature and lead to cellular senescence. The activity of p53 is regulated by a number of proteins, including those implicated in aging and longevity, such as SIRT1, which deacetylates p53. Activated p53 can transcriptionally regulate aging-associated genes such as SIRT1 and p66^{Shc}. The ability of p53 to induce cell cycle arrest, senescence, and apoptosis in response to stress is critical for its role in suppressing cancer. Thus, as a tumor suppressor, p53 is a central longevity-assurance gene. An important remaining question is whether these anti-proliferative functions of p53 can also affect the organismal aging process.

rapidly following DNA damage. For example, the DNA damage-induced ataxia-telangiectasia and Rad3-related (ATR) and ataxia-telangiectasia mutated (ATM) kinases directly phosphorylate p53 at serine 15 and indirectly phosphorylate p53 at serine 20 through activation of the intermediary kinase Chk1 (Appella & Anderson, 2001). Phosphorylation of p53 at some sites has been correlated to increases in transcriptional activity of p53, but the exact importance of all phosphorylation sites remains undetermined (Dohoney *et al.*, 2004). Some phosphorylation sites have been shown to affect the binding of p53 to Mdm2, a negative regulator of p53 that facilitates its degradation (Fuchs *et al.*, 1998; Moll & Petrenko, 2003). Post-translational phosphorylation increases the stability of p53, which

can enhance the activity of p53. p53 is also acetylated on several lysines in the carboxy-terminus of the protein (Appella & Anderson, 2001). Acetylation has been linked to transcriptional activation of the protein, and histone deacetylase activity has been shown to play a role in downregulation of p53 activity (Gu *et al.*, 2004; Juan *et al.*, 2000). Interestingly, one deacetylase that acts on p53 is the SIRT1 deacetylase (Vaziri *et al.*, 2001). SIRT1 has been shown to antagonize p53-mediated cellular senescence (Langley *et al.*, 2002) and may regulate metabolic pathways that play an important role in the aging process (Blander & Guarente, 2004; Hekimi & Guarente, 2003; Langley *et al.*, 2002).

The two major biological consequences of p53 activation are cell cycle arrest and apoptosis. p53 induces cell cycle arrest by transactivation of one of its most well-characterized target genes, p21^{CIP1} (el-Deiry *et al.*, 1993). p21^{CIP1} is a cyclin-dependent kinase inhibitor whose activation results in G1 arrest (Harper *et al.*, 1993). The induction of cell cycle arrest by p53 following DNA damage or stress allows the cell sufficient time to repair the damage through DNA repair pathways (which p53 also promotes) prior to re-entry into the cell cycle. This prevents the propagation of damaged DNA templates to daughter cells and thus precludes the fixation of mutations or abnormal chromosome complements (Lane, 1992).

In some contexts, such as excessive or irreparable DNA damage, it may be advantageous to kill the damaged cell rather than arrest it. In this scenario, p53 may induce apoptosis via transcriptional regulation of numerous pro- and anti-apoptotic genes (Fridman & Lowe, 2003). p53 can also influence apoptosis in a non-transcriptional manner by translocation to the mitochondria, where it induces caspase 3 activation (Erster *et al.*, 2004). Thus, apoptosis prevents the survival of damaged cells that might ultimately turn cancerous.

The induction of cell cycle arrest by p53 can be transient, allowing time for DNA damage to be repaired, but sometimes p53-mediated arrest is terminal and the cell never re-enters the cell cycle (Itahana et al., 2001; Serrano et al., 1997). This terminal cell cycle arrest mediated by p53 appears to be similar to cellular replicative senescence. The association of p53 with cellular senescence was among the first clues that p53 could potentially play a role in aging. A more detailed description of regulation of cellular senescence by p53 is described in the next section. In much of this chapter, a major emphasis will be on the examination of the role of p53 in organismal aging through the use of genetically engineered mouse models.

II. p53 and Cellular Senescence

The ability of p53 to induce transient cell cycle arrest, apoptosis, and/or senescence in response to cellular stress is crucial for the prevention of tumorigenesis (Itahana et al., 2001). In contrast to transient cell cycle arrest and apoptosis, which allow for the repair and removal of damaged cells from tissues, respectively, senescence does not remove cells. Thus, cells may be permanently retained that are dysfunctional, or potentially neoplastic (Campisi, 2003a). There is mounting evidence that senescent cells accumulate in mammalian tissues with age (Campisi, 2003a; Choi et al., 2000; Dimri et al., 1995; Krishnamurthy et al., 2004; Melk et al., 2003; Paradis et al., 2001; Vasile et al., 2001). This evidence is based largely on increased levels of markers believed to be specific for senescent cells, such as beta-galactosidase staining at pH 6.0 and increased levels of p16^{INK4a}. If these markers are reliable indicators of senescent cells, it will be important to establish that accumulation of senescent cells contributes substantially to organismal

aging phenotypes (Bird et al., 2003). It has been hypothesized that senescent cells in vivo contribute to aging by actively disrupting the integrity, function, and/or homeostasis of the organs in which they accumulate (Campisi, 2003a).

Cellular senescence was first identified over four decades ago, when Hayflick described replicative senescence in human fibroblasts as the irreversible loss of the proliferative capacity of cells with the maintenance of metabolic functions sufficient for cell survival (Hayflick, 1965). Since then, many types of cells from a variety of species have been shown to undergo cellular senescence (Campisi, 2001). Cellular senescence is defined by an irreversible arrest of cell division. Senescent cells permanently arrest in G$_1$ and do not enter S phase in response to mitogenic signals (Goldstein, 1990). Despite this permanent arrest, senescent cells remain metabolically active, and some cell types (e.g., human fibroblasts and T lymphocytes) become resistant to the induction of apoptosis (Seluanov et al., 2001). In addition to irreversible arrest, senescent cells also exhibit an enlarged, flattened morphology, increased lysosomal and mitochondrial size, and expression of a β-galactosidase, which can be used as a marker of senescence (senescence associated β-galactosidase staining) when cells are stained at pH 6.0 (Bird et al., 2003; Dimri et al., 1995). Senescent fibroblasts also exhibit a secretory matrix degrading phenotype, but this appears to be cell-type specific (Krtolica et al., 2001).

Cellular senescence is initiated in response to a variety of cellular stressors, including shortened telomeres, DNA damage, abnormal mitogenic signals, and the disruption of chromatin (Campisi, 2003a). Telomere shortening in particular has been shown to play an important role in the induction of senescence in human cells (Wright & Shay, 2002). Telomeres are repetitive 10 to 20 kilobase (kb) DNA sequences at the end of chromosomes that ensure chromosomal integrity by preventing end-to-end fusions (Ben-Porath & Weinberg, 2004; Smogorzewska & de Lange, 2004). Human somatic cells lack telomerase, the enzyme required to maintain telomeric length, and lose 50 to 200 basepairs (bp) of telomere sequence with each cell division (Campisi *et al.*, 2001; Klapper *et al.*, 2001). Human fibroblasts typically reach senescence with an average telomere length of only 5 to 10 kb (Ben-Porath & Weinberg, 2004; Harley *et al.*, 1994). Evidence suggests that the p53 kinase ATM, which is able to transduce DNA damage signals, is also capable of signaling telomere loss to p53. In response to telomere loss, ATM activates p53 through phosphorylation, leading to the induction of senescence (Herbig *et al.*, 2004; Itahana *et al.*, 2004). The ectopic expression of telomerase in presenescent human cells leads to an immortal phenotype and demonstrates that if telomere length is maintained, cells can divide indefinitely and avoid senescence (Bodnar *et al.*, 1998; Vaziri & Benchimol, 1998).

Despite the link between telomere length and senescence in human cells, it is clear that reduction in telomere length is not responsible for the induction of senescence in all cell types. Murine embryonic fibroblasts (MEFs) undergo senescence in culture while retaining very long telomeres, typically greater than 50 kb (Kipling *et al.*, 1999). It has also been shown that other cellular stressors, such as DNA damage, mitogenic signals, oxidative stress, the expression of oncogenes (e.g., Ras), and the disruption of chromatin, can all induce senescence in a variety of species and cell types, including human cells (Campisi, 2003a; Serrano *et al.*, 1997; Sherr & DePinho, 2000; Zhu *et al.*, 1998). A recent study suggests that MEFs are particularly susceptible to senescence induced by oxidative stress (Parrinello *et al.*, 2003).

When cultured in standard conditions (20 percent atmospheric oxygen), MEFs begin to senesce after 8 to 10 population doublings. However, under physiological oxygen levels (3 percent), MEFs did not enter senescence as early as under 20 percent oxygen conditions. This suggests that oxidative stress-induced DNA damage may play an important role in the induction of senescence in MEFs (Parrinello *et al.*, 2003; Sherr & DePinho, 2000).

Several tumor suppressor proteins such as p53, retinoblastoma (Rb), promyelocytic leukemia (PML), p19^{ARF}, and p16^{INK4a} are implicated in the induction of senescence through both telomere-dependent and -independent mechanisms (Bringold & Serrano, 2000; Ferbeyre, 2002; Ferbeyre *et al.*, 2002; Itahana *et al.*, 2003). In this chapter, particular emphasis will be placed on the role of p53. A number of observations have linked p53 to cellular senescence. For example, MEFs null for p53 bypass the induction of senescence and rapidly immortalize, directly demonstrating that p53-mediated senescence can suppress immortalization (Harvey *et al.*, 1993b). Induction of senescence in human and rodent fibroblasts by the overexpression of Ras is p53-dependent, and cells exposed to Ras in the absence of p53 become transformed (Serrano *et al.*, 1997). Despite an extended life span, human fibroblasts lacking p53 will eventually arrest in a state of high genomic instability, known as *cellular crisis* (Harley *et al.*, 1994). Cells with active p53 will arrest before cellular crisis is reached, preventing the propagation of genomic rearrangements and mutations. The inactivation of p53, through lentiviral suppression or microinjection of anti-p53 antibodies, is sufficient to extend the replicative life span of human cells and can release both human and murine cells from a senescent growth arrest (Dirac & Bernards, 2003; Gire & Wynford-Thomas, 1998). Moreover, human diploid fibroblasts obtained from individuals with the familial cancer predisposition Li-Fraumeni syndrome contain a defective p53 allele and are prone to immortalization after emerging from crisis (Bischoff *et al.*, 1990). These data indicate that the presence of active p53 is required for the induction, and in some cases the maintenance of, senescence in several cell types.

Although p53 has been shown to play an important role in the induction of senescence, there are conflicting reports about the status of p53 protein levels in senescent cells. One report demonstrates that p53 protein levels do not appear to increase during senescence (Vaziri *et al.*, 1997). However, both human and murine cells that become senescent in response to oxidative stress or the overexpression of Ras show a transient spike in p53 protein levels, with p53 returning to pre-senescent levels (Ferbeyre *et al.*, 2002). It is possible that p53 protein is transiently induced during replicative senescence. However, this change may be difficult to detect, possibly because cells in culture and tissue become senescent in an asynchronous manner.

Despite the debate about p53 protein levels, there is clearly a detectable increase in p53 activity in senescent cells. Both p53 DNA binding ability and transcriptional activity increase during senescence (Atadja *et al.*, 1995). A p53 target gene, p21^{CIP1}, a cyclin-dependent kinase inhibitor, shows elevated levels at both the transcriptional and protein level in several types of senescent cells (Alcorta *et al.*, 1996; Noda *et al.*, 1994; Tahara *et al.*, 1995). This suggests that p53 is able to induce senescence in part through the induction of p21, a critical mediator of the G_1 arrest typical of senescent cells. p53-mediated induction of p21 expression prevents the phosphorylation of Rb and halts progression through the cell cycle, leading to a G_1 arrest (Bringold & Serrano, 2000). The elevation of p21 levels during senescence is transient, although the interval of elevated p21

expression is relatively long (Alcorta *et al.*, 1996). Senescent human fibroblasts show a gradual decline in p21 several weeks after becoming senescent, which is concurrent with an increase in levels of p16^{INK4a}, a tumor suppressor protein that can induce G_1 arrest by preventing the phosphorylation of Rb (Alcorta *et al.*, 1996). Inactivation of p53 in senescent human cells re-stimulated robust growth, but only if p16 levels were low (Beausejour *et al.*, 2003). This suggests that p53 can initiate senescence through the induction of p21 and that an increase in p16 may maintain the senescent growth arrest (Beausejour *et al.*, 2003).

Post-translational modifications of the p53 protein are critical for its stabilization and activation in response to cellular stressors. Both the phosphorylation and acetylation of p53 appear to play an important role in its ability to mediate the induction of cellular senescence. Concurrent with an increase in activity, p53 is phosphorylated in senescent cells. However, the pattern of modification is distinct from that seen in response to DNA damage (Webley *et al.*, 2000). In both senescent and damaged cells, there is an increase in Ser15 phosphorylation. However, senescent cells show an increase in Thr18 and Ser376 and a decrease in Ser392 phosphorylation (Webley *et al.*, 2000). p53 is also acetylated in senescent MEFs (Pearson *et al.*, 2000). A conserved yeast nicotinamide adenine dinucleotide (NAD)-dependent histone deacetylase, Sir2, has been shown to modulate life span extension in yeast and worms (Guarente, 2000; Sinclair, 2002). The human Sir2 homolog, SIRT1, has been shown to negatively regulate p53 through deacetylation (Langley *et al.*, 2002). SIRT1 null cells exhibit higher levels of acetylated p53 that is more active in apoptosis induction (Cheng *et al.*, 2003; McBurney *et al.*, 2003). Overexpression of SIRT1 in MEFs antagonizes PML-induced cellular senescence, which is dependent on the activation of p53 (Langley *et al.*, 2002). This suggests that the deacetylation and inactivation of p53 inhibit the induction of cellular senescence. These specific modifications of p53 in senescent cells support a direct role of p53 in the signaling pathway of senescence.

Senescent fibroblasts have been shown to secrete growth factors, cytokines, extracellular matrix, and degradative enzymes that can disrupt tissue structure and function and can also promote neoplastic transformation (Krtolica *et al.*, 2001; Rinehart & Torti, 1997). These secreted factors are responsible, at least in part, for the ability of senescent human fibroblasts to stimulate both premalignant and malignant epithelial cells to proliferate in culture and *in vivo* (Krtolica *et al.*, 2001). Interestingly, although senescent fibroblasts stimulated preneoplastic epithelial cells, they had had no effect on normal epithelial cells when grown together in culture (Krtolica *et al.*, 2001). When a combination of preneoplastic epithelial cells and senescent fibroblasts were injected into immunocompromised mice, these mice developed epithelial-based tumors. Thus, an increase in senescent cells in an aged individual may promote the development of cancer through a combination of genetic changes and changes in the microenvironment caused by the secretion of soluble and insoluble factors by the senescent cells. Although this mechanism could contribute to the increase in cancer incidence seen in older individuals, it doesn't account for the fact that cancer death rates actually decline in extreme old age (Horiuchi *et al.*, 2003; Smith, 1996).

III. Linkage of IGF-1, Sir2, and p53 Signaling

Reduction in calorie intake increases longevity in yeast, worms, flies, and mice (Barger *et al.*, 2003; Longo & Finch, 2003).

Deficiencies in the insulin like growth factor 1 (IGF-1)/insulin pathway in worms and flies and growth hormone/IGF-1 signaling in mice also extend life span, although this is accompanied by reduced body size (Longo & Finch, 2003). Calorie restriction may extend longevity at least in part through its effects in reducing the activity of the IGF-1 signaling pathway, although recent evidence suggests IGF-1-independent mechanisms may also operate (Bartke *et al.*, 2001). Another longevity-extending molecule in yeast and worms, Sir2, has been shown to interact with the IGF-1 signaling pathway in worms and human cells (Cohen *et al.*, 2004; Hekimi & Guarente, 2003). Moreover, the mammalian homologue of Sir2, SIRT1, has been shown to be induced in calorie-restricted rodents (Cohen *et al.*, 2004). SIRT1 appears to regulate the cellular response to stress by the Foxo family of transcription factors, including Foxo3a, which is a component of the insulin/IGF-1 signaling pathway (Cohen *et al.*, 2004). SIRT1 also deacetylates and represses the activity of Foxo3a (Motta *et al.*, 2004). The discovery that Sir2 deacetylates and reduces p53 activity was the first linkage of p53 to well-established longevity pathways (Luo *et al.*, 2001; Vaziri *et al.*, 2001). Recently, Finkel and colleagues have demonstrated that nutrient deprivation *in vitro* (somewhat analogous to calorie restriction *in vivo*) augments expression of SIRT1 in mammalian cells (Nemoto *et al.*, 2004). Nutrient removal also activates Foxo3a expression and induces its relocalization from the cytoplasm to the nucleus. SIRT1 upregulation by nutrient scarcity was found to be dependent on Foxo3a levels, indicating that Foxo3a transcriptionally reglates SIRT1. Remarkably, SIRT1 transcriptional upregulation was dependent on the presence of two p53 response elements in the SIRT1 promoter, and that a physical interaction between nuclear Foxo3a and p53 occurs (Nemoto *et al.*,

2004). SIRT1 expression could not be induced by overnight starvation in tissues of p53 null mice, indicating that calorie-restriction-dependent SIRT1 upregulation is dependent on p53. These findings integrate three key pathways implicated in aging and nutrient sensing in a very intriguing way (see Figure 6.2). Foxo3a and p53 both upregulate SIRT1 in starved cells, yet SIRT1 deacetylates and suppresses these two transcription factors in what appears to be a negative feedback regulatory loop. Figure 6.2 shows a model for how calorie restriction could affect aging and longevity through IGF-1, Foxo3a, SIRT1, and p53 signaling. In conditions of nutrient abundance, IGF-1 signaling is enhanced and Foxo3a is localized primarily in the cytoplasm. SIRT1 is consequently expressed at low levels and is not able to downregulate p53. Reduced SIRT1 results in low expression of SIRT1-regulated stress response genes and higher activity of p53, ultimately resulting in higher levels of cellular senescence and apoptosis that could contribute to aging phenotypes. In contrast to this nutrient abundance scenario, calorie restriction produces reduced activity in IGF-1 signaling and increased Foxo3a nuclear localization. Nuclear Foxo3a and p53 would combine to activate SIRT1 transcription. Enhanced SIRT1 expression would result in an enhanced response to reactive oxygen species (ROS) and reduced p53 activity through deacetylation. Reduced cellular senescence and apoptosis in somatic cells would likely enhance longevity. It will be of great interest to test the validity of this model in mice through the appropriate assays, crosses, and longevity studies.

IV. Mouse Models of Aging

Cell culture–based senescence models have obvious limitations if the goal is to understand the aging of whole multicellular organisms. The last decade has seen a dramatic increase in research devoted to understanding the mechanisms behind organismal aging. Much of the recent work on the genetics of longevity in yeast, nematodes, and flies demonstrated the importance of certain signaling pathways and genes in regulation of life span (Fabrizio & Longo, 2003; Guarente & Kenyon, 2000; Helfand & Rogina, 2003). The nematode *C. elegans* and *Drosphila melanogaster* possess many advantages for aging studies, including very well-understood biology and genetics, ease of genetic manipulability, and relatively short life spans. However, the use of model organisms whose somatic cells are all post-mitotic may provide limitations in their applicability to mammalian systems. There is growing evidence that the somatic stem cells in more long-lived organisms with renewable tissue compartments play an important role in aging (Campisi, 2003a; Donehower, 2002; Pelicci, 2004; Sharpless & DePinho, 2004; Van Zant & Liang, 2003). Currently, the most widely used mammalian aging model is the laboratory mouse (*Mus musculus*). It has many of the advantages of the nematode and fly systems, particularly with respect to its well-understood genetics and the availability of advanced genetic manipulation tools. The close evolutionary relationship of men and mice gives mouse aging studies obvious relevance to human aging. The life span of 2 to 3 years for most inbred laboratory strains is among the shortest of all mammalian species, though it is hardly an advantage when compared to the life spans of worms (3 weeks) and flies (3 months). Yet despite the exponential increases in time, labor, and costs associated with mouse longevity studies, many important insights into aging have recently been provided. One exciting outcome of the mouse studies was the revelation that some of the longevity-associated genes in the lower organisms

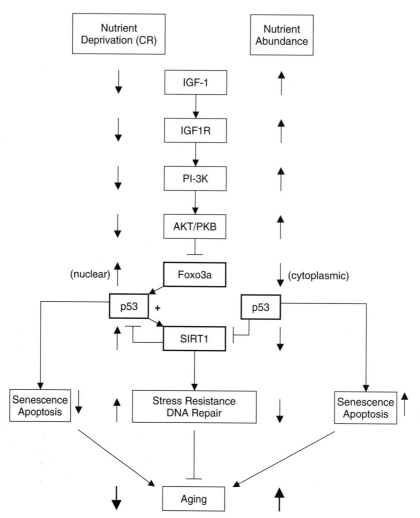

Figure 6.2 Differential aging-associated effects of interacting IGF-1, SIRT1, and p53 signaling components in conditions of nutrient abundance or scarcity. The model illustrates how nutrient conditions could affect IGF-1 signaling and Foxo3a function to influence the aging process. In conditions of ample nutrients, IGF-1 signaling is enhanced and Foxo3a remains cytoplasmic, allowing p53 to transcriptionally repress SIRT1 expression. Reduced SIRT1 and active p53 could lead to aging phenotypes through a reduced stress response and enhanced formation of senescent or apoptotic cells, respectively. Under conditions of nutrient scarcity, reduced IGF-1 signaling results in nuclear Foxo3a translocation. Nuclear Foxo3a and p53 can transcriptionally activate SIRT1. Augmented expression of SIRT1 represses p53 through deacetylation. Increased SIRT1 enhances stress-response pathways and DNA repair, whereas reduced p53 activity could result in fewer senescent or apoptotic cells, outcomes that could contribute to the delayed aging phenotypes associated with calorie restriction.

were also important in determining longevity in mammalian models (Guarente & Kenyon, 2000; Tatar *et al.*, 2003). However, equally important was the discovery of new longevity-regulating genes that might be specific for vertebrate or mammalian organisms (de Boer *et al.*, 2002; Migliaccio *et al.*, 1999; Tyner *et al.*, 2002; Vogel *et al.*, 1999). Many of these altered mouse longevity models are deficient for genes that maintain genomic integrity. These will be described below. Given the established importance of p53 in cellular senescence and the maintenance of genomic stability, we will place particular emphasis on mouse models with altered p53 activity, which is the focus of our own laboratory.

Organismal aging models can be subdivided into two general categories: those exhibiting extended longevity and those exhibiting reduced longevity and accelerated aging compared to their normal counterparts. There has been some controversy over whether accelerated aging and reduced longevity models actually reflect real alterations in the intrinsic aging process, as opposed to pathological defects unrelated to aging (Harrison, 1997; Miller, 2004a). The arguments pro and con with respect to accelerated aging models have been forcefully presented by Hasty and Vijg (Hasty & Vijg, 2004a,b) and Miller (Miller, 2004a,b). Given that our laboratory has generated a mouse model that exhibits aspects of accelerated aging, it should be obvious where our sympathies lie. Thus, accelerated aging models will be discussed below because we and many others believe they do provide important insights into the mechanisms of aging (Donehower, 2002; Hasty & Vijg, 2004a; Warner & Sierra, 2003).

Mouse aging models can also be categorized by how they were generated. Such models can be produced by both environmental and genetic interventions. The major environmental intervention is through calorie restriction, in which nutrients are maintained at high levels but total calories ingested are 30 to 50 percent lower than *ad lib* caloric intake. Calorie-restricted mice often show remarkable extensions of life span, up to 50 percent beyond those of mice fed *ad libitum* (Masoro, 2000; Sohal & Weindruch, 1996). The mechanisms responsible for longevity extension by calorie restriction are discussed below and elsewhere in this volume. Genetic interventions to produce altered longevity have utilized a number of approaches. Selective inbreeding of AKR/J mice by Japanese scientists has led to the development of the senescence-accelerated mouse (SAM). There are 14 senescence-prone inbred strains (SAM-P) and 4 senescence-resistant strains (SAM-R) (Takeda, 1999). Each of the SAM-P lines exhibits a specific constellation of accelerated aging phenotypes. However, the genetics of the SAM-P mice remain undefined, so genotype–phenotype correlations are difficult.

A number of mouse aging models were discovered as spontaneous mutations or as a result of random mutagenesis approaches. These include the Snell and Ames dwarf mice with extended longevity and the accelerated aging *Klotho* mouse that was identified as a result of inactivation by transgene insertion (Andersen *et al.*, 1995; Kuro-o *et al.*, 1997; Li *et al.*, 1990). In the last several years, a more targeted genetic engineering approach has generated a number of useful mouse aging models (Misra & Duncan, 2002). Many of these models are the result of embryonic stem cell gene targeting or standard transgenic methods and exhibit either accelerated or delayed aging phenotypes (Anisimov, 2003; Donehower, 2002; Hasty *et al.*, 2003; Liang *et al.*, 2003). The remainder of this review will focus primarily on the insights that these genetically altered mice have given us with respect to aging and longevity.

Before delving into genetic models of aging, it is important to examine what to look for, answering the question, "How do you know whether you have a mouse with accelerated or delayed aging?" Fortunately, with the close evolutionary relationship of mice and men, murine aging and human aging share many characteristics. These include the appearance of such aging phenotypes as osteoporosis; arteriosclerosis; cataracts; decreased wound healing and stress tolerance; cachexia (wasting); hair-graying and alopecia; increased cancer incidence; hunching of the spine (lordokyphosis); muscle, skin, and generalized organ atrophy and pathology; and more (Arking, 1998; Mohr *et al.*, 1996). Observation of many or all of these phenotypes in conjunction with a shortened life span in a mouse model should satisfy the definition of premature aging. Moreover, these premature aging phenotypes should only appear after complete adult maturation. The appearance of one or a few early aging phenotypes is clearly insufficient to make a strong argument for an accelerated aging model. Conversely, a mutant mouse can be said to have delayed aging if it lives significantly longer than its wildtype littermates of the same genetic background. A delayed onset of aging phenotypes is also a useful indicator.

Another confirmatory tool is a statistical demonstration of aging by Gompertz analysis of mouse survival data. The Gompertz equation can measure age-specific increases in mortality rates, which may represent the rate of aging (Arking, 1998; Pletcher *et al.*, 2000). If a putative aging model ages differently from its normal counterpart, it should exhibit a significantly different slope in the plot of age-specific mortality (plotted logarithmically) versus age over most, if not all, of its life span. A recent summary of accelerated and delayed aging mouse models indicates that the majority do not exhibit the expected divergence in mortality rate doubling times (de Magalhaes *et al.*, 2004). The failure of these models to display different rates of aging could be due to a number of factors, including inadequate sample size, inadequate control populations, and experimental artifacts such as housing conditions, faulty reporting, and diet. Alternatively, the models may display segmental aging phenotypes that do not alter mortality rates sufficiently to show up as significant in the Gompertz analysis. Alternatively, the models may not be displaying altered rates of aging; consequently other nonaging related pathologies may play a primary role in mortality. However, the fact that even some extended longevity models fail to exhibit altered rates of aging by Gompertz analysis raises a concern about this approach. A complete analysis utilizing an array of statistical, biological, pathological, and biochemical approaches may be necessary to reach a more definitive conclusion that a particular model does indeed exhibit altered aging.

Recent research indicates that many of the genes that affect organismal aging and longevity are involved in stress management and DNA repair metabolism (Finkel & Holbrook, 2000; Hasty *et al.*, 2003; Hekimi & Guarente, 2003; Lehmann, 2002). This indicates that aging may result from genetic activity stimulated by exogenous (DNA damaging agents) and endogenous (metabolic oxidation, DNA replication errors, and stalled replication forks) sources. Studies using *lacI* and *lacZ* reporter mice have shown old mice accumulate DNA damage with age. The spectrum of damage varies with the type of tissue observed, but the general trend is an increase in point mutations, large deletions, and/or rearrangements in nuclear DNA (Dolle *et al.*, 2000; Dolle *et al.*, 2002; Hill *et al.*, 2004; Vijg & Dolle, 2002). These data suggest that the possibility that genetic alterations that increase the age-associated mutation rates could also influence the aging process. Thus, mice with defects in genes that regulate genomic stability might occasionally be expected to show accelerated aging phenotypes, and recent genetically engineered mouse models bear this out. A number of these models are described below. The aging phenotypes in these models are supportive of the idea that DNA damage plays an initiating role in organismal aging processes.

V. Mouse Models of Accelerated Aging

A mouse model of defective transcription-associated nucleotide excision repair was created by mutating one of the xeroderma pigmentosum (XP) genes, XPD, as a model of trichothiodystrophy (TTD), a disorder in humans characterized by postnatal growth failure, progressive neurological dysfunction, skeletal abnormalities, and a reduced life expectancy (de Boer et al., 2002). TTD mice have impaired transcription and mildly impaired nucleotide excision repair (NER). They develop normally but exhibit many aspects of accelerated aging, including osteoporosis, early graying, cachexia, and infertility. Interestingly, when the TTD mice were crossed to xeroderma pigmentosum group A (XPA)-deficient mice, the bi-deficient mice showed an even greater acceleration of the aging phenotypes compared to the TTD mice. It was concluded that the data strongly supports the DNA damage theory of aging, and a model was invoked in which increased unrepaired damage in the TTD mice in conjunction with transcription defects resulted in increased apoptosis and depletion of cell renewal capacity and subsequent accelerated aging (de Boer et al., 2002).

Some mouse models exhibiting accelerated aging are the products of mutations in chromosomal integrity pathways. Ku80 is a component of the complex involved in non-homologous end-joining (NHEJ) repair of double strand breaks (DSBs) (Lieber et al., 2003). Homozygous deletion of this allele presumably results in increased DSBs in vivo. These mice prematurely exhibit a number of aging phenotypes, including lordokyphosis and osteoporosis, decreased wound healing, reduced muscle cellularity, and reduced subdermal adipose levels (Vogel et al., 1999). Surprisingly, these mice have a reduced tumor incidence compared to control mice. The incidence of tumors was 27.6 percent and 2.2 percent for Ku80 wildtype and null mice, respectively, although increased life span in the control mice may account for some of this difference. On a cellular level, Ku80 null mouse embryonic fibroblasts exhibit early passage senescence, decreased colony size, and hypersensitivity to ionizing radiation and oxidative stress (Lim et al., 2000). All of these cellular observations were shown to be dependent on the tumor suppressor p53. Additionally, reducing the p53 dose in vivo dramatically increased the tumor incidence and altered spectrum. Curiously, it was shown that Ku80 null mice exhibit a decrease in both point mutations and large genomic rearrangements (Rockwood et al., 2003). This was concluded to be the result of a more active p53 response, whereby the presumptive increase in DSBs leads to apoptosis and clearing of affected cells.

The breast cancer susceptibility gene BRCA1 is a tumor suppressor with cell cycle checkpoint and DNA repair functions (Venkitaraman, 2002). Homozygous deletion of Brca1 results in early embryonic lethality (Gowen et al., 1996; Hakem et al., 1996). A homozygous deletion of only Brca1 exon 11 results in embryonic lethality that can be rescued by making the Brca1-deficient mice heterozygous for p53 (Xu et al., 2001). The unrescued Brca1$^{\Delta 11/\Delta 11}$ embryos exhibit a massive increase in p53-dependent senescence as measured by the senescence-associated β-galactosidase staining assay (Cao et al., 2003). Interestingly, the rescued Brca1$^{\Delta 11/\Delta 11}$ p53$^{+/-}$ mice show a large number of early aging phenotypes by 8 months of age. Longevity was reduced to about one year. The loss of intact Brca1 was associated with increased p53 levels, and fibroblasts from Brca1$^{\Delta 11/\Delta 11}$ embryos showed greatly increased rates of senescence that could be reduced by removal of p53. These studies further support the idea that DNA repair deficiencies can contribute to aging, in this case through activation of p53-mediated senescence pathways.

Another genome maintenance model of accelerated aging is the BubR1 hypomorphic mouse (Baker et al., 2004). BubR1 is a spindle assembly checkpoint protein important in the faithful segregation of chromosomes during mitosis and meiosis (Chan & Yen, 2003). Complete loss of *BubR1* gene function results in embryonic lethality, but the hypomorph is viable yet exhibits progressive aneuploidy, shortened longevity, and a number of premature aging phenotypes (Baker *et al.*, 2004). Reduced BubR1 in embryo fibroblasts is also associated with early senescence as well as aneuploidy. Finally, expression of *BubR1* is decreased in multiple aged tissues, suggesting it may serve as a useful aging marker.

Telomere shortening in human cells has been closely correlated with replicative senescence (Ben-Porath & Weinberg, 2004; Wright & Shay, 2002). Each time a eukaryotic cell divides, due to the nature of DNA polymerase replication and linear chromosomes, a portion of the ends of the chromosome (telomere) is lost. Since the telomere provides a protective barrier to the coding regions of the chromosome, their gradual erosion is believed to be the primary factor for the Hayflick Limit of human diploid fibroblast division in culture (Ben-Porath & Weinberg, 2004; Hayflick, 1965; Wright & Shay, 2002). Telomerase null cells can escape this replicative senescence by immortalization. This is associated with chromosome instability, characterized by end–end fusions of chromosomes lacking their telomeres (Mathieu *et al.*, 2004).

The importance of telomeres in affecting organismal aging has also been demonstrated by the telomerase knockout mice (Rudolph *et al.*, 1999). Inbred mice have much longer telomeres than humans (Kim Sh *et al.*, 2002). Consequently, knocking out the RNA component of telomerase, *Terc*, requires mice to proceed through at least four generations of intercrossing to sufficiently shrink their telomeres *in vivo* before showing accelerated aging phenotypes (Rudolph *et al.*, 1999). Phenotypes in these mice develop primarily in tissues that undergo many divisions during the life span of the animal, particularly the skin and gametes. p53 levels were increased in the late-generation telomerase knockout mice, and introducing a defective p53 allele into the *Terc* null background resulted in attenuation of a number of the accelerated aging phenotypes.

Terc deletion also facilitates Werner's syndrome phenotypes in a mouse model. Ablation of the gene encoding the Werner helicase alone does not produce anything resembling the accelerated aging phenotypes of Werner's patients at the organismal level (Lebel & Leder, 1998). However, by crossing the *Wrn* null background into late-generation *Terc* null animals, the bi-deficient offspring exhibit all the phenotypes found in Werner's patients (e.g., osteoporosis, cataracts, and dysfunctional insulin metabolism) in addition to those of the *Terc* null animals, but earlier and more severely (Chang *et al.*, 2004; Du *et al.*, 2004). These results indicate that the Werner (WRN) helicase has a telomere maintenance function and further support the notion that genomic instability plays a causative role in mammalian aging.

In addition to genomic instability, other types of DNA damage have been shown to influence aging. A premature mouse aging model whereby a single gene, *Klotho*, was disrupted may fall into this category (Kuro-o *et al.*, 1997). The primary pathways found to be affected by this deletion involve vitamin D metabolism and calcium homeostasis, which have not been shown to have any effect on the aging phenotype (Nabeshima, 2002). *Klotho* deficient mice accrue heightened levels of oxidized DNA adducts, which follows the oxidative stress/free-radical theory of aging, but the mechanism of this vulnerability remains a mystery (Nagai *et al.*, 2003). Moreover, one potential problem with the *klotho* mouse as an aging model is the extreme reduction in longevity and the appearance of aging phenotypes before full maturity of the mouse is reached.

A verified target of oxidative stress is the mitochondrial genome (mtDNA), which accumulates deletions, point mutations, and oxidative adducts with age (Khaidakov *et al.*, 2003; Richter *et al.*, 1988; Tanhauser & Laipis, 1995; Yakes & Van Houten, 1997). These data were entirely correlative until a mouse model lacking the proofreading function of the mitochondrial DNA polymerase, PolgA, was generated (Jacobs, 2003; Trifunovic *et al.*, 2004). These mutated mice accumulated up to five times the point mutations and accelerated the appearance of large deletions as compared to wildtype mice. Interestingly, these PolgA-deficient mice exhibited reduced longevity and many symptoms of accelerated aging, suggesting that progressive mitochondrial dysfunction is not merely an aging correlate but may also play a causative role in aging phenotypes.

The recurring theme of the above accelerated aging mouse models is that the maintenance of genomic stability is a critical aspect of longevity assurance. Although mouse models with defective DNA repair and even enhanced DNA repair can exhibit normal life spans, this does not negate the theory that the damage response influences life span (Walter *et al.*, 2001). DNA repair is a complex system involving hundreds of genes such that compensating mechanisms may obscure aging phenotypes. As seen above, only the more drastic changes in DNA damage response may result in accelerated aging.

VI. Mouse Models of Delayed Aging

In contrast to the above models of accelerated aging in mice, several mouse models have been generated with increased life span, some of which are resistant to stress and damaging agents. Before murine molecular genetic manipulation

techniques were developed, the only intervention resulting in life extension in mammals was calorie restriction (CR). McCay and colleages showed that by reducing the amount of food but maintaining adequate nutrition, rats lived significantly longer (McCay *et al.*, 1989). Over the years, research has focused on mechanisms of longevity extension by CR (Koubova & Guarente, 2003; Masoro, 2000). Simplistically, CR causes an organism to think food availability is low such that it needs to protect itself molecularly to ensure, when food supplies return, the organism will live to reproduce. This may be achieved by a combination of altered gene silencing, gene activation, chaperone activation, and increased resistance to oxidative and other forms of stress (Lee *et al.*, 1999, Lee & Yu, 1990, Lin *et al.*, 2000, Um *et al.*, 2003).

Several genetic models of increased life span were serendipitously discovered involving mice characterized by hereditary dwarfism: the Ames and Snell dwarf mice. Snell mice have a spontaneous point mutation in the pituitary-specific transcription factor 1 (*Pit1*) gene (Li *et al.*, 1990), and Ames mice have a point mutation in *Prop*-1, a gene directly upstream of *Pit-1* activation (Andersen *et al.*, 1995). Because these mutations occur in the same pathway, these two dwarf strains exhibit many of the same phenotypes: dwarfism as a result of the inability to secrete growth hormone, thyroid-stimulatory hormone, and prolactin (Li *et al.*, 1990). Mice with mutations in this pathway exhibit dramatic increases in mean and maximal life span of up to 68 and 50 percent, respectively (Brown-Borg *et al.*, 1996). Although the study of these enhanced longevity models has been very informative, the many pleiotropic effects of reduced hormone levels may make it more difficult to identify the critical genes and pathways central to the aging process.

Targeted gene ablation experiments have been recently exploited to identify novel genes associated with extended longevity. The protein p66[Shc] is a splice isoform of the mammalian *Shc* locus involved in cytoplasmic signal transduction (Migliaccio *et al.*, 1997). It is differentially tyrosine or serine phosphorylated depending on stimulation by epidermal growth factor (EGF) or oxidative stress (Migliaccio *et al.*, 1999). The Pelicci group targeted a mutation of the unique collagen-homology domain CH2 of the *Shc* locus resulting in the deletion of the p66[Shc] isoform (Migliaccio *et al.*, 1999). Mice carrying this deletion showed an inverse relationship between p66[Shc] dose and life span/oxidative stress resistance. Homozygous knockouts of p66[Shc] produced mice that lived 30 percent longer and were 50 percent more resistant to the powerful oxidizer paraquat. These mice had reduced levels of oxidized DNA adducts and enhanced mtDNA integrity in a variety of tissues with age as compared to wildtype littermates (Trinei *et al.*, 2002). MEFs derived from null animals exhibit enhanced resistance to H_2O_2 and ultraviolet radiation in addition to a 50 percent decrease in steady-state ROS levels in a p53 dependent manner (Trinei *et al.*, 2002). p53 was shown to be an upstream regulator of p66[Shc] expression and function (Trinei *et al.*, 2002). Additionally, p66[Shc] null cells exhibit increased activity of the mammalian forkhead homolog FHKR1, drawing a parallel to the DAF-16 life span regulation pathway in *C. elegans* (Murphy *et al.*, 2003; Nemoto & Finkel, 2002).

Another mouse model of increased life span is the IGF-1 receptor (IGF-1R) heterozygous knockout mouse (Holzenberger *et al.*, 2003). Female *Igf1r*[+/−] mice appeared normal but had a 33 percent extended life span over their wildtype counterparts. Molecular analysis revealed a broad array of altered intracellular signaling, particularly with regard to stress responses. In addition to the expected 50 percent reduction in IGF-1R levels and of its substrate IRS-1, downstream targets such as p66[Shc] were also negatively regulated. This reduction in p66[Shc] levels and phosphorylation correlates with oxidative stress resistance. Indeed, these animals were resistant to paraquat injections, and their cells were resistant to H_2O_2 administration, albeit in a sex-dependent manner. Collectively, these studies emphasize the importance of oxidative stress resistance in life-span extension, though there are likely to be other factors responsible for extended longevity (Liang *et al.*, 2003). Moreover, issues of sample size, animal husbandry procedures, and aging-related pathology need to be more completely addressed for some of these models before definitive conclusions on aging can be obtained (Liang *et al.*, 2003).

VII. Links to p53 in Mouse Aging Models

In the mouse models discussed above, a few salient themes emerge. It is evident that alterations in responses to DNA damage and oxidative stress can elicit significant alterations in longevity and aging processes. However, it is also clear that cell signaling pathways that are not directly involved in DNA metabolism or damage repair can be important mediators of aging and longevity. For example, hormonal signaling pathway alterations typified by the Ames and Snell dwarf mice and the IGF-1 receptor heterozygotes aren't generally thought of as being directly involved in the DNA damage response. However, downstream targets of some of these pathways may monitor DNA integrity. This is also evident with the p66[Shc−/−] mice, which have an enhanced response to oxidative stress (Migliaccio *et al.*, 1999). Such findings suggest that the response to DNA damage rather than the damage *per se* is the critical factor in influencing aging and longevity. Thus, it could be argued that those mutant animals with mutations in DNA maintenance genes (e.g., the TTD, $Ku80^{-/-}$, and late generation $Terc^{-/-}$ mice) exhibit aging phenotypes not because of stochastic increases in genetic lesions but because these lesions elicit an augmented signaling response in cell cycle checkpoint and apoptotic pathways. We hypothesize that the more active DNA damage response in the mutant animals could lead to increased rates of terminal cell cycle arrest (senescence). Thus, with aging in these mutant mice, organs would more rapidly accumulate poorly functioning or nonfunctioning senescent cells that could not only inhibit organ function, but might also facilitate the formation of cancers. In addition, the mutant animals could show augmented apoptosis that would more rapidly deplete organs of critical stem and progenitor cells. It should be emphasized that this model is still speculative in nature and far from established.

One central damage response molecule is the tumor suppressor p53. As described above, following an array of different cell stresses, p53 can execute various cellular anti-proliferative or apoptotic responses. Several of the aging models described above clearly have altered p53 function. These include the $Ku80^{-/-}$, $p66^{Shc}-/-$, and $Brca^{\Delta 11/\Delta 11}$ $p53^{+/-}$, and late generation $Terc^{-/-}$ mice. $Ku80^{-/-}$ MEFs prematurely senesce, and null animals age prematurely while exhibiting a decreased tumor incidence (Lim et al., 2000). Deletion of p53 in the $Ku80$ null background restores the proliferation of MEFs, releasing them from G1/S checkpoint arrest. $Ku80^{-/-}p53^{-/-}$ MEFs are also more sensitive to irradiation and oxidative stress than are $p53^{-/-}$ MEFs. $Ku80$ null mice that are heterozygous for p53 have a broad spectrum of tumors and an increased incidence from 2.2 to 20 percent; double null mice have a 100 percent incidence of lymphoma. The absence of

the p53 damage response in the context of increased DNA lesions in the $Ku80$ null mice dramatically increases cancer frequency. Together these data suggest that both $Ku80$ null mice and cells incur increased DNA damage in the form of DSBs that activate p53-mediated cell cycle checkpoints. This checkpoint activation may be responsible for the senescent phenotype observed in $Ku80^{-/-}$ cells and possibly some of the observed aging phenotypes.

$p66^{Shc}-/-$ mice have an increased life span owing directly to an increased resistance to oxidative stress (Migliaccio et al., 1999). These data were verified in another pathway where $p66^{Shc}$ is negatively regulated (Holzenberger et al., 2003). It was shown that $p66^{Shc}$ is downstream of p53's response to oxidative stress and is required for p53-mediated induction of apoptosis by ROS in MEFs (Trinei et al., 2002). Consequently, the converse may also be true: a heightened p53 response may increase the $p66^{Shc}$-mediated ROS response, leading to increased oxidative stress and premature aging. $Brca^{\Delta 11/\Delta 11}$ mice require a reduction in the p53 dose to survive, rescuing embryos from premature senescence but developing premature aging phenotypes (Cao et al., 2003). The data suggest that p53 is activated by an increase in genomic instability due to the $Brca^{\Delta 11/\Delta 11}$ mutation. The increased p53 activation results in premature cellular senescence, and accelerated aging in the viable adults.

The ataxia telangiectasia mutated (Atm) gene has been shown to encode a critical kinase that detects DNA damage and initiates cell cycle arrest and DNA repair responses (Shiloh, 2003). Humans with two mutant Atm alleles are afflicted with ataxia telangiectasia, a syndrome that is characterized by immunodeficiency, progressive cerebellar ataxia, defective spermatogenesis, and oculocutaneous telangiectasia, lymphoma susceptibility, and aspects of premature aging (Perlman *et al.*, 2003). Interestingly, the Atm protein is an upstream regulator of p53 by directly phosphorylating it, assisting in p53 stabilization and activation (Canman *et al.*, 1998). In addition, Atm may contribute to telomere maintenance because Atm-deficient cells exhibit accelerated telomere loss and increased end-to-end chromosome fusions (Metcalfe *et al.*, 1996; Pandita, 2002). Analysis of Atm$^{-/-}$ mice has shown that they recapitulate some of the corresponding human ataxia telangiectasia phenotypes, such as lymphoma susceptibility, but neuronal and premature aging phenotypes are relatively muted (Barlow *et al.*, 1996; Elson *et al.*, 1996, Xu *et al.*, 1996). However, when Terc$^{-/-}$ mice were crossed to Atm$^{-/-}$ mice over several generations, the resulting bi-deficient offspring showed accelerated telomere loss, a reduction in lymphoma incidence, premature aging, and reduced longevity (Wong *et al.*, 2003). These late-generation Terc$^{-/-}$ Atm$^{-/-}$ mice also exhibited a generalized proliferation defect in cells of many tissues that extended to multiple tissue stem cell and progenitor compartments. Bone-marrow-colony-forming units were reduced in late generation Terc$^{-/-}$ Atm$^{-/-}$ compared to their Terc$^{-/-}$ Atm$^{+/+}$ counterparts. The stem cell compartment of the brain in late generation Terc$^{-/-}$ showed reduced proliferation in the absence of Atm compared to normal controls (Wong *et al.*, 2003). *In vitro* differentiation and survival of Terc$^{-/-}$ neural stem cells was also more deficient in the absence of Atm. This study is particularly noteworthy for its linkage of reduced stem cell/progenitor function with accelerated appearance of aging phenotypes.

VIII. Mutant Mouse p53 Models, Aging, and Cancer

Many of the genetically engineered mouse aging models discussed above implicate p53 in some aspects of the aging process, particularly those related to the DNA damage and stress responses. However, a direct test for p53 involvement in aging would entail alteration of p53 dosage or activity itself and monitoring for altered aging phenotypes. Based on the data described above, a simplistic prediction is that any genetic intervention that increases p53 levels would accelerate aging, while a reduction of p53 dosage might delay the aging process. Unfortunately, the reality is more complicated. Our laboratory and other laboratories have shown that reduction of p53 dosage by inactivation of germ line p53 dramatically shortens longevity due to early cancers (Donehower *et al.*, 1992). Mice with two null p53 alleles (p53$^{-/-}$) have a median cancer incidence and longevity of 4.5 months, whereas mice with one defective allele (p53$^{+/-}$) have a median longevity of 18 months due to cancers, versus a 30-month longevity for wildtype littermates, about half of which succumb to cancer (Donehower, 1996; Harvey *et al.*, 1993a). An intriguing question is whether reduction of p53 dosage could promote enhanced longevity if early cancers could somehow be prevented or reduced in their incidence.

The recent data regarding longevity and aging in mice with increased dosages of p53 is also complicated by differing results. Initial attempts to generate transgenic mice overexpressing wildtype p53 failed, presumably because dramatically increased p53 levels inhibited proliferation during development, resulting in embryonic lethality (Choi & Donehower, 1999). In 2002, our laboratory published results documenting the production of a mouse with hyperactive p53, the p53 +/m mouse (Tyner *et al.*, 2002). We reported that these heightened levels of p53 activity suppressed spontaneous tumor formation and, more interestingly, also produced accelerated aging-associated phenotypes. Two other recent papers have described mice with increases in p53, although they exhibited different phenotypes. These were the "super p53" mice (Garcia-Cao et al., 2002) and the p44 transgenic mice (Maier et al., 2004) discussed below.

Our p53+/m mouse contains one wild-type (WT) and one mutant (m) p53 allele. The mutant allele was serendipitously engineered while trying to introduce a single point mutation at codon 245 (Arg245Trp) of p53 (Tyner et al., 2002). The point mutation was successfully introduced, but in doing so, exons 1 through 6 of the p53 gene were deleted, as well as an area of upstream sequence. The 3' exons 7–11 of p53 gene sequence are transcribed and translated into a truncated C-terminal p53 protein by a heterologous upstream promoter. We have shown this C-terminal p53 m protein to interact with wildtype p53 in the cell, altering its stability and transactivational activity. Consistent with increased p53 activity, the p53+/m mouse does exhibit increased tumor resistance, as only 2 of 35 (6 percent) p53+/m mice displayed cancers compared to 27 of 56 (48 percent) $p53^{+/+}$ littermates (Tyner et al., 2002).

Following careful characterization, the p53+/m mouse was shown to have developed numerous traits consistent with premature aging, including decreased life span (median of 96 weeks compared to 118 weeks for wildtype littermates), decreased organ mass and cellularity (documented in the liver, kidney, spleen, skeletal muscle, and skin), decreased bone mineral density (BMD), an associated kyphosis of the spine, and a decrease tissue regenerative response (skin wound healing, hair re-growth, and recovery from hematopoietic progenitor ablation). It is of importance to mention that some premature aging traits were not observed in the p53+/m mouse. These included liver pathologies, hair graying or alopecia, intestinal atrophy, skin ulceration, amyloid plaques, brain atrophy, arthrosclerosis, and cataracts.

Current evidence supports our hypothesis that the aging phenotypes seen in this mouse are due to a hyperactive p53 status. How the augmented p53 activity in the p53+/m mouse might affect aging and longevity will be discussed in the next section.

The production of a mutant mouse with increased wildtype p53 dosage was described by the Serrano laboratory (Garcia-Cao et al., 2002). This model, designated the "super p53 mouse," was generated by transgenic introduction of one or two extra copies of p53 encoded on bacterial artificial chromosomes (BAC). The BAC approach was employed in an attempt to bypass longstanding problems associated with the nonphysiological regulation of traditional transgene constructions that are not located within the appropriate genomic context. Serrano and colleagues reported the production of two mice; the $p53^{+/+;tg/\cdot}$ mouse, which contained one 130 kb genomic fragment with one copy of p53, and the $p53^{+/+;tg/tg}$ mouse, which is transgenic for two copies of a 175 kb genomic fragment that flanks and includes the p53 gene. Most of the phenotypic characterization reported in the paper was based on the $p53^{+/+;tg/\cdot}$ model. Analysis of the two models, however, confirmed observations that genes introduced within their genomic context function more similarly to the endogenous gene, and furthermore, they function independently of the integration site and in proportion to the gene dosage.

Phenotypically, the $p53^{+/+;tg/\cdot}$ mice display an enhanced resistance to DNA damage and exhibit elevated p21 levels and increased apoptosis following whole-body irradiation (Garcia-Cao et al., 2002). The mice also appear relatively resistant to chemically induced carcinogenesis. For example, the mice were exposed to two chemical agents, 3-methylcholanthrene (3MC) and N-butyl-N(4-hydroxybutyl) nitrosamine (BBN), which cause fibrosarcoma and urinary bladder cancer, respectively. Although 92 percent of WT mice developed fibrosarcoma, only 33 percent of p53$^{+/+;tg/}$ did. On exposure to BBN, 57 percent of WT mice developed multiple bladder tumors, whereas the p53$^{+/+;tg/}$ tumors occurred with longer latency and were mostly monofocal, although percentages of wildtype and transgenic tumor-affected animals did not differ greatly. Only 1 out of 6 super p53 mice died from a spontaneous tumor. These tumor-resistant phenotypes are consistent with those observed in the p53+/m mouse. However, the longevity of the super p53 mouse was not different from that of wildtype control mice. Moreover, the mice did not possess any traits consistent with accelerated aging, such as reduced fertility, hair growth, enhanced skin atrophy, or signs of osteoporosis and lordokyphosis.

In general, the super p53 mouse exhibits the increased tumor suppression one might expect from a mouse encoding additional copies of p53 regulated in a WT manner. More interesting was that the elevated tumor suppression activity could be achieved without any apparent sacrifice of longevity, though this transgenic mouse needs to be characterized in more depth. This is in contradiction to the p53+/m model, which did show accelerated aging. These differences have been ascribed to differential regulation of p53 in the two models (Klatt & Serrano, 2003). Normally regulated p53 is stabilized and activated only following stress so that in the unstressed super p53 mice, p53 levels were not greatly different from those of normal mice. When tissues or cells of the super p53 mice were subjected to DNA damaging agents, the p53 response was augmented in the super p53 mice compared to normal mice. We have also observed an increased stress response in the p53+/m mice, but we have hypothesized that the C-terminal truncated p53 m protein in the p53+/m mice may exhibit a chronic low level p53 activation during unstressed periods (Donehower, 2002; Tyner et al., 2002). A number of previous studies have shown that C-terminal p53 peptides and fragments can interact with wildtype and mutant p53 protein to increase its functional activities (Jayaraman & Prives, 1995; Selivanova et al., 1997, Selivanova et al., 1999). Consistent with this, we have shown that p53 m protein can bind to wildtype p53 and increase p53 transactivation of the p21 promoter, a prototypical p53 transcription target (Tyner et al., 2002).

Recently, the production of another truncated p53 expressing mouse, the "p44 transgenic mouse," was described (Maier et al., 2004). This mouse contained the two endogenous copies of p53 and, in addition, a transgene expressing a truncated p53 that initiates at codon 41 (in exon 4) and results in the production of a 44kD p53 protein. This p44 protein is a naturally occurring short isoform of p53, and the experiment was designed to determine its biological role. Two transgenic lines were produced and designated P and Q. Line P expressed moderate levels of p44 and did not seem to have altered p53 levels, whereas line Q had markedly high levels of p44 in addition to elevated p53 levels. Most of the described analysis was performed on the P line. The effect of cellular stress on p53 levels was not investigated.

The p44 transgenic (tg) mouse was found to be smaller in size than its wildtype littermates; in fact, the tg$^{+/+}$ mice were approximately half the size of the tg$^{+/-}$ and wildtype mice (Maier et al., 2004). This growth deficit could be restored when the tg$^{+/+}$ mouse was crossed to a p53$^{-/-}$ mouse, suggesting the phenotype to be p53 dependent. Upon further characterization, this size deficit was observed both pre- and postnatally. In addition, the tg$^{+/+}$ mouse was reported to be relatively tumor resistant, had a shortened life span (at 60 weeks an average of 15 percent tg$^{+/+}$ alive versus 90 percent of wild type), and a host of phenotypes consistent with premature aging. These phenotypes began at 4 months and included a reduced reproductive life span (with males more severely affected), reduced bone mineral density, lordokyphosis, decreased trabecular bone content, reduced osteoblast number, and an overall reduction in bone turnover. In addition, detailed analysis of transcriptional targets of p53 revealed that in the presence of p44, there was upregulation of the p53-responsive genes p21, mdm2, and IGFBP-3. Conversely, GADD45 and IGF-1R were shown to be downregulated.

The authors went on to elucidate the underlying molecular mechanism of the small size, slower growth rate, and reduced life span of the p44tg mouse. Of particular interest in growth mutants with altered longevity is the growth hormone (GH) and IGF-1 signaling axis. The p44tg mice were shown to have no perturbation in GH secretion, and the mice did not respond to treatment with GH. However, the levels of IGF-1 and IGF-1R were shown to be elevated in the old p44tg mouse (no increase in young). The study showed directly, by transfection of wildtype MEFs with p44, that p44 promoted an increase in IGF-1R and phosphorylation of Akt/PKB, a downstream target of IGF. Furthermore, they analyzed downstream signal transduction events and showed an exaggerated forkhead response in p44tg embryos, which results in activation of p53. The authors argued that it was these alterations to the IGF signaling pathway that facilitate the aging phenotypes, and that the IGF pathway aberrations are driven by selective transactivation and suppression of p53 by the p44 isoform (Maier et al., 2004).

Direct comparison of these three mutant p53 mice is difficult as they were all uniquely engineered and the resulting phenotypes are somewhat varied.

However, there are several important similarities. First, it appears possible to increase tumor resistance by increasing the gene dosage (or activity) of p53. The super p53 mouse illustrates that this tumor suppression can be achieved without deleterious side-effects when the additional p53 gene is located within its correct genomic context (Garcia-Cao et al., 2002; Klatt & Serrano, 2003). This is important because the aging phenotypes reported in the p53+/m mouse initially raised concerns regarding the use of elevated p53 in therapies to combat cancer (Ferbeyre & Lowe, 2002). Second, it appears that increasing the activity and stability of p53 via the use of a C-terminal p53 protein is problematic. Although serving to reduce cancer incidence, there is the unfortunate side-effect of premature aging and reduced life span (Maier et al., 2004; Tyner et al., 2002). This is potentially an important observation because these C-terminal p53 proteins are naturally occurring and may serve a biological role in cellular aging. Numerous similarities exist between the p53+/m and the p44 transgenic mouse (more so than with either of these mice and the super p53). Both mice share the heightened tumor suppression and concomitant premature aging phenotypes. We believe these phenotypes are driven by the presence of the shorter p53 isoforms and the effects these short isoforms have on WT p53. Scrable and colleagues suggested that the C-terminal p44 dimerizes with WT p53, altering the tetramer conformation and thus affecting the transactivational activity of p53 (Maier et al., 2004). This is supported by the fact that various transcription levels of p53 target genes are augmented in the presence of p44. We have limited evidence to suggest a similar situation in the p53+/m mouse; various promoter elements of p53 targets have been tested in the presence of m and were shown to be altered (C. Gatza, unpublished data).

We hypothesize that alterations in p53 transactivation may drive the downstream effects of altered gene expression and consequently altered cellular outcomes, perhaps contributing to increased cell senescence or apoptosis. It is these cellular outcomes that may be responsible for the organismal aging seen in the mouse models.

IX. Influence of p53 on Longevity in Humans

That p53 has an important effect on human longevity is illustrated by affected members of families with Li-Fraumeni syndrome. These individuals inherit a single mutant p53 allele and are profoundly susceptible to early cancers. Half of all Li-Fraumeni patients develop cancer by the age of 30 versus a 1 percent incidence of this disease in the general population (Malkin *et al.*, 1990). By the age of 70, 90 percent of affected Li-Fraumeni individuals have been diagnosed with cancer. By preventing early incidence of cancer, p53 clearly qualifies as a longevity-assurance gene. Yet in earlier sections of this chapter, we have cited examples of mouse models with enhanced p53 activity that seem to suppress longevity, at least in later stages of the mouse life span. We attempted to reconcile this paradox through the principle of "antagonistic pleiotropy," the concept that genes with beneficial effects during early life span stages can be deleterious later in the life span.

A remarkable recent report by Van Heemst and collaborators supports the notion that p53 in humans is a gene that exhibits antagonistic pleiotropy (Van Heemst *et al.*, 2005). These investigators examined a polymorphic variation of p53 in humans at codon 72. The allele frequency of Arg at this codon in the general Caucasian population is roughly 70 percent, whereas the allele frequency of

Pro is 30 percent and is produced by single G to C nucleotide change (Weston & Godbold, 1997). A number of studies suggest that individuals with codon 72 Pro homozygosity have a modestly elevated cancer risk, though there is some controversy about the significance of that risk (Matakidou *et al.*, 2003; Weston & Godbold, 1997). Molecular analyses show that the Pro variant is partially defective in p53 anti-proliferative functions. The p53 codon 72 Pro form is less efficient than its Arg counterpart in induction of apoptosis, suppression of cancer cell proliferation, and suppression of Ras-induced transformation (Dumont *et al.*, 2003; Thomas *et al.*, 1999). Such modest deficiencies in p53 tumor suppressor function would be consistent with increased tumor susceptibility in the codon 72 Pro/Pro carriers. Van Heemst and colleagues performed a meta-analysis of cancer susceptibility data from 61 study populations in which the p53 codon 72 variant had been identified (Van Heemst *et al.*, 2005). Their analysis indicated a modestly increased cancer risk estimate of 1.30 ($p < 0.05$) for p53 Pro/Pro individuals compared to Arg/Arg carriers.

If the p53 Pro variant is a weaker tumor suppressor than its Arg counterpart, this might be manifested in increased cancer risks and a consequent under-representation of Pro/Pro genotypes in the oldest cohorts of the general population. However, an association of Pro/Pro individuals with reduced life expectancy has not been observed (Bonafe *et al.*, 1999). It appears that the potential increase in cancer rates attributed to the Pro allele does not deleteriously affect longevity. Van Heemst and collaborators pursued this issue further through a powerful prospective study. Two cohorts of 1,226 individuals 85 or older were genotyped for the p53 codon 72 polymorphism and were followed for specific causes of death. Proportional cancer mortality was 29 percent for Pro/Pro individuals versus 14 percent for Arg/Arg subjects, a significant difference that agreed with their earlier meta-analysis of the relevant literature. The surprising result was that, despite an increased cancer mortality, the Pro/Pro individuals had a 1.41-fold relative survival compared to Arg/Arg carriers (P = 0.032). The Arg/Pro genotype conferred no apparent survival advantage over the Arg/Arg genotype. Deaths from general exhaustion and frailty occurred in 21 percent of the Arg/Arg subjects but only 6 percent of the Pro/Pro individuals. It appears that the Pro/Pro genotype confers a significant survival benefit that outweighs the deleterious effects of enhanced cancer susceptibility. Such results are consistent with our hypothesis derived from p53 mutant mouse models that p53 is a longevity assurance gene early in life, but may become a longevity suppressor gene later in life.

X. How Might p53 Influence Organismal Aging?

Genes that respond to cellular stresses and damage have been shown to be key regulators of aging and longevity (Finkel & Holbrook, 2000; Sohal & Weindruch, 1996). The cellular pathways that maintain genomic stability are likely to be of great importance in assuring the normal longevity of a species (Hasty et al., 2003). It is well established that p53 is a critical stress response protein and a longevity assurance gene; its absence results in dramatically reduced longevity due to early tumors (Donehower et al., 1992). What is less well established is whether p53 can under some circumstances be a longevity-suppression gene. A gene can promote survival early in life and inhibit longevity in late life if it exhibits antagonistic pleiotropy (Campisi, 2003b; Kirkwood & Rose, 1991). Such a gene

may protect a young organism in its reproductive years when selective forces are highly active, but in post-reproductive years, the absence of selective forces may result in that same gene having deleterious effects. Such could be the case for p53 (Campisi, 2003a; Donehower, 2002). The same anti-proliferative functions of p53 that benefit the young organism by suppressing cancers may in old age promote aging phenotypes.

How might p53 influence aging in older organisms? We know that p53 can induce cell cycle arrest or apoptosis when it is activated by stress. In some cases, p53 can promote a terminal cell cycle arrest, or senescence. Both cellular senescence and apoptosis processes have been shown to be altered in the aging mammal (Campisi, 2003a). It is likely that some of the age-associated cellular senescence and apoptosis result from p53 effects. Consistent with this we have observed dramatic age-associated increases in senescent cell numbers in several mouse organs as measured by the senescence-associated beta-galactosidase assay (C. Gatza, unpublished data). Interestingly, the older p53+/m mice show even higher levels of senescent cells than their wildtype p53$^{+/+}$ counterparts (C. Gatza, unpublished data).

p53 is also likely to be at least partially responsible for the stress-induced apoptosis that occurs in the aging organism. p53 transactivates an array of pro-apoptotic genes and has also been shown to directly mediate apoptosis through protein–protein interactions (Fridman & Lowe, 2003). Apoptosis of damaged cells or cells that have initiated aberrant oncogenic signaling protects the organism from accumulation of nonfunctional cells and cancerous cells and obviously provides a major selective advantage. However, as the organism ages, the elimination of dysfunctional stem or progenitor cells could have the cumulative effect of reducing the regenerative capacity that maintains organ homeostasis. The result could be age-related losses in organ cellularity, functionality, and stress response capacities. The simultaneous accumulation of poorly functioning or nonfunctioning senescent cells could also contribute to organ atrophy and reduced capacity.

Although p53-induced apoptosis and senescence may affect post-mitotic differentiated cells, we postulate that it has a more profound effect on the mitotic cells of an aging organism, in particular the tissue stem cells. These cells are primarily responsible for maintaining organ homeostasis by their ability to self-renew and differentiate into progeny cells that eventually compose the mature cells in each organ. Accumulating evidence suggests that stem cells are fundamentally important in longevity and aging. Although there remains some controversy, a number of studies have indicated that stem cell functionality declines with age (Campisi, 2003a; Donehower, 2002; Ito *et al.*, 2004; Pelicci, 2004; Sharpless & DePinho, 2004; Van Zant & Liang, 2003; Wong *et al.*, 2003). This reduced functionality likely contributes to the organ atrophies and reduced regenerative responses so characteristic of aged individuals.

The age-associated failure of stem cells may be directly linked to damage induced by oxidative stress. It has recently been shown that Atm has a direct role in the self-renewal and differentiation of hematopoietic stem cells (HSCs) through its ability to suppress ROS (Ito *et al.*, 2004). Atm$^{-/-}$ mice showed a progressive bone marrow failure that correlated with increased levels of ROS. Interestingly, the defective hematopoiesis of older Atm$^{-/-}$ HSCs could be reversed by anti-oxidants, indicating that the reduced HSC functional capacity was a direct result of increased ROS levels (Ito *et al.*, 2004). The increased ROS in the Atm$^{-/-}$ stem cells was associated with increased levels of

tumor suppressors p16^{INK4a} and p19^{ARF}. Thus, suppression of ROS in stem cells by Atm suppresses tumor suppressor function and allows for stem cell self-renewal. These results demonstrate that the accumulation of age-associated ROS damage occurs not only in post-mitotic somatic cells, but also in mitotic stem cells. Whereas ROS damage to single post-mitotic cells is likely to have limited effects on the organism, ROS damage to the stem cells may be much more consequential, resulting in loss of large numbers of progeny cells through loss of self-renewal and differentiation capacity.

We have hypothesized that p53 plays an important role in regulating stem cell functionality through its anti-proliferative activities (Donehower, 2002). For example, we and others have shown that stem cells derived from p53-deficient mice have higher proliferative activities than their wildtype counterparts (M. Dumble, unpublished data). Moreover, p53+/m mice exhibit reduced stem cell numbers, proliferation, and reconstitution potential in transplantation experiments (M. Dumble, unpublished data).

While there are multiple stress response pathways, we have placed most of our focus on the p53 response pathway because of its central role in the damage response. It is likely that stochastic ROS-induced stresses are important initiators of aging, but we believe that the cellular damage generated by these and other stressors has less importance than the signaling response that they evoke. The damage response signaling pathways may be of primary importance because of the many biological outcomes they execute. These signaling pathways repair the damage (sometimes imperfectly), arrest (sometimes terminally) the dividing stem or progenitor cell, or induce apoptosis. Although these pathways may be functioning in most cells of the organism, the most profound effects may be in the tissue stem cells. The gradual reduction in stem cell functionality through these anti-proliferative stress responses is not a factor during the youth of the organism because of excess stem cell reserves. However, with age and accumulated stresses, stem cell function may be reduced to the point where the stem cells can no longer replenish sufficient numbers of mature cells, and organ atrophy and functional decline sets in, leading to the aging phenotypes described above.

The senescence and apoptosis pathways induced by stress are critical for preventing cancer, but the stress response pathways appear less effective in older organisms as tumors begin to appear more frequently. This may be due to a variety of factors, including fixation of mutations following DNA repair, or perhaps a less efficient stress response. Moreover, as the Campisi laboratory has shown, senescent fibroblasts secrete factors that may induce a hyperproliferative response in adjacent epithelial cells, ultimately leading to cancer (Krtolica *et al.*, 2001). Thus, senescence may be a mixed blessing, preventing cancer in some contexts and promoting it in others.

The model described above is primarily focused on the role of one signaling pathway (p53) on one type of cell (the stem cell). Therefore, it is certainly incomplete with respect to aging in the entire organism. However, we do believe it has explanatory value for important components of the aging process. Ongoing experiments in our laboratory and other laboratories may help determine the validity of the model. At the very least, we hope to establish that p53 has a significant regulatory role in the aging process.

Acknowledgments

The authors thank Scott Pletcher and Steve Helfand for helpful discussions. This work is supported by a grant to L. Donchower (R01 AG019693) and a training grant award to G. Hinkal (T32 AG000183) from the National Institute of Aging.

References

Alcorta, D. A., Xiong, Y., Phelps, D., Hannon, G., Beach, D., & Barrett, J. C. (1996). Involvement of the cyclin-dependent kinase inhibitor p16 (INK4a) in replicative senescence of normal human fibroblasts. *Proceedings of the National Academy of Sciences of the USA, 93*, 13742–13747.

Andersen, B., Pearse, R. V., 2nd, Jenne, K., Sornson, M., Lin, S. C., Bartke, A., & Rosenfeld, M. G. (1995). The Ames dwarf gene is required for Pit-1 gene activation. *Developmental Biology, 172*, 495–503.

Anisimov, V. N. (2003). Aging and cancer in transgenic and mutant mice. *Frontiers in Bioscience, 8*, s883–s902.

Appella, E., & Anderson, C. W. (2001). Post-translational modifications and activation of p53 by genotoxic stresses. *European Journal of Biochemistry, 268*, 2764–2772.

Arking, R. (1998). *The biology of aging* (p. 570). Sunderland, MA: Sinauer Associates, Inc.

Ashcroft, M., & Vousden, K. H. (1999). Regulation of p53 stability. *Oncogene, 18*, 7637–7643.

Atadja, P., Wong, H., Garkavtsev, I., Veillette, C., & Riabowol, K. (1995). Increased activity of p53 in senescing fibroblasts. *Proceedings of the National Academy of Sciences of the USA, 92*, 8348–8352.

Baker, D. J., Jeganathan, K. B., Cameron, J. D., Thompson, M., Juneja, S., Kopecka, A., Kumar, R., Jenkins, R. B., de Groen, P. C., Roche, P., & van Deursen, J. M. (2004). BubR1 insufficiency causes early onset of aging-associated phenotypes and infertility in mice. *Nature Genetics, 36*, 744–749.

Barger, J. L., Walford, R. L., & Weindruch, R. (2003). The retardation of aging by caloric restriction: its significance in the transgenic era. *Experimental Gerontology, 38*, 1343–1351.

Barlow, C., Hirotsune, S., Paylor, R., Liyanage, M., Eckhaus, M., Collins, F., Shiloh, Y., Crawley, J. N., Ried, T., Tagle, D., & Wynshaw-Boris, A. (1996). Atm-deficient mice: a paradigm of ataxia telangiectasia. *Cell, 86*, 159–171.

Bartke, A., Wright, J. C., Mattison, J. A., Ingram, D. K., Miller, R. A., & Roth, G. S. (2001). Extending the lifespan of long-lived mice. *Nature, 414*, 412.

Beausejour, C. M., Krtolica, A., Galimi, F., Narita, M., Lowe, S. W., Yaswen, P., & Campisi, J. (2003). Reversal of human cellular senescence: roles of the p53 and p16 pathways. *Embo Journal,* 22, 4212–4222.

Ben-Porath, I., & Weinberg, R. A. (2004). When cells get stressed: an integrative view of cellular senescence. *Journal of Clinical Investigation,* 113, 8–13.

Bird, J., Ostler, E. L., & Faragher, R. G. (2003). Can we say that senescent cells cause ageing? *Experimental Gerontology,* 38, 1319–1326.

Bischoff, F. Z., Yim, S. O., Pathak, S., Grant, G., Siciliano, M. J., Giovanella, B. C., Strong, L. C., & Tainsky, M. A. (1990). Spontaneous abnormalities in normal fibroblasts from patients with Li-Fraumeni cancer syndrome: aneuploidy and immortalization. *Cancer Research,* 50, 7979–7984.

Blander, G., & Guarente, L. (2004). The Sir2 family of protein deacetylases. *Annual Review of Biochemistry,* 73, 417–435.

Bode, A. M., & Dong, Z. (2004). Post-translational modification of p53 in tumorigenesis. *Nature Reviews Cancer,* 4, 793–805.

Bodnar, A. G., Ouellette, M., Frolkis, M., Holt, S. E., Chiu, C. P., Morin, G. B., Harley, C. B., Shay, J. W., Lichtsteiner, S., & Wright, W. E. (1998). Extension of life-span by introduction of telomerase into normal human cells. *Science,* 279, 349–352.

Bonafe, M., Olivieri, F., Mari, D., Baggio, G., Mattace, R., Berardelli, M., Sansoni, P., De Benedictis, G., De Luca, M., Marchegiani, F., Cavallone, L., Cardelli, M., Giovagnetti, S., Ferrucci, L., Amadio, L., Lisa, R., Tucci, M. G., Troiano, L., Pini, G., Gueresi, P., Morellini, M., Sorbi, S., Passeri, G., Barbi, C., & Valensin, S. (1999). p53 codon 72 polymorphism and longevity: additional data on centenarians from continental Italy and Sardinia. *American Journal of Human Genetics,* 65, 1782–1785.

Bringold, F., & Serrano, M. (2000). Tumor suppressors and oncogenes in cellular senescence. *Experimental Gerontology,* 35, 317–329.

Brooks, C. L., & Gu, W. (2003). Ubiquitination, phosphorylation and acetylation: the molecular basis for p53 regulation. *Current Opinion in Cell Biology,* 15, 164–171.

Brown-Borg, H. M., Borg, K. E., Meliska, C. J., & Bartke, A. (1996). Dwarf mice and the ageing process. *Nature,* 384, 33.

Campisi, J. (2001). From cells to organisms: can we learn about aging from cells in culture? *Experimental Gerontology,* 36, 607–618.

Campisi, J. (2003a). Cancer and ageing: rival demons? *Nature Reviews Cancer,* 3, 339–349.

Campisi, J. (2003b). Cellular senescence and apoptosis: how cellular responses might influence aging phenotypes. *Experimental Gerontology,* 38, 5–11.

Campisi, J., Kim, S. H., Lim, C. S., & Rubio, M. (2001). Cellular senescence, cancer and aging: the telomere connection. *Experimental Gerontology,* 36, 1619–1637.

Canman, C. E., Lim, D. S., Cimprich, K. A., Taya, Y., Tamai, K., Sakaguchi, K., Appella, E., Kastan, M. B., & Siliciano, J. D. (1998). Activation of the Atm kinase by ionizing radiation and phosphorylation of p53. *Science,* 281, 1677–1679.

Cao, L., Li, W., Kim, S., Brodie, S. G., & Deng, C. X. (2003). Senescence, aging, and malignant transformation mediated by p53 in mice lacking the Brca1 full-length isoform. *Genes & Development,* 17, 201–213.

Chan, G. K., & Yen, T. J. (2003). The mitotic checkpoint: a signaling pathway that allows a single unattached kinetochore to inhibit mitotic exit. *Progress in Cell Cycle Research,* 5, 431–439.

Chang, S., Multani, A. S., Cabrera, N. G., Naylor, M. L., Laud, P., Lombard, D., Pathak, S., Guarente, L., & DePinho, R. A. (2004). Essential role of limiting telomeres in the pathogenesis of Werner syndrome. *Nature Genetics,* 36, 877–882.

Cheng, H. L., Mostoslavsky, R., Saito, S., Manis, J. P., Gu, Y., Patel, P., Bronson, R., Appella, E., Alt, F. W., & Chua, K. F. (2003). Developmental defects and p53 hyperacetylation in Sir2 homolog (SIRT1)-deficient mice. *Proceedings of the National Academy of Sciences of the USA,* 100, 10794–10799.

Choi, J., & Donehower, L. A. (1999). p53 in embryonic development: maintaining a fine balance. *Cell and Molecular Life Sciences*, 55, 38–47.

Choi, J., Shendrik, I., Peacocke, M., Peehl, D., Buttyan, R., Ikeguchi, E. F., Katz, A. E., & Benson, M. C. (2000). Expression of senescence-associated beta-galactosidase in enlarged prostates from men with benign prostatic hyperplasia. *Urology*, 56, 160–166.

Cohen, H. Y., Miller, C., Bitterman, K. J., Wall, N. R., Hekking, B., Kessler, B., Howitz, K. T., Gorospe, M., de Cabo, R., & Sinclair, D. A. (2004). Calorie restriction promotes mammalian cell survival by inducing the SIRT1 deacetylase. *Science*, 305, 390–392.

de Boer, J., Andressoo, J. O., de Wit, J., Huijmans, J., Beems, R. B., van Steeg, H., Weeda, G., van der Horst, G. T., van Leeuwen, W., Themmen, A. P., Meradji, M., & Hoeijmakers, J. H. (2002). Premature aging in mice deficient in DNA repair and transcription. *Science*, 296, 1276–1279.

de Magalhaes, J. P., Cabral, J., & Magalhaes, D. (2005). The influence of genes on the aging process of mice: a statistical assessment of the genetics of aging. *Genetics*, 169, 265–274.

Dimri, G. P., Lee, X., Basile, G., Acosta, M., Scott, G., Roskelley, C., Medrano, E. E., Linskens, M., Rubelj, I., Pereira-Smith, O., Peacocke, M., & Campisi, J. (1995). A biomarker that identifies senescent human cells in culture and in aging skin in vivo. *Proceedings of the National Academy of Sciences of the USA*, 92, 9363–9367.

Dirac, A. M., & Bernards, R. (2003). Reversal of senescence in mouse fibroblasts through lentiviral suppression of p53. *Journal of Biological Chemistry*, 278, 11731–11734.

Dohoney, K. M., Guillerm, C., Whiteford, C., Elbi, C., Lambert, P. F., Hager, G. L., & Brady, J. N. (2004). Phosphorylation of p53 at serine 37 is important for transcriptional activity and regulation in response to DNA damage. *Oncogene*, 23, 49–57.

Dolle, M. E., Snyder, W. K., Dunson, D. B., & Vijg, J. (2002). Mutational fingerprints of aging. *Nucleic Acids Research*, 30, 545–549.

Dolle, M. E., Snyder, W. K., Gossen, J. A., Lohman, P. H., & Vijg, J. (2000). Distinct spectra of somatic mutations accumulated with age in mouse heart and small intestine. *Proceedings of the National Academy of Sciences of the USA*, 97, 8403–8408.

Donehower, L. A. (1996). The p53-deficient mouse: a model for basic and applied cancer studies. *Seminars in Cancer Biology*, 7, 269–278.

Donehower, L. A. (2002). Does p53 affect organismal aging? *Journal of Cellular Physiology*, 192, 23–33.

Donehower, L. A., Harvey, M., Slagle, B. L., McArthur, M. J., Montgomery, C. A., Jr., Butel, J. S., & Bradley, A. (1992). Mice deficient for p53 are developmentally normal but susceptible to spontaneous tumours. *Nature*, 356, 215–221.

Du, X., Shen, J., Kugan, N., Furth, E. E., Lombard, D. B., Cheung, C., Pak, S., Luo, G., Pignolo, R. J., DePinho, R. A., Guarente, L., & Johnson, F. B. (2004). Telomere shortening exposes functions for the mouse Werner and Bloom syndrome genes. *Molecular and Cellular Biology*, 24, 8437–8446.

Dumont, P., Leu, J. I., Della Pietra, A. C. 3rd, George, D. L., & Murphy, M. (2003). The codon 72 polymorphic variants of p53 have markedly different apoptotic potential. *Nature Genetics*, 33, 357–365.

el-Deiry, W. S., Tokino, T., Velculescu, V. E., Levy, D. B., Parsons, R., Trent, J. M., Lin, D., Mercer, W. E., Kinzler, K. W., & Vogelstein, B. (1993). WAF1, a potential mediator of p53 tumor suppression. *Cell*, 75, 817–825.

Elson, A., Wang, Y., Daugherty, C. J., Morton, C. C., Zhou, F., Campos-Torres, J., & Leder, P. (1996). Pleiotropic defects in ataxia-telangiectasia protein-deficient mice. *Proceedings of the National Academy of Sciences of the USA*, 93, 13084–13089.

Erster, S., Mihara, M., Kim, R. H., Petrenko, O., & Moll, U. M. (2004). In vivo mitochondrial p53 translocation triggers a rapid first wave of cell death in response to DNA damage that can precede p53 target gene activation. *Molecular and Cellular Biology*, 24, 6728–6741.

Fabrizio, P., & Longo, V. D. (2003). The chronological life span of Saccharomyces cerevisiae. *Aging Cell*, 2, 73–81.

Ferbeyre, G. (2002). PML a target of translocations in APL is a regulator of cellular senescence. *Leukemia*, 16, 1918–1926.

Ferbeyre, G., & Lowe, S. W. (2002). The price of tumour suppression? *Nature*, 415, 26–27.

Ferbeyre, G., de Stanchina, E., Lin, A. W., Querido, E., McCurrach, M. E., Hannon, G. J., & Lowe, S. W. (2002). Oncogenic ras and p53 cooperate to induce cellular senescence. *Molecular and Cellular Biology*, 22, 3497–3508.

Finkel, T., & Holbrook, N. J. (2000). Oxidants, oxidative stress and the biology of ageing. *Nature*, 408, 239–247.

Fridman, J. S., & Lowe, S. W. (2003). Control of apoptosis by p53. *Oncogene*, 22, 9030–9040.

Fuchs, S. Y., Adler, V., Buschmann, T., Wu, X., & Ronai, Z. (1998). Mdm2 association with p53 targets its ubiquitination. *Oncogene*, 17, 2543–2547.

Garcia-Cao, I., Garcia-Cao, M., Martin-Caballero, J., Criado, L. M., Klatt, P., Flores, J. M., Weill, J. C., Blasco, M. A., & Serrano, M. (2002). "Super p53" mice exhibit enhanced DNA damage response, are tumor resistant and age normally. *Embo Journal*, 21, 6225–6235.

Giaccia, A. J., & Kastan, M. B. (1998). The complexity of p53 modulation: emerging patterns from divergent signals. *Genes & Development*, 12, 2973–2983.

Gire, V., & Wynford-Thomas, D. (1998). Reinitiation of DNA synthesis and cell division in senescent human fibroblasts by microinjection of anti-p53 antibodies. *Molecular and Cellular Biology*, 18, 1611–1621.

Goldstein, S. (1990). Replicative senescence: the human fibroblast comes of age. *Science*, 249, 1129–1133.

Gowen, L. C., Johnson, B. L., Latour, A. M., Sulik, K. K., & Koller, B. H. (1996). Brca1 deficiency results in early embryonic lethality characterized by neuroepithelial abnormalities. *Nature Genetics*, 12, 191–194.

Gu, W., Luo, J., Brooks, C. L., Nikolaev, A. Y., & Li, M. (2004). Dynamics of the p53 acetylation pathway. *Novartis Foundation Symposium*, 259, 197–205; discussion 205–207, 223–225.

Guarente, L. (2000). Sir2 links chromatin silencing, metabolism, and aging. *Genes & Development*, 14, 1021–1026.

Guarente, L., & Kenyon, C. (2000). Genetic pathways that regulate ageing in model organisms. *Nature*, 408, 255–262.

Hakem, R., de la Pompa, J. L., Sirard, C., Mo, R., Woo, M., Hakem, A., Wakeham, A., Potter, J., Reitmair, A., Billia, F., Firpo, E., Hui, C. C., Roberts, J., Rossant, J., & Mak, T. W. (1996). The tumor suppressor gene Brca1 is required for embryonic cellular proliferation in the mouse. *Cell*, 85, 1009–1023.

Harley, C. B., Kim, N. W., Prowse, K. R., Weinrich, S. L., Hirsch, K. S., West, M. D., Bacchetti, S., Hirte, H. W., Counter, C. M., Greider, C. W., Piatyszek, M. A., Wright, W. E., & Shay, J. W. (1994). Telomerase, cell immortality, and cancer. *Cold Spring Harbor Symposium of Quantitative Biology*, 59, 307–315.

Harper, J. W., Adami, G. R., Wei, N., Keyomarsi, K., & Elledge, S. J. (1993). The p21 Cdk-interacting protein Cip1 is a potent inhibitor of G1 cyclin-dependent kinases. *Cell*, 75, 805–816.

Harrison, D. E. (1997). Animal models showing "accelerated aging" are more likely to be useful for pathology than for mechanisms of aging. *Growth, Development, and Aging*, 61, 167–168.

Harvey, M., McArthur, M. J., Montgomery, C. A. Jr., Butel, J. S., Bradley, A., & Donehower, L. A. (1993a). Spontaneous and carcinogen-induced tumorigenesis in p53-deficient mice. *Nature Genetics*, 5, 225–229.

Harvey, M., Sands, A. T., Weiss, R. S., Hegi, M. E., Wiseman, R. W., Pantazis, P., Giovanella, B. C., Tainsky, M. A., Bradley, A., & Donehower, L. A. (1993b). In vitro growth characteristics of embryo fibroblasts isolated from p53-deficient mice. *Oncogene*, 8, 2457–2467.

Hasty, P., & Vijg, J. (2004a). Accelerating aging by mouse reverse genetics: a rational approach to understanding longevity. *Aging Cell*, 3, 55–65.

Hasty, P., & Vijg, J. (2004b). Rebuttal to Miller: 'accelerated aging': a primrose path to insight?' *Aging Cell*, 3, 67–69.

Hasty, P., Campisi, J., Hoeijmakers, J., van Steeg, H., & Vijg, J. (2003). Aging and genome maintenance: lessons from the mouse? *Science*, 299, 1355–1359.

Hayflick, L. (1965). The limited in vitro lifetime of human diploid cell strains. *Experimental Cell Research*, 37, 614–636.

Hekimi, S., & Guarente, L. (2003). Genetics and the specificity of the aging process. *Science*, 299, 1351–1354.

Helfand, S. L., & Rogina, B. (2003). Genetics of aging in the fruit fly, *Drosophila melanogaster*. *Annual Review of Genetics*, 37, 329–348.

Herbig, U., Jobling, W. A., Chen, B. P., Chen, D. J., & Sedivy, J. M. (2004). Telomere shortening triggers senescence of human cells through a pathway involving Atm, p53, and p21(CIP1), but not p16(INK4a). *Molecular Cell*, 14, 501–513.

Hill, K. A., Buettner, V. L., Halangoda, A., Kunishige, M., Moore, S. R., Longmate, J., Scaringe, W. A., & Sommer, S. S. (2004). Spontaneous mutation in Big Blue mice from fetus to old age: tissue-specific time courses of mutation frequency but similar mutation types. *Environmental Molecular Mutagenesis*, 43, 110–120.

Holzenberger, M., Dupont, J., Ducos, B., Leneuve, P., Geloen, A., Even, P. C., Cervera, P., & Le Bouc, Y. (2003). IGF-1 receptor regulates lifespan and resistance to oxidative stress in mice. *Nature*, 421, 182–187.

Horiuchi, S., Finch, C. E., Mesle, F., & Vallin, J. (2003). Differential patterns of age-related mortality increase in middle age and old age. Journals of Gerontology Series A: Biological and Medical Sciences, 58, 495–507.

Itahana, K., Campisi, J., & Dimri, G. P. (2004). Mechanisms of cellular senescence in human and mouse cells. *Biogerontology*, 5, 1–10.

Itahana, K., Dimri, G., & Campisi, J. (2001). Regulation of cellular senescence by p53. *European Journal of Biochemistry*, 268, 2784–2791.

Itahana, K., Zou, Y., Itahana, Y., Martinez, J. L., Beausejour, C., Jacobs, J. J., Van Lohuizen, M., Band, V., Campisi, J., & Dimri, G. P. (2003). Control of the replicative life span of human fibroblasts by p16 and the polycomb protein Bmi-1. *Molecular and Cellular Biology*, 23, 389–401.

Ito, K., Hirao, A., Arai, F., Matsuoka, S., Takubo, K., Hamaguchi, I., Nomiyama, K., Hosokawa, K., Sakurada, K., Nakagata, N., Ikeda, Y., Mak, T. W., & Suda, T. (2004). Regulation of oxidative stress by ATM is required for self-renewal of haematopoietic stem cells. *Nature*, 431, 997–1002.

Jacobs, H. T. (2003). The mitochondrial theory of aging: dead or alive? *Aging Cell*, 2, 11–17.

Jayaraman, J., & Prives, C. (1995). Activation of p53 sequence-specific DNA binding by short single strands of DNA requires the p53 C-terminus. *Cell*, 81, 1021–1029.

Juan, L. J., Shia, W. J., Chen, M. H., Yang, W. M., Seto, E., Lin, Y. S., & Wu, C. W. (2000). Histone deacetylases specifically down-regulate p53-dependent gene activation. *Journal of Biology Chemistry*, 275, 20436–20443.

Khaidakov, M., Heflich, R. H., Manjanatha, M. G., Myers, M. B., & Aidoo, A. (2003). Accumulation of point mutations in mitochondrial DNA of aging mice. *Mutation Research*, 526, 1–7.

Kim Sh, S. H., Kaminker, P., & Campisi, J. (2002). Telomeres, aging and cancer: in search of a happy ending. *Oncogene*, 21, 503–511.

Kipling, D., Wynford-Thomas, D., Jones, C. J., Akbar, A., Aspinall, R., Bacchetti, S., Blasco, M. A., Broccoli, D., DePinho, R. A., Edwards, D. R., Effros, R. B., Harley, C. B., Lansdorp, P. M., Linskens, M. H., Prowse, K. R., Newbold, R. F., Olovnikov, A. M., Parkinson, E. K., Pawelec, G., Ponten, J., Shall, S., Zijlmans, M., & Faragher, R. G. (1999). Telomere-dependent senescence. *Nature Biotechnology*, 17, 313–314.

Kirkwood, T. B., & Rose, M. R. (1991). Evolution of senescence: late survival sacrificed for reproduction. *Philosophical Transactions of the Royal Society of London: B Biological Sciences*, 332, 15–24.

Klapper, W., Parwaresch, R., & Krupp, G. (2001). Telomere biology in human aging and aging syndromes. *Mechanisms of Ageing and Development*, 122, 695–712.

Klatt, P., & Serrano, M. (2003). Engineering cancer resistance in mice. *Carcinogenesis*, 24, 817–826.

Koubova, J., & Guarente, L. (2003). How does calorie restriction work? *Genes & Development*, 17, 313–321.

Krishnamurthy, J., Torrice, C., Ramsey, M. R., Kovalev, G. I., Al-Regaiey, K., Su, L., & Sharpless, N. E. (2004). Ink4a/Arf expression is a biomarker of aging. *Journal of Clinical Investigation*, 114, 1299–1307.

Krtolica, A., Parrinello, S., Lockett, S., Desprez, P. Y., & Campisi, J. (2001). Senescent fibroblasts promote epithelial cell growth and tumorigenesis: a link between cancer and aging. *Proceedings of the National Academy of Sciences of the USA*, 98, 12072–12077.

Kuro-o, M., Matsumura, Y., Aizawa, H., Kawaguchi, H., Suga, T., Utsugi, T., Ohyama, Y., Kurabayashi, M., Kaname, T., Kume, E., Iwasaki, H., Iida, A., Shiraki-Iida, T., Nishikawa, S., Nagai, R., & Nabeshima, Y. I. (1997). Mutation of the mouse klotho gene leads to a syndrome resembling ageing. *Nature*, 390, 45–51.

Lane, D. P. (1992). Cancer. p53, guardian of the genome. *Nature*, 358, 15–16.

Lane, D. P., & Crawford, L. V. (1979). T antigen is bound to a host protein in SV40-transformed cells. *Nature*, 278, 261–263.

Langley, E., Pearson, M., Faretta, M., Bauer, U. M., Frye, R. A., Minucci, S., Pelicci, P. G., & Kouzarides, T. (2002). Human SIR2 deacetylates p53 and antagonizes PML/p53-induced cellular senescence. *Embo Journal*, 21, 2383–2396.

Lebel, M., & Leder, P. (1998). A deletion within the murine Werner syndrome helicase induces sensitivity to inhibitors of topoisomerase and loss of cellular proliferative capacity. *Proceedings of the National Academy of Sciences of the USA*, 95, 13097–13102.

Lee, C. K., Klopp, R. G., Weindruch, R., & Prolla, T. A. (1999). Gene expression profile of aging and its retardation by caloric restriction. *Science*, 285, 1390–1393.

Lee, D. W., & Yu, B. P. (1990). Modulation of free radicals and superoxide dismutases by age and dietary restriction. *Aging (Milano)*, 2, 357–362.

Lehmann, A. (2002). Ageing: repair and transcription keep us from premature ageing. *Current Biology*, 12, R550–R551.

Levine, A. J. (1997). p53, the cellular gatekeeper for growth and division. *Cell*, 88, 323–331.

Levine, A. J., Finlay, C. A., & Hinds, P. W. (2004). P53 is a tumor suppressor gene. *Cell*, 116, S67–S69, 1 p following S69.

Li, S., Crenshaw, E. B. 3rd, Rawson, E. J., Simmons, D. M., Swanson, L. W., & Rosenfeld, M. G. (1990). Dwarf locus mutants lacking three pituitary cell types result from mutations in the POU-domain gene pit-1. *Nature*, 347, 528–533.

Liang, H., Masoro, E. J., Nelson, J. F., Strong, R., McMahan, C. A., & Richardson, A. (2003). Genetic mouse models of extended lifespan. *Experimental Gerontology*, 38, 1353–1364.

Lieber, M. R., Ma, Y., Pannicke, U., & Schwarz, K. (2003). Mechanism and regulation of human non-homologous DNA end-joining. *Nature Reviews Molecular and Cellular Biology*, 4, 712–720.

Lim, D. S., Vogel, H., Willerford, D. M., Sands, A. T., Platt, K. A., & Hasty, P. (2000). Analysis of ku80-mutant mice and cells with deficient levels of p53. *Molecular and Cellular Biology*, 20, 3772–3780.

Lin, S. J., Defossez, P. A., & Guarente, L. (2000). Requirement of NAD and SIR2 for life-span extension by calorie restriction in Saccharomyces cerevisiae. *Science*, 289, 2126–2128.

Linzer, D. I., & Levine, A. J. (1979). Characterization of a 54K Dalton cellular SV40 tumor antigen present in SV40-transformed cells and uninfected embryonal carcinoma cells. *Cell*, 17, 43–52.

Ljungman, M. (2000). Dial 9–1–1 for p53: mechanisms of p53 activation by cellular stress. *Neoplasia*, 2, 208–225.

Longo, V. D., & Finch, C. E. (2003). Evolutionary medicine: from dwarf model systems to healthy centenarians? *Science*, 299, 1342–1346.

Lozano, G., & Elledge, S. J. (2000). p53 sends nucleotides to repair DNA. *Nature*, 404, 24–25.

Luo, J., Nikolaev, A. Y., Imai, S., Chen, D., Su, F., Shiloh, A., Guarente, L., & Gu, W. (2001). Negative control of p53 by Sir2alpha promotes cell survival under stress. *Cell*, 107, 137–148.

Maier, B., Gluba, W., Bernier, B., Turner, T., Mohammad, K., Guise, T., Sutherland, A., Thorner, M., & Scrable, H. (2004). Modulation of mammalian life span by the short isoform of p53. *Genes & Development*, 18, 306–319.

Malkin, D., Li, F. P., Strong, L. C., Fraumeni, J. F., Jr., Nelson, C. E., Kim, D. H., Kassel, J., Gryka, M. A., Bischoff, F. Z., & Tainsky, M. A. (1990). Germ line p53 mutations in a familial syndrome of breast cancer, sarcomas, and other neoplasms. *Science*, 250, 1233–1238.

Masoro, E. J. (2000). Caloric restriction and aging: an update. *Experimental Gerontology*, 35, 299–305.

Matakidou, A., Eisen, T., & Houlston, R. S. (2003). TP53 polymorphisms and lung cancer risk: a systematic review and meta-analysis. *Mutagenesis*, 18, 377–385.

Mathieu, N., Pirzio, L., Freulet-Marriere, M. A., Desmaze, C., & Sabatier, L. (2004). Telomeres and chromosomal instability. *Cellular and Molecular Life Sciences* 61, 641–656.

McBurney, M. W., Yang, X., Jardine, K., Hixon, M., Boekelheide, K., Webb, J. R., Lansdorp, P. M., & Lemieux, M. (2003). The mammalian SIR2alpha protein has a role in embryogenesis and gametogenesis. *Molecular and Cellular Biology*, 23, 38–54.

McCay, C. M., Crowell, M. F., & Maynard, L. A. (1989). The effect of retarded growth upon the length of life span and upon the ultimate body size. 1935. *Nutrition*, 5, 155–171; discussion, 172.

Melk, A., Kittikowit, W., Sandhu, I., Halloran, K. M., Grimm, P., Schmidt, B. M., & Halloran, P. F. (2003). Cell senescence in rat kidneys in vivo increases with growth and age despite lack of telomere shortening. *Kidney International*, 63, 2134–2143.

Metcalfe, J. A., Parkhill, J., Campbell, L., Stacey, M., Biggs, P., Byrd, P. J., & Taylor, A. M. (1996). Accelerated telomere shortening in ataxia telangiectasia. *Nature Genetics*, 13, 350–353.

Migliaccio, E., Giorgio, M., Mele, S., Pelicci, G., Reboldi, P., Pandolfi, P. P., Lanfrancone, L., & Pelicci, P. G. (1999). The p66Shc adaptor protein controls oxidative stress response and life span in mammals. *Nature*, 402, 309–313.

Migliaccio, E., Mele, S., Salcini, A. E., Pelicci, G., Lai, K. M., Superti-Furga, G., Pawson, T., Di Fiore, P. P., Lanfrancone, L., & Pelicci, P. G. (1997). Opposite effects of the p52Shc/p46Shc and p66Shc splicing isoforms on the EGF receptor-MAP kinase-fos signalling pathway. *Embo Journal*, 16, 706–716.

Miller, R. A. (2004a). 'Accelerated aging': a primrose path to insight? *Aging Cell*, 3, 47–51.

Miller, R. A. (2004b). Rebuttal to Hasty and Vijg: 'Accelerating aging by mouse reverse genetics: a rational approach to understanding longevity'. *Aging Cell*, 3, 53–54.

Misra, R. P., & Duncan, S. A. (2002). Gene targeting in the mouse: advances in introduction of transgenes into the genome by homologous recombination. *Endocrine*, 19, 229–238.

Mohr, U., Dungworth, D. L., Capen, C. C., Carlton, W. W., Sundberg, J. P., and Ward, J. M. (1996). *Pathobiology of the aging mouse* (p. 1032). Washington, D.C.: ILSI Press.

Moll, U. M., & Petrenko, O. (2003). The MDM2–p53 interaction. *Molecular Cancer Research*, 1, 1001–1008.

Motta, M. C., Divecha, N., Lemieux, M., Kamel, C., Chen, D., Gu, W., Bultsma, Y., McBurney, M., & Guarente, L. (2004). Mammalian SIRT1 represses forkhead transcription factors. *Cell*, 116, 551–563.

Murphy, C. T., McCarroll, S. A., Bargmann, C. I., Fraser, A., Kamath, R. S., Ahringer, J., Li, H., & Kenyon, C. (2003). Genes that act downstream of DAF-16 to influence the lifespan of *Caenorhabditis elegans*. *Nature*, 424, 277–283.

Nabeshima, Y. (2002). Klotho: a fundamental regulator of aging. *Ageing Research Reviews*, 1, 627–638.

Nagai, T., Yamada, K., Kim, H. C., Kim, Y. S., Noda, Y., Imura, A., Nabeshima, Y., & Nabeshima, T. (2003). Cognition impairment in the genetic model of aging klotho gene mutant mice: a role of oxidative stress. *Faseb Journal*, 17, 50–52.

Nemoto, S., & Finkel, T. (2002). Redox regulation of forkhead proteins through a p66Shc-dependent signaling pathway. *Science*, 295, 2450–2452.

Nemoto, S., Fergusson, M. M., & Finkel, T. (2004). Nutrient availability regulates SIRT1 through a forkhead-dependent pathway. *Science*, 306, 2105–2108.

Noda, A., Ning, Y., Venable, S. F., Pereira-Smith, O. M., & Smith, J. R. (1994). Cloning of senescent cell-derived inhibitors of DNA synthesis using an expression screen. *Experimental Cell Research*, 211, 90–98.

Oren, M. (2003). Decision making by p53: life, death and cancer. *Cell Death and Differentiation*, 10, 431–442.

Pandita, T. K. (2002). ATM function and telomere stability. *Oncogene*, 21, 611–618.

Paradis, V., Youssef, N., Dargere, D., Ba, N., Bonvoust, F., Deschatrette, J., & Bedossa, P. (2001). Replicative senescence in normal liver, chronic hepatitis C, and hepatocellular carcinomas. *Human Pathology, 32*, 327–332.

Parrinello, S., Samper, E., Krtolica, A., Goldstein, J., Melov, S., & Campisi, J. (2003). Oxygen sensitivity severely limits the replicative lifespan of murine fibroblasts. *Nature Cell Biology, 5*, 741–747.

Pearson, M., Carbone, R., Sebastiani, C., Cioce, M., Fagioli, M., Saito, S., Higashimoto, Y., Appella, E., Minucci, S., Pandolfi, P. P., & Pelicci, P. G. (2000). PML regulates p53 acetylation and premature senescence induced by oncogenic Ras. *Nature, 406*, 207–210.

Pelicci, P. G. (2004). Do tumor-suppressive mechanisms contribute to organism aging by inducing stem cell senescence? *Journal of Clinical Investigation, 113*, 4–7.

Perlman, S., Becker-Catania, S., & Gatti, R. A. (2003). Ataxia-telangiectasia: diagnosis and treatment. *Seminars in Pediatric Neurology, 10*, 173–182.

Pletcher, S. D., Khazaeli, A. A., & Curtsinger, J. W. (2000). Why do life spans differ? Partitioning mean longevity differences in terms of age-specific mortality parameters. *Journals of Gerontology, Series A, Biological Sciences and Medical Sciences, 55*, B381–B389.

Richter, C., Park, J. W., & Ames, B. N. (1988). Normal oxidative damage to mitochondrial and nuclear DNA is extensive. *Proceedings of the National Academy of Sciences of the USA, 85*, 6465–6467.

Rockwood, L. D., Nussenzweig, A., & Janz, S. (2003). Paradoxical decrease in mutant frequencies and chromosomal rearrangements in a transgenic lacZ reporter gene in *Ku80* null mice deficient in DNA double strand break repair. *Mutation Research, 529*, 51–58.

Rudolph, K. L., Chang, S., Lee, H. W., Blasco, M., Gottlieb, G. J., Greider, C., & DePinho, R. A. (1999). Longevity, stress response, and cancer in aging telomerase-deficient mice. *Cell, 96*, 701–712.

Selivanova, G., Iotsova, V., Okan, I., Fritsche, M., Strom, M., Groner, B., Grafstrom, R. C., & Wiman, K. G. (1997). Restoration of the growth suppression function of mutant p53 by a synthetic peptide derived from the p53 C-terminal domain. *Nature Medicine, 3*, 632–638.

Selivanova, G., Ryabchenko, L., Jansson, E., Iotsova, V., & Wiman, K. G. (1999). Reactivation of mutant p53 through interaction of a C-terminal peptide with the core domain. *Molecular and Cellular Biology, 19*, 3395–3402.

Seluanov, A., Gorbunova, V., Falcovitz, A., Sigal, A., Milyavsky, M., Zurer, I., Shohat, G., Goldfinger, N., & Rotter, V. (2001). Change of the death pathway in senescent human fibroblasts in response to DNA damage is caused by an inability to stabilize p53. *Molecular and Cellular Biology, 21*, 1552–1564.

Serrano, M., Lin, A. W., McCurrach, M. E., Beach, D., & Lowe, S. W. (1997). Oncogenic ras provokes premature cell senescence associated with accumulation of p53 and p16INK4a. *Cell, 88*, 593–602.

Sharpless, N. E., & DePinho, R. A. (2004). Telomeres, stem cells, senescence, and cancer. *Journal of Clinical Investigation, 113*, 160–168.

Sherr, C. J., & DePinho, R. A. (2000). Cellular senescence: mitotic clock or culture shock? *Cell, 102*, 407–410.

Shiloh, Y. (2003). ATM and related protein kinases: safeguarding genome integrity. *Nature Reviews Cancer, 3*, 155–168.

Sinclair, D. A. (2002). Paradigms and pitfalls of yeast longevity research. *Mechanisms of Ageing and Development, 123*, 857–867.

Smith, D. W. (1996). Cancer mortality at very old ages. *Cancer, 77*, 1367–1372.

Smogorzewska, A., & de Lange, T. (2004). Regulation of telomerase by telomeric proteins. *Annual Review of Biochemistry, 73*, 177–208.

Sohal, R. S., & Weindruch, R. (1996). Oxidative stress, caloric restriction, and aging. *Science, 273*, 59–63.

Tahara, H., Sato, E., Noda, A., & Ide, T. (1995). Increase in expression level of p21sdi1/cip1/waf1 with increasing division age in both normal and SV40-transformed human fibroblasts. *Oncogene, 10*, 835–840.

Takeda, T. (1999). Senescence-accelerated mouse (SAM): a biogerontological resource in aging research. *Neurobiology of Aging*, 20, 105–110.

Tanhauser, S. M., & Laipis, P. J. (1995). Multiple deletions are detectable in mitochondrial DNA of aging mice. *Journal of Biological Chemistry*, 270, 24769–24775.

Tatar, M., Bartke, A., & Antebi, A. (2003). The endocrine regulation of aging by insulin-like signals. *Science*, 299, 1346–1351.

Thomas, M., Kalita, A., Labrecque, S., Pim, D., Banks, L., & Matlashewski, G. (1999). Two polymorphic variants of wild-type p53 differ biochemically and biologically. *Molecular and Cellular Biology*, 19, 1092–1100.

Trifunovic, A., Wredenberg, A., Falkenberg, M., Spelbrink, J. N., Rovio, A. T., Bruder, C. E., Bohlooly, Y. M., Gidlof, S., Oldfors, A., Wibom, R., Tornell, J., Jacobs, H. T., & Larsson, N. G. (2004). Premature ageing in mice expressing defective mitochondrial DNA polymerase. *Nature*, 429, 417–423.

Trinei, M., Giorgio, M., Cicalese, A., Barozzi, S., Ventura, A., Migliaccio, E., Milia, E., Padura, I. M., Raker, V. A., Maccarana, M., Petronilli, V., Minucci, S., Bernardi, P., Lanfrancone, L., & Pelicci, P. G. (2002). A p53-p66Shc signalling pathway controls intracellular redox status, levels of oxidation-damaged DNA and oxidative stress-induced apoptosis. *Oncogene*, 21, 3872–3878.

Tyner, S. D., Venkatachalam, S., Choi, J., Jones, S., Ghebranious, N., Igelmann, H., Lu, X., Soron, G., Cooper, B., Brayton, C., Hee Park, S., Thompson, T., Karsenty, G., Bradley, A., & Donehower, L. A. (2002). p53 mutant mice that display early ageing-associated phenotypes. *Nature*, 415, 45–53.

Um, J. H., Kim, S. J., Kim, D. W., Ha, M. Y., Jang, J. H., Chung, B. S., Kang, C. D., & Kim, S. H. (2003). Tissue-specific changes of DNA repair protein Ku and mtHSP70 in aging rats and their retardation by caloric restriction. *Mechanisms of Ageing and Development*, 124, 967–975.

Van Heemst, D., Mooijaart, S. P., Beekman, M., Schreuder, J., de Craen, A. J. M., Brandt, B. W., Slagboom, P. E., Westendorp, R. G. J., Long Life Study Group (2005). Variation in the human TP53 gene affects old age survival and cancer mortality. *Experimental Gerontology*, 40, 11–15.

Van Zant, G., & Liang, Y. (2003). The role of stem cells in aging. *Experimental Hematology*, 31, 659–672.

Vasile, E., Tomita, Y., Brown, L. F., Kocher, O., & Dvorak, H. F. (2001). Differential expression of thymosin beta-10 by early passage and senescent vascular endothelium is modulated by VPF/VEGF: evidence for senescent endothelial cells in vivo at sites of atherosclerosis. *Faseb Journal*, 15, 458–466.

Vaziri, H., & Benchimol, S. (1998). Reconstitution of telomerase activity in normal human cells leads to elongation of telomeres and extended replicative life span. *Current Biology*, 8, 279–282.

Vaziri, H., Dessain, S. K., Ng Eaton, E., Imai, S. I., Frye, R. A., Pandita, T. K., Guarente, L., & Weinberg, R. A. (2001). hSIR2(SIRT1) functions as an NAD-dependent p53 deacetylase. *Cell*, 107, 149–159.

Vaziri, H., West, M. D., Allsopp, R. C., Davison, T. S., Wu, Y. S., Arrowsmith, C. H., Poirier, G. G., & Benchimol, S. (1997). ATM-dependent telomere loss in aging human diploid fibroblasts and DNA damage lead to the post-translational activation of p53 protein involving poly(ADP-ribose) polymerase. *Embo Journal*, 16, 6018–6033.

Venkitaraman, A. R. (2002). Cancer susceptibility and the functions of BRCA1 and BRCA2. *Cell*, 108, 171–182.

Vijg, J., & Dolle, M. E. (2002). Large genome rearrangements as a primary cause of aging. *Mechanisms of Ageing and Development*, 123, 907–915.

Vogel, H., Lim, D. S., Karsenty, G., Finegold, M., & Hasty, P. (1999). Deletion of Ku86 causes early onset of senescence in mice. *Proceedings of the National Academy of Sciences of the USA*, 96, 10770–10775.

Vousden, K. H. (2002). Activation of the p53 tumor suppressor protein. *Biochimica et Biophysica Acta*, 1602, 47–59.

Vousden, K. H., & Lu, X. (2002). Live or let die: the cell's response to p53. *Nature Reviews Cancer*, 2, 594–604.

Walter, C. A., Zhou, Z. Q., Manguino, D., Ikeno, Y., Reddick, R., Nelson, J., Intano, G., Herbert, D. C., McMahan, C. A., & Hanes, M. (2001). Health span and life span in transgenic mice with modulated DNA repair. *Annals of the New York Academy of Sciences*, 928, 132–140.

Warner, H. R., & Sierra, F. (2003). Models of accelerated ageing can be informative about the molecular mechanisms of ageing and/or age-related pathology. *Mechanisms of Ageing and Development*, 124, 581–587.

Webley, K., Bond, J. A., Jones, C. J., Blaydes, J. P., Craig, A., Hupp, T., & Wynford-Thomas, D. (2000). Posttranslational modifications of p53 in replicative senescence overlapping but distinct from those induced by DNA damage. *Molecular and Cellular Biology*, 20, 2803–2808.

Weston, A., & Godbold, J. H. (1997). Polymorphisms of H-ras-1 and p53 in breast cancer and lung cancer: a meta-analysis. *Environmental Health Perspectives*, 105 Supplement 4, 919–926.

Wong, K. K., Maser, R. S., Bachoo, R. M., Menon, J., Carrasco, D. R., Gu, Y., Alt, F. W., & DePinho, R. A. (2003). Telomere dysfunction and Atm deficiency compromises organ homeostasis and accelerates ageing. *Nature*, 421, 643–648.

Wright, W. E., & Shay, J. W. (2002). Historical claims and current interpretations of replicative aging. *Nature Biotechnology*, 20, 682–688.

Xu, X., Qiao, W., Linke, S. P., Cao, L., Li, W. M., Furth, P. A., Harris, C. C., & Deng, C. X. (2001). Genetic interactions between tumor suppressors Brca1 and p53 in apoptosis, cell cycle and tumorigenesis. *Nature Genetics*, 28, 266–271.

Xu, Y. (2003). Regulation of p53 responses by post-translational modifications. *Cell Death and Differentiation*, 10, 400–403.

Xu, Y., Ashley, T., Brainerd, E. E., Bronson, R. T., Meyn, M. S., & Baltimore, D. (1996). Targeted disruption of ATM leads to growth retardation, chromosomal fragmentation during meiosis, immune defects, and thymic lymphoma. *Genes and Development*, 10, 2411–2422.

Yakes, F. M., & Van Houten, B. (1997). Mitochondrial DNA damage is more extensive and persists longer than nuclear DNA damage in human cells following oxidative stress. *Proceedings of the National Academy of Sciences of the USA*, 94, 514–519.

Zhu, J., Woods, D., McMahon, M., & Bishop, J. M. (1998). Senescence of human fibroblasts induced by oncogenic Raf. *Genes & Development*, 12, 2997–3007.

Chapter 7

Complex Genetic Architecture of *Drosophila* Longevity

Trudy F. C. Mackay, Natalia V. Roshina, Jeff W. Leips, and Elena G. Pasyukova

I. Introduction

Limited life span and senescence are near-universal phenomena and are quantitative traits controlled by genetic and environmental factors whose interactions both limit life span and generate variation in life span among individuals, populations, and species. Recently, there has been considerable progress toward understanding the environmental factors and genetic pathways that regulate life span across diverse taxa (Finch & Ruvkun, 2001; Guarente & Kenyon, 2000; Partridge & Gems, 2002; Tatar *et al.*, 2003). For example, caloric restriction extends life span in mammals (Weindruch & Walford, 1988), *Drosophila melanogaster* (Pletcher *et al.*, 2002), and yeast (Lin *et al.*, 2000), whereas reproduction shortens longevity in humans (Westendorp & Kirkwood, 1998), *D. melanogaster* (Chapman *et al.*, 1995; Partridge & Farquar, 1981; Partridge *et al.*, 1987), and *Caenorhabditis elegans* (Gems & Riddle, 1996). Similarly, mutations in evolutionarily conserved genes encoding components of the insulin or insulin-like

signaling pathway confer increased longevity in yeast (Fabrizio *et al.*, 2001; *C. elegans* (Kimura *et al.*, 1997; Lin *et al.*, 1997), *D. melanogaster* (Clancy *et al.*, 2001; Glannakou *et al.*, 2004; Hwangbo *et al.*, 2004; Tatar *et al.*, 2001), and mice (Blüher *et al.*, 2003; Brown-Borg *et al.*, 1996; Flurkey *et al.*, 2001; Holzenberger *et al.*, 2003).

Pleiotropic effects of mutations causing extended longevity often (but not universally) include increased resistance to oxidative and other stresses (Clancy *et al.*, 2001; Fabrizio *et al.*, 2001; Lin *et al.*, 1998; Migliaccio *et al.*, 1999; Tatar *et al.*, 2001), as well as reduced fertility (Clancy *et al.*, 2001; Tatar *et al.*, 2001). Evidence that life span is indeed limited by accumulation of toxic superoxide radicals and peroxides comes from observations that mutations in genes required for the detoxification of reactive oxygen species (ROS) are associated with reduced life span in *C. elegans* (Ishii *et al.*, 1998), *D. melanogaster* (Griswold *et al.*, 1993), and also in humans, where mutations in Cu/Zn Superoxide dismutase (SOD) cause motor neuron

Handbook of the Biology of Aging, Sixth Edition

degeneration in amyotrophic lateral sclerosis (Wong *et al.*, 1998). Superoxide dismutase/catalase mimetics increase *C. elegans* life span (Melov *et al.*, 2000), and overexpression of these genes has been associated with increased life span in *D. melanogaster* (Parkes *et al.*, 1998; Sun *et al.*, 2002). Consistent with the central role of mitochondria in metabolism and the production of ROS, mutational and RNAi inactivation of genes required for mitochondrial function prolongs *C. elegans* life span (Dillin *et al.*, 2002; Lee *et al.*, 2003).

Other pathways directly implicated in the regulation of longevity include intermediary metabolism (Branicky *et al.*, 2000; Rogina *et al.*, 2000), sensory perception (Apfeld & Kenyon, 1999), serotonin signaling (Sze *et al.*, 2000), chromatin silencing (Defossez *et al.*, 2001), DNA repair (de Boer *et al.*, 2002), and the heat-shock response (Verbeke *et al.*, 2001). Given the plethora of genes for which expression is altered in aging mice (Lee *et al.*, 1999) and *Drosophila* (Pletcher *et al.*, 2002; Zou *et al.*, 2000), it is becoming clear that a substantial fraction of the genome could be involved in the regulation of life span.

There is considerable segregating variation in longevity in natural populations of most organisms, including humans. Estimates of heritability of life span are of the order of 10 to 30 percent (Finch & Tanzi, 1997), and it is easy to artificially select for long-lived strains of *Drosophila* (Luckinbill *et al.*, 1984; Partridge & Fowler, 1992; Rose, 1984; Zwaan *et al.*, 1995). However, in contrast to the wealth of accumulating knowledge regarding the loci and pathways regulating life span, virtually nothing is known about the genes causing naturally occurring variation in longevity. Are these a subset of the genes identified by analysis of mutations and candidate genes implicated from changes of gene expression with aging, or will analysis of naturally occurring variation for life span uncover additional loci and novel pathways? Is the genetic architec-

ture of natural variation in longevity simple, with relatively few genes with large additive effects contributing to most of the variation, or is it more complex, with variation attributable to many epistatically interacting loci? In this chapter, we summarize recent progress in dissecting the genetic architecture of natural variation in life span of *D. melanogaster*. We show that genetic variation for longevity is indeed complex, but that analysis of natural variants with subtle effects indeed reveals novel loci affecting life span not yet implicated by mutational analyses.

II. Genome Scan for Quantitative Trait Loci (QTLs)

Identifying genes affecting segregating variation for life span is an iterative processes, the first step of which is to localize genomic regions containing one or more quantitative trait loci (QTLs) affecting variation in longevity. QTL mapping in *Drosophila* requires two inbred strains that vary genetically for life span, and a polymorphic molecular marker linkage map. One can then assess the longevity and multi-locus genotype for individuals in a segregating mapping population (backcross, F_2 or recombinant inbred lines, RILs) derived from the two parental strains. QTLs are mapped by linkage to the molecular markers; if there is a significant statistical difference in longevity between genotype classes for a particular marker, one infers a QTL affecting longevity is linked to the marker (Falconer & Mackay, 1996; Lynch & Walsh, 1998).

QTLs affecting *Drosophila* longevity have been mapped in a population of 98 RILs derived from *Oregon* (*Ore*), a standard wildtype strain, and *2b*, a strain selected for low male mating activity (Pasyukova & Nuzhdin, 1993). The RILs were genotyped for insertion sites of polymorphic *roo* transposable element markers, giving a 3.2 cM marker map (Nuzhdin *et al.*, 1997).

The RIL line design is particularly useful for mapping QTLs affecting traits with low heritabilities, such as life span, because assessing multiple individuals from each line gives a more accurate estimate of the genotypic values of each line than single backcross or F₂ individuals (Soller & Beckmann, 1990). Further, each line needs to be genotyped only once, and the same lines can be grown in multiple environments, affording an opportunity to evaluate environment-specific effects on longevity. Longevity was assessed for virgin flies from each of the homozygous RILs under several different environmental conditions: standard culture conditions (25 °C), flies housed singly (Nuzhdin *et al.*, 1997); standard culture conditions, flies maintained in single-sex groups of 10 individuals (Vieira *et al.*, 2000); and in single-sex groups of 10 individuals under conditions of starvation stress, a brief 37 °C heat shock early in life, and chronic heat (29 °C) and cold (14 °C) stress (Vieira *et al.*, 2000). Each of the RILs was also crossed separately to *Ore* and to *2b*, and life span of the resulting 196 genotypes assessed under high and low larval density conditions for virgin flies reared at 25 °C, in groups of five single-sex individuals (Leips & Mackay, 2000), and under high larval density conditions for mated flies reared at 25 °C in groups of three males and three females (Leips & Mackay, 2002). Map positions and effects of QTLs affecting life span were estimated using composite interval mapping (Zeng, 1994) for each of these experiments. Table 7.1 summarizes the locations of all QTLs affecting longevity at 25 °C. The same general regions were detected in most studies, although the exact borders vary.

Table 7.1
QTL Affecting Variation in Life Span Between *Ore* and *2b* at 25 °C

QTL	Sex[a]	Location[b]	Reference
1B;3E	F	1B-3E	Vieira *et al.*, 2000
6E;10D	F	6E-10D	Vieira *et al.*, 2000
17C;19A	F	17C-19A	Vieira *et al.*, 2000
	M	30D-38E	Leips & Mackay, 2002
	F	33E-34E	Nuzhdin *et al.*, 1997
	F	35B-38E	Leips & Mackay, 2000
	M	35B-43A	Leips & Mackay, 2000
	F&M	38E-43A	Vieira *et al.*, 2000
	M	38E-46C	Nuzhdin *et al.*, 1997
30D;49D			
	M	46C-49D	Leips & Mackay, 2000
	M	65D-67D	Nuzhdin *et al.*, 1997
	F	67D-68C	Leips & Mackay, 2000
	F	68B-69D	Vieira *et al.*, 2000
	F	69D-87B	Leips & Mackay, 2000
	M	72A-85F	Nuzhdin *et al.*, 1997
	M	72A-77A	Leips & Mackay, 2000
	M	73D-87B	Vieira *et al.*, 2000
65D;89B	M	87B-89B	Leips & Mackay, 2002
	M	96F-97E	Leips & Mackay, 2002
	F&M	97E-99A	Leips & Mackay, 2002
	F	99A-100A	Leips & Mackay, 2002
96F;100A	M	99B-100A	Nuzhdin *et al.*, 1997

[a]Female (F), Male (M)
[b]2 LOD support interval

Curtsinger and Khazaeli (2002) used a similar experimental design to map QTLs affecting variation in life span between inbred derivatives of lines selected for postponed senescence (Luckinbill & Clare, 1985) and their unselected controls. It is encouraging that two of the three QTLs detected in this mapping population (at 34F;45D and 66A;68D) coincided with those affecting variation between *Ore* and *2b*. Because the two sets of strains are completely unrelated, this suggests that naturally occurring variation in life span could be caused by alleles at intermediate frequency. Forbes and colleagues (2004) and Valenzuela and colleagues (2004) mapped QTLs affecting variation in life span between inbred derivatives of a different set of lines selected for postponed senescence (Rose, 1984) and found a minimum of 10 QTLs. However, these experiments had low power, and the QTLs spanned the majority of the genome.

A. Genotype × Sex and Genotype × Environment Interactions

QTLs affecting variation in longevity are often sex-specific, but the degree to which QTLs affect both sexes can vary according to mating status and culture conditions. In quantitative genetics, the cross-sex genetic correlation (r_{GS}) is a measure of the degree to which the same genes affect both sexes. If $r_{GS} = 1$, the same genes affect variation in longevity in the same direction in males and females; if $r_{GS} = -1$, the same genes affect variation in longevity in males and females, but in opposite directions (i.e., sexually antagonistic); if $r_{GS} = 0$, different loci affect variation in life span in the two sexes. Estimates of r_{GS} from analysis of longevity of the RILs derived from *Ore* and *2b* for virgin males and females, reared under standard culture conditions, were approximately 0.2, and the estimated QTL effects were highly sex-

specific (see Table 7.1, Leips & Mackay, 2000; Nuzhdin *et al.*, 1997; Vieira *et al.*, 2000). However, estimates of r_{GS} for longevity in the same set of lines increase when the flies are mated and/or reared under stressful conditions (Leips & Mackay, 2002; Reiwitch & Nuzhdin, 2002; Vieira *et al.*, 2000), and increasing numbers of QTLs affect both sexes. Curtsinger and Khazaeli (2002) and Forbes and colleagues (2004) mapped QTLs affecting variation in life span of mated flies between inbred derivatives of lines selected for postponed selection and the unselected control. In the former case, the same QTLs affected life span in both sexes, whereas in the latter case, half of the QTLs were sex-specific. One possible explanation of sex-specific QTL effects is the low power of many mapping experiments (Curtsinger, 2002). However, the quantitative genetic analysis of longevity among the *Ore* and *2b* RILs revealed highly significant line-by-sex interactions (Leips & Mackay, 2000; 2002; Nuzhdin *et al.*, 1997; Vieira *et al.*, 2000), which can only occur if $r_{GS} < 1$. Further, one of the first analyses of natural variation in life span (Maynard Smith, 1958) showed there was a low correlation in longevity between males and females among inbred strains derived from nature. Indeed, sex-specific or sex-biased effects appear to be a common feature of alleles affecting quantitative traits in *Drosophila* (Mackay, 2001).

QTL effects on longevity are exquisitely sensitive to rearing environment. All of the 17 QTLs detected by Vieira and colleagues (2000) and five of the six QTLs mapped by Leips and Mackay (2000) exhibited significant genotype × environment interactions. Some life span QTLs were both sex- and environment-specific (Leips & Mackay, 2000; Vieira *et al.*, 2000). Sex- and environment-specific QTL effects were attributable to both conditional neutrality (Nuzhdin *et al.*, 1997) and antagonistic pleiotropy. In the study of Vieira and colleagues (2000), three QTLs had opposite effects in males and females, four had opposite effects in two environments, and three had sexually antagonistic effects in one environment and antagonistic pleiotropic effects in two environments that were expressed only in one sex. Similarly, Leips and Mackay (2000) observed four interactions of longevity QTLs with density and one QTL × sex interaction attributable to changes in the direction of homozygous effects. In this study, the degree of dominance of life span QTLs also depended on density and sex. These data provide support for the hypothesis that variation for longevity might be maintained by opposing selection pressures in males and females and variable environments. On the other hand, QTL effects that are highly conditional on sex and environment seriously complicate efforts to understand the genetic basis of variation in longevity because results will be specific to the particular environment in which the experiment was conducted.

B. Epistasis (Genotype × Genotype Interactions)

To what extent do effects of QTLs on life span depend on the genotype at other loci—that is, exhibit epistasis? Leips and Mackay (2000; 2002) tested for epistatic interactions between QTLs with main effects on longevity by fitting models that included the single markers closest to the QTL peaks for all QTLs with main effects, and one pair-wise marker by marker interaction. Leips and Mackay (2000) found four significant interactions, involving five QTLs, after correcting for multiple tests (38E × 76B, 48D × 76B, 50D × 68B and 50D × 76B). In the analysis of mated flies, only one interaction term (87F × 97D) was significant. However, this analysis is conservative and does not examine whether epistasis occurs between QTLs with main effects

and markers that do not themselves have main effects on life span, or even between two markers that do not have significant marginal effects.

We performed whole genome screens for pair-wise interactions affecting life span for the data of Vieira and colleagues (2000) and Leips and Mackay (2000). All possible pairs of markers were evaluated, separately for each treatment, sex and cross (where relevant), using the two-way factorial ANOVA model $Y = \mu + M_i + M_j + M_i \times M_j + Er$, where M denotes a polymorphic marker ($i \neq j$), and Er is the within line variance. Vieira and colleagues (2000) used 76 markers, giving 2,850 possible pair-wise comparisons to test in each epistasis screen. Thus, we expect 142, 28.5, 2.85, and 0.285 interactions to be significant by chance at $P \leq 0.05$, ≤ 0.01, ≤ 0.001, and ≤ 0.0001, respectively. Leips and Mackay (2000; 2002) used 80 markers, giving 3,160 possible interactions. Here we expect 158, 31.6, 3.16, and 0.316 significant interactions by chance at $P \leq 0.05$, ≤ 0.01, ≤ 0.001, and < 0.0001, respectively. The results of these analyses are given in Table 7.2. Clearly, far more significant interactions were observed than expected by chance, illustrating the ubiquity of epistatic interactions.

The nature of these interactions is illustrated in Figure 7.1, which shows the pattern of epistasis for longevity in the high-density treatment of Leips and Mackay (2000). The same features were observed in the other analyses. The first feature to note is that the pattern of epistasis is both cross- and sex-specific, with far more significant interactions observed for females in the cross to *Ore* (see Figure 7.1a, below diagonal) and for males in the cross to *2b* (Figure 7.1b, above diagonal). Second, the vast majority of interactions do not involve QTLs with main effects but rather occur between pairs of markers without significant marginal effects. Nevertheless,

Table 7.2
Significant Interactions from Pair-Wise Tests for Epistasis

Treatment	$0.01 \leq P \leq 0.05$	$0.001 \leq P \leq 0.01$	$0.0001 \leq P \leq 0.001$	$P \leq 0.0001$	Total
Control Male[a]	352	324	214	358	1248
Control Female[a]	342	319	191	404	1256
HS Male[a]	469	318	166	294	1247
HS Female[a]	417	309	160	275	1161
HT Male[a]	373	297	136	224	1030
HT Female[a]	368	308	205	292	1173
LT Male[a]	367	336	221	492	1416
LT Female[a]	440	300	168	170	1078
Starvation Male[a]	358	295	184	587	1424
Starvation Female[a]	334	354	180	483	1351
Ore HD Male[b]	360	242	63	89	754
Ore HD Female[b]	435	309	175	244	1163
2b LD Male[b]	440	408	202	312	1362
2b HD Male[b]	437	321	175	242	1175
2b HD Female[b]	355	184	41	11	591

[a] Vieira *et al.*, 2000. HS, Heat Shock; HT, High Temperature; LT, Low Temperature
[b] Leips & Mackay, 2000. LD, Low Density; HD, High Density
Note that epistasis was not evaluated for Ore LD males and females, and 2b LD females, because genetic variation for longevity was not significant in these cross/treatment combinations.

it is encouraging that three of the four interactions between QTLs detected by Leips and Mackay (2000) were also recapitulated in this analysis (between 48D×76B, 50D×68B, and 50D×76B). Third, the pattern of interactions is highly non-random, with the same markers participating in multiple interactions. For example, in the analysis of females in the cross to *Ore* (see Figure 7.1, below diagonal), there are highly significant interactions between 1B and/or 3E at the tip of the *X* chromosome with the *X* chromosome markers 9A-11D, 33EF-38A and 57C-57F on chromosome 2, and 85F-87F and 98A-100A on chromosome 3. The 9A-11D markers interact with 29F-30D, 57F, 61A-65A, and 85F-87F. In turn, 87F interacts with markers 96F-100A at the end of chromosome 3. Examples of similar blocks of interactions in the analysis of males in the cross to *2b* (see Figure 7.1b, above diagonal) include one or markers in the 94D-100A interval with the *X* chromosome markers in the 1B-9A and 14C-19A

intervals, the region from 33E-43E on chromosome 2, and the 89B-93B interval on chromosome 3. One or more markers in the 73D-87E region interact with 1B, 10D-12E, 17C-19A, 48D-50F, and 85A-85F. Thus, it is possible that the hundreds of highly significant interactions observed are actually attributable to a manageable number of interacting loci, and that adjacent markers are in linkage disequilibrium with one QTL or a small number of linked QTLs.

The presence of epistasis confounds QTL mapping. Detecting QTLs by linkage to molecular markers is based on the marginal effects of the markers on the trait, and estimates of the main QTL effects are biased in the face of epistasis. Sophisticated statistical methods such as multiple interval mapping (Kao *et al.*, 1999) are capable of fitting main and interacting QTL effects simultaneously, and iteratively converging on a best-fitting model. These methods require large sample sizes for successful implementation, however; with 98 RILs

A

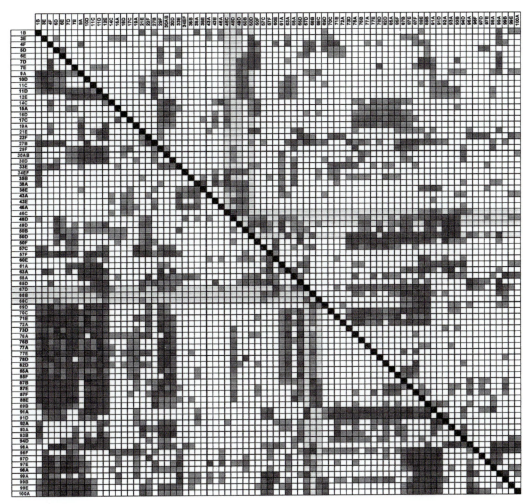

Figure 7.1 Results of tests for epistatic interactions from the data of Leips and Mackay (2000). The numbers and letters refer to cytogenetic insertion sites of polymorphic *roo* element markers. Results for males are given above the diagonal and for females below the diagonal. ■ $0.01 \leq P \leq 0.05$; ■ $0.001 \leq P \leq 0.01$; ■ $0.0001 \leq P \leq 0.001$; ■ $P < 0.0001$. QTL regions are highlighted (■). (a) Cross to *Ore*, high-density treatment.

and 80 markers, the models quickly become overparameterized and unstable. Nevertheless, we note that many of the regions detected as interacting epistatically in our analyses were identified as main effect QTLs in other composite interval mapping analyses of longevity under control (25 °C and high density) conditions (see Table 7.1).

III. Deficiency Complementation Mapping

QTLs defined by recombination mapping are not genetic loci but chromosomal regions containing one or more loci affecting the trait. For example, the average size of intervals containing *Drosophila* QTLs affecting longevity and other quantitative

B

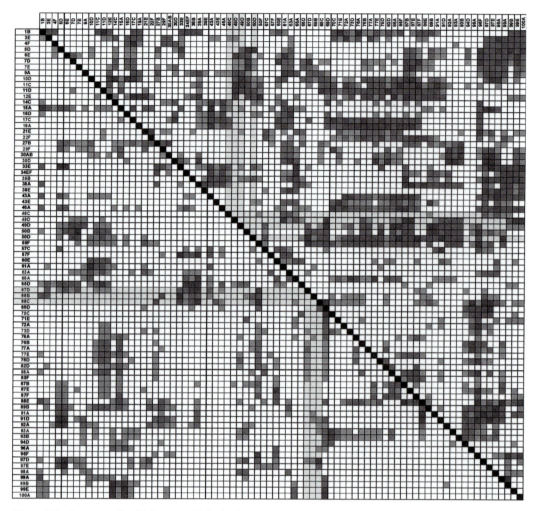

Figure 7.1 (*continued*) (b) Cross to *2b*, high-density treatment.

traits segregating between *Ore* and *2b* was 8.9.cM and 4459 kilobases (kb). Given that an average *Drosophila* gene is 8.8 kb, an average QTL therefore encompasses over 500 genes. The challenge is to map these QTLs to the level of individual genes. In *Drosophila*, complementation tests to deficiency (*Df*) chromosomes, in each of which a small region of the genome has been deleted, are typically used to map mutations to sub-cM regions. This technique can be extended to map QTLs with high resolution (Pasyukova

et al., 2000). The method requires that a minimum of two parental strains (e.g., *Ore*, *2b*) containing different QTL alleles are crossed to a set of deficiency chromosomes (*Df/Bal*, where *Bal* is a balancer chromosome) with overlapping breakpoints, and the quantitative trait phenotype is scored on F_1 individuals of each of the four resulting genotypes (*Df/Ore*, *Df/2b*, *Bal/Ore*, and *Bal/2b*). The data for each deficiency are analyzed by factorial ANOVA, partitioning the variance between lines (*L*; *Ore* and *2b*), genotypes

(*G*, *Df*, and *Bal*) and the *L*×*G* interaction. If the *L*×*G* interaction term is not significant, then the difference in phenotype between the *Ore* and *2b* strains is the same in the *Df* and *Bal* chromosome backgrounds, and complementation is inferred (i.e., the contrast [*Df/Ore-Df/2b*] – [*Bal/Ore-Bal/2b*] is not significantly different from zero). If the *L*×*G* interaction is significant, then the difference in phenotype between the *Ore* and *2b* strains varies between the *Df* and *Bal* chromosome backgrounds, the contrast [*Df/Ore-Df/2b*] – [*Bal/Ore-Bal/2b*] is significantly different from zero, and failure to complement is inferred. The location of the QTL is then delineated by the region of non-overlap of deficiencies complementing the trait phenotype with those that fail to complement the trait phenotype.

As for all genetic complementation tests, there are two possible interpretations of quantitative failure to complement: (1) the deficiency uncovers a QTL in the parental strains with different allelic effects on the trait or (2) there is epistasis between QTLs in the parental strains with other QTLs on the *Df* or *Bal* chromosome. To minimize the effects of epistatic failure to complement, we impose the constraint that the difference between the parental strains must be significant in the deficiency background but not the balancer chromosome background, and uncover the same genetic regions with independent deficiencies in different backgrounds where this is possible.

We have used deficiency complementation to map QTLs affecting variation in longevity between *Ore* and *2b* with high resolution (De Luca *et al.*, 2003; Pasyukova *et al.*, 2000; see Figure 7.2). The experimental design and analysis was as described above, with one additional criterion. The *Ore* and *2b* strains do not differ significantly in life span under standard rearing conditions, but there is significant variation in life span among their recombinant derivatives. Thus, loci affecting variation in life span between these strains are in dispersion: at some loci, the *Ore* allele confers increased life span relative to the *2b* allele, whereas at others the reverse is true. If a deficiency uncovers a "plus" allele in one line relative to a "minus" allele in the other, and all other loci affecting the trait do not contribute a net difference in life span between the strains, there could be a difference in life span between the *Df* hemizygotes but not the *Bal* heterozygotes. This could lead to a significant main effect of *L* in the ANOVA, but not necessarily an *L*×*G* interaction, if the effect is small. Thus, in this special case, a significant *L* effect was also interpreted as quantitative failure to complement, provided the contrast [*Df/Ore-Df/2b*] was significantly different from zero and the contrast [*Bal/Ore-Bal/2b*] was not significantly different from zero.

A. Chromosome 1

Vieira and colleagues (2000) mapped a female-specific QTL to the 6E;10D region of the *X* chromosome. We crossed *Ore* and *2b* to a total of 15 deficiencies spanning the regions from 6E2;10F9 (see Figure 7.2). We measured the longevity of 25 females of each of the four genotypes per deficiency, with five females in each of five replicate vials per genotype (escapees reduced the total number in some vials, so the total number scored was 1,434 rather than 1,500). Only one deficiency, *Df(1)Sxl-ra*, satisfied the criteria for quantitative failure to complement, localizing the QTL to the 233-kb 7A6;7B2 cytological region, containing 18 genes that have been mapped to the sequence.

B. Chromosome 2

The results of recombination mapping indicate at least two QTL between 30D and 49D (see Table 7.1). We crossed *Ore*

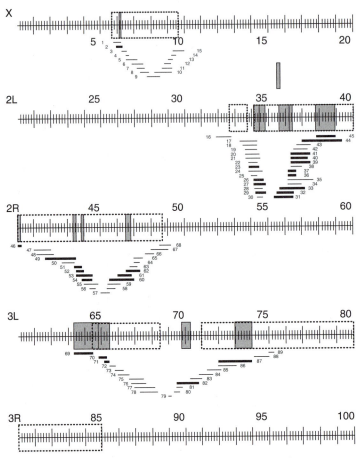

Figure 7.2 Deficiency mapping of QTLs affecting variation in life span between *Ore* and *2b*. The five major chromosome arms and major cytological divisions are depicted. The dashed lines indicate positions of QTLs from recombination mapping and the grey boxes the QTL locations determined by deficiency complementation mapping. The numbers denote the deficiencies used, and the horizontal lines show the locations of the deficiencies. Wide bars indicate deficiencies that failed to complement *Ore* and *2b* life span QTLs. Deficiency genotypes (and cytological locations of the deficiency breakpoints) are: **(1)** *Df(1)Sxl-bt*, *y¹/FM7c*, *wᵃ snˣ² vᴼᶠ g⁴ B¹* (6E2; 7A6). **(2)** ***Df(1)Sxl-ra, y¹ w¹ sn³/FM7c*, *wᵃ snˣ² vᴼᶠ g⁴ B¹*** (6F5; 7B3) **(F)**. **(3)** *Df(1)ct4 b1*, *y¹/FM7c*, *wᵃ snˣ² vᴼᶠ g⁴ B¹* (7B2; 7C4). **(4)** *Df(1)C128/FM6*, *y³¹ᵈ sc⁸ dm B* (7D1; 7D5). **(5)** *Df(1)RA2/FM7c*, *wᵃ snˣ² vᴼᶠ g⁴ B¹* (7D18–22; 8A4). **(6)** *Df(1)KA14/FM7c*, *wᵃ snˣ² vᴼᶠ g⁴ B¹* (7F1; 8C6). **(7)** *Df(1)lz-90b24*, *y² wᵃ/FM7c*, *wᵃ snˣ² vᴼᶠ g⁴ B¹* (8B5–8; 8D8–9). **(8)** *Df(1)9a4-5*, *y¹ cv¹ v¹ f¹ car¹/FM7c*, *wᵃ snˣ² vᴼᶠ g⁴ B¹* (8C7–8; 8E1–2). **(9)** *Df(1)C52, flwᶜ⁵²/FM7c*, *wᵃ snˣ² vᴼᶠ g⁴ B¹* (8E4; 9C4). **(10)** *Df(1)v-L15/ FM7c*, *wᵃ snˣ² vᴼᶠ g⁴ B¹* (9B1; 10A4). **(11)** *Df(1)vᴺ¹²⁴ᴮ/FM7c*, *wᵃ snˣ² vᴼᶠ g⁴ B¹* (9E3–F3; 10A1–8). **(12)** *Df(1)v-L2/FM7c*, *wᵃ snˣ² vᴼᶠ g⁴ B¹* (9F13; 10A1). **(13)** *Df(1)RA37/FM7c*, *wᵃ snˣ² vᴼᶠ g⁴ B¹* (10A7; 10B12). **(14)** *Df(1)GA112/FM7c*, *wᵃ snˣ² vᴼᶠ g⁴ B¹* (10B1; 10C2). **(15)** *Df(1)HA85/FM7c*, *wᵃ snˣ² vᴼᶠ g⁴ B¹* (10C2; 10F9). **(16)** *Df(2L)Prl/CyO* (32F1–3; 33F1–2). **(17)** *Df(2L)fn30*, *pr¹ cn¹/CyO* (34C6–7; 35B9–11). **(18)** *Df(2L)64j, L²/CyO*, *Cy¹ dp¹ᵛ¹ pr¹ cn²* (34D1; 35B9–C1). **(19)** *Df(2L)fn7*, *pr¹ cn¹/CyO*, *Cy¹ dp¹ᵛ¹ pr¹ cn²* (34E1–2; 35B3–5). **(20)** *Df(2L)A376, b¹ cn¹ bw¹/CyO*, *Cy¹ dp¹ᵛ¹ pr¹ cn²* (34E3; 35C4–5). **(21)** *Df(2L)A263, b¹ cn¹ bw¹/CyO*, *Cy¹ dp¹ᵛ¹ pr¹ cn²* (34E5–F1; 35C3). **(22)** *Df(2L)A217, b¹ cn¹ bw¹/In(2lr)Gla, Gla¹ l(2)34De² l(2)35Bb⁶* (34F5; 35B3). **(23)** ***Df(2L) fn5*, *pr¹ cn¹/CyO*, *Cy¹ dp¹ᵛ¹ pr¹ cn²*** (34F5; 35C3) **(F)**. **(24)** *Df(2L)fn1/CyO*, *Cy¹ dp¹ᵛ¹ pr¹ cn²* (34F4–35A1; 35D5–7). **(25)** *Df(2L)A245, b¹ cn¹ bw¹/CyO*, *Cy¹ dp¹ᵛ¹ pr¹ cn²* (35A4; 35B2). **(26)** ***Df(2L)TE35BC-8, pr¹ cn¹ sp¹/CyO*, *Cy¹ dp¹ᵛ¹ pr¹ cn²*** (35B1; 35E1) **(B)**. **(27)** ***Df(2L)osp29, Adhᵁᶠ pr¹ cn¹/CyO*** (35B1–3; 35E6) **(F)**. **(28)** *Df(2L)TE35BC-34, b¹ pr¹ pk¹ cn¹ sp¹/CyO*, *Cy¹ dp¹ᵛ¹ pr¹ cn²* (35B4; 35D4). **(29)** ***Df(2L)TE35BC-24, b¹ pr¹ pk¹ cn¹ sp¹/CyO*, *Cy¹ dp¹ᵛ¹ pr¹ cn²*** (34B4–6; 35E1–2) **(M)**. **(30)** *Df(2L)TE35BC-3, b¹ pr¹ pk¹ cn¹ sp¹/CyO*, *Cy¹ dp¹ᵛ¹ pr¹ cn²* (35C1; 35D3–7). **(31)** ***Df(2L)TW137, cn¹ bw¹/CyO*** (36C2–4; 37B9–C1) **(B)**.

and *2b* to 53 deficiencies spanning the region from 32F1–3 to 50A2 (De Luca *et al.*, 2003; Pasyukova *et al.*, 2000; see Figure 7.2). We measured the longevity of 20 males and 20 females for each of the four genotypes per deficiency, with five individuals in each of four replicate vials per sex and genotype, for a total of over 8,400 individuals scored. These data reveal from 10 to 12 QTLs affecting variation in longevity between *Ore* and *2b* in this region.

Failure of *Df(2l)fn5*, *Df(2L)TE35BC-8*, *Df(2L)osp29*, and *Df(2L)TE35BC-24* to complement the life span phenotypes of *Ore* and *2b* QTL indicates there is at least one QTL affecting variation in life span between *Ore* and *2b* in the 35B-E region. However, it is necessary to postu-late three QTLs in this region to account for the significant variation in the direction and sex-specificities of the complementation effects, and observation of complementation for other deficiencies uncovering this region. Specifically, all the data can be accounted for if there are two closely linked female-specific QTLs at 35B9-C3 (for which the *Ore* allele increases longevity relative to *2b*) and 35C3 (for which the *2b* allele increases longevity relative to *Ore*), and a third QTL at 35D5-E1, which has variable sex-specific effects depending on the genetic background (Pasyukova *et al.*, 2000). The 35B9-C3 QTL encompasses 168 kb and contains nine genes. The 35C3 QTL spans 62.5 kb, in which only one pre-dicted gene has been mapped to the

---

Figure 7.2 *(continued)*   **(32) *Df(2L)VA18*, *m¹ pr¹*/CyO, Cy¹ dp^{lv1} pr¹ cn²** (36D1; 37C2–5) **(B)**. **(33) *Df(2L)TW50*, *cn¹*/CyO** (36E4–F1; 38A6–8) **(F)**. **(34)** *Df(2L)TW158*, *cn¹ bw¹*/CyO (37B2–8; 37E2–F1). **(35)** *Df(2L)pr-A16*, *cn¹ bw¹*/CyO (37B2–12; 38D2–5). **(36) *Df(2L)VA23*, *noc^{Sco} pr¹*/CyO** (37B9–10; 37D5) **(M)**. **(37) *Df(2L)TW130*, *cn¹ bw¹*/CyO** (37B9–C1; 37D1–2) **(M)**. **(38) *Df(2L)VA17*, *Ddc^{VA17} pr¹*/CyO** (37C1–4; 37F5). **(39) *Df(2L)VA12*, *cn¹ bw¹*/CyO** (37C2–5; 38B2–C) **(F)**. **(40) *Df(2L)VA19*, *noc^{Sco} rdo¹ pr¹*/CyO, Cy¹ dp^{lv1} pr¹ cn²** (37C2–7; 38A6–B1) **(B)**. **(41) *Df(2L)Sd77*/CyO** (37C2–7; 38C1–2) **(B)**. **(42)** *Df(2L)Sd37*/SM5 (37D2–5; 38A6–B2). **(43)** *Df(2L)TW9*, *Tft¹ cn¹*/CyO (37E2–F1; 38B5–C1). **(44) *Df(2L)TW161*, *cn¹ bw¹*/CyO** (38A6–B1; 40A4–B1) **(M)**. **(45) *Df(2L)DS6*, *b¹ pr¹ cn¹*/CyO** (38F5; 39E7–F1) **(B)**. **(46) *Df(2R)rl10a*, *lt¹ cn¹*/In(2LR)bw^{V1}** (41A) **(M)**. **(47)** *Df(2R)nap9*/In(2LR)Gla (42A1–2; 42E6–F1). **(48)** *Df(2R)cn87e*/In(2LR)bw^{V1}, *b¹* (42B4–C1; 43F–44A). **(49) *Df(2R)cn9*/SM6b, Cy¹ Roi¹** (42E; 44C) **(M)**. **(50)** *Df(2R)CA53*/CyO (43E6; 44B6). **(51) *Df(2R)44CE*, *al¹ dp^{ov1} b¹ pr¹*/CyO** (44C4–5; 44E2–4) **(M)**. **(52) *Df(2R)H3E1*/CyO, Cy¹ dp^{lv1} pr¹ cn²** (44D1–4; 44F12) **(M)**. **(53) *Df(2R)Np3*, *bw¹*/CyO, Cy¹ dp^{lv1} pr¹ cn²** (44D2; 45B8–C1) **(M)**. **(54) *Df(2R)Np1*, *bw¹*/CyO, Cy¹ dp^{lv1} pr¹ cn²** (44F2–3; 45C6) **(M)**. **(55)** *Df(2R)w45-30n*, *cn¹*/CyO (45A6–7; 45E2–3). **(56)** *Df(2R)wun-GL*/CyO (45C8; 45D8). **(57)** *Df(2R)B5*, *px¹ sp¹*/CyO, Adh^{nB} (46A1–4; 46C3–12). **(58)** *Df(2R)X3*/CyO, Adh^{nB} (46C1–2; 46E1–2). **(59)** *Df(2R)X1*/CyO, Adh^{nB} (46C2; 47A1). **(60) *Df(2R)stan1*, *P{ry^{+t7.2}}42D cn¹ sp¹*/CyO** (46D7–9; 47F15–17) **(M)**. **(61) *Df(2R)E3363*/CyO-CR2**, *P{sevRas1.V12}* (47A3; 47E) **(M)**. **(62) *Df(2R)en-A*/CyO** (47D3; 48B5) **(M)**. **(63)** *Df(2R)en-B*, *b¹ pr¹*/CyO (47E3; 48A4). **(64)** *Df(2R)en-SFX31*/CyO (48A1; 48B5). **(65)** *Df(2R)en30*/SM5, *al² Cy¹ cn² sp²* (48A3; 48C6–8). **(66)** *Df(2R)CB21*/CyO (48E; 49A). **(67)** *Df(2R)vg-C*/CyO, *P{sevRas1.V12}* (49A4; 49E7–F1). **(68)** *Df(2R)vg-B*/SM5 (49D3–4; 50A2). **(69) *Df(3L)ZN47*, *ry^{506}*/TM3** (64C; 65C) **(F)**. **(70) *Df(3L)pbl-X1*/TM6B** (65F3; 66B10) **(M)**. **(71) *Df(3L)66C-G28*/TM3** (66B8–9; 66C9–10) **(M)**. **(72)** *Df(3L)h-i22*, *Ki¹ roe¹ p^p*/TM3 (66D10–11; 66E1–2). **(73)** *Df(3L)29A6*, *ri¹ p^p*/TM3 (66F5; 67B1). **(74)** *Df(3L)AC1*, *roe¹ p^p*/TM3 (67A2; 67D11–13). **(75)** *Df(3L)lxd6*/TM3, *y^+ Sb¹ e¹ Ser¹* (67E1–2; 68C1–2). **(76)** *Df(3L)vin2*/TM3 (67F2–3; 68D6). **(77)** *Df(3L)vin5*, *ru¹ h¹ gl² e⁴ ca¹*/TM3, *Sb¹ Ser¹* (68A2–3; 69A1–3). **(78)** *Df(3L)vin7*, *e¹*/TM3 (68C8–11; 69B4–5). **(79)** *Df(3L)Ly*, *mvh¹*/TM1, *jv* (70A2–3; 70A5–6). **(80)** *Df(3L)fz-GF36*/TM6B (70C1–2; 70D4–5). **(81)** *Df(3L)fz-GS1a*, *P{w[+tAR] ry[+t7.2AR]* = *wA[R]}66E*/TM3 (70D2; 70E4–5). **(82) *Df(3L)fz-M21*/TM6** (70D2; 71E4–5) **(B)**. **(83)** *Df(3L)BK10*, *ru¹ red¹ cv-c¹ Sb^{sbd-1} sr¹ e¹*/TM3 (71C; 71F). **(84)** *Df(3L)brm11*/TM6C, *cu¹ Sb¹ e¹ ca¹* (71F1–4; 72D1–10). **(85)** *Df(3L)st-f13*, *Ki¹ roe¹ p^p*/TM6B (72C1–D1; 73A3–4). **(86)** *Df(3L)st7*, *e¹*/TM3, *Sb¹ Ser¹* (73A3–4; 74A3). **(87) *Df(3L)81k19*/TM6B** (73A3; 74F) **(F)**. **(88)** *Df(3L)Cat*, *ri e*/TM6, *Hn^p ss^{aP88} Ubx^{bx-34l} e¹* (75B8; 75F1). **(89)** *Df(3L)VW3*/TM3 (76A3; 76B2). Deficiencies that failed to complement *Ore* and *2b* QTLs are indicated in **bold font**. **(F)**, **(M)** and **(B)** denote failure to complement for females, males, or both sexes, respectively. Results of quantitative complementation mapping using Deficiencies 16–51 and 69–89 have been reported in Pasyukova *et al.* (2000) and De Luca *et al.* (2003).

sequence. At least three additional genes have been mapped to the region, but not the sequence. The 35D5-E1 QTL is a 188-kb region including 18 genes (14 predicted) that have been mapped to the sequence.

There are at least two QTLs affecting variation in life span between *Ore* and *2b* in the region between 36E4 (the left breakpoint of *Df(2L)TW50*) and 37D1–2 (the right breakpoint of *Df(2L)TW130*). Since *Df(2L)TW137* and *Df(2L)TW130* do not overlap, one QTL is between 36E4;37B9 (a 550-kb region containing 70 genes mapped to the sequence), and the other is between 37B9;37D1–2 (a 371-kb region containing 45 genes mapped to the sequence). However, four QTLs must be invoked to account for complementation of *Df(2L)pr-16* and *Df(2L)TW158* and sex-specific complementation effects. For three of these QTLs (36E4;37B2, 37B9;37C1–2, and 37C5;37D1–2) the hemizygous longevity of the *Ore* allele is greater than that of the *2b* allele, whereas the fourth QTL (37B9) is postulated to have the opposite effect (De Luca *et al.*, 2003).

Failure of *Df(2L)TW161* and *Df(2L)DS6* to complement the *Ore* and *2b* longevity QTLs defines a QTL at 38F5;39E7-F1, a 12.6-kb region containing only two predicted genes. *Df(2R)r110a* also fails to complement and defines a QTL at the heterochromatic 41A region. There are at least two QTLs affecting variation in longevity between *Ore* and *2b* in the region from 42E;45A because deficiencies *Df(2R)cn9* and *Df(2R)H3E1*, which both failed to complement, are non-overlapping. The most parsimonious interpretation is a male-specific QTL at 44C1–5, the presumed region of overlap of *Df(2R)cn9* and *Df(2R)44CE*, and a male-specific QTL at 44F2–12, the region of overlap of *Df(2R)H3E1*, *Df(2R)Np3*, and *Df(2R)Np1*. The 44C1–5 QTL is a 221-kb region with 26 genes mapped to the sequence, and the 44F2–12 QTL

encompasses a 123-kb region containing 29 genes mapped to the sequence.

Finally, male-specific failure to complement for *Df(2R)stan1*, *Df(2R)E3363*, and *Df92R)en-A*, and complementation for *Df(2R)en-B*, all of which overlap, defines a QTL from 47D3;E3. This 208-kb region contains 41 genes that have been mapped to the sequence.

C. Chromosome 3

The results of recombination mapping indicate at least two QTLs between 65D and 77A (see Table 7.1). We crossed *Ore* and *2b* to 21 deficiencies spanning the region from 65C to 76B2 (Pasyukova *et al.*, 2000; see Figure 7.2). We measured the longevity of 20 males and 20 females for each of the four genotypes per deficiency, with five individuals in each of four replicate vials per sex and genotype, for a total of 3,360 individuals scored. These data reveal from four to five QTLs affecting variation in longevity between *Ore* and *2b* in this region.

The first QTL is defined by failure of *Df(3L)ZN47* to complement *Ore* and *2b* QTLs. This deficiency uncovers 64C;65C, a large (2,024-kb) region containing 201 genes mapped to the sequence, and does not overlap with the other chromosome 3 deficiencies tested.

Df(3L)pbl-X1 and *Df(3L)66C-G28* both exhibit male-specific failure to complement the *Ore* and *2b* longevity QTLs, but the complementation effects are in opposite directions, and the difference between them is highly significant (Pasyukova *et al.*, 2000). There are two possible interpretations of this result. First, there may be two male-specific QTLs located in the non-overlapping regions of these deficiencies: one at 65F;66B8–9 and the other at 66B10;66C9–10. Alternatively, there may be one male-specific QTL at 66B8–10, and the opposite effects on longevity are caused by epistatic effects attributable to the uncontrolled genetic background of the deficiency chromosomes. To be conservative, we consider the region from 65F;66C10 to harbor one or two QTLs. This 1,167-kb interval contains 170 genes that have been mapped to the sequence.

Df(3L)fz-M21 fails to complement *Ore* and *2b* longevity QTLs in males and females, whereas *Df(3L)81k19* exhibits female-specific failure to complement. The overlapping flanking deficiencies define these QTLs as 70E4–5;71C and 74A3-F. The 70E4–5;71C is a 23-kb region in which only two genes have been mapped to the sequence, and the 74A3-F interval spans 436 kb, in which 51 genes have been mapped to the sequence.

IV. Complementation Tests to Mutations at Positional Candidate Genes

Deficiency complementation tests have revealed at least 14 QTLs affecting variation in life span between *Ore* and *2b*. On average, the QTLs have been localized to 413-kb regions containing 49 genes: a vast improvement over recombination mapping. This is a minimum number because deficiency mapping has not been applied yet to four QTL regions (1B;3E, 17C;19A, 76B;89B, and 96F;100A).

All genes in the QTL regions specified by deficiency mapping are positional candidate genes that could correspond to the QTL. It is sobering that the vast majority of these candidate genes are predicted only. Table 7.3 lists the confirmed candidate genes within the QTL regions uncovered by deficiencies, as well as their molecular function and biological process gene ontologies. Many are obvious attractive QTLs for life span. If mutations in these candidate genes are available (and for most, they are not), we can perform quantitative complementation tests of the mutations to *Ore* and *2b*, exactly as was done for quantitative complementation to deficiencies. To date, we have performed

quantitative complementation tests to 24 mutations at 11 positional candidate genes: *inactive* (*iav*), *shuttle craft* (*stc*), *reduced* (*rd*), *Fasciclin 3* (*Fas3*), *tailup* (*tup*), *Catecholamines up* (*Catsup*), *Diphenol oxidase A2* (*Dox-A2*), *Dopa decarboxylase* (*Ddc*), *a methyl dopa-resistant* (*amd*), *Lim3*, and *pale* (*ple*). Sample sizes ranged from 20 to 25 flies per sex per genotype, or 160 to 200 flies per mutant allele tested. Complementation was observed for *iav¹*, *rd¹*, *Fas3^E25^*, *amd¹*, *amd⁶*, *amd⁹*, and *ple⁴*. The remaining six loci are candidate genes affecting variation in life span between *Ore* and *2b*.

stc encodes an RNA polymerase II transcription factor that is the only known homologue of human transcription factor NF-X1 (Stroumbakis *et al.*, 1996). *stc* is expressed in the embryonic central nervous system, where it is required for motor neuron development, as well as in larvae, pupae, and adults, where expression is greatest in ovaries (Stroumbakis *et al.*, 1996). We performed complementation tests to four *stc* alleles (*stc³*, *stc⁶*, *stc^k11112^*, and *stc^05441^*). The *stc⁶* allele is associated with an inversion with one breakpoint within *stc* and is probably the most severe alteration of the gene. *stc^k11112^* is likely a gene disruption caused by *P*-element excision. *stc^05441^* is associated with a *P*-element insertion in the putative regulatory region 2 kb upstream of the gene. The nature of the lesion in *stc³* is unknown but is probably a point mutation because it was generated by EMS mutagenesis.

We evaluated the complementation effects of these mutations in three different genetic backgrounds: (1) the "random" genetic backgrounds in which the mutations were derived, crossed to *Ore* and *2b*; (2) second chromosomes bearing the *stc* alleles substituted into the highly inbred *Samarkand* (*Sam*) background, crossed to *Ore* and *2b*; and (3) second chromosome bearing the *stc* alleles substituted into the highly inbred *Sam*

Table 7.3
Positional Candidate Genes Affecting Variation in Longevity Between *Ore* and *2b*

QTL	Gene	Location[a]	Molecular Function	Biological Process
7A6-B2	unc-119	7B1(S)	receptor activity	chemosensory perception
	brinker	7B1(S)	RNA polymerase II transcription factor activity; transcriptional repressor activity	negative regulation of transcription from Pol II promoter; regulation of BMP signaling pathway; transforming growth factor beta receptor signaling pathway
	sarcoplasmic calcium-binding protein	7B2	calcium ion binding	
	agametic	7A5-C1(R)		pole cell, gonad development
	inactive	7A5-C1(R)	ion channel activity	perception of sound; response to heat; courtship; locomotion
35B9-C3	crinkled	35B8–9(S)	actin binding; motor activity; structural constituent of cytoskeleton; ATPase activity, coupled	intracellular protein transport; perception of sound; vesicle-mediated transport; visual perception
	RNA polymerase II elongation factor	35B9–10(S)	RNA polymerase II transcription factor activity; transcriptional elongation regulator activity	RNA elongation from Pol II promoter
	vasa	35B10-C1(S)	RNA helicase activity; nucleic acid binding; ATP-dependent helicase activity	dorsal appendage formation; oogenesis (sensu Insecta); pole plasm RNA localization; pole plasm assembly
	vasa intronic gene	35B10-C1(S)	RNA binding	RNA interference
	shuttle craft	35C2(S)	single-stranded DNA binding; RNA polymerase II transcription factor activity	regulation of transcription
35C3	reduced	35C3(R)		
35D5-E1	Tektin-A	35D5(S)	microtubule binding; structural constituent of cytoskeleton	microtubule-based process
	Thiolester containing protein I	35D6(S)		antibacterial humoral response (sensu Invertebrata)
	beaten path Ib	35D6–7(S)		axon choice point recognition; cell adhesion; defasciculation of motor neuron
	beaten path Ic	35E1(S)		axon choice point recognition; cell adhesion; defasciculation of motor neuron

(continues)

Table 7.3 (*Cont'd*)

QTL	Gene	Location[a]	Molecular Function	Biological Process
36E4;37B9	*Fasciclin 3*	36F2–4(S)		axon guidance; synaptic target recognition
	Phosphodiesterase 11	36F6(S)	cGMP-specific phosphodiesterase activity; cAMP-specific phosphodiesterase activity	cyclic nucleotide metabolism; signal transduction
	absent MD neurons and olfactory sensilla	36F6(S)	transcription factor activity	sensory organ determination
	Misexpression suppressor of ras 3	36F7–9(S)		
	Cyp310a1	36F8(S)	electron transporter activity; oxidoreductase activity	steroid metabolism
	tosca	36F11(S)	exodeoxyribonuclease I activity; nuclease activity; nucleic acid binding	DNA repair
	male-specific lethal 1	36F11–37A1(S)	chromatin binding; DNA binding; protein binding	dosage compensation
	Inwardly rectifying potassium channel 3	37A1(S)	inward rectifier potassium channel activity	cation transport
	Sterol carrier protein X-related thiolase	37B1(S)	phospholipid transporter activity; sterol carrier protein X-related thiolase activity; carrier activity	phospholipid transport
	mitochondrial ribosomal protein L13	37B1(S)	structural constituent of ribosome; nucleic acid binding	protein biosynthesis
	tailup	37B1(S)	specific RNA polymerase II transcription factor activity	ectoderm development; regulation of transcription from Pol II promoter; terminal region determination; torso signaling pathway
	Nedd8	37B7(S)	protein binding	regulation of proteolysis and peptidolysis
	Numb-associated kinase	37B7(S)	protein serine/threonine kinase activity; receptor signaling protein serine/threonine kinase activity	asymmetric cytokinesis
	Ribosomal protein L30	37B9(S)	structural constituent of ribosome; nucleic acid binding	peripheral nervous system development; protein biosynthesis
	robl37BC	37B9(S)	ATPase activity, coupled	microtubule-based movement
	similar to Deadpan	37B9–10(S)	transcription factor activity	cell proliferation; ectoderm development; neurogenesis; regulation of transcription; regulation of transcription from Pol II promoter

(*continues*)

Table 7.3   *(Cont'd)*

QTL	Gene	Location[a]	Molecular Function	Biological Process
	hamlet	37A2–3(R)	transcription factor activity	regulation of transcription from Pol II promoter; sensory organ development
37B9-D2	*hook*	37B10(S)	structural constituent of cytoskeleton; microtubule binding	endocytosis; intracellular protein transport
	Catecholamines up	37B11(S)		nurse cell/oocyte transport (sensu Insecta); regulation of catecholamine metabolism
	lethal (2) 37Bb	37B12(S)	oxidoreductase activity	metabolism
	Diphenol oxidase A2	37B12(S)	endopeptidase activity; enzyme activator activity	proteolysis and peptidolysis
	Lim3	37B13-C1(S)	specific RNA polymerase II transcription factor activity	ectoderm development; regulation of transcription from Pol II promoter; regulation of transcription, DNA-dependent
	a methyl dopa-resistant	37C1(S)	carboxy-lyase activity; aromatic-L-amino-acid decarboxylase activity	amino acid metabolism
	Dopa decarboxylase	37C1(S)	aromatic-L-amino-acid decarboxylase activity	dopamine biosynthesis from tyrosine; serotonin biosynthesis from tryptophan
	lethal (2) 37Cc	37C1(S)		DNA replication; regulation of cell cycle
	brain tumor	37C1–6(S)	translation regulator activity; transcription regulator activity	cell proliferation; regulation of transcription from Pol II promoter; transport
	?-Tubulin at 37C	37C7(S)	structural constituent of cytoskeleton; tubulin binding	cell motility; chromosome segregation; intracellular protein transport; mitosis
	derailed	37C7(S)	transmembrane receptor protein tyrosine kinase activity; protein-tyrosine kinase activity	Wnt receptor signaling pathway; cell-cell signaling; ectoderm development; protein amino acid phosphorylation; transmembrane receptor protein tyrosine kinase signaling pathway
	doughnut on 2	37D2(S)	transmembrane receptor protein tyrosine kinase activity; protein-tyrosine kinase activity	cell-cell signaling; ectoderm development; protein amino acid phosphorylation; transmembrane receptor protein tyrosine kinase signaling pathway
44C1–5	*deadpan*	44C2(S)	RNA polymerase II transcription factor activity; specific RNA polymerase II transcription factor activity	cell proliferation; regulation of transcription from Pol II promoter; sex determination, establishment of X:A ratio

(continues)

Table 7.3   *(Cont'd)*

QTL	Gene	Location[a]	Molecular Function	Biological Process
	peanut	44C2(S)	actin binding; microtubule binding; structural constituent of cytoskeleton; small monomeric GTPase activity; hydrolase activity	cytokinesis; mitosis
44F2–12	*Ryanodine receptor 44F*	44F1–2(S)	ryanodine-sensitive calcium-release channel activity; receptor activity	calcium ion transport; muscle contraction
	Dynamitin	44F3(S)	structural constituent of cytoskeleton	microtubule-based movement; mitosis
	sec31	44F3(S)		exocytosis; intracellular protein transport
	G protein ? 1	44F3–5(S)	heterotrimeric G-protein GTPase activity	G-protein coupled receptor protein signaling pathway
	Phosphoglucose isomerase	44F6(S)	phosphogluconate dehydrogenase (decarboxylating) activity; glucose-6-phosphate isomerase activity	gluconeogenesis; glycolysis
	lines	44F6–7(S)		terminal region determination; torso signaling pathway
	baboon	44F11–12(S)	G-protein coupled receptor kinase activity; protein serine/threonine kinase activity; protein kinase activity; type I transforming growth factor beta receptor activity; hematopoietin/ interferon-class (D200-domain) cytokine receptor activity; activin binding; type I activin receptor activity	cytokine and chemokine mediated signaling pathway; eye-antennal disc metamorphosis; mesoderm development; skeletal development
47D3-E3	*luna*	47D1–3(S)	transcription factor activity	regulation of transcription
	schnurri	47D6-E1(S)	RNA polymerase II transcription factor activity	wing morphogenesis
	Syntaxin 6	47E1(S)	t-SNARE activity	intracellular protein transport; synaptic vesicle docking
	skiff	47E1(S)	guanylate kinase activity	asymmetric protein localization; protein targeting; signal transduction
	Odorant receptor 47a	47E1–2(S)	olfactory receptor activity	perception of smell
	Troponin C at 47D	47E3(S)	calcium ion binding; calmodulin binding	calcium-mediated signaling; muscle contraction

(continues)

Table 7.3   *(Cont'd)*

QTL	Gene	Location[a]	Molecular Function	Biological Process
	von Hippel-Lindau	47E3(S)		cytoskeleton organization and biogenesis; tracheal system development (sensu Insecta)
	Monoamine oxidase	47D-E(R)	amine oxidase (flavin-containing) activity	
64C;65C	*Dynein heavy chain 64C*	64C1(S)	microtubule motor activity; motor activity; structural constituent of cytoskeleton; ATPase activity, coupled	cell motility; intracellular protein transport; microtubule-based movement; vesicle-mediated transport
	Connectin	64C2–4(S)	structural molecule activity	signal transduction
	mitochondrial alanyl-tRNA synthetase	64C7(S)	alanine-tRNA ligase activity; RNA binding	alanyl-tRNA aminoacylation
	Signal recognition particle protein 54k	64C7(S)	signal sequence binding; 7S RNA binding; RNA binding	SRP-dependent cotranslational membrane targeting; protein targeting
	Kinesin-like protein at 64D	64C13(S)	structural constituent of cytoskeleton; microtubule motor activity	microtubule-based movement; protein t argeting
	Leucokinin receptor	64D2(S)	neuropeptide receptor activity; leucokinin receptor activity; neuropeptide Y receptor activity; tachykinin receptor activity	tachykinin signaling pathway; transmission of nerve impulse
	sinuous	64D3(S)		septate junction assembly; tracheal system development (sensu Insecta)
	Sucb	64D3(S)	succinate-CoA ligase (GDP-forming) activity	tricarboxylic acid cycle
	severas	64D3(S)	prenyl protein specific endopeptidase activity	proteolysis and peptidolysis
	methuselah-like 2	64D6(S)	G-protein coupled receptor activity	G-protein coupled receptor protein signaling pathway; determination of adult life span; response to stress
	Separase	64E1(S)		mitotic sister chromatid separation
	still life	64E1–5(S)	Rho guanyl-nucleotide exchange factor activity; guanyl-nucleotide exchange factor activity	ectoderm development; intracellular signaling cascade; neurogenesis
	DnaJ-like-1	64E5(S)	chaperone activity; heat shock protein activity	defense response; protein folding; response to stress
	Ubiquitin-specific protease 64E	64E5–6(S)	ubiquitin-specific protease activity; ubiquitin thiolesterase activity	protein deubiquitination; proteolysis and peptidolysis
	Thioredoxin-like	64E6–7(S)	thiol-disulfide exchange intermediate activity	protein folding; sulfur metabolism

(continues)

Table 7.3 *(Cont'd)*

QTL	Gene	Location[a]	Molecular Function	Biological Process
	Myt1	64E7(S)	protein threonine/ tyrosine kinase activity	mitosis; protein amino acid phosphorylation; regulation of cell cycle
	Cellular retinaldehyde binding protein	64E8(S)	retinal binding; carrier activity	coenzyme and prosthetic group metabolism; vitamin/cofactor transport
	RPS6-p70-protein kinase	64E8–11(S)	ribosomal protein S6 kinase activity; receptor signaling protein serine/ threonine kinase activity	MAPKKK cascade; cell cycle
	vein	64E12-F2(S)	epidermal growth factor receptor binding	brain development; cell projection biogenesis; epidermal growth factor receptor signaling pathway; notum morphogenesis; wing morphogenesis
	Bj1 protein	65A1(S)	chromatin binding; Ran guanyl-nucleotide exchange factor activity	chromosome condensation; mRNA processing; nucleobase, nucleoside, nucleotide and nucleic acid transport
	yippee interacting protein 7	65A3(S)	chymotrypsin activity; serine-type endopeptidase activity	proteolysis and peptidolysis
	tantalus	65A4(S)		pigmentation; sensory organ development
	Laminin A	65A8–9(S)	structural molecule activity	cell-cell adhesion; cell-matrix adhesion; signal transduction
	Multiple drug resistance 65	65A10(S)	multidrug transporter activity; xenobiotic-transporting ATPase activity	defense response; extracellular transport; response to toxin
	Ecdysone-inducible gene L3	65A11(S)	L-lactate dehydrogenase activity	glycolysis
	smell impaired 65A	65A(R)		olfactory behavior; response to chemical substance
	sulfateless	65B3–4(S)	heparin N-deacetylase/ N-sulfotransferase activity	defense response
	nudel	65B5(S)	serine-type peptidase activity; peptidase activity; serine-type endopeptidase activity; trypsin activity	defense response; protein processing
	zero population growth	65B5(S)	innexin channel activity	germ-cell development; signal transduction
	Glutamate receptor I	65C1(S)	alpha-amino-3-hydroxy-5-methyl-4-isoxazole propionate selective glutamate receptor activity; glutamate-gated ion channel activity	cation transport; nerve-nerve synaptic transmission

(continues)

Table 7.3   (*Cont'd*)

QTL	Gene	Location[a]	Molecular Function	Biological Process
	Gustatory receptor 65a	65C1(S)	taste receptor activity	perception of taste
	pale	65C3(S)	tyrosine 3-monooxygenase activity	amino acid catabolism; catecholamine metabolism; signal transduction
	ventral veins lacking	65C5(S)	DNA binding; protein binding; RNA polymerase II transcription factor activity	ectoderm development; regulation of transcription from Pol II promoter
65F; 66C10	*RpL18*	65F1(S)	structural constituent of ribosome; nucleic acid binding	protein biosynthesis
	Neosin	65F1(S)	RNA binding	
	mitochondrial ribosomal protein L50	65F1–2(S)	structural constituent of ribosome	
	meiotic P22	65F2(S)		meiotic recombination
	Cdc27	65F2(S)		mitosis
	Trap36	65F2(S)	RNA polymerase II transcription mediator activity	transcription initiation from Pol II promoter
	unc-13–4A	65F2(S)		neurotransmitter secretion; synaptic vesicle priming
	RhoGEF4	65F4(S)	Rho guanyl-nucleotide exchange factor activity; signal transducer activity	
	lark	65F5(S)	RNA binding	circadian rhythm; nucleobase, nucleoside, nucleotide and nucleic acid metabolism
	Signal recognition particle protein 19	65F5(S)	7S RNA binding; RNA binding	SRP-dependent cotranslational membrane targeting; protein biosynthesis; protein complex assembly; protein targeting
	quemao	65F5–6(S)	farnesyltranstransferase activity; geranyltranstransferase activity; dimethylallyltranstransferase activity; acyltransferase activity	
	CTCF	65F6(S)	transcription factor activity	cell proliferation; regulation of transcription from Pol II promoter
	smallminded	65F9–10(S)	ATPase activity	exocytosis; intracellular protein transport; mitosis
	Rac2	66A1(S)	Rho small monomeric GTPase activity; small monomeric GTPase activity	G-protein coupled receptor protein signaling pathway; tracheal outgrowth (sensu Insecta); tracheal system development (sensu Insecta)

(*continues*)

Table 7.3   (*Cont'd*)

QTL	Gene	Location[a]	Molecular Function	Biological Process
	methuselah-like 6	66A2(S)	G-protein coupled receptor activity	G-protein coupled receptor protein signaling pathway; determination of adult life span; response to stress
	Cyp316a1	66A2(S)	electron transporter activity; oxidoreductase activity	steroid metabolism
	Cytochrome P450–4d8	66A2(S)	electron transporter activity; oxidoreductase activity	steroid metabolism
	liquid facets	66A4–5(S)		intracellular protein transport; intracellular signaling cascade; receptor mediated endocytosis; visual perception
	PGRP-SD	66A8(S)	peptidoglycan recognition activity	defense response; immune response
	Ank2	66A10(S)	cytoskeletal protein binding; structural constituent of cytoskeleton; receptor binding; actin binding	ectoderm development; neurogenesis
	Henna	66A12(S)	phenylalanine 4-monooxygenase activity; tryptophan 5-monooxygenase activity	eye pigment biosynthesis; signal transduction; phenylalanine catabolism
	Clock	66A12(S)	DNA binding; RNA polymerase II transcription factor activity	positive regulation of transcription, DNA-dependent
	PAR-domain protein 1	66A14–17(S)	DNA binding; transcription factor activity; protein homodimerization activity	circadian rhythm; mesoderm development; regulation of transcription from Pol II promoter
	pebble	66A18–19(S)	guanyl-nucleotide exchange factor activity; Rho guanyl-nucleotide exchange factor activity	cytokinesis
	sunday driver	66A20(S)	kinesin binding; kinase regulator activity	intracellular signaling cascade
	extra-extra	66A21(S)	transcription factor activity	regulation of transcription; central nervous system development
	Ribonuclease X25	66A21(S)	endoribonuclease activity; nucleic acid binding	RNA catabolism
	nemo	66A22-B3(S)	protein serine/threonine kinase activity; receptor signaling protein serine/threonine kinase activity	MAPKKK cascade; anti-apoptosis; cell proliferation; ommatidial rotation
	farinelli	66B6(S)		intracellular protein transport; synaptic transmission; vesicle-mediated transport

(*continues*)

Table 7.3 *(Cont'd)*

QTL	Gene	Location[a]	Molecular Function	Biological Process
	Actin-related protein 66B	66B6(S)	structural constituent of cytoskeleton; actin binding	cell cycle dependent actin filament reorganization; cytoskeleton organization and biogenesis; pseudocleavage (sensu Insecta)
	moleskin	66B6(S)	RAN protein binding; protein carrier activity; small GTPase regulatory/interacting protein activity	epidermal growth factor receptor signaling pathway; protein-nucleus import; transmembrane receptor protein tyrosine kinase signaling pathway
	Smt3 activating enzyme 2	66B7(S)	ubiquitin activating enzyme activity; SUMO activating enzyme activity; ubiquitin-like activating enzyme activity; ligase activity	SMT3-dependent protein catabolism; ubiquitin cycle
	CDP diglyceride synthetase	66B7(S)	phosphatidate cytidylyltransferase activity	phospholipid metabolism; phototransduction
	RecQ4	66B10(S)	helicase activity; DNA helicase activity; nucleic acid binding; ATP dependent DNA helicase activity	DNA recombination; DNA replication
	N-myristoyl transferase	66B10(S)	glycylpeptide N-tetradecanoyl-transferase activity	N-terminal protein myristoylation; dorsal closure
	methuselah-like 7	66B10–11(S)	G-protein coupled receptor activity	G-protein coupled receptor protein signaling pathway; determination of adult life span; response to stress
	estrogen-related receptor	66B11(S)	ligand-dependent nuclear receptor activity; transcription regulator activity	female gamete generation; hormone secretion; signal transduction; transcription from Pol II promoter; transmission of nerve impulse
	Trap100	66B11–12(S)	RNA polymerase II transcription mediator activity	transcription from Pol II promoter; transcription initiation from Pol II promoter
	Rab-related protein 3	66C5(S)	GTP binding; hydrolase activity, acting on acid anhydrides, in phosphorus-containing anhydrides; Rab GTPase activator activity; small monomeric GTPase activity	endocytosis; intracellular protein transport; regulation of exocytosis
	Gustatory receptor 66a	66C5(S)	taste receptor activity	perception of taste

(continues)

Table 7.3   *(Cont'd)*

QTL	Gene	Location[a]	Molecular Function	Biological Process
	DNA polymerase a 50kD	66C7–8(S)	DNA primase activity; nucleic acid binding; alpha DNA polymerase activity	DNA replication; DNA replication, priming
	Isocitrate dehydrogenase	66C8(S)	isocitrate dehydrogenase (NADP+) activity	glyoxylate cycle; tricarboxylic acid cycle
	Ecdysone-inducible gene E1	66C8(S)	lipoprotein binding	imaginal disc eversion
	mutagen-sensitive 301	65F3–66B10(R)		oocyte cell fate determination (sensu Insecta); oogenesis (sensu Insecta)
70E4;71C	*shade*	70E4(S)	electron transporter activity; oxidoreductase activity	steroid metabolism
74A3-F	*Odorant receptor 74a*	74A4(S)	olfactory receptor activity	perception of smell
	Myoinhibiting peptide precursor	74A5(S)	hormone activity; neuropeptide hormone activity; ecdysiostatic hormone activity; myoinhibitory hormone activity	neuropeptide signaling pathway
	target of Poxn	74A5(S)	specific RNA polymerase II transcription factor activity	cell proliferation; ectoderm development
	Cad74A	74A5–6(S)		calcium-dependent cell-cell adhesion; signal transduction
	bloated tubules	74B1–2(S)	neurotransmitter transporter activity	morphogenesis of an epithelium; transport
	fringe connection	74B4(S)	pyrimidine nucleotide sugar transporter activity; UDP-galactose transporter activity; NOT GDP-fucose transporter activity; NOT GDP-mannose transporter activity; NOT UDP-galactose transporter activity; NOT UDP-glucose transporter activity; UDP-N-acetylglucosamine transporter activity; UDP-glucose transporter activity; UDP-glucuronic acid transporter activity; UDP-xylose transporter activity	carbohydrate metabolism
	Nedd4	74D2–3(S)	ubiquitin-protein ligase activity	axon guidance; proteolysis and peptidolysis

(continues)

Table 7.3 *(Cont'd)*

QTL	Gene	Location[a]	Molecular Function	Biological Process
	Cyclin T	74D4(S)	transcriptional elongation regulator activity; [RNA-polymerase]-subunit kinase activity; positive transcription elongation factor activity; kinase activator activity; cyclin-dependent protein kinase regulator activity	RNA elongation from Pol II promoter; regulation of transcription from Pol II promoter; response to heat; transcription
	Ecdysone-induced protein 74EF	74E2–4(S)	transcription factor activity; specific RNA polymerase II transcription factor activity	mesoderm development; regulation of transcription from Pol II promoter; regulation of transcription, DNA-dependent
	Keren	74F1(S)	growth factor activity; epidermal growth factor receptor binding	MAPKKK cascade; positive regulation of epidermal growth factor receptor activity

[a](S) refers to genes that have been mapped to the sequence; (R) refers to genes that have been mapped to the region, but not to the sequence.

background, crossed to *Ore* and *2b* second chromosomes that had also been substituted into the *Sam* background (Pasyukova *et al.*, 2004). There was sex- and genetic-background-specific failure of *stc* alleles to complement *Ore* and *2b* longevity QTLs: *stc*[6] had a female-specific effect in the "random" and homozygous *Sam* backgrounds; *stc*[k11112] had a female-specific effect in the random and heterozygous *Sam* backgrounds; and *stc*[3] and *stc*[05441] had male-specific effects in the sensitized homozygous *Sam* background only (Pasyukova *et al.*, 2004, see Figure 7.3).

tup (also known as *l(2)37Aa* and *islet*, *isl*) encodes a specific RNA polymerase II transcription factor and is a member of the LIM homeodomain family of transcriptional regulators implicated in the transcriptional control of motor neuronal differentiation in vertebrates and invertebrates. In embryos, *tup* is expressed in the heart and aorta, the pharynx and the amnioserosa, the brain, and in a subset of developing motor neurons and interneurons in the ventral nerve cord, including the dopaminergic and serotonergic cells of the ventral nerve cord (Thor & Thomas, 1997). *tup*-expressing interneurons and motor neurons exhibit pathfinding defects in *tup* mutants. Further, *tup* mutants have no detectable tyrosine hydroxylase (TH) expression and little or no expression of serotonin or dopa decarboxylase in the ventral nerve cord (Thor & Thomas, 1997). Thus, *tup* is required for both axonal pathfinding and neurotransmitter production. We performed complementation tests to *tup*[1] and *tup*[isl-1] mutations. *tup*[1] mutant phenotypes are manifest in the amnioserosa, cephalopharyngeal skeleton, contracted and extended germ band stages, embryonic head, latticed process, and vertical bridge. The *tup*[isl-1] mutant has largely neural effects, including the dendrite, dopamine, serotonin, and motor neurons; Class I and II interneurons; and Class III local interneurons. The *tup*[1] mutation complemented the longevity effects of *Ore* and *2b* QTLs, but the *tup*[isl-1] exhibited a male-specific failure to complement (see Figure 7.3).

Ddc, *Catsup* (*l(2)37Bc*), *Dox-A2*, and *Lim3* (*l(2)37Bd*) are members of the *Ddc* gene cluster, which contains at least 21 genes tightly packed in a 162.5-kb region (Stathakis *et al.*, 1995). Mutations in many of the genes in this cluster show defects in cuticle formation, sclerotinization (hardening) or melanization of the cuticle, and formation of melanotic pseudotumors, all of which are hallmarks of abnormal catecholamine metabolism (Wright, 1996). In *Drosophila* as well as vertebrates, the first and rate-limiting step in catecholamine biosynthesis is the hydroxylation of L-tyrosine into 3–4-dihydroxy-L-phenylalanine (DOPA), a reaction catalyzed by TH (Kumar & Vrana, 1996). In *Drosophila*, TH is encoded by the *ple* locus (Neckameyer & White, 1993). *Ddc* encodes Dopa decarboxylase, which catalyzes the decarboxylation of DOPA to dopamine (DA) and 5-hydroxytryptophan to serotonin (Blenau & Baumann, 2001). Ddc is required for the production of dopamine and serotonin in the central nervous system and in the hypoderm, where it is necessary for sclerotinization and melanization of the cuticle (Stathakis *et al.*, 1999). We performed quantitative complementation tests for three *Ddc* alleles, *Ddc*[27], *Ddc*[43], and *Ddc*[lol]. *Ddc*[27] and *Ddc*[43] are homozygous lethal, and *CyO/Ddc* heterozygotes have specific Ddc activities of 44 percent and 57.8 percent, respectively, relative to *CyO/+* controls. *Ddc*[lol] is a viable hypomorphic allele; *CyO/Ddc*[lol] heterozygotes have 77 percent wildtype-specific Ddc activity. Again, we observed sex- and allele-specific failure to complement. *Ddc*[27] and *Ddc*[lol] did not complement the longevity phenotype of *Ore* and *2b* QTLs in males, and *Ddc*[43] did not complement the longevity phenotype of *Ore* and *2b* QTLs in females (De Luca *et al.*, 2003; see Figure 7.3).

Catsup is a negative regulator of TH (Stathakis *et al.*, 1999). Catsup encodes a transmembrane protein and is a putative zinc transporter. It has extended histidine repeats in two predicted extracellular domains with the potential for binding heavy metal ions, including nickel and zinc, and three membrane-spanning domains with predicted zinc transport function based on similarity to known zinc transporters in yeast and mammals (J. O'Donnell *et al.*, 2002). We performed complementation tests to *Catsup*[1], *Catsup*[cs1], and *Catsup*[cs2]. *Catsup*[1] is a homozygous larval lethal. *Catsup*[cs1] and *Catsup*[cs2] are lethal at 18° C and have greatly reduced viability at 22° C; escaper females are sterile, and heterozygous adults have melanotic pseudotumors (Stathakis *et al.*, 1999). All three mutations exhibited male-specific failure to complement the *Ore* and *2b* longevity QTLs.

Dox-A2 encodes the structural gene for the A2 component of the phenol oxidase enzyme complex, which is involved in the sclerotinization of the cuticle and egg shell, in wound healing and melanization, defense against pathogens, and catecholamine metabolism (Pentz *et al.*, 1986; Pentz & Wright, 1986; 1991). This enzyme complex converts catecholamines to their respective quinones, which are then further metabolized to either form melanin (from DOPA and DA) or crosslink proteins in sclerotonin (from N-acetyldopamine and N-β-alanyldopamine) (Pentz & Wright, 1991; Stathakis *et al.*, 1999). We used three *Dox-A2* alleles, *Dox-A2*[1], *Dox-A2*[2], and *Dox-A2*[mfs1]. *Dox-A2*[1] and *Dox-A2*[2] are homozygous larval lethal, and heterozygotes have phenol oxidase activity of 48 percent and 64 percent of wild type, respectively (Pentz *et al.*, 1986). *Dox-A2*[mfs1] is viable but sterile, with normal diphenol oxidase activity. All three mutations exhibited male-specific failure

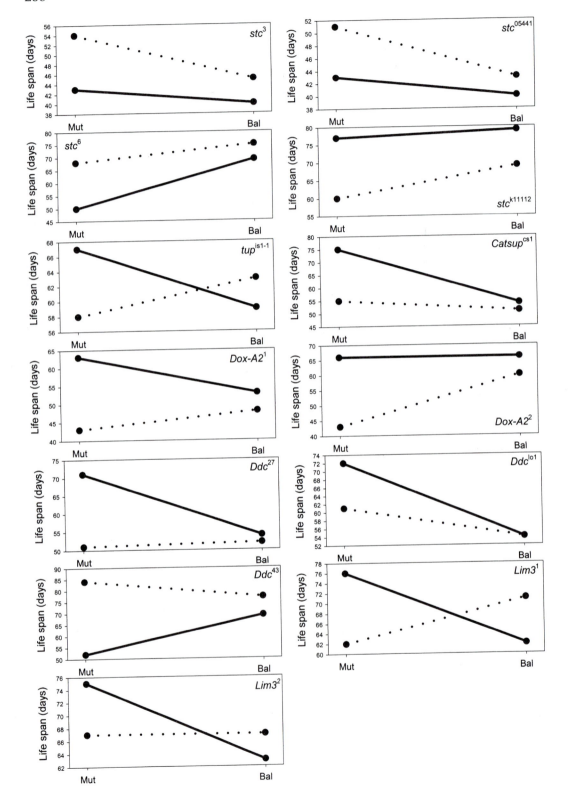

to complement the *Ore* and *2b* longevity QTLs (see Figure 7.3).

Lim3 (*l(2)37Bd*) encodes another specific RNA polymerase II transcription factor and member of the LIM homeodomain protein family and is required for motor neuron development (Thor *et al.*, 1999). Embryonic expression of *Lim3* is similar to that of *tup*, as it is expressed in a subset of interneurons and motor neurons. Although *Lim3* and *tup* are not coexpressed in the same interneurons, they are coexpressed in a subset of motor neurons and could act together to specify distinct motor neuron identities (Thor *et al.*, 1999). We performed complementation tests to *Lim3*[1] and *Lim3*[2] mutations. All *Lim3*-expressing interneurons and motor neurons show pathfinding defects in *Lim3*[1] mutants (Thor *et al.*, 1999). *Lim3*[2] mutations are larval lethal, with occasional survival to pharate adults with incomplete sclerotization (Stathakis *et al.*, 1995). Both mutations exhibited male-specific failure to complement the longevity effects of *Ore* and *2b* QTLs (see Figure 7.3).

V. Linkage Disequilibrium (LD) Mapping

Observing genetic failure of a mutation at a positional candidate gene to complement QTL alleles nominates the gene for further study but does not constitute formal proof that the gene corresponds to the QTL (see below). We have used linkage disequilibrium (LD) mapping to corroborate that

candidate genes correspond to QTLs (Mackay, 2001) and to begin to define the molecular signature of QTL alleles.

LD refers to the correlation of allele frequencies at two (or more) polymorphic loci (Falconer & Mackay, 1996; Hartl & Clark, 1997). When a new mutation occurs at a QTL allele, it is initially in complete LD with all other polymorphic loci in the genome. Recombination quickly dissipates LD between the new mutation and unlinked loci, but equilibrium is restored more slowly between closely linked loci. The length of the genomic fragment containing loci in LD with the original mutation depends on the average amount of recombination per generation experienced by that region of the genome, the number of generations that have passed since the mutation occurred, and the effective population size (Falconer & Mackay, 1996; Hartl & Clark, 1997; Hill & Robertson, 1968; Weir, 1996). For old mutations in large populations, strong LD is expected to extend over distances of the order of a few kb or less, whereas larger tracts of LD are expected in populations derived from a recent founder event or in population isolates with small effective population size. Nevertheless, the additional historical recombination considerably increases the power to map QTLs to genes or regions of the genome containing a few candidate genes (Risch & Merikangas, 1996), and there is great excitement about using the millions of single nucleotide polymorphisms (SNPs)

Figure 7.3 Sex- and allele-specific failure of mutations at candidate genes to complement *Ore* (solid lines) and *2b* (dashed lines) longevity QTLs. In all cases, either the L or $L \times G$ term from two-way ANOVA was significant (see text for explanation), the contrast [*mut/Ore -mut/2b*] was significant, and the contrast [*Bal/Ore-Bal/2b*] was not significant. *stc*[3]: male-specific failure to complement, homozygous *Sam* background. *stc*[05441]: male-specific failure to complement, homozygous *Sam* background. *stc*[6]: female-specific failure to complement, random background. *stc*[k11112]: female-specific failure to complement, random background. *tup*[isl-1]: male-specific failure to complement. *Catsup*[cs1]: male-specific failure to complement. *Dox-A2*[1]: male-specific failure to complement. *Dox-A2*[2]: male-specific failure to complement. *Ddc*[27]: male-specific failure to complement. *Ddc*[lo1]: male-specific failure to complement. *Ddc*[43]: female-specific failure to complement. *Lim3*[1]: male-specific failure to complement. *Lim3*[2]: male-specific failure to complement.

that are the fruit of the human genome project (The International SNP Map Working Group, 2001) in LD mapping paradigms to identify candidate genes affecting complex traits in humans.

LD decays rapidly with physical distance in *Drosophila* regions of normal recombination (Long *et al.*, 1998; Miyashita & Langley, 1990), which is a favorable scenario for identifying the actual polymorphisms (quantitative trait nucleotides, or QTNs) causing the differences in trait phenotype between QTL alleles. The requirements for LD mapping are simple and analogous to QTL mapping. One needs a sample of alleles from a single random mating population (population admixture generates spurious LD) (Falconer & Mackay, 1996; Hartl & Clark, 1997); genotypes of each allele for polymorphic markers in the candidate gene (or candidate gene region) of interest; and a measure of the trait phenotype for each allele. One then groups the population sample by marker (or haplotype) genotype and conducts a statistical test to assess whether there is a difference in trait mean between marker genotype classes. If so, the QTN is in LD with the marker.

LD mapping requires large samples—at least 500 individuals are necessary to detect a QTN contributing 5 percent of the total phenotypic variance with 80 percent power (Long & Langley, 1999; Luo *et al.*, 2000). The ability to construct *Drosophila* chromosome substitution lines, in which single chromosomes sampled from nature are made isogenic (homozygous) and substituted into a highly inbred background, greatly increases the power of LD mapping. First, genetic variance attributable to chromosomally unlinked loci is eliminated. Second, the ability to measure multiple individuals per substitution line increases the accuracy in estimating the genotypic value of each line, which is particularly useful for low heritability traits such as longevity. And third, all markers are homozygous, circumventing the problem of inferring haplotypes in the presence of heterozygotes in outbred populations.

We nominated *Ddc* as a positional candidate gene affecting variation in longevity between *Ore* and *2b* based on deficiency mapping and quantitative failure of *Ddc* mutants to complement the life span phenotype of *Ore* and *2b* alleles (De Luca *et al.*, 2003). *Ddc* is an attractive candidate gene because dopamine and serotonin affect insect mating behavior, fertility, circadian rhythms, endocrine secretion, aggression, and learning and memory (Blenau & Baumann, 2001). We constructed 173 second chromosome substitution lines from a single contemporaneous sample from the Raleigh population and measured the longevity of each. There was significant genetic variation in longevity among these lines, with a heritability of 0.14. We sequenced 14 *Ddc* alleles and identified 36 common polymorphisms, for which the entire sample was genotyped.

After Bonferroni correction for multiple tests, three SNPs were highly significantly associated with variation in life span, consistent with the inference that *Ddc* indeed corresponds to a life span QTL. T420C is in the promoter and could be associated with regulatory elements required for the expression of Ddc in the central nervous system. C1685A is an amino acid polymorphism in the exon that is translated only in the nervous system. T2738G is intronic but is the only SNP associated with longevity among the Raleigh alleles that is also polymorphic between *Ore* and *2b*. These SNPs were in strong global LD, forming six common haplotypes that accounted for 15.5 percent of the genetic and 2.2 percent of the phenotypic variance in longevity attributable to chromosome 2. Further, the SNPs showed evidence of epistatic gene action. For example, there was a significant difference in longevity between haplotypes

TAT and TCT (the letters denote the allele for each of the three significant SNPs, in order), but not between haplotypes TAG and TCG. Similarly, haplotypes TAT and TAG had different mean longevities, but haplotypes TCT and TCG did not. That is, whether a particular SNP is associated with variation in life span depends on the genotype of the other contributing SNPs (De Luca *et al.*, 2003).

VI. Conclusions and Future Prospects

How many loci affect variation in life span? We have used recombination mapping followed by deficiency complementation mapping to show that there are at least 14 QTLs affecting variation in life span between the two laboratory strains, *Ore* and *2b*. Single QTLs identified by recombination mapping are confirmed by more precise deficiency mapping but tend to fractionate into multiple linked QTLs. Complementation tests to mutations show that multiple closely linked genes within a single QTL can be associated with variation in life span. For example, four genes in the 37B9-D2 QTL failed to complement the life span phenotype of *Ore* and *2b* alleles. Clearly, a large number of loci potentially contribute to naturally occurring variation in longevity because *Ore* and *2b* represent only a small sample of possible genes contributing to natural variation in life span. In addition, our fine-mapping analysis was only conducted under control culture conditions, and longevity QTLs display remarkable genotype by environment interactions (Leips & Mackay, 2000; Vieira *et al.*, 2000), such that different QTLs are expressed in different environments. Future experiments must address the issue of genetic sampling, either by screening inbred lines recently derived from nature for particularly long-lived lines, or by using lines selected for increased life span in mapping

experiments (e.g., Forbes *et al.*, 2004). Further, fine-mapping efforts must be extended to QTLs expressed in multiple environments.

We have repeatedly observed sex-specific effects of longevity QTLs, whether detected by recombination mapping, deficiency complementation mapping, or complementation to mutations. This suggests that mechanisms underlying variation in aging could be different in males and females, which has important evolutionary consequences as well as implications for human health. This phenomenon is not likely to be a peculiar property of the *Ore* and *2b* genotypes. Geiger-Thornsberry and Mackay (2004) evaluated complementation effects of candidate genes/gene regions affecting longevity in crosses to 10 inbred lines derived from a natural population and found the line-by-sex interaction term was typically highly significant, indicative of sex-specific effects of life span QTLs in natural populations. The life span extension of homozygous *chico*[1] mutations is female-specific (Clancy *et al.*, 2001), as is the extension in life span conferred by overexpressing dFOXO in the adult fat body (Glannakou *et al.*, 2004). More generally, sex-specific effects have been observed in *Drosophila* for *P*-element-induced insertional mutations (Anholt *et al.*, 1996; Harbison *et al.*, 2004; Lyman *et al.*, 1996; Norga *et al.*, 2003) and QTLs (Dilda *et al.*, 2002; Fanara *et al.*, 2002; Harbison *et al.*, 2004) affecting sensory bristle number, olfactory behavior, and resistance to starvation stress. Sex-specific effects on enzyme activity have been observed for polymorphisms in *Esterase-6* (Game & Oakeshott, 1990) and for polymorphisms associated with variation in sensory bristle number in *Delta* (Long *et al.*, 1998) and *achaete-scute* (Long *et al.*, 2000). Thus, variation in expression of QTLs between the sexes appears to be a general feature of complex traits in *Drosophila*, and by extension in other organisms, including humans (De Benedictis *et al.*, 1998; Templeton, 1999).

We observed considerable epistasis for longevity, most often between pairs of markers that did not have significant marginal effects on life span. In the future, it will be necessary to perform QTL mapping studies with greatly increased sample sizes to be able to take full account of epistasis using sophisticated statistical models which jointly fit main and interaction effects (Kao *et al.*, 1999). Further, pervasive epistasis complicates the interpretation of complementation tests to deficiencies and mutations. As for all complementation tests, quantitative or qualitative, failure to complement cannot unambiguously be attributed to an interaction between the *Df* and QTL alleles in the region uncovered by the *Df* (allelism), or to an interaction between the *Df* and QTL alleles elsewhere in the genome (epistasis). However, it is important to note that this does not invalidate the approach. In either case, the QTLs (genes) mapped in this manner affect variation in the trait between the strains tested; it just cannot be said whether their effect is direct or through interaction with another locus. One solution to this problem would be to utilize near-isoallelic lines (which contain a single QTL from one strain introgressed into the pure background of the other) in complementation tests. In this case, epistasis between genes outside the QTL region can be eliminated as a confounding interpretation.

Deficiency complementation mapping has the potential for rapidly mapping QTLs to small genomic regions. However, until recently, the approach has been limited because there are gaps in deficiency coverage, and the breakpoints have only been ascertained cytologically. More importantly, deficiencies have been induced in a heterogeneous collection of genetic backgrounds and are often marked with recessive and dominant mutations, and the Balancer chromosome is from an unrelated genetic background with additional mutations. The heterogeneous genetic backgrounds pose a problem for comparing effects across overlapping deficiencies because variable effects could be due to multiple linked QTLs or differences in genetic background. These problems have been solved by the recent release of the DrosDel and Exelixis deficiencies to the *Drosophila* research community. These deficiencies have been generated in co-isogenic backgrounds without additional mutations and have molecularly defined breakpoints (Parks *et al.*, 2004).

Quantitative complementation tests of naturally occurring variants with subtle effects on life span to mutations at positional candidate genes can identify new candidate genes and pathways important in the regulation of life span. The studies reported here have implicated genes involved in catecholamine and bioamine biosynthesis, as well as genes involved in motor neuron development, affecting variation in longevity between *Ore* and *2b*. This approach is currently compromised because mutations exist for so few positional candidate genes embraced by a QTL (ideally, one would like to perform complementation tests to all positional candidate genes), and because those that exist are not typically derived in an isogenic background. The Exelixis collection of co-isogenic *P* and *piggyBac* insertions that has been recently released (Thibault *et al.*, 2004) will be a boon for future mutant complementation studies, and the effort to mutate all *Drosophila* genes is progressing well (Bellen *et al.*, 2004).

Nominating a novel candidate gene via quantitative complementation tests to mutations is only the first step towards understanding its direct effects on longevity, which will require analysis of adult viable mutations induced in an isogenic background, characterizing their effects on longevity relative to the co-isogenic control, demonstrating functional rescue, and assessing the effects of overexpression and/or knockout in defined tissues. Formal proof that the *Ore* and *2b* alleles of a candidate gene indeed cause a difference in life span will require a functional test. Ideally, one would replace the *Ore* allele with its *2b* counterpart (or vice versa) while maintaining the *Ore* (or *2b*) isogenic background (Rong *et al.*, 2002), but standard transgenic rescue of a null mutation with *Ore* and *2b* alleles should suffice, provided position effects of the transgene insertions are accounted for by assessing multiple insertion sites of each allele (Stam & Laurie, 1996).

Mapping genes contributing to variation in longevity between two strains conveys no information on gene frequency, and knowledge of gene frequency of causal QTNs gives insight regarding the evolutionary mechanisms maintaining variation for life span in nature. Naturally occurring genetic variation for longevity will occur at some loci due to a balance between the introduction of deleterious alleles by mutation and their elimination by natural selection (Houle *et al.*, 1996). One expects the mutant allele to be rare at these loci. At other loci, evolutionary theory predicts alleles will be maintained at intermediate frequency, either because mutations have late-age-specific effects and are effectively neutral during early life where natural selection is most effective (Medawar, 1952), or because there is balancing selection on the opposite effects of alleles early and late in life (Kirkwood & Rose, 1991; Rose & Charlesworth, 1980; Williams, 1957). To address this question, we have used LD mapping to determine the molecular polymorphisms(s) associated with natural variation in longevity at *Ddc*, one of the candidate genes implicated by high-resolution mapping and mutant complementation tests. Three polymorphisms at intermediate frequency were associated with variation in life span. These results

corroborate that *Ddc* is indeed a novel longevity gene and suggest that variation is maintained because the alleles have late-age specific effects on life span or are under balancing selection.

One caveat regarding LD mapping studies is that the cost of genotyping combined with the requirement for genotyping large numbers of alleles typically constrains studies to sample molecular polymorphisms across the gene that have been predetermined to be at intermediate frequency. In this case, observed associations may not be causal but in LD with the true causal polymorphism(s) that were not genotyped in the sample. Further, associations with rare alleles are not tested. In order to exclude the possibility of hidden causal polymorphisms and evaluate the contribution of rare mutations with large effects, it will be necessary to obtain complete sequence data for each candidate gene, extending sufficiently 3′ and 5′ of the target region for LD to decay across the sequenced region. Again, formal proof that natural alleles cause variation in life span will ultimately require functional tests, either by gene replacement (Rong *et al.*, 2002) or transgenic rescue of a null mutation (Stam & Laurie, 1996). Finally, we observed that several genes involved in catecholamine and biogenic amine synthesis are associated with variation in longevity between *Ore* and *2b*. The challenge for future association studies will be to incorporate all relevant candidate genes simultaneously, to evaluate interactions between loci, and to determine functional correlates of naturally occurring polymorphisms.

Acknowledgements

We thank Luz Tello and Saritha Pasham for technical assistance. This work was supported by National Institutes of Health grant P01 GM 45146 to T. F. C. M. and E. G. P, the Russian Fund for Basic research grants 00–04–48770 and 03–04–48605 to E. G. P., and NSF grant DEB-0349856 to J. W. L.

References

Anholt, R. R. H., Lyman, R. F., & Mackay, T. F. C. (1996). Effects of single *P* element insertions on olfactory behavior in *Drosophila melanogaster. Genetics*, 143, 293–301.

Apfeld, J., & Kenyon, C. (1999). Regulation of lifespan by sensory perception in *Caenorhabditis elegans. Nature*, 402, 804–809.

Bellen, H. J., Levis, R. W., Liao, G., He, Y., Carlson, J. W., Tsang, G., Evans-Holm, M., Hiesinger, P. R., Schulze, K. L., Rubin, G. M., Hoskins, R. A., & Spradling, A. C. (2004). The BDGP gene disruption project: single transposon insertions associated with 40% of *Drosophila* genes. *Genetics*, 167, 761–781.

Blenau, W., & Baumann, A. (2001). Molecular and pharmacological properties of insect bioamine receptors: lessons from *Drosophila melanogaster* and *Apis mellifera. Archives of Insect Biochemistry and Physiology*, 48, 13–38.

Blüher, M., Kahn, B. B., & Kahn, C. R. (2003). Extended longevity in mice lacking the insulin receptor in adipose tissue. *Science*, 299, 572–574.

Branicky, R., Benard, C., & Hekimi, S. (2000). *clk-1*, mitochondria, and physiological rates. *BioEssays*, 22, 48–56.

Brown-Borg, H. M., Borg, K. E., Meliska, C. J., & Bartke, A. (1996). Dwarf mice and the ageing process. *Nature*, 384, 33–39.

Chapman, T., Liddle, L. F., Kalb, J. M., Wolfner, M. F., & Partridge, L. (1995). Cost of mating in *Drosophila melanogaster* females is mediated by male accessory gland products. *Nature*, 373, 241–244.

Clancy, D. J., Gems, D., Harshman, L. G., Oldham, S., Stocker, H., Hafen, E., Leevers, S. J., & Partridge, L. (2001). Extension of life-span by loss of CHICO, a *Drosophila* insulin receptor substrate protein. *Science*, 292, 104–106.

Curtsinger, J. W. (2002). Sex-specificity, lifespan QTLs, and statistical power. *Journal of Gerontology*, 57, B409–B414.

Curtsinger, J. W., & Khazaeli, A. A. (2002). Lifespan, age-specificity, and pleiotropy in *Drosophila. Mechanisms of Ageing and Development*, 123, 82–93.

De Benedictis, G., Carotenuto, L., Carrieri, G., De Luca, M., Falcone, E., Rose, G.,

Cavalcanti, S., Corsonello, F., Feraco, E., Baggio, G., Bertolini, S., Mari, D., Mattace, R., Yashin, A. I., Bonafe, M., & Franceschi, C. (1998). Gene/longevity association studies at four autosomal loci (*REN, THO, PARP, SOD2*). *European Journal of Human Genetics*, 6, 534–541.

de Boer, J., Andressoo, J. O., de Wit, J., Huijmans, J., Beems, R. B., van Steeg, H., Weeda, G., van der Horst, G. T., van Leeuwen, W., Themmen, A. P., Meradji, M., & Hoeijmakers, J. H. (2002). Premature aging in mice deficient in DNA repair and transcription. *Science*, 296, 1276–1279.

Defossez, P. A., Lin, S. J., & McNabb, D. (2001). Sound silencing: the Sir2 protein and cellular senescence. *BioEssays*, 23, 327–332.

De Luca, M., Roshina, N. V., Geiger-Thornsberry, G. L., Lyman, R. F., Pasyukova, E. G., & Mackay, T. F. C. (2003). *Dopa-decarboxylase* affects variation in *Drosophila* longevity. *Nature Genetics*, 34, 429–433.

Dilda, C. L., & Mackay, T. F. C. (2002). The genetic architecture of *Drosophila* sensory bristle number. *Genetics*, 162, 1655–1674.

Dillin, A., Hsu, A. L., Arantes-Oliveira, N., Lehrer-Graiwer, J., Hsin, H., Fraser, A. G., Kamath, R. S., Ahringer, J., & Kenyon, C. (2002). Rates of behavior and aging specified by mitochondrial function during development. *Science*, 298, 2398–2401.

Fabrizio, P., Pozza, F., Pletcher, S. D., Gendron, C. M., & Longo, V. D. (2001). Regulation of longevity and stress resistance by Sch9 in yeast. *Science*, 292, 288–290.

Falconer, D. S. F., & Mackay, T. F. C. (1996). *Introduction to Quantitative Genetics* (4th ed). Harlow, Essex: Addison Wesley Longman.

Fanara, J. J., Robinson, K. O., Rollmann, S. M., Anholt, R. R. H., & Mackay, T. F. C. (2002). *Vanaso* is a candidate quantitative trait gene for *Drosophila* olfactory behavior. *Genetics*, 162, 1321–1328.

Flurkey, K., Papaconstantinou, J., Miller, R. A., & Harrison, D. E. (2001). Lifespan extension and delayed immune and collagen aging in mutant mice with defects in growth hormone production. *Proceedings of the National Academy of Sciences of the USA*, 98, 6736–6741.

Finch, C. E., & Ruvkun, G. (2001). The genetics of aging. *Annual Reviews of Genomics and Human Genetics*, 2, 435–362.

Finch, C. E., & Tanzi, R. E. (1997). Genetics of aging. *Science*, 278, 407–411.

Forbes, S. N., Valenzuela, R. K., Keim, P., & Service, P. M. (2004). Quantitative trait loci affecting life span in replicated populations of *Drosophila melanogaster*. I. Composite interval mapping. *Genetics*, 168, 301–311.

Game, A. Y., & Oakeshott, J. G. (1990). The association between restriction site polymorphism and enzyme activity variation for Esterase 6 in *Drosophila melanogaster*. *Genetics*, 139, 907–920.

Gems, D., & Riddle, D. L. (1996). Longevity in *Caenorhabditis elegans* reduced by mating but not gamete production. *Nature*, 379, 723–725.

Geiger-Thornsberry, G. L., & Mackay, T. F. C. (2004). Quantitative trait loci affecting natural variation in *Drosophila* longevity. *Mechanisms of Ageing and Development*, 125, 179–189.

Glannakou, M. E., Goss, M., Jünger, M. A., Hafen, E., Leevers, S. J., & Partridge, L. (2004). Long-lived *Drosophila* with over-expressed dFOXO in adult fat body. *Science*, 305, 361.

Griswold, C. M., Matthews, A. L., Bewley, K. E., & Mahaffey, J. W. (1993). Molecular characterization and rescue of acatalasemic mutants of *Drosophila melanogaster*. *Genetics*, 134, 781–788.

Guarente, L., & Kenyon, C. (2000). Genetic pathways that regulate ageing in model organisms. *Nature*, 408, 255–262.

Harbison, S. T., Yamamoto, A. H., Fanara, J. J., Norga, K. K., & Mackay, T. F. C. (2004). Quantitative trait loci affecting starvation resistance in *Drosophila melanogaster*. *Genetics*, 166, 1807–1823.

Hartl, D. L., & Clark, A. G. (1997). *Principles of Population Genetics* (3rd ed.). Sunderland, MA: Sinauer.

Hill, W. G., & Robertson, A. (1968). Linkage disequilibrium in finite populations. *Theoretical and Applied Genetics*, 38, 226–231.

Holzenberger, M., Dupont, J., Ducos, B., Leneuve, P., Geloen, A., Even, P. C., Cervera, P., & Le Bouc, Y. (2003). IGF-1 receptor regulates lifespan and resistance to oxidative stress in mice. *Nature*, 421, 182–186.

Houle, D., Morikawa, B., & Lynch, M. (1996). Comparing mutational variabilities. *Genetics*, 143, 1467–1483.

Hwangbo, D. S., Gersham, B., Tu, M. P., Palmer, M., & Tatar, M. (2004). *Drosophila* dFOXO controls lifespan and regulates insulin signalling in brain and fat body. *Nature*, 429, 562–566.

Ishii, N., Fujii, M., Hartman, P. S., Tsuda, M., Yasuda, K., Senoo-Matsuda, N., Yanase, S., Ayusawa, D., & Suzuki, K. (1998). A mutation in succinate dehydrogenase cytochrome b causes oxidative stress and ageing in nematodes. *Nature*, 394, 694–697.

Kao, C. H., Zeng, Z. B., & Teasdale, R. (1999). Multiple interval mapping for quantitative trait loci. *Genetics*, 152, 1203–1216.

Kimura, K. D., Tissenbaum, H. A., Liu, Y., & Ruvkun, G. (1997). *daf-2*, an insulin receptor-like gene that regulates longevity and diapause in *Caenorhabditis elegans*. *Science*, 277, 942–946.

Kirkwood, T. B. L., & Rose, M. R. (1991). Evolution of senescence: late survival sacrificed for reproduction. *Philosophical Transactions of the Royal Society of London, Series B*, 332, 15–24.

Kumar, S. C., & Vrana, K. E. (1996). Intricate regulation of tyrosine hydroxylase activity and gene expression. *Journal of Neurochemistry*, 67, 443–462.

Lee, C. K., Klopp, R. G., Weindruch, R., & Prolla, T. A. (1999). Gene expression profile of aging and its retardation by caloric restriction. *Science*, 285, 1390–1393.

Lee, S. S., Lee, R. Y. N., Fraser, A. G., Kamath, R. S., Ahringer, J., & Ruvkun, G. (2003). A systematic RNAi screen identifies a critical role for mitochondria in *C. elegans* longevity. *Nature Genetics*, 33, 40–48.

Leips, J., & Mackay, T. F. C. (2000). Quantitative trait loci for life span in *Drosophila melanogaster*: interactions with genetic background and larval density. *Genetics*, 155, 1773–1788.

Leips, J., & Mackay, T. F. C. (2002). The complex genetic architecture of *Drosophila* life span. *Experimental Aging Research*, 28, 361–390.

Lin, K., Dorman, J. B., Rodan, A., & Kenyon, C. (1997). *daf-16*: An HNF-3/forkhead family member that can function to double the life-span of *Caenorhabditis elegans*. *Science*, 278, 1319–1322.

Lin, S. J., Defossez, P., & Guarente, L. (2000). Requirement of NAD and *SIR2* for life-span extension by calorie restriction in *Saccharomyces cerevisiae*. *Science*, 289, 2126–2128.

Lin, Y. J., Seroude, L., & Benzer, S. (1998). Extended life-span and stress resistance in the *Drosophila* mutant *methuselah*. *Science*, 282, 943–946.

Long, A. D., & Langley, C. H. (1999). Power of association studies to detect the contribution of candidate genetic loci to complexly inherited phenotypes. *Genome Research*, 9, 720–731.

Long, A. D., Lyman, R. F., Langley, C. H., & Mackay, T. F. (1998). Two sites in the *Delta* gene region contribute to naturally occurring variation in bristle number in *Drosophila melanogaster*. *Genetics*, 149, 999–1017.

Long, A. D., Lyman, R. F., Morgan, A. H., Langley, C. H., & Mackay, T. F. C. (2000). Both naturally occurring insertions of transposable elements and intermediate frequency polymorphisms at the *achaete-scute* complex are associated with variation in bristle number in *Drosophila melanogaster*. *Genetics*, 154, 1255–1269.

Luckinbill, L. S., & Clare, M. J. (1985). Selection for life span in *Drosophila melanogaster*. *Heredity*, 55, 9–18.

Luckinbill, L. S., Arking, R., Clare, M. J., Cirocco, W. C., & Buck, S. A. (1984). Selection of delayed senescence in *Drosophila melanogaster*. *Evolution*, 38, 996–1003.

Luo, Z. W., Tao, S. H., & Zeng, Z. B. (2000). Inferring linkage disequilibrium between a polymorphic marker locus and a trait locus in natural populations. *Genetics*, 156, 457–4667.

Lyman, R. F., Lawrence, F., Nuzhdin, S. V., & Mackay, T. F. C. (1996). Effects of single *P*-element insertions on bristle number and viability in *Drosophila melanogaster*. *Genetics*, 143, 277–292.

Lynch, M., & Walsh, J. B. (1998). *Genetics and Analysis of Quantitative Traits*. Sunderland, MA: Sinauer.

Mackay, T. F. C. (2001). The genetic architecture of quantitative traits. *Annual Reviews of Genetics*, 35, 303–339.

Maynard Smith, J. (1958). Sex limited inheritance of longevity in *Drosophila subobscura*. *Journal of Genetics*, 56, 227–235.

Medawar, P. B. (1952). *An Unsolved Problem of Biology*. London: H. K. Lewis.

Melov, S., Ravenscroft, J., Malik, S., Gill, M. S., Walker, D. W., Clayton, P. E., Wallace, D. C., Malfroy, B., Doctrow, S. R., & Lithgow, G. J. (2000). Extension of life-span with superoxide dismutase/catalase mimetics. *Science*, 289, 1567–1569.

Migliaccio, E., Giorgio, M., Mele, S., Pelicci, G., Reboldi, P., Pandolfi, P. P., Lanfrancone, L., & Pelicci, P. G. (1999). The p66[shc] adaptor protein controls oxidative stress response and life span in mammals. *Nature*, 402, 309–313.

Miyashita, N., & Langley, C. H. (1990). Molecular and phenotypic variation of the *white* locus region in *Drosophila melanogaster*. *Genetics*, 120, 199–212.

Neckameyer, W. S., & White, K. (1993). *Drosophila* tyrosine hydroxylase is encoded by the *pale* locus. *Journal of Neurogenetics*, 8, 189–199.

Norga, K. K., Gurganus, M. C., Dilda, C. L., Yamamoto, A., Lyman, R. F., Patel, P. H., Rubin, G. M., Hoskins, R. A., Mackay, T F C., & Bellen, H. J. (2003). Quantitative analysis of bristle number in *Drosophila* mutants identifies genes involved in neural development. *Current Biology*, 13, 1388–1397.

Nuzhdin, S. V., Pasyukova, E. G., Dilda, C. L., Zeng, Z. B., & Mackay, T. F. C. (1997). Sex-specific quantitative trait loci affecting longevity in *Drosophila melanogaster*. *Proceedings of the National Academy of Sciences of the USA*, 94, 9734–9739.

O'Donnel, J. M., Stathakis, D. G., Burton, D., & Chen, Z. (2002). Catecholamines-up, a negative regulator of tryrosine hydroxylase and GTP cyclohydrolase I in *Drosophila melanogaster*. In G. K. S. Milstein, R. A. Levine, & B. Shane (Eds.), *Chemistry and Biology of Pteridines and Folates*, pp. 211–215. Boston, MA: Kluwer.

Parkes, T. L., Elia, A. J., Dickinson, D., Hilliker, A. J., Phillips, J. P., & Boulianne, G. L. (1998). Extension of *Drosophila* life span by over-expression of human SOD1 in motorneurons. *Nature Genetics*, 19, 226–231.

Parks, A. L., Cook, K. R., Belvin, M., Dompe, N. A., Fawcett, R., Huppert, K., Tan, L. R., Winter, C. G., Bogart, K. P.,

Deal, J. E., Deal-Herr, M. E., Grant, D., Marcinko, M., Miyazaki, W. Y., Robertson, S., Shaw, K. J., Tabios, M., Vysotskaia, V., Zhao, L., Andrade, R. S., Edgar, K. A., Howie, E., Killpack, K., Milash, B., Norton, A., Thao, D., Whittaker, K., Winner, M. A., Friedman, L., Margolis, J., Singer, M. A., Kopczynski, C., Curtis, D., Kaufman, T. C., Plowman, G. D., Duyk, G., & Francis-Lang, H. L. (2004). Systematic generation of high-resolution deletion coverage of the *Drosophila melanogaster* genome. *Nature Genetics*, 36, 288–292.

Partridge, L., & Farquhar, M. (1981). Sexual activity reduces longevity of male fruitflies. *Nature*, 294, 580–582.

Partridge, L., & Fowler, K. (1992). Direct and correlated responses to selection on age of reproduction in *Drosophila melanogaster*. *Evolution*, 46, 76–91.

Partridge, L., & Gems, D. (2002). Mechanisms of ageing: public or private? *Nature Reviews Genetics*, 3, 165–175.

Partridge, L., Green, A., & Fowler, K. (1987). Effects of egg production and of exposure to males on female survival in *Drosophila melanogaster*. *Journal of Insect Physiology*, 33, 745–749.

Pasyukova, E. G., & Nuzhdin, S. V. (1993). *Doc* and *copia* instability in an isogenic *Drosophila melanogaster* stock. *Molecular and General Genetics*, 240, 302–306.

Pasyukova, E. G., Roshina, N. V., & Mackay, T. F. C. (2004). *Shuttle craft*: a candidate quantitative trait gene for *Drosophila* lifespan. *Aging Cell*, 3, 297–307.

Pasyukova, E. G., Vieira, C., & Mackay, T. F. C. (2000). Deficiency mapping of quantitative trait loci affecting longevity in *Drosophila melanogaster*. *Genetics*, 156, 1129–1146.

Pentz, E. S., & Wright, T. R. F. (1986). A diphenol oxidase gene is part of a cluster of genes involved in catecholamine metabolism and sclerotization in *Drosophila*. II. Molecular characterization of the *Dox-A2* coding region. *Genetics*, 112, 843–859.

Pentz, E. S., & Wright, T. R. F. (1991). *Drosophila melanogaster* diphenol oxidase A2: gene structure and homology with the mouse mast-cell tum⁻ transplantation antigen, P91A. *Gene*, 103, 239–242.

Pentz, E. S., Black, B. C., & Wright, T. R. F. (1986). A diphenol oxidase gene is part of a cluster of genes involved in catecholamine metabolism and sclerotization in *Drosophila*. I. Identification of the biochemical defect in *Dox-A2 [l(2)37Bf]* mutants. *Genetics*, 112, 823–841.

Pletcher, S. D., Macdonald, S. J., Marguerie, R., Certa, U., Stearns, S. C., Goldstein, D. B., & Partridge, L. (2002). Genome-wide transcript profiles in aging and calorically restricted *Drosophila melanogaster*. *Current Biology*, 12, 712–723.

Reiwitch, S. G., & Nuzhdin, S. V. (2002). Quantitative trait loci for lifespan of mated *Drosophila melanogaster* affect both sexes. *Genetical Research*, 80, 225–230.

Risch, N., & Merikangas, K. (1996). The future of genetic studies of complex human diseases. *Science*, 273, 1516–1517.

Rogina, B., Reenan, R. A., Nilsen, S. P., & Helfand, S. L. (2000). Extended life-span conferred by co-transporter gene mutations in *Drosophila*. *Science*, 290, 2137–2140.

Rong, Y. S., Titen, S. W., Xie, H. B., Golic, M. M., Bastiani, M., Bandyopadhyay, P., Olivera, B. M., Brodsky, M., Rubin, G. M., & Golic, K. G. (2002). Targeted mutagenesis by homologous recombination in *D. melanogaster*. *Genes and Development*, 16, 1658–1581.

Rose, M. R. (1984). Laboratory evolution of postponed senescence in *Drosophila melanogaster*. *Evolution*, 38, 1004–1010.

Rose, M. R., & Charlesworth, B. (1980). A test of evolutionary theories of senescence. *Nature*, 287, 141–142.

Soller, M., & Beckmann, J. S. (1990). Marker-based mapping of quantitative trait loci using replicated progenies. *Theoretical and Applied Genetics*, 80, 205–208.

Stam, L. F., & Laurie, C. C. (1996). Molecular dissection of a major gene effect on a quantitative trait: the level of alcohol dehydrogenase expression in *Drosophila melanogaster*. *Genetics*, 144, 1559–1564.

Stathakis, D. G., Burton, D. Y., McIvor, W. E., Krishnakumar, S., Wright, T. R. F., & O'Donnell, J. (1999). The Catecholamines up (Catsup) protein of *Drosophila melanogaster* functions as a negative regulator of tyrosine hydroxylase activity. *Genetics*, 153, 361–382.

Stathakis, D. G., Pentz, E. S., Freeman, M. E., Kullman, J., Hankins, G. R., Pearlson, N. J., & Wright, T. R. F. (1995). The genetic and molecular organization of the *Dopa decarboxylase* gene cluster of *Drosophila melanogaster. Genetics,* 141, 629–655.

Stroumbakis, N. D., Li, Z., & Tolias, P. P. (1996). A homolog of human transcription factor NF-X1 encoded by *Drosophila shuttle craft* gene is required in the embryonic central nervous system. *Molecular and Cell Biology,* 16, 192–201.

Sun, J., Folk, D., Bradley, T. J., & Tower, J. (2002). Induced overexpression of mitochondrial Mn-superoxide dismutase extends the life span of adult *Drosophila melanogaster. Genetics,* 161, 661–672.

Sze, J. Y., Victor, M., Loer, C., Shi, Y., & Ruvkun, G. (2000). Food and metabolic signaling defects in a *Caenorhabditis elegans* serotonin synthesis mutant. *Nature,* 403, 560–564.

Tatar, M., Bartke, A., & Antebi, A. (2003). The endocrine regulation of aging by insulin-like signals. *Science,* 299, 1346–1351.

Tatar, M., Kopelman, A., Epstein, D., Tu, M. P., Yin, C. M., & Garofalo, R. S. (2001). A mutant *Drosophila* insulin receptor homolog that extends life-span and impairs neuroendocrine function. *Science,* 292, 107–110.

Templeton, A. (1999). Uses of evolutionary theory in the human genome project. *Annual Reviews of Ecology and Systematics,* 30, 23–49.

The International SNP Map Working Group. (2001). A map of human genome sequence variation containing 1.42 million single nucleotide polymorphisms. *Nature,* 409, 928–933.

Thibault, S. T., Singer, M. A., Miyazaki, W. Y., Milash, B., Dompe, N. A., Singh, C. M., Buchholz, R., Demsky, M., Fawcett, R., Francis-Lang, H. L., Ryner, L., Cheung, L. M., Chong, A., Erickson, C., Fisher, W. W., Greer, K., Hartouni, S. R., Howie, E., Jakkula, L., Joo, D., Killpack, K., Laufer, A., Mazzotta, J., Smith, R. D., Stevens, L. M., Stuber, C., Tan, L. R., Ventura, R., Woo, A., Zakrajsek, I., Zhao, L., Chen, F., Swimmer, C., Kopczynski, C., Duyk, G., Winberg, M. L., & Margolis, J. (2004). A complementary transposon tool kit for *Drosophila melanogaster* using *P* and *piggyBac. Nature Genetics,* 36, 283–287.

Thor, S., & Thomas, J. B. (1997). The *Drosophila islet* gene governs axon pathfinding and neurotransmitter identity. *Neuron,* 18, 397–409.

Thor, S., Andersson, S. G. E., Tomlinson, A., & Thomas, J. B. (1999). A LIM-homeodomain combinatorial code for motor-neuron pathway selection. *Nature,* 397, 76–80.

Valenzuela, R. K., Forbes, S. N., Keim, P, & Service, P. M. (2004). Quantitative trait loci affecting life span in replicated populations of *Drosophila melanogaster.* II. Response to selection. *Genetics,* 168, 313–324.

Verbeke, P., Fonager, J., Clark, B. F. C., & Rattan, S. I. S. (2001). Heat shock response and ageing: mechanisms and applications. *Cell Biology International,* 25, 845–857.

Vieira, C., Pasyukova, E. G., Zeng, Z. B., Hackett, J. B., Lyman, R. F., & Mackay, T. F. C. (2000). Genotype-environment interaction for quantitative trait loci affecting life span in *Drosophila melanogaster. Genetics,* 154, 213–227.

Weindruch, R., & Walford, R. L. (1988). *The Retardation of Aging and Disease by Dietary Restriction.* Springfield, IL: Thomas.

Weir, B. S. (1996). *Genetic data analysis II.* Sunderland, MA: Sinauer.

Westendorp, R. J., & Kirkwood, T. B. L. (1998). Human longevity and the cost of reproductive success. *Nature,* 396, 743–746.

Williams, G. C. (1957). Pleiotropy, natural selection, and the evolution of senescence. *Evolution,* 11, 398–411.

Wong, P. C., Rothstein, J. D., & Price, D. L. (1998). The genetic and molecular mechanisms of motor neuron disease. *Current Opinion in Neurobiology,* 8, 791–799.

Wright, T. R. F. (1996). Phenotypic analysis of the *Dopa decarboxylase* gene cluster in *Drosophila melanogaster. Journal of Heredity,* 87, 175–190.

Zeng, Z. B. (1994). Precision mapping of quantitative trait loci. *Genetics,* 136, 1547–1468.

Zou, S., Meadows, S., Sharp, L., Jan, L. Y., & Jan, Y. N. (2000). Genome-wide study of aging and oxidative stress response in *Drosophila melanogaster. Proceedings of the National Academy of Sciences of the USA,* 97, 13726–13731.

Zwaan, B. J., Bijlsma, R., Hoekstra, R. F. (1995). Direct selection on lifespan in *Drosophila melanogaster. Evolution,* 49, 649–659.

Chapter 8

Evolutionary Biology of Aging: Future Directions

Daniel E. L. Promislow, Kenneth M. Fedorka, and Joep M. S. Burger

I. Introduction

Over the past two decades, we have seen extraordinary progress in evolutionary studies of senescence. Beginning with the early quantitative genetic tests of theories of senescence (Edney & Gill, 1968; Luckinbill *et al.*, 1984; Rose & Charlesworth, 1980), we have progressed to the point where evolutionary biologists rely on state-of-the-art molecular tools, and the ties between evolutionary and molecular approaches in the study of senescence are often seamless. More than perhaps any other research area in evolutionary ecology, molecular biologists working on senescence appreciate how evolutionary biology contributes to our understanding of senescence. Many will tell you about George Williams' antagonistic pleiotropy theory of senescence (Williams, 1957), or perhaps Tom Kirkwood's disposable soma theory (Kirkwood, 1977), and the especially well-rounded researcher might mention that molecular biologists have identified individual genes that appear to exhibit antagonistic pleiotropic effects (Campisi, 2003).

Serious effort has been expended in testing these classic evolutionary theories of senescence (e.g., Hughes & Charlesworth, 1994; Promislow *et al.*, 1996; Rose & Charlesworth, 1980). The field is now moving beyond tests of existing hypotheses, but what exactly is the future direction for the evolutionary studies of aging? We do not have a scientific crystal ball, and making definite predictions places us somewhere between hubris and folly. Nevertheless, with this caveat in mind, we hope that the ideas presented here may spur the next generation of biogerontologists to consider evolutionary studies of senescence.

What differentiates evolutionary studies of aging from studies that take a strictly molecular, physiological, or demographic approach? One distinction is that non-evolutionary biologists frequently ask proximate questions (e.g., how do specific biological processes change with age, and how do genes affect these changes?), whereas evolutionary biologists are

Handbook of the Biology of Aging, Sixth Edition

interested in ultimate questions (why has aging evolved, and why have particular genes evolved to influence longevity?). The molecular biologist is trying to identify the mechanisms that cause aging. The evolutionary biologist is trying to place those mechanisms in a broader perspective, asking why those mechanisms and not others are important to aging, and how those mechanisms are shaped by other forces—mutation, selection, genetic drift—acting over evolutionary time.

In the past few years, the lines between these two fields have begun to blur. Molecular geneticists working on aging have used evolutionary theory to motivate studies of single genes (Campisi, 2003; Walker et al., 2000), and evolutionary biologists have embraced techniques that are firmly rooted in modern molecular biology (e.g., Pletcher et al., 2002; Tatar et al., 2001).

Although evolutionary biologists now rely on 21st-century techniques, the greatest evolutionary contributions to aging studies date back half a century. Until the middle of the 20th century, the standard argument for the evolution of aging was that it was good for the species (Weismann, 1891). In the 1940s, we began to move beyond that argument, which we now recognize as fallacious. Following from the insights of Fisher (1930) and Haldane (1941), in 1946, Medawar argued that because the strength of selection declines with age, senescence will arise as an inevitable consequence of this decline (Medawar, 1946). Consider a novel, germline mutation that reduces survival at just one age. If it reduces survival before the age at maturity, then the probability of surviving to produce offspring at any age is uniformly reduced. Such a deleterious mutation would experience strong negative selection and eventually be lost from the population. In contrast, a mutation that reduces survival at some late age, after most individuals in the population had died, would experience only very

weak selection and could spread through random genetic drift. Over evolutionary time, early-acting deleterious mutations will continually be removed by selection, whereas late-acting ones will accumulate. According to Medawar's mutation accumulation theory, it is inevitable that we carry a relatively high load of late-acting deleterious mutations inherited from our ancestors. As we age, we experience the effects of these mutations, which cause a decrease in rates of survival and/or fertility.

A decade later, George Williams developed his antagonistic pleiotropy theory, in which he argued that senescence would arise if late-acting deleterious mutations were actually favored by selection due to their early-acting beneficial effects (Williams, 1957). In this case, senescence evolves due to tradeoffs between early-age benefits and late-age costs, an idea that was further developed by Tom Kirkwood in his disposable soma theory (Kirkwood, 1977). A half-century after Medawar and Williams, evolutionary biologists are still trying to determine which of these theories provides the best explanation for senescence (Charlesworth, 2001; Charlesworth & Hughes, 1996; Hughes et al., 2002; Partridge & Gems, 2002a; Snoke & Promislow, 2003). More recently, molecular gerontologists have begun to embrace these ideas, with a particular interest in finding genes with antagonistic pleiotropic effects (Campisi, 2003; Walker et al., 2000).

The current focus in the evolutionary biology of aging encompasses three main areas:

1. Ongoing studies are trying to characterize the genetic architecture of aging (see Chapter 7, Mackay et al.), asking not only which model can explain genetic variation for senescence, but also whether genes that have been found to extend life span in the lab (so called "aging genes") show allelic variation that

correlates with longevity in wild-caught isolates, and whether the effect of aging genes depends on the sex or external environment in which they are expressed (Fry *et al.*, 1998; Leips & Mackay, 2000; Nuzhdin *et al.*, 1997).

2. A second body of work has focused specifically on the shape of mortality trajectories (see Chapter 1, Gavrilov and Gavrilova), asking why mortality curves increase exponentially with age (Abrams & Ludwig, 1995; Charlesworth, 2001) and why mortality rates appear to decelerate late in life in some cases (Mueller *et al.*, 2003; Mueller & Rose, 1996; Service, 2000; Vaupel *et al.*, 1998, but see Finch & Pike, 1996; Linnen *et al.*, 2001).

3. Finally, many evolutionary biologists have become interested in the central role that the endocrine system may play in determining the evolution of the suite of traits that make up an individual's "life history strategy," including development time, age at maturity, growth rate, body size, fecundity, and, of course, life span (Tatar *et al.*, 2003). The evolution of aging in general, and these three subjects in particular, have all been reviewed recently in other sources (e.g., Promislow & Bronikowski, in press; Tatar *et al.*, 2003) and in this book (see Chapter 15, Tu *et al*; Chapter 19, Miller and Austad; Chapter 20, Carter and Sonntag). Accordingly, rather than going over well-tilled ground, in the rest of this chapter, we will look at five areas that are less studied at present but which we think may provide fertile soil for the growth of future evolutionary studies of aging. These include (1) molecular evolution and gene networks; (2) the intersection of physiology and demography; (3) parasites and immunity; (4) sexual selection and sexual conflict; and (5) genetic variation in natural populations.

The rationale for focusing on these particular areas comes from our thinking about early models of aging. The first

mathematical model for the evolution of senescence was developed by W. D. Hamilton (1966). Hamilton started with the well-known Euler-Lotka equation (Euler, 1760; Lotka, 1925):

$$1 = \Sigma e^{-rx}l(x)m(x) \qquad (1)$$

in which r is the intrinsic rate of increase in a population (also called the *Malthusian parameter*, and used as a measure of Darwinian fitness), $l(x)$ is the probability of surviving from birth to age x, and $m(x)$ is the number of daughters that a female produces at age x. Hamilton's model used this equation to provide exact descriptions of how the strength of selection acting on rates of mortality or fecundity would change with age. One can think of the strength of selection as a measure of how fast a new mutation will be fixed or lost in a population. In particular, the strength of selection acting on $P(x)$, the survival rate from age x to $x + 1$, is given by

$$\frac{\partial r}{\partial \ln p(x)} = \frac{\sum\limits_{y=x+1}^{\infty} e^{-ry}l(y)m(y)}{\Sigma x e^{-rx}l(x)m(x)} \qquad (2)$$

The strength of selection acting on fecundity is given by

$$\frac{\partial r}{\partial m(x)} = \frac{e^{-rx}l(x)}{\Sigma x e^{-rx}l(x)m(x)} \qquad (3)$$

The important point that these equations illustrate is that the demographic parameters themselves determine the rate at which selection declines with age. We show how the strength of selection declines for one particular set of values for age-specific survival and fecundity in Figure 8.1. These equations do not include information about such factors as social behavior (e.g., mate choice, parent-offspring conflict), host-parasite interactions, variation in the environment, physiology, or the underlying

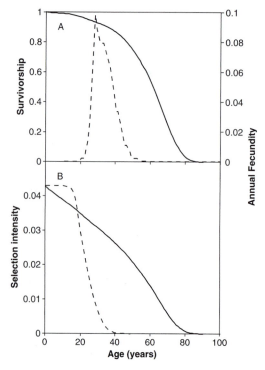

Figure 8.1 (a) Age-specific fecundity (dashed line) and survivorship (solid line) for a hypothetical human population. (b) Intensity of selection acting on a mutation that decreases age-specific fecundity (dashed line) or survival (solid line) for a single age class. Note the dramatic decline in the intensity of selection on survival after age at maturity, eventually reaching zero after the last age at reproduction.

genetic architecture of these demographic traits. All of these factors could alter the shape of the curves described by equations (2) and (3).

Researchers interested in the evolution of aging have begun to develop ways to extend Hamilton's equations, enhancing both biological realism and predictive power. For example, Peter Abrams showed that if one adds density dependence to classic models for the evolution of aging, in some cases extrinsic mortality rates no longer influence the evolution of rates of senescence (Abrams, 1993). Ron Lee has developed models that incorporate interactions between parents and their offspring into models of aging; these models make impressively accurate

predictions about the shape of human mortality curves (Lee, 2003). And most recently, Jim Vaupel and colleagues have created models to demonstrate that species with indeterminate growth (i.e., no asymptotic size as adults) may evolve "negative senescence," where mortality rates actually decline with age (Vaupel et al., 2004). In the following sections, we explore a range of biological phenomena that may allow us to further extend classic models of aging. Clearly there is much work to be done, and we are optimistic that as we unite new molecular tools and new evolutionary ideas, the coming years will bring a more comprehensive understanding of the evolution of senescence.

II. Genetics of Senescence

For almost 20 years, evolutionary biologists and molecular biologists working on the biology of aging appeared to be working on utterly different problems, with little communication between the two groups (perhaps not unlike the gap between those working on cellular senescence and those working on aging in animal models; Campisi, 2001). This has changed in the past few years, with evolutionary biologists now embracing the newest molecular techniques, and molecular biologists starting to test evolutionary hypotheses. For example, a collaborative effort among evolutionary and molecular biologists led to the first large-scale microarray analysis of patterns of gene transcription associated with senescence in the entire fly genome (Pletcher et al., 2002). The sequencing of entire genomes has made it extremely easy to identify genes associated with aging that occur across taxonomically diverse organisms (and so, by inference, to identify aging processes that have deep evolutionary roots). George Martin wondered whether genes associated with aging were likely to be specific to each species ("private" mechanisms) or constant across evolutionary time ("public" mechanisms) (Martin, 1997). At least two gene pathways associated with aging—sirtuins and insulin signaling—appear to be public mechanisms (Partridge & Gems, 2002b; Tissenbaum & Guarente, 2001).

Current work on the molecular genetics of aging is focused on characterizing the function of the genes and gene pathways that have already been identified, and on finding new genes (see Chapter 7, Mackay et al.). Clearly, this is where the action is. So where does evolutionary biology fit within this decidedly molecular enterprise? In the introduction, we discussed how the strength of selection changes with age. One challenge is to determine how the strength of selection acts not only on demographic traits, but also on the individual genes that shape those demographic traits. If we can do this, we may be able to develop an evolutionary genetic model of aging that allows us to actually predict what kinds of genes should be associated with aging. A more refined analysis of selection at the level of individual genes and genomes will come about in two ways—first, by combining molecular evolutionary studies of gene sequences or genome structure with analyses of life span, and second, through the study of gene- and protein-interaction networks.

A. Molecular Evolution and Aging

Molecular evolutionists study the process of evolution by analyzing variation in DNA and protein sequences within and among species. Many workers in the field have focused on the historical and current patterns of selection that act on genes—an area of inquiry that began in earnest with the debate over whether most genetic variation was due to selection or had occurred in the absence of selection due to the effects of random drift of neutral or nearly neutral mutations (Kimura, 1968). In some ways, the history of the neutralist–

selectionist debate in molecular evolution mirrors that of the mutation accumulation–antagonistic pleiotropy debate in senescence. After a long argument between neutralists and selectionists, most evolutionary biologists now accept that some genes have evolved under a neutral scenario whereas others have evolved due primarily to selective forces. Nevertheless, the debate started by Kimura fueled decades of exciting and productive research. Similarly, in the world of evolutionary gerontology, it will likely turn out that some genes have evolved due to mutation accumulation and others due to antagonistic pleiotropy, but the debate over which is the better explanatory hypothesis has sparked invaluable research progress.

However, we see the parallel between molecular evolution and aging research as having far more than just historical interest. Molecular evolution has led to fundamental advances in the way that we understand the biology of organisms, and some of these advances could inform future studies in the biology of aging.

Work on the genomes of a diversity of organisms has found that substantial portions of the genome are often made up of transposable elements (TEs). These "jumping genes" can function as parasites in the genomes of their host and can lead to substantial increases in background mutation rates (McDonald, 1993). To the extent that aging is affected by age-related increases in somatic mutation rates, TEs may turn out to play an important role in the aging process. Surprisingly, relatively few studies have examined the relationship between TEs and aging (Nikitin & Shmookler Reis, 1997; Woodruff & Nikitin, 1995). One study makes the interesting (and cautionary) point that when genes associated with longevity in *Drosophila* are identified by knocking the gene out with a P-element (a type of TE found in flies), the P-element insertion alone may influence life span, independent of the effects of the target gene (Kaiser *et al.*, 1997). It would be useful to quantify the extent to which age-related accumulation of somatic mutations accounts for the aging process and to examine the role that TEs play in this process.

Molecular studies have found that over evolutionary history, some genes have experienced periods of very strong selection, whereas others appear to have been strongly shaped by drift (Li, 1997). Might this variation in selection translate to differences not just among genes but also among tissues? Early studies examined age-related declines in specific tissues, such as the early 20th-century work of Krumbiegel (1929) on fat body in aging *Drosophila*. More recent studies have found that the age-related rate of decline varies among tissue types. For example, in nematodes, muscle cells appear to age at a much faster rate than nerve cells (Herndon *et al.*, 2002). Furthermore, the effect of gene signaling on longevity is often tissue-specific (Hwangbo *et al.*, 2004; Libina *et al.*, 2003). One obvious challenge is to determine whether tissues differ in their rate of aging because of different patterns of selection acting on different tissues. For example, the fitness consequences of a cell failing to produce hair follicles are likely to be quite different than the consequences of a pancreatic cell failing to produce insulin. If tissue-specific variation in rates of aging (what we might call "senescent heterochrony"—the opposite of the "one hoss shay" effect[1]) turns out to have

deep evolutionary roots, it would be of interest to look for common genetic or epigenetic causes of this pattern.

Finally, comparisons of whole genomes across species have been used to infer physiological process from genetic pattern. For example, Eisen and Hanawalt (1999) determined the presence or absence of various DNA repair genes across more than 20 species of microbes. On the basis of their "phylogenomic" analysis, they were able not only to determine the degree of ubiquity of different repair genes or gene pathways, but also to predict the repair phenotypes of different microbes based on their underlying genotypes. Interestingly, they found that although some repair processes, such as those associated with the *recA* gene, are strikingly constant across taxa, others have evolved relatively recently. The genetic basis of repair differs among species, and in some cases, specific repair mechanisms have evolved convergently in different taxa. These findings should serve as a warning to biogerontologists. Although some aging genes, such as those in the insulin signaling pathway, may have deep evolutionary roots, our current focus on these ubiquitous pathways may lead us to overlook many others that evolve rapidly and are highly variable among species. We are confident that "phylogenomic" approaches will lead to profound insights into the evolutionary history of genetic mechanisms of aging in the coming years.

---

[1]The observed patterns of senescent heterochrony contrast with the classic example of the "One Hoss Shay," made famous in Oliver Wendel Holmes' "The Deacon's Masterpiece":

> The poor old chaise in a heap or mound,
> As if it had been to the mill and ground!
> You see, of course, if you're not a dunce,
> How it went to pieces all at once, –
> All at once, and nothing first, –
> Just as bubbles do when they burst.

B. Gene Networks

Classic studies of aging relied on forward or reverse genetic techniques to identify individual genes that extended longevity. But a one-gene/one-trait perspective is clearly an oversimplification (Lewontin & White, 1960; Wright, 1932). The past few years have given us a new appreciation for the complex interactions among genes and proteins that affect the formation of the final phenotype (Gibson & Honeycutt, 2002; Wolf *et al.*, 2000). Already, studies have shown that in worms (Shook & Johnson, 1999) and flies (Jackson *et al.*, 2002; Leips & Mackay, 2000), the way in which a particular allele affects longevity can depend on the presence of specific alleles at other loci (Spencer *et al.*, 2003).

However, the shift from thinking about single genes to epistatic interactions between pairs of loci is still an oversimplification. We need to begin thinking about age-related changes to whole networks of interacting elements. Recent studies have shown that when genes or proteins interact within a complex network, the network structure itself can make the network resilient to damage in a way that would not be possible if all the elements in the network were operating independently (Albert *et al.*, 2000; Flatt, 2005; Maslov *et al.*, 2004; Siegal & Bergman, 2002; Wagner, 2000).

Networks can describe a wide array of interactions, from the regulatory interactions among genes, to social interactions among individuals, to transfer of electricity from power stations to users. In general, networks consist of "nodes" or "vertices" connected to each other by "edges." The number of edges that a particular node has is called its "degree" or "connectivity," and the frequency distribution of connectivity across all nodes in a network is the network's degree distribution (Albert & Barabási, 2002). Biological networks typically have a degree distribution that approximates a power law (Albert & Barabási, 2002), such that the majority of nodes have just one or two edges, but some may have tens or hundreds of edges. Studies on network robustness illustrate that the strength of selection acting on a single gene depends largely on the network context within which that gene functions. For example, we might

hypothesize that more highly connected genes or proteins are under stronger selection. This idea is supported by findings that more highly connected proteins evolve more slowly (Fraser *et al.*, 2002), that genes that produce these proteins are more likely to have a lethal phenotype when knocked out (Jeong *et al.*, 2001), and that these genes are less likely to be lost over evolutionary time (Krylov *et al.*, 2003).

In light of these studies, we might expect that the structure of gene- and protein-interaction networks may influence which genes are associated with senescent decline (Sozou & Kirkwood, 2001). In a study of the yeast protein–protein interaction network, Promislow (2004) found that proteins with relatively high connectivity were more likely to be associated with replicative aging than proteins with fewer interactions. Furthermore, aging genes tended to have a higher degree of functional pleiotropy than expected by chance. Although Promislow (2004) argues that these results are consistent with the antagonistic pleiotropy theory of senescence, just why we observe these patterns is still an open question.

Molecular studies have identified complex pathways that affect senescence, best exemplified by work on the insulin-like/insulin growth factor signaling pathway in *C. elegans* and *D. melanogaster* (see Chapter 13, Henderson *et al.*; Chapter 15, Tu *et al.*). We now face the exciting challenge of using classical genetics approaches (Van Swinderen and Greenspan, 2005) and microarray studies to describe the larger networks of interacting genes that might affect aging. At the same time, we need theoretical models to predict how the network of nodes with which a single gene interacts can be used to predict (1) whether this gene will be associated with longevity and (2) how likely the gene is to fail as the organism ages.

III. From Physiology to Demography

In his book on the evolution of aging, Michael Rose defines senescence as "a persistent decline in the age-specific fitness components of an organism *due to internal physiological deterioration*" (our italics, page 20, Rose, 1991). Most evolutionary biologists studying senescence have focused on the decline in age-specific fitness components (mortality and fecundity). Whereas physiologists have focused on age-related changes in a wide array of physiological systems (Masoro, 1995), much less attention has been devoted to testing the hypothesis that demographic senescence is due to internal physiological deterioration (see Williams, 1999), or to exploring the possibility that physiological homeostasis may even limit the senescent decline in survival or fecundity (Kowald & Kirkwood, 1996).

In standard evolutionary models, the currency that measures how likely a gene is to make it into subsequent generations is made up solely of age-specific survival and fecundity (Equation 1). Evolutionary biologists are interested in changes in gene frequencies over time, so it seems logical to measure senescence by observing age-specific declines in survival and fecundity. Until recently, the physiological factors that are presumably the proximate cause of age-related changes in survival or fecundity have been considered of secondary importance among evolutionary gerontologists. In fact, some models suggest demographic senescence may evolve even in the absence of physiological decline. Houston and McNamara (1999) showed that mortality rates can increase with age solely as a result of how individuals optimize reproductive effort, and without any age-related deterioration in physiological state. Where evolutionary biologists have looked at both demographic and physiological parameters, the results have sometimes been counterintuitive. Recently, Reznick et al. (2004) found that guppies from high-predation environments had higher rates of decline in neuromuscular function, but they lived longer and had lower rates of reproductive aging than guppies from low-predation environments. Thus, there may not be a simple one-to-one relationship between physiological senescence and demographic decline.

The task of mapping out the relationship between genotype, physiological senescence and demographic senescence is no small challenge, but drawing these connections is crucially important. In the coming decades, the social and medical costs associated with physiological decline in aging humans will increase rapidly. We may gain most if we turn at least some of our attention from demographic quantity of life to physiological quality of life in evolutionary studies of aging. We see three primary areas where a more integrated approach, one that unites demography and physiology, can lead to a more comprehensive understanding of the biology of aging. In particular, we need to (1) develop more physiologically based theoretical models of senescence; (2) use classical quantitative genetic approaches to determine whether the genes that determine rates of physiological decline are the same ones that determine rates of demographic decline; and (3) include both physiological and demographic measures in molecular studies that are searching for specific genes and gene pathways that can slow the aging process. In the following section, we use the term *physiology* in its broadest sense—that is, the overall functioning of an organism. This includes organ performance, system function such as immunity (see Section IV), cell morphology, organismal behavior, and so forth. We need a broad definition as these non-demographic traits may overlap and interact in complex ways to ultimately determine the fitness parameters of age-specific fertility, fecundity, and survival.

A. Physiological Models of Senescence

Within the theoretical literature on aging, not all studies have ignored physiology. For example, Mangel (2001) incorporated an organism's energy level and the accumulated level of metabolic damage as physiological states into life-history models. These models predict how caloric restriction and reproduction affect the shape of the mortality curve. A physiologically structured model by Mangel and Bonsall (2004) predicts that the actual shape of the mortality curve can depend on physiological processes, such as growth and the level of repair. As information becomes available about the genetic control of declining organ function (e.g., Wessells *et al.*, 2004), we should be able to construct ever-more realistic models for the way in which physiological senescence relates to demographic senescence.

B. Quantitative Genetic Analyses of Physiology and Demography

We discussed earlier the need to develop a more complex and subtle model for the genetic architecture of aging. We would further suggest that a complete understanding of the genetics of demographic aging must include physiology. But the genetic relationship between physiological and demographic senescence may be complicated. Physiological senescence may be the functional intermediary between so-called "longevity genes" and demographic senescence (see Figure 8.2a). Alternatively, the same genes may regulate rates of senescence in both demography and certain physiological processes independently, such that the demographic decline may not be specifically caused by those physiological processes (see Figure 8.2b). Last, the two processes

could be both functionally and genetically independent (see Figure 8.2c). In a study on age-related changes in heart failure rate in *Drosophila*, Wessells and colleagues (2004) showed that long-lived insulin signaling mutants had much lower rates of heart failure. Although this study demonstrates that a gene that influences mortality rates also affects a physiological parameter, we do not know if heart failure plays any causal role in aging and/or death in fruit flies (the case illustrated in Figure 8.2b).

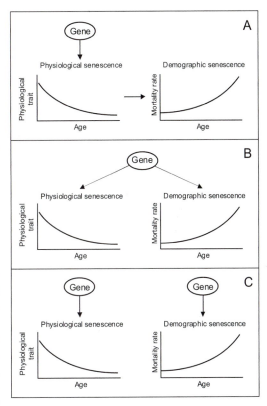

Figure 8.2 The influence of physiology in the genetics of senescence. The figure presents a schematic for three possible scenarios: (a) Genes influence physiological processes, which then lead to downstream effects on demographic senescence in mortality or fecundity. (b) The same genes that influence senescence in physiological processes independently determine rates of senescence in demographic traits. (c) Different genes determine rates of senescence in physiological and demographic processes.

Quantitative genetic studies have demonstrated that there is genetic variation for the rate of decline in age-specific survival (Hughes & Charlesworth, 1994; Promislow et al., 1996) and fecundity (Tatar et al., 1996). There is ample evidence to suggest that there is genetic variation for physiological traits in diverse taxa, from dairy cattle to *Drosophila* (Kiddy, 1979; Zera & Harshman, 2001). And we also know that genetic variation in longevity is correlated with underlying physiological differences (e.g., Djawdan *et al.*, 1998; Gibbs et al., 1997). But information about genetic variation for the age-related rate of decline in physiological function is rare (Wessells et al., 2004), and we know little about the genetic correlation with longevity and mortality parameters.

To map the relation between genotype and physiological and demographic senescence, we need to address a series of specific questions: Do genotypes that show a fast decline in physiological traits also have a higher rate at which intrinsic mortality increases with age? If an intervention extends life span through a decrease in the rate of increase in age-specific mortality rate, does it also decrease the rate of physiological deterioration? Alternatively, if an intervention extends life span through a decrease in the initial mortality rate, does the rate of physiological deterioration remain the same (see Chapter 1, Gavrilov and Gavrilova)? Is there a shared regulatory system that mediates the rate of deterioration for all physiological traits as predicted by Williams (1957), or is the genetic basis for the rate at which one trait deteriorates independent of the genetic basis for the rate at which another trait deteriorates? And finally, if the link between physiology and demography is not as straightforward as generally assumed, how does the shape of the selection curve change when physiological processes are incorporated into Hamilton's (1966) theoretical model?

C. Molecular Genetic Analyses of Physiology and Demography

As with evolutionary geneticists, molecular biologists working on aging have also tended to focus on demographic traits. This has been motivated in large part by the search for genes that will make organisms live longer, no matter what the physiological state of the animal. Of course, most biogerontologists hope to find ways to increase not only the quantity of life, but also the quality of life at late ages (Arantes-Oliveira et al., 2003). But to do this, we need a balanced research program that includes both demographic and physiological perspectives.

Fortunately, we are beginning to see just such a shift in focus. For example, Huang and colleagues (2004) found that the age-related decline in pharyngeal pumping and body movement in *C. elegans* was positively correlated with life span among a series of mutants. This suggests either that the decline in physiological processes causes a reduction in survival probability (see Figure 8.2a), or that the declines in physiological function and survival are regulated by a shared mechanism (see Figure 8.2b). Future work should focus on attempts to test these two hypotheses explicitly and should include demographic parameters other than longevity. Interestingly, Huang and colleagues (2004) found that the age-related decline in pharyngeal pumping and body movement were not correlated with self-fertile reproductive span. The authors speculate that other measures of reproductive aging may correlate with physiological decline. Alternatively, genes that affect aging may have pleiotropic effects on body movement and survival, but not on fecundity.

We are also likely to see substantial progress from studies of cellular physiology. Using a histological approach to study aging in *C. elegans*, Herndon and colleagues (2002) found that long-lived *age-1* mutants showed a slower rate of deterioration in cell ultrastructure. Interestingly, these lower rates were only seen in certain cell types.

Taken together, these two studies in *C. elegans* show that physiology is correlated with some but not all demographic traits (Huang *et al.*, 2004), and that demography is correlated with some but not all physiological traits (Herndon *et al.*, 2002). The challenge now before us is for theoretical, quantitative, and molecular geneticists to develop an integrated research program that incorporates genetics, physiology and demography to create a more integrated research program in biogerontology.

IV. Parasites and Immune Function

In the previous section, we argue that a critical challenge for evolutionary gerontologists is to bridge the gap between physiology and demography in studies of aging, and we propose some explicit ways in which this might be accomplished. One candidate for a ubiquitous factor that might tie together physiological senescence and demographic senescence is parasites.

We all have first-hand experience of the deleterious effects of parasites, and not surprisingly, there is abundant evidence for their life-shortening effects in model organisms. Likewise, when individuals are deprived of their normal bacterial flora they often show increased life span (e.g., Croll *et al.*, 1977; Garigan *et al.*, 2002; Houthoofd *et al.*, 2002; Larsen & Clarke, 2002; Min & Benzer, 1997). Recently, researchers have begun to identify molecular pathways that appear to have overlapping effects on survival and immune function. For instance, the secretion of juvenile hormone (JH) is crucial for several important reproductive pathways in insects, including gametogenesis and spermatophore production (Wigglesworth, 1965). However, increased JH titers have been shown to decrease immune function in the mealworm beetle (Rantala *et al.*, 2003; Rolff & Siva-Jothy, 2002) and to decrease longevity in monarch butterflies (Herman & Tatar, 2001). This apparent physiological antagonism between reproduction, immune function, and survivorship may play an important role in how insects age.

Although the proximate effects of parasites on longevity are often clear and straightforward, there are more subtle and interesting relationships between hosts and their parasites that may develop over evolutionary time. Parasites may play an important role in the evolution of a striking variety of biological traits, including the existence of sexual reproduction (Hamilton, 1980); the dramatic, dimorphic coloration in birds (Hamilton & Zuk, 1982); and the ability of organisms to invade novel habitats (Torchin *et al.*, 2003; Wolfe, 2002). And recent work on parasites and life-history strategies (Rolff & Siva-Jothy, 2003; Williams & Day, 2001) suggests that parasites may influence the way that natural selection shapes patterns of senescence.

A. From Immunosenescence to Demographic Senescence

We discussed the possibility that physiological decline may give rise to decline in fitness traits. One potentially important physiological factor is the age-related decline in immunocompetence, or "immunosenescence" (Walford, 1969). We have a pretty good idea of the proximate causes of immunosenescence in humans. For example, the thymus, where T cells mature, exhibits degenerative changes throughout life. Consequently, thymic tissue loses the capacity to influence a variety of important immune functions, including the repopulation of T cells in the lymph nodes (Hirokawa & Makinodan, 1975). Similarly, the sources of B cells, which fine-tune an antigen match for invading pathogens, begin to disappear over time (Leslie, 2004). This decline, coupled with a change in T-cell population with age, may lead to a decreased antibody response to most antigens (Weksler & Schwab, 1992). These age-specific changes in the immune system mark a dramatic physiological decline late in life that may greatly contribute to patterns of demographic senescence.

The cellular details differ, but this general pattern of immunosenescence is seen across an impressively broad array of species, including fish, birds, and reptiles (Torroba & Zapata, 2003). Insect species, including bumble bees, crickets, and dragonflies, also exhibit a marked age-related change in a variety of immune components, often leading to increased rates of parasitism and mortality (Adamo *et al.*, 2001; Doums *et al.*, 2002; Rolff, 2001). Even in the nematode, *C. elegans*, a positive association between age and susceptibility to bacterial infection is found (Laws *et al.*, 2004). Whether a causal relationship exists between immunosenescence and the age-specific decline in fitness, however, is currently unknown.

Immune senescence could contribute to a general physiological decline if, as the immune system ages, it requires increased resources to maintain the status quo. Consequently, there may be fewer resources available for other costly physiological systems. For example, in the collared flycatcher (*Ficedula albicollis*), older females tend to suffer from a decline both in humoral immune function and offspring size (Cichon *et al.*, 2003). However, more work is needed to determine whether the decline in offspring size is due to the increased energy demands of an aging immune system. Alternatively, the immune changes seen late in life may merely be a superficial marker of other underlying causes of aging. If so, then immunosenescence may serve as a useful biomarker of physiological age for future studies.

B. Immunocompetence Tradeoffs

Hamilton showed that the age-related decline in the strength of selection can be predicted solely on the basis of age-specific survival and fecundity (see Equations 2 and 3). Previous models have argued that these two traits should be negatively correlated because the amount of resources that can be invested in both is finite (de Jong & van Noordwijk, 1992). This tradeoff underlies Kirkwood's disposable soma theory for the evolution of senescence (Kirkwood, 1977). However, this framework may be incomplete. We suggest here that in addition to investment in survival and reproduction, it may be worth considering other intermediate physiological components as distinct model elements, such as neuron, circulatory, or immune function. For instance, if investment in immune function is directly correlated with both age-specific reproduction and age-specific survival (e.g., if the physiological costs of immunity affect fecundity and survival simultaneously), immune function may account for the correlation between fecundity and survival. This, in turn, will influence the age-related decline in the strength of selection.

To avoid parasites, potential hosts invest in a variety of defenses, some of which prevent infection in the first place and others of which fight off the parasite once an infection has taken hold. But these defenses can be costly. For example, increasing investment in immunity is often paid for with lower fecundity (Zuk & Stoehr, 2002). Conversely, among individuals who increase their investment in reproduction, we see a decrease not only in survivorship (Partridge & Harvey, 1985), but also in immunocompetence (e.g.,

Fedorka *et al.*, 2004). Most examples of these immune costs of reproduction come from insects. However, a recent study in women from 18th- and 19th-century Finland (Helle *et al.*, 2004) found that women who had born twins at some time in their reproductive life span were more likely to succumb to an infectious disease after menopause than women who had only given birth to singletons. This result held even after controlling for the total number of offspring born to each woman.

There is still much work to be done as we try to sort out how costs of parasitism and immunity are translated into the currency of demographic senescence. One important problem will be to determine how the physiological costs of mounting an immune response and the mortality costs of being parasitized change with age. Such changes can have complicated and nonintuitive consequences on mortality rates. In traditional models of either host–parasite coevolution or senescence, as background mortality rates increase, virulence and rates of aging also increase, respectively. In two separate theoretical studies, Williams and Day (2001; 2003) demonstrate that when extrinsic sources of mortality interact with the host's physiological state in a nonadditive fashion, virulence and rates of aging may actually decrease as background mortality rates increase. We now need theory that combines Williams and Day's models of parasitism (Williams & Day, 2001) and senescence (Williams & Day, 2003) and empirical tests of the existing theory. Such models should help us determine how selection should shape patterns of age-specific investment in immunity and age-specific survival, and how the two may interact.

C. Parasites and the Genetics of Aging

Studies of aging and immunity may also further our understanding of the genetic architecture of senescence. Recent stud-

ies have shown that many of the genes that affect longevity play an integral role in immune defense (Caruso *et al.*, 2001; Garsin *et al.*, 2003; Ivanova *et al.*, 1998; Lagaay *et al.*, 1991; Laws *et al.*, 2004). In some cases, immunity may be the proximate mechanism that gives rise to genes with antagonistic pleiotropic effects. For example, human centenarian studies have uncovered a strong association between Major Histocompatibility Complex (MHC) haplotypes and life span (Caruso *et al.*, 2001; Ivanova *et al.*, 1998; Lagaay *et al.*, 1991). At least one human leukocyte antigen haplotype, 8.1 AH, may provide a selective advantage in early infancy by providing protection from infectious disease (Caruso *et al.*, 2000). However, this haplotype is also associated with susceptibility to several autoimmune disorders that occur during reproductive adulthood, such as sarcoidosis and systemic lupus erythematosus (Lio *et al.*, 1997; Price *et al.*, 1999). Interestingly, this haplotype also provides a late-life, sex-specific advantage for male carriers, whereas female carriers continue to suffer from early morbidity and mortality late in life (Caruso *et al.*, 2000).

Such tradeoffs may turn out to be quite common for genes associated with immune function. Another example comes from the MHC mutation C28Y. This mutation increases the intestinal absorption of iron, which is crucial in many immune pathways (Salter-Cid *et al.*, 2000). However, the mutation is also associated with haemochromatosis in homozygotes, a disease characterized by a reduced life expectancy due to an excess accumulation of iron in the organs and concomitant reduction in immunity (Waheed *et al.*, 1997). Researchers have also suggested relationships between tuberculosis and Tay-Sachs disease (Spyropoulos, 1988), and cholera and cystic fibrosis (Gabriel *et al.*, 1994). In the past few years, biologists have begun to focus on the evolutionary consequences of immunity-related tradeoffs (reviewed in DeVeale *et al.*, 2004), although a detailed connection to senescence has yet to be made. Just how common these tradeoffs are, and whether some tradeoffs show age-specificity consistent with the antagonistic pleiotropy theory of senescence, remains to be seen. Finding such genes will provide an interesting challenge for those interested in developing an evolutionary perspective on immunosenescence.

Parasites may turn out to influence the genetics of aging in an even more general fashion. A recent study found that the ability of some genes to increase longevity depended on the presence of the bacterial flora (Brummel et al., 2004). For example, flies carrying the DJ817 mutant, which are normally long-lived, lost their life span advantage when treated with antibiotics. The same study showed that D. melanogaster males deprived of their normal bacterial complement in early adulthood suffered a significant reduction in life expectancy. In light of this interesting set of results, we should now set out to determine how many genes associated with longevity depend on the presence of bacteria for their phenotype, and of the many bacteria found in Drosophila, which ones are early-age symbionts and why.

D. Parasites and Sex Differences in Longevity

Finally, studies of parasites, immunity, and senescence may help us to understand why males and females often have quite different patterns of aging. Studies of immunosenescence have found that many of the MHC haplotypes associated with longevity are sex-dependent (Lagaay et al., 1991; Lio et al., 2002). Ivanova and colleagues (1998) found that of the three MHC alleles linked to human longevity in their study, two had a sex-dependent effect. Similarly, Lio and colleagues (2002) found a male-biased pattern among centenarians for polymorphisms in the promoter region of the IL-10 gene. IL-10

inhibits the pro-inflammatory immune response, which is believed to contribute substantially to mortality in late life. These patterns are not surprising considering that sex differences in immune function are widespread. Male mammals often have a lower level of immunocompetence (e.g., Klein & Nelson, 1997) and a higher rate of parasitic infection when compared to females (Moore & Wilson, 2002). Invertebrate males show a similar pattern (Adamo et al., 2001; Kurtz & Sauer, 2001; Kurtz et al., 2000; Radhika et al., 1998; Rolff, 2001), although due to the complex nature of life-history tradeoffs, sex differences in immune defense are often difficult to predict (Doums et al., 2002; Moret & Schmid-Hempel, 2000; Zuk et al., 2004; Zuk & Stoehr, 2002). These sex-specific patterns suggest that the selection pressures that influence immunity and longevity are different for males and females.

We have suggested here that sex-specific differences in immune function may account, in part, for sex differences in longevity. In the following section, we move away from immunity and explore causes of sex-related differences in longevity in greater detail.

V. Sex, Sexual Selection, and Sexual Conflict

Sex differences in longevity are common. Female mammals generally live longer than their male counterparts (Promislow, 1992), with a few interesting exceptions, such as among anthropoid primates with extended paternal care, where males live longer than females (Allman et al., 1998). Conversely, in birds (Promislow et al., 1992) and nematodes (McCulloch & Gems, 2003), males tend to outlive females. Many specific mechanisms have been proposed to account for these patterns, from differences in hormon profiles (e.g., testosterone levels in males) to differences in predation risk (e.g., vulnerability of nesting females).

It is likely that at least part of these differences is due to a basic disparity in reproductive strategies. A female's optimal reproductive strategy may be very different than that of her male partner (Rice, 1996). These differences may lead to very different age-specific selection pressures acting on the two sexes. We are only beginning to understand the full implications of these differences. In the following section, we describe three specific areas that could further our understanding of sex-specific patterns of senescence, including costs of reproduction, the proximate and evolutionary consequences of female choice, and intersexual conflict.

A. Cost of Reproduction

Reproduction can increase the mortality rate in many organisms (e.g., Fedorka et al., 2004; Sgrò & Partridge, 1999), but these costs can differ dramatically between the sexes in a range of organisms (Lyons & Dunne, 2003; Michener & Locklear, 1990; Rocheleau & Houle, 2001). Males and females may differ in the resources they allocate to gamete production, parental care, and mating effort. Dissimilar reproductive investment can, in turn, lead to differences in the risk of predation or sexually transmitted disease, or in the resources available for somatic maintenance. The evolution of sexually dimorphic traits through female choice or male competition exemplifies these sex-specific costs. To attract females or outcompete other males for access to mates, males often develop exaggerated secondary sexual characteristics, such as bright plumage or coloration, conspicuous calling songs, or large antlers. However, these traits may also attract predators or encumber the male when trying to escape from harm. Furthermore, these traits come at a large physiological cost and may reduce the resources that are available for immune defense or other traits, leading to reduced survival (Andersson, 1994). These changes in survival rates can then lead to sex-specific differences in the declining force of selection with age. At this point, we need sex-specific models to help us determine how sex differences in the risk of mortality might lead to sex differences in rates of aging.

B. Female Mate Choice

There is extensive evidence from different species suggesting that females will often choose to mate with males based on their genetic quality (Andersson, 1994). In so doing, choosy females may affect the evolution of senescence. For instance, according to Hamilton and Zuk (1982), female birds may use a male's bright coloration to assess his underlying ability to resist parasitic infection. If female choice thereby increases immunocompetence in the population, mean survival rates may increase, and selection on senescence will change accordingly.

Female choice may have a more direct effect on senescence in a population if females prefer to mate with males of a particular age. Some theoretical studies have suggested that females might choose to mate with older males because they have proven their ability to live long (Beck & Powell, 2000; but see Hansen & Price, 1995; Kokko, 1998). In their computer simulations, Beck and colleagues (2002) found that when females were allowed to choose males based on their age, they typically evolved a preference for older males. In a genetically heterogeneous population, older males will have a higher proportion of alleles associated with increased life span than younger males. Thus, female preference for older males leads not only to lower mortality rates in the choosy female's offspring, but will actually increase mean life span in the entire cohort over evolutionary time.

The theoretical findings that choosiness can lead to increased longevity are consistent with experimental studies in *Drosophila*. Promislow and colleagues (1998) compared mortality rates in strains that were maintained under enforced monogamy for multiple generations with strains where female choice and male–male competition were allowed. They found that the strains with higher levels of sexual selection evolved lower mortality rates. Similarly, among birds, female survival rates are highest in those species that appear to have been under stronger sexual selection (Promislow *et al.*, 1992). Further empirical work is needed to determine whether female preference for older males, in particular, can alter patterns of senescence in natural populations.

C. Sexual Conflict

Sexual conflict has also been suggested as playing a significant role in the evolution of senescence (Promislow, 2003; Svensson & Sheldon, 1998). Sexual conflict arises when the optimal reproductive strategy differs between the sexes. For example, a female may enhance her fitness by mating multiple times with different males, but this may reduce the fitness of each of her mates by diluting his sperm with those of his rivals. These conflicts can give rise to a situation where males, in an effort to maximize their fitness, evolve the capacity to dramatically reduce female fitness.

We have long known that male behavior can be detrimental to females: Parker and Thompson (1980) observed that, in the quest for mating opportunities, competing male dung flies (*Scatophaga stercoraria*) would often drown potential mates, leading to an obvious conflict of interest between the dying female and the overzealous male. Similarly, male bed bugs (*Cimex lectularius*) forcibly inseminate females by piercing their abdominal wall with needle-like genitalia, leading to high rates of female mortality (Stutt & Siva-Jothy, 2001). Conflict can even take place at a molecular level. In *Drosophila* spp., males pass accessory gland proteins (Acps) during copulation that may decrease a female's sexual receptivity, incapacitate previously donated sperm, prevent future sperm displacement (see Chapman *et al.*, 1995, and references therein), and increase the rate of oviposition (Heifetz *et al.*, 2000). Moreover, Acps tend to decrease a female's overall life expectancy in a dose-dependent manner (Chapman *et al.*, 1995; Lung *et al.*, 2002). And tying Acps more directly to longevity, Moshitzky and colleagues (1996) have shown that one of the sex peptides, a protein found in the male ejaculate, can induce the biosynthesis of juvenile hormone, which is associated with longevity (see Chapter 15, Tu *et al.*).

Further experiments are needed to determine whether sexual conflict can affect rates of senescence and differences in patterns of senescence between the sexes. Are rates of aging higher in species with greater sexual conflict? Do species with higher levels of conflict show greater sex-differences in rates of aging than species with lower levels of conflict? And are genes associated with conflict (such as Acps in *Drosophila*) also associated with variation in longevity in either sex?

VI. Genetic Variation in Natural Populations

In a separate chapter in this volume, Brunet-Rossinni and Austad (see Chapter 9) examine evidence for senescence in natural populations. Both lab and natural populations generally show similar Gompertz-like increases in mortality. However, several studies have shown that when we bring organisms into a lab environment, we often inadvertently expose them to novel selection pressures that lead to shorter life span [Sgrò & Partridge, 2000; Linnen *et al.*, 2001]. Thus, what we learn about the genetics of aging in the lab may not always transfer to the wild.

For many years, senescence was assumed to be rare in the wild (Comfort, 1979) because organisms were most likely to die by accident before they would have a chance to senesce. However, later studies demonstrated that senescence is not an artifact created by ideal laboratory conditions but is actually common in natural populations of mammals (Promislow, 1991) and birds (Ricklefs, 1998; 2000). We even see evidence for senescence in natural populations of insects. Bonduriansky and Brassil (2002) demonstrated aging in wild populations of very short-lived male antler flies, and Carey (2002) was even able to find evidence of aging in the famously short-lived mayfly. These new studies on aging in nature in short-lived animals suggest the possibility for developing free-living model systems to study the genetics of aging.

A few studies have demonstrated a genetic basis to variation in rates of aging in natural populations (e.g., Bronikowski *et al.*, 2002; Reznick *et al.*, 2004; Tatar *et al.*, 1997). Not surprisingly, most of what we know about the genetics of aging comes from lab studies. But we need to be especially cautious in assuming that what we learn in the lab translates directly to the field. We usually assume that an allele that increases longevity in a lab incubator will also increase longevity in the wild. Unfortunately, when we introduce natural populations into the lab, the change in environment can select for quite dramatic changes in demographic characteristics. Lab-adapted organisms typically mature earlier and have increased early-age fecundity and greatly shortened life span (Clark, 1987; Houle & Rowe, 2003; Miller *et al.*, 2002; Promislow & Tatar, 1998; Sgrò & Partridge, 2000). One might argue that the life-extending effects of novel mutants or artificial selection simply restore short-lived lab strains to the longevity of their wild relatives (Linnen *et al.*, 2001).

Recent studies from worms and flies point to two specific factors that we need to consider before assuming that lab results necessarily apply to wild populations. First, the effect of a mutation can depend on the environment in which an organism lives, due to gene by environment (G × E) interaction. The importance of G × E interactions in the genetics of longevity has been explored in great detail by Mackay and her co-workers (Chapter 7, Mackay *et al.*). Second, some studies appear to find life extension at no cost. For instance, the *daf-2* mutation in *C. elegans* can greatly extend longevity in the laboratory without apparent loss of fertility or activity (Kenyon *et al.*, 1993). However, when the long-lived *daf-2* mutant is combined with the wildtype strain in the same culture, the long-lived mutant is always outcompeted (Jenkins *et al.*, 2004). In general, it may turn out that when placed in a natural environment, genes that extend life span in the lab may have unanticipated negative consequences for fitness.

Several studies have now tried to determine whether alleles associated with longevity in the lab have similar functions in natural populations. Schmidt and colleagues (2000) showed that there is geographic variation in the frequency of *methuselah*, a *Drosophila* gene that can substantially increase longevity (Lin *et al.*, 1998). However, clinal variation in longevity was not correlated with clinal variation in single nucleotide polymorphisms at the *methuselah* gene. Other studies have had greater luck in applying lab-based results to field populations. Geiger-Thornsberry and Mackay (2004) studied genetic variation for genes associated with aging in the lab in wild-derived inbred strains of *Drosophila*.

Using quantitative complementation tests (see Chapter 7, Mackay *et al.*), they found that there was standing genetic variation at these loci in natural populations, and that this genetic variation was correlated with variation in longevity among strains. We now need to determine whether Geiger-Thornsberry and Mackay's findings with the *InR* and *Adh* genes are the exception or the rule, and how selection has shaped these loci over evolutionary time.

It is clearly important to determine whether genes identified in lab-reared populations of flies are effective at extending life span in natural populations. But an even greater challenge beckons. Can we translate lab-based findings to natural populations of different taxa? Can the genetic results for flies or worms in the lab be applied to natural populations of vertebrates? Researchers have suggested that various fish species, including killifish (Herrera & Jagadeeswaran, 2004), zebrafish (Gerhard, 2003; Gerhard & Cheng, 2002), and guppies (Reznick, 1997), may be ideal model systems to help bridge the gap between invertebrate and mammalian taxa in studies of aging. Reznick recently used a natural population of guppies to test the hypothesis that rates of senescence should be highest in populations with high extrinsic mortality (Reznick *et al.*, 2004). Interestingly, the data did not support this classic hypothesis, which reiterates the point we made earlier in this chapter that we need more biologically realistic models for the evolution of senescence.

Researchers have also argued that birds (Holmes *et al.*, 2001), bats (Wilkinson & South, 2002), and other "slow-aging" organisms (Austad, 2001) may be valuable model systems for the study of senescence. By extending the range of taxa that we use to study aging, we should be able to determine the extent to which mechanisms of aging are shared among taxa. Although there are distinct advantages to studying short-lived species, studying long-lived organisms in the wild (or the lab, for that matter) could add a new dimension to aging research (Holmes & Ottinger, 2003).

VII. Conclusions

The most important conceptual advances in our understanding of the evolution of senescence came from the initial models (Medawar, 1946; 1952; Williams 1957). Since the time of Medawar's and Williams's pioneering efforts, a half-century of evolutionary research has led to extraordinary advances in our understanding of evolutionary patterns and processes, from adaptation to altruism, from speciation to sex ratios. However, with few exceptions, these enormous conceptual advances have occurred independently of evolutionary studies of aging.

In this chapter, we have explored five areas that have excellent potential to further our understanding of the evolution of senescence. These include the genetic architecture of senescence, the relationship between physiological and demographic decline, the importance of parasites and the immune system, sex differences in behavior and aging, and studies of aging in the wild. Some of these areas include those in which we have already seen important advances by evolutionary biologists working outside of the field of aging. All are linked by the general problem of which forces will shape the age-related decline in the force of selection.

We hope that the questions that we have posed here will encourage more evolutionary biologists to take on the problem of the evolution of senescence. In the meantime, most of the action in biogerontological research appears to be found in the molecular labs, where new genes and gene pathways that affect aging are being uncovered at an extraordinary rate. One might ask, then, whether there is still a need for an evolutionary perspective in this fast-paced world of sequenced genomes and microarrays. We believe that the most exciting challenge facing all of us is to develop an integrated research program, where molecular and evolutionary biologists work hand in hand—molecular biologists asking evolutionary questions, evolutionary biologists using state-of-the-art molecular tools. With such an integration, as old problems are solved, new and interesting questions will arise at an even faster rate, ensuring that the study of aging continues to be exciting and enlightening.

Acknowledgements

We thank Thomas Flatt and members of the Promislow lab for thoughtful discussions. Richard Miller, Steve Austad, Edward Masoro, and one anonymous reviewer provided valuable comments on a previous draft of this manuscript. This work was supported by an NSF Minority post-doctoral fellowship from the National Science Foundation (KF) and a grant from the Ellison Medical Foundation (DP).

References

Abrams, P. A. (1993). Does increased mortality favor the evolution of more rapid senescence? *Evolution*, 47, 877–887.

Abrams, P. A., & Ludwig, D. (1995). Optimality theory, Gompertz' law, and the disposable-soma theory of senescence. *Evolution*, 49, 1055–1066.

Adamo, S. A., Jensen, M., & Younger, M. (2001). Changes in lifetime immunocompetence in male and female *Gryllus texensis* (formerly *G. integer*): trade-offs between immunity and reproduction. *Animal Behaviour*, 62, 417–425.

Albert, R., & Barabási, A.-L. (2002). Statistical mechanics of complex networks. *Reviews of Modern Physics*, 74, 47–97.

Albert, R., Jeong, H., & Barabasi, A. L. (2000). Error and attack tolerance of complex networks. *Nature*, 406, 378–382.

Allman, J., Rosin, A., Kumar, R., & Hasenstaub, A. (1998). Parenting and survival in anthropoid primates: caretakers live longer. *Proceedings of the National Academy of Sciences of the USA*, 95, 6866–6869.

Andersson, M. (1994). *Sexual selection: monographs in behavior and ecology*. Princeton, NJ: Princeton University Press.

Arantes-Oliveira, N., Berman, J. R., & Kenyon, C. (2003). Healthy animals with extreme longevity. *Science*, 302, 611.

Austad, S. N. (2001). An experimental paradigm for the study of slowly-aging organisms. *Experimental Gerontology*, 36, 599–605.

Beck, C. W., & Powell, L. A. (2000). Evolution of female mate choice based on male age: are older males better mates? *Evolutionary Ecology Research*, 2, 107–118.

Beck, C. W., Shapiro, B., Choksi, S., & Promislow, D. E. L. (2002). A genetic algorithm approach to study the evolution of female preference based on male age. *Evolutionary Ecology Research*, 4, 275–292.

Bonduriansky, R., & Brassil, C. E. (2002). Rapid and costly ageing in wild male flies. *Nature*, 420, 377–377.

Bronikowski, A. M., Alberts, S. C., Altmann, J., Packer, C., Carey, K. D., & Tatar, M. (2002). The aging baboon: comparative demography in a non-human primate. *Proceedings of the National Academy of Sciences of the USA*, 99, 9591–9595.

Brummel, T., Ching, A., Seroude, L., Simon, A. F., & Benzer, S. (2004). *Drosophila* life span enhancement by exogenous bacteria. *Proceedings of the National Academy of Sciences of the USA*, 101, 12974–12979.

Campisi, J. (2001). From cells to organisms: can we learn about aging from cells in culture? *Experimental Gerontology*, 36, 607–618.

Campisi, J. (2003). Cellular senescence and apoptosis: how cellular responses might influence aging phenotypes. *Experimental Gerontology*, 38, 5–11.

Carey, J. R. (2002). Longevity minimalists: life table studies of two species of northern Michigan adult mayflies. *Experimental Gerontology*, 37, 567–570.

Caruso, C., Candore, G., Colonna Romano, G., Lio, D., Bonafe, M., Valensin, S., & Franceschi, C. (2000). HLA, aging, and longevity: a critical reappraisal. *Human Immunology*, 61, 942–949.

Caruso, C., Candore, G., Romano, G. C., Lio, D., Bonafe, M., Valensin, S., & Franceschi, C. (2001). Immunogenetics of longevity. Is major histocompatibility complex polymorphism relevant to the control of human longevity? A review of literature data. *Mechanisms of Ageing and Development*, 122, 445–462.

Chapman, T., Liddle, L. F., Kalb, J. M., Wolfner, M. F., & Partridge, L. (1995). Cost of mating in *Drosophila melanogaster* is mediated by male accessory gland products. *Nature*, 373, 241–244.

Charlesworth, B. (2001). Patterns of age-specific means and genetic variances of mortality rates predicted by the mutation accumulation theory of aging. *Journal of Theoretical Biology*, 210, 47–65.

Charlesworth, B., & Hughes, K. A. (1996). Age-specific inbreeding depression and components of genetic variance in relation to the evolution of senescence. *Proceedings of the National Academy of Sciences of the USA*, 93, 6140–6145.

Cichon, M., Sendecka, J., & Gustafsson, L. (2003). Age-related decline in humoral immune function in Collared Flycatchers. *Journal of Evolutionary Biology*, 16, 1205–1210.

Clark, A. G. (1987). Senescence and the genetic correlation hang-up. *American Naturalist*, 129, 932–940.

Comfort, A. (1979). *The biology of senescence*. Edinburgh: Churchill Livingstone.

Croll, N. A., Smith, J. M., & Zuckerman, B. M. (1977). Behavioral parameters in aging of *C. elegans. Journal of Nematology*, 9, 266–267.

de Jong, G., & van Noordwijk, A. J. (1992). Acquisition and allocation of resources—genetic (co)variances, selection, and life histories. *American Naturalist*, 139, 749–770.

DeVeale, B., Brummel, T., & Seroude, L. (2004). Immunity and aging: the enemy within? *Aging Cell*, 3, 195–208.

Djawdan, M., Chippindale, A. K., Rose, M. R., & Bradley, T. J. (1998). Metabolic reserves and evolved stress resistance in *Drosophila melanogaster*. *Physiological Zoology*, 71, 584–594.

Doums, C., Moret, Y., Benelli, E., & Schmid-Hempel, P. (2002). Senescence of immune defense in *Bombus* workers. *Ecological Entomology*, 27, 138–144.

Edney, E. B., & Gill, R. W. (1968). Evolution of senescence and specific longevity. *Nature*, 220, 281–282.

Eisen, J. A., & Hanawalt, P. C. (1999). A phylogenomic study of DNA repair genes, proteins, and processes. *Mutation Research*, 435, 171–213.

Euler, L. (1760). Rechèrches générales sur la mortalité et la multiplication. *Mémoires de l'Académie Royale des Sciences et Belles Lettres*, 16, 144–164.

Fedorka, K. M., Zuk, M., & Mousseau, T. A. (2004). Immune suppression and the cost of reproduction in the ground cricket, *Allonemobius socius. Evolution*, 58, 2478–2485.

Finch, C. E., & Pike, M. C. (1996). Maximum life span predictions from the Gompertz mortality model. *Journal of Gerontology Series A Biological Sciences and Medical Sciences*, 51, B183–B194.

Fisher, R. A. (1930). *The genetical theory of natural selection*. Oxford: Clarendon Press.

Flatt, T. (2005). The evolutionary genetics of canalization. *Quarterly Review of Biology*, 80, 287–316.

Fraser, H. B., Hirsh, A. E., Steinmetz, L. M., Scharfe, C., & Feldman, M. W. (2002). Evolutionary rate in the protein interaction network. *Science*, 296, 750–752.

Fry, J. D., Nuzhdin, S. V., Pasyukova, E. G., & Mackay, T. F. (1998). QTL mapping of genotype-environment interaction for fitness in *Drosophila melanogaster*. *Genetics Research*, 71, 133–141.

Gabriel, S. E., Brigman, K. N., Koller, B. H., Boucher, R. C., & Stutts, M. J. (1994). Cystic fibrosis heterozygote resistance to cholera toxin in the cystic fibrosis mouse model. *Science*, 266, 107–109.

Garigan, D., Hsu, A. L., Fraser, A. G., Kamath, R. S., Ahringer, J., & Kenyon, C. (2002). Genetic analysis of tissue aging in *C. elegans*: a role for heat-shock factor and bacterial proliferation. *Genetics*, 161, 1101–1112.

Garsin, D. A., Villanueva, J. M., Begun, J., Kim, D. H., Sifri, C. D., Calderwood, S. B., Ruvkun, G., & Ausubel, F. M. (2003). Long-lived *C. elegans* daf-2 mutants are resistant to bacterial pathogens. *Science*, 300, 1921.

Geiger-Thornsberry, G. L., & Mackay, T. F. C. (2004). Quantitative trait loci affecting natural variation in *Drosophila* longevity.

Mechanisms of Ageing and Development, 125, 179–189.

Gerhard, G. S. (2003). Comparative aspects of zebrafish (*Danio rerio*) as a model for aging research. *Experimental Gerontology*, 38, 1333–1341.

Gerhard, G. S., & Cheng, K. C. (2002). A call to fins! Zebrafish as a gerontological model. *Aging Cell*, 1, 104–111.

Gibbs, A. G., Chippindale, A. K., & Rose, M. R. (1997). Physiological mechanisms of evolved desiccation resistance in *Drosophila melanogaster*. *Journal of Experimental Biology*, 200, 1821–1832.

Gibson, G., & Honeycutt, E. (2002). The evolution of developmental regulatory pathways. *Current Opinions in Genetics and Development*, 12, 695–700.

Haldane, J. B. S. (1941). *New paths in genetics*. London: Allen and Unwin.

Hamilton, W. D. (1966). The moulding of senescence by natural selection. *Journal of Theoretical Biology*, 12, 12–45.

Hamilton, W. D. (1980). Sex versus non-sex versus parasite. *Oikos*, 35, 282–290.

Hamilton, W. D., & Zuk, M. (1982). Heritable true fitness and bright birds: a role for parasites? *Science*, 218, 384–387.

Hansen, T. F., & Price, D. K. (1995). Good genes and old age: do old mates provide superior genes? *Journal of Evolutionary Biology*, 8, 759–778.

Heifetz, Y., Lung, O., Frongillo, E. A., Jr., & Wolfner, M. F. (2000). The *Drosophila* seminal fluid protein Acp26Aa stimulates release of oocytes by the ovary. *Current Biology*, 10, 99–102.

Helle, S., Lummaa, V., & Jokela, J. (2004). Accelerated immunosenescence in preindustrial twin mothers. *Proceedings of the National Academy of Sciences of the USA*, 101, 12391–12396.

Herman, W. S., & Tatar, M. (2001). Juvenile hormone regulation of longevity in the migratory monarch butterfly. *Proceedings of the Royal Society of London Series B Biological Sciences*, 268, 2509–2514.

Herndon, L. A., Schmeissner, P. J., Dudaronek, J. M., Brown, P. A., Listner, K. M., Sakano, Y., Paupard, M. C., Hall, D. H., & Driscoll, M. (2002). Stochastic and genetic factors influence tissue-specific decline in ageing *C. elegans*. *Nature*, 419, 808–814.

Herrera, M., & Jagadeeswaran, P. (2004). Annual fish as a genetic model for aging. *Journals of Gerontology Series A-Biological Sciences and Medical Sciences*, 59, 101–107.

Hirokawa, K., & Makinodan, T. (1975). Thymic involution: effect on T cell differentiation. *Journal of Immunology*, 114, 1659–1664.

Holmes, D. J., & Ottinger, M. A. (2003). Birds as long-lived animal models for the study of aging. *Experimental Gerontology*, 38, 1365–1375.

Holmes, D. J., Fluckiger, R., & Austad, S. N. (2001). Comparative biology of aging in birds: an update. *Experimental Gerontology*, 36, 869–883.

Houle, D., & Rowe, L. (2003). Natural selection in a bottle. *American Naturalist*, 161, 50–67.

Houston, A. I., & McNamara, J. M. (1999). *Models of adaptive behaviour*. Cambridge, UK: Cambridge University Press.

Houthoofd, K., Braeckman, B. P., Lenaerts, I., Brys, K., De Vreese, A., Van Eygen, S., & Vanfleteren, J. R. (2002). Axenic growth up-regulates mass-specific metabolic rate, stress resistance, and extends life span in *C. elegans*. *Experimental Gerontology*, 37, 1371–1378.

Huang, C., Xiong, C. J., & Kornfeld, K. (2004). Measurements of age-related changes of physiological processes that predict lifespan of *C. elegans*. *Proceedings of the National Academy of Sciences of the USA*, 101, 8084–8089.

Hughes, K. A., & Charlesworth, B. (1994). A genetic analysis of senescence in *Drosophila*. *Nature*, 367, 64–66.

Hughes, K. A., Alipaz, J. A., Drnevich, J. M., & Reynolds, R. M. (2002). A test of evolutionary theories of aging. *Proceedings of the National Academy of Sciences of the USA*, 99, 14286–14291.

Hwangbo, D. S., Gersham, B., Tu, M. P., Palmer, M., & Tatar, M. (2004). *Drosophila* dFOXO controls lifespan and regulates insulin signalling in brain and fat body. *Nature*, 429, 562–566.

Ivanova, R., Henon, N., Lepage, V., Charron, D., Vicaut, E., & Schachter, F. (1998). HLA-DR alleles display sex-dependent effects on survival and discriminate between individual and familial longevity. *Human Molecular Genetics*, 7, 187–194.

Jackson, A. U., Galecki, A. T., Burke, D. T., & Miller, R. A. (2002). Mouse loci associated with life span exhibit sex-specific and epistatic effects. *Journal of Gerontology Series A Biological Sciences and Medical Sciences*, 57, B9–B15.

Jenkins, N. L., McColl, G., & Lithgow, G. J. (2004). Fitness cost of extended lifespan in *C. elegans*. *Proceedings of the Royal Society of London Series B Biological Sciences*, 271, 2523–2526.

Jeong, H., Mason, S. P., Barabasi, A. L., & Oltvai, Z. N. (2001). Lethality and centrality in protein networks. *Nature*, 411, 41–42.

Kaiser, M., Gasser, M., Ackermann, R., & Stearns, S. C. (1997). P-element inserts in transgenic flies—A cautionary tale. *Heredity*, 78, 1–11.

Kenyon, C., Chang, J., Gensch, E., Rudner, A., & Tabtiang, R. (1993). A *C. elegans* mutant that lives twice as long as wild type. *Nature*, 366, 461–464.

Kiddy, C. A. (1979). Review of research on genetic variation in physiological characteristics related to performance in dairy cattle. *Journal of Dairy Science*, 62, 818–824.

Kimura, M. (1968). Evolutionary rate at the molecular level. *Nature*, 217, 624–626.

Kirkwood, T. B. L. (1977). Evolution and ageing. *Nature*, 270, 301–304.

Klein, S. L., & Nelson, R. J. (1997). Sex differences in immunocompetence differ between two *Peromyscus* species. *American Journal of Physiology*, 273, R655–R660.

Kokko, H. (1998). Good genes, old age and life-history trade-offs. *Evolutionary Ecology*, 12, 739–750.

Kowald, A., & Kirkwood, T. B. (1996). A network theory of ageing: the interactions of defective mitochondria, aberrant proteins, free radicals and scavengers in the ageing process. *Mutation Research*, 316, 209–236.

Krumbiegel, I. (1929). Untersuchungen über die Einwirkung der fortpflanzung auf Altern und Lebensdauer der Insekten: Carabas und *Drosophila*. *Zoologische Jahrbuch (Anatomie und Ontogenie der Tiere)*, 51, 111–162.

Krylov, D. M., Wolf, Y. I., Rogozin, I. B., & Koonin, E. V. (2003). Gene loss, protein sequence divergence, gene dispensability, expression level, and interactivity are correlated in eukaryotic evolution. *Genome Research*, 13, 2229–2235.

Kurtz, J., & Sauer, K. P. (2001). Gender differences in phenoloxidase activity of *Panorpa vulgaris* hemocytes. *Journal of Invertebrate Pathology*, 78, 53–55.

Kurtz, J., Wiesner, A., Gotz, P., & Sauer, K. P. (2000). Gender differences and individual variation in the immune system of the scorpionfly *Panorpa vulgaris* (Insecta: Mecoptera). *Developmental and Comparative Immunology*, 24, 1–12.

Lagaay, A. M., D'Amaro, J., Ligthart, G. J., Schreuder, G. M., van Rood, J. J., & Hijmans, W. (1991). Longevity and heredity in humans. Association with the human leukocyte antigen phenotype. *Annals of the New York Academy of Sciences*, 621, 78–89.

Larsen, P. L., & Clarke, C. F. (2002). Extension of life-span in *C. elegans* by a diet lacking coenzyme Q. *Science*, 295, 120–123.

Laws, T. R., Harding, S. V., Smith, M. P., Atkins, T. P., & Titball, R. W. (2004). Age influences resistance of *C. elegans* to killing by pathogenic bacteria. *FEMS Microbiology Letters*, 234, 281–287.

Lee, R. D. (2003). Rethinking the evolutionary theory of aging: transfers, not births, shape senescence in social species. *Proceedings of the National Academy of Sciences of the USA*, 100, 9637–9642.

Leips, J., & Mackay, T. F. (2000). Quantitative trait loci for life span in *Drosophila melanogaster*: interactions with genetic background and larval density. *Genetics*, 155, 1773–1788.

Leslie, M. (2004). All pain, no gain. *Science of Aging Knowledge Environment*, 27, 1–4.

Lewontin, R. C., & White, M. J. D. (1960). Interaction between inversion polymorphisms and two chromosome pairs in the grasshopper, *Moraba scurra*. *Evolution*, 14, 116–129.

Li, W.-H. (1997). *Molecular evolution*. Sunderland, MA: Sinauer Associates.

Libina, N., Berman, J. R., & Kenyon, C. (2003). Tissue-specific activities of *C. elegans* DAF-16 in the regulation of lifespan. *Cell*, 115, 489–502.

Lin, Y. J., Seroude, L., & Benzer, S. (1998). Extended life-span and stress resistance in the *Drosophila* mutant methuselah. *Science*, 282, 943–946.

Linnen, C., Tatar, M., & Promislow, D. E. L. (2001). Cultural artifacts: a comparison of senescence in natural, lab-adapted and artificially selected lines of *Drosophila melanogaster*. *Evolutionary Ecology Research*, 3, 877–888.

Lio, D., Candore, G., Romano, G. C., D'Anna, C., Gervasi, F., Di Lorenzo, G., Modica, M. A., Potestio, M., & Caruso, C. (1997). Modification of cytokine patterns in subjects bearing the HLA-B8,DR3 phenotype: implications for autoimmunity. *Cytokines Cell Mol. Ther.* 3, 217–224.

Lio, D., Scola, L., Crivello, A., Colonna-Romano, G., Candore, G., Bonafe, M., Cavallone, L., Franceschi, C., & Caruso, C. (2002). Gender-specific association between -1082 IL-10 promoter polymorphism and longevity. *Genes Immun*, 3, 30–33.

Lotka, A. J. (1925). *Elements of physical biology*. Baltimore, MD: Williams & Watkins.

Luckinbill, L. S., Arking, R., Clare, M. J., Cirocco, W. J., & Buck, S. A. (1984). Selection for delayed senescence in *Drosophila melanogaster*. *Evolution*, 38, 996–1003.

Lung, O., Tram, U., Finnerty, C. M., Eipper-Mains, M. A., Kalb, J. M., & Wolfner, M. F. (2002). The *Drosophila melanogaster* seminal fluid protein Acp62F is a protease inhibitor that is toxic upon ectopic expression. *Genetics*, 160, 211–224.

Lyons, D. O., & Dunne, J. J. (2003). Reproductive costs to male and female worm pipefish. *Journal of Fish Biology*, 62, 767–773.

Mangel, M. (2001). Complex adaptive systems, aging and longevity. *Journal of Theoretical Biology*, 213, 559–571.

Mangel, M., & Bonsall, M. B. (2004). The shape of things to come: using models with physiological structure to predict mortality trajectories. *Theoretical Population Biology*, 65, 353–359.

Martin, G. M. (1997). The Werner mutation: does it lead to a "public" or "private" mechanism of aging? *Molecular Medicine*, 3, 356–358.

Maslov, S., Sneppen, K., Eriksen, K. A., & Yan, K. K. (2004). Upstream plasticity and downstream robustness in evolution of molecular networks. *BMC Evolutionary Biology*, 4, 9.

Masoro, E. J. (Ed.) (1995). *Handbook of Physiology* (Section 11: Aging). New York: Oxford University Press.

McCulloch, D., & Gems, D. (2003). Evolution of male longevity bias in nematodes. *Aging Cell*, 2, 165–173.

McDonald, J. F. (1993). Evolution and consequences of transposable elements. *Current Opinions in Genetics and Development*, 3, 855–864.

Medawar, P. B. (1946). Old age and natural death. *Modern Quarterly*, 2, 30–49.

Medawar, P. B. (1952). *An unsolved problem in biology*. London: H. K. Lewis.

Michener, G. R., & Locklear, L. (1990). Differential costs of reproductive effort for male and female Richardsons ground-squirrels. *Ecology*, 71, 855–868.

Miller, R. A., Harper, J. M., Dysko, R. C., Durkee, S. J., & Austad, S. N. (2002). Longer life spans and delayed maturation in wild-derived mice. *Experimental Biology and Medicine*, 227, 500–508.

Min, K. T., & Benzer, S. (1997). *Wolbachia*, normally a symbiont of *Drosophila*, can be virulent, causing degeneration and early death. *Proceedings of the National Academy of Sciences of the USA*, 94, 10792–10796.

Moore, S. L., & Wilson, K. (2002). Parasites as a viability cost of sexual selection in natural populations of mammals. *Science*, 297, 2015–2018.

Moret, Y., & Schmid-Hempel, P. (2000). Survival for immunity: the price of immune system activation for bumblebee workers. *Science*, 290, 1166–1168.

Moshitzky, P., Fleischmann, I., Chaimov, N., Saudan, P., Klauser, S., Kubli, E., & Applebaum, S. W. (1996). Sex-peptide activates juvenile hormone biosynthesis in the *Drosophila melanogaster corpus allatum*. *Archives of Insect Biochemistry and Physiology*, 32, 363–374.

Mueller, L. D., Drapeau, M. D., Adams, C. S., Hammerle, C. W., Doyal, K. M., Jazayeri, A. J., Ly, T., Beguwala, S. A., Mamidi, A. R., & Rose, M. R. (2003). Statistical tests of demographic heterogeneity theories. *Exp Gerontol*, 38, 373–386.

Mueller, L. D., & Rose, M. R. (1996). Evolutionary theory predicts late-life mortality plateaus. *Proceedings of the National Academy of Sciences of the USA*, 93, 15249–15253.

Nikitin, A. G., & Shmookler Reis, R. J. (1997). Role of transposable elements in age-related genomic instability. *Genetics Research*, 69, 183–195.

Nuzhdin, S. V., Pasyukova, E. G., Dilda, C. L., Zeng, Z.-B., & Mackay, T. F. C. (1997). Sex-specific quantitative trait loci affecting longevity in *Drosophila melanogaster*. *Proceedings of the National Academy of Sciences of the USA*, 94, 9734–9739.

Parker, G. A., & Thompson, E. A. (1980). Dung fly struggles—a test of the war of attrition. *Behavioral Ecology and Sociobiology*, 7, 37–44.

Partridge, L., & Gems, D. (2002a). The evolution of longevity. *Current Biology*, 12, R544–R546.

Partridge, L., & Gems, D. (2002b). Mechanisms of ageing: public or private? *Nature Reviews Genetics*, 3, 165–175.

Partridge, L., & Harvey, P. (1985). Costs of reproduction. *Nature*, 316, 20.

Pletcher, S. D., Macdonald, S. J., Marguerie, R., Certa, U., Stearns, S. C., Goldstein, D. B., & Partridge, L. (2002). Genome-wide transcript profiles in aging and calorically restricted *Drosophila melanogaster*. *Current Biology*, 12, 712–723.

Price, P., Witt, C., Allcock, R., Sayer, D., Garlepp, M., Kok, C. C., French, M., Mallal, S., & Christiansen, F. (1999). The genetic basis for the association of the 8.1 ancestral haplotype (A1, B8, DR3) with multiple immunopathological diseases. *Immunol Rev*, 167, 257–274.

Promislow, D. E. L. (1991). Senescence in natural populations of mammals: a comparative study. *Evolution*, 45, 1869–1887.

Promislow, D. E. L. (1992). Costs of sexual selection in natural populations of mammals. *Proceedings of the Royal Society (London): Biological Sciences*, 247, 203–210.

Promislow, D. E. L. (2003). Mate choice, sexual conflict, and evolution of senescence. *Behavioral Genetics*, 33, 191–201.

Promislow, D. E. L. (2004). Protein networks, pleiotropy and the evolution of senescence.

Proceedings of the Royal Society Series B (London), 271, 1225–1234.

Promislow, D. E. L., & Bronikowski, A. M. (in press). Evolutionary genetics of senescence. In C. W. Fox and J. B. Wolf (Eds.), *Evolutionary genetics: concepts and case studies*. Oxford: Oxford University Press.

Promislow, D. E. L., & Tatar, M. (1998). Mutation and senescence: where genetics and demography meet. *Genetica*, 102/103, 299–314.

Promislow, D. E. L., Montgomerie, R. D., & Martin, T. E. (1992). Mortality costs of sexual dimorphism in birds. *Proceedings of the Royal Society (London): Biological Sciences*, 250, 143–150.

Promislow, D. E. L., Smith, E. A., & Pearse, L. (1998). Adult fitness consequences of sexual selection in *Drosophila melanogaster*. *Proceedings of the National Academy of Sciences of the USA*, 95, 10687–10692.

Promislow, D. E. L., Tatar, M., Khazaeli, A., & Curtsinger, J. W. (1996). Age-specific patterns of genetic variance in *Drosophila melanogaster*. I. Mortality. *Genetics*, 143, 839–848.

Radhika, M., Abdul Nazar, A. K., Munuswamy, N., & Nellaippan, K. (1998). Sex-linked differences in phenoloxidase in the fairy shrimp *Streptocephalus dichotomous* Baird and their possible role (Crustacea: Anostraca). *Hydrobiologia*, 377, 161–164.

Rantala, M. J., Vainikka, A., & Kortet, R. (2003). The role of juvenile hormone in immune function and pheromone production trade-offs: a test of the immunocompetence handicap principle. *Proceedings of the Royal Society of London Series B Biological Sciences*, 270, 2257–2261.

Reznick, D. N. (1997). Life history evolution in guppies (*Poecila reticulata*): guppies as a model for studying the evolutionary biology of aging. *Experimental Gerontology*, 32, 245–258.

Reznick, D. N., Bryant, M. J., Roff, D., Ghalambor, C. K., & Ghalambor, D. E. (2004). Effect of extrinsic mortality on the evolution of senescence in guppies. *Nature*, 431, 1095–1099.

Rice, W. R. (1996). Sexually antagonistic male adaptation triggered by experimental arrest of female evolution. *Nature*, 381, 232–234.

Ricklefs, R. E. (1998). Evolutionary theories of aging: confirmation of a fundamental prediction, with implications for the genetic basis and evolution of life span. *American Naturalist*, 152, 24–44.

Ricklefs, R. E. (2000). Intrinsic aging-related mortality in birds. *Journal of Avian Biology*, 31, 103–111.

Rocheleau, A. F., & Houle, G. (2001). Different cost of reproduction for the males and females of the rare dioecious shrub *Corema conradii* (Empetraceae). *American Journal of Botany*, 88, 659–666.

Rolff, J. (2001). Effects of age and gender on immune function of dragonflies (Odonata, Lestidae) from a wild population. *Canadian Journal of Zoology*, 12, 2176–2180.

Rolff, J., & Siva-Jothy, M. T. (2002). Copulation corrupts immunity: a mechanism for a cost of mating in insects. *Proceedings of the National Academy of Sciences of the USA*, 99, 9916–9918.

Rolff, J., & Siva-Jothy, M. T. (2003). Invertebrate ecological immunology. *Science*, 301, 472–475.

Rose, M. R. (1991). *Evolutionary biology of aging*. Oxford: Oxford University Press.

Rose, M. R., & Charlesworth, B. (1980). A test of evolutionary theories of senescence. *Nature*, 287, 141–142.

Salter-Cid, L., Peterson, P. A., & Yang, Y. (2000). The major histocompatibility complex-encoded HFE in iron homeostasis and immune function. *Immunology Research*, 22, 43–59.

Schmidt, P. S., Duvernell, D. D., & Eanes, W. F. (2000). Adaptive evolution of a candidate gene for aging in *Drosophila*. *Proceedings of the National Academy of Sciences of the USA*, 97, 10861–10865.

Service, P. M. (2000). Heterogeneity in individual mortality risk and its importance for evolutionary studies of senescence. *American Naturalist*, 156, 1–13.

Sgrò, C. M., & Partridge, L. (1999). A delayed wave of death from reproduction in *Drosophila*. *Science*, 286, 2521–2524.

Sgrò, C. M., & Partridge, L. (2000). Evolutionary responses of the life history of wild-caught *Drosophila melanogaster* to two standard methods of laboratory culture. *American Naturalist*, 156, 341–353.

Shook, D. R., & Johnson, T. E. (1999). Quantitative trait loci affecting survival and fertility-related traits in *C. elegans* show genotype-environment interactions,

pleiotropy and epistasis. *Genetics*, 153, 1233–1243.

Siegal, M. L., & Bergman, A. (2002). Waddington's canalization revisited: developmental stability and evolution. *Proceedings of the National Academy of Sciences of the USA*, 99, 10528–10532.

Snoke, M. S., & Promislow, D. E. (2003). Quantitative genetic tests of recent senescence theory: age-specific mortality and male fertility in *Drosophila melanogaster*. *Heredity*, 91, 546–556.

Sozou, P. D., & Kirkwood, T. B. (2001). A stochastic model of cell replicative senescence based on telomere shortening, oxidative stress, and somatic mutations in nuclear and mitochondrial DNA. *Journal of Theoretical Biology*, 213, 573–586.

Spencer, C. C., Howell, C. E., Wright, A. R., & Promislow, D. E. L. (2003). Testing an 'aging gene' in long-lived *Drosophila* strains: increased longevity depends on sex and genetic background. *Aging Cell*, 2, 123–130.

Spyropoulos, B. (1988). Tay-Sachs carriers and tuberculosis resistance. *Nature*, 331, 666.

Stutt, A. D., & Siva-Jothy, M. T. (2001). Traumatic insemination and sexual conflict in the bed bug Cimex lectularius. *Proceedings of the National Academy of Sciences of the USA*, 98, 5683–5687.

Svensson, E., & Sheldon, B. C. (1998). The social context of life history evolution. *Oikos*, 83, 466–477.

Tatar, M., Bartke, A., & Antebi, A. (2003). The endocrine regulation of aging by insulin-like signals. *Science*, 299, 1346–1351.

Tatar, M., Gray, D. W., & Carey, J. R. (1997). Altitudinal variation for senescence in *Melanoplus* grasshoppers. *Oecologia*, 111, 357–364.

Tatar, M., Kopelman, A., Epstein, D., Tu, M. P., Yin, C. M., & Garofalo, R. S. (2001). A mutant *Drosophila* insulin receptor homolog that extends life-span and impairs neuroendocrine function. *Science*, 292, 107–110.

Tatar, M., Promislow, D. E. L., Khazaeli, A., & Curtsinger, J. W. (1996). Age-specific patterns of genetic variance in *Drosophila melanogaster*. II. Fecundity and its genetic correlation with age-specific mortality. *Genetics*, 143, 849–858.

Tissenbaum, H. A., & Guarente, L. (2001). Increased dosage of a sir-2 gene extends lifespan in *C. elegans*. *Nature*, 410, 227–230.

Torchin, M. E., Lafferty, K. D., Dobson, A. P., McKenzie, V. J., & Kuris, A. M. (2003). Introduced species and their missing parasites. *Nature*, 421, 628–630.

Torroba, M., & Zapata, A. G. (2003). Aging of the vertebrate immune system. *Microscopy Research and Technique*, 62, 477–481.

van Swinderen, B., & Greenspan, R. J. (2005). Flexibility in a gene network affecting a simple behavior in *Drosophila melanogaster*. *Genetics*, 169, 2151–2163.

Vaupel, J. W., Baudisch, A., Dolling, M., Roach, D. A., & Gampe, J. (2004). The case for negative senescence. *Theoretical Population Biology*, 65, 339–351.

Vaupel, J. W., Carey, J. R., Christensen, K., Johnson, T. E., Yashin, A. I., Holm, N. V., Iachine, I. A., Kannisto, V., Khazaeli, A. A., Liedo, P., Longo, V. D., Zeng, Y., Manton, K. G., & Curtsinger, J. W. (1998). Biodemographic trajectories of longevity. *Science*, 280, 855–860.

Wagner, A. (2000). Robustness against mutations in genetic networks of yeast. *Nature Genetics*, 24, 355–361.

Waheed, A., Parkkila, S., Zhou, X. Y., Tomatsu, S., Tsuchihashi, Z., Feder, J. N., Schatzman, R. C., Britton, R. S., Bacon, B. R., & Sly, W. S. (1997). Hereditary hemochromatosis: effects of C282Y and H63D mutations on association with beta2-microglobulin, intracellular processing, and cell surface expression of the HFE protein in COS-7 cells. *Proceedings of the National Academy of Sciences of the USA*, 94, 12384–12389.

Walford, R. L. (1969). *The immunological theory of aging*. Copenhagen: Munksgaard.

Walker, D. W., McColl, G., Jenkins, N. L., Harris, J., & Lithgow, G. J. (2000). Evolution of lifespan in *C. elegans*. *Nature*, 405, 296–297.

Weismann, A. (1891). *Essay on heredity and kindred biological problems* (2nd ed., Vol. 1.). Oxford: Clarendon Press.

Weksler, M. E., & Schwab, R. (1992). The immunogenetics of immune senescence. *Experimental and Clinical Immunogenetics*, 9, 182–187.

Wessells, R. J., Fitzgerald, E., Cypser, J. R., Tatar, M., & Bodmer, R. (2004). Insulin regulation of heart function in aging fruit flies. *Nature Genetics*, 36, 1275–1281.

Wigglesworth, V. B. (1965). Juvenile hormone. *Nature*, 208, 522.

Wilkinson, G. S., & South, J. M. (2002). Life history, ecology and longevity in bats. *Aging Cell*, 1, 124–131.

Williams, G. C. (1957). Pleiotropy, natural selection, and the evolution of senescence. *Evolution*, 11, 398–411.

Williams, G. C. (1999). The Tithonus error in modern gerontology. *Quarterly Review of Biology*, 74, 405–415.

Williams, P. D., & Day, T. (2001). Interactions between sources of mortality and the evolution of parasite virulence. *Proceedings of the Royal Society London Series B Biological Sciences*, 268, 2331–2337.

Williams, P. D., & Day, T. (2003). Antagonistic pleiotropy, mortality source interactions, and the evolutionary theory of senescence. *Evolution*, 57, 1478–1488.

Wolf, J. B., Brodie, E. D. I., & Wade, M. J. (2000). *Epistasis and the evolutionary process*. Oxford: Oxford University Press.

Wolfe, L. M. (2002). Why alien invaders succeed: support for the escape-from-enemy hypothesis. *American Naturalist*, 160, 705–711.

Woodruff, R. C., & Nikitin, A. G. (1995). P DNA element movement in somatic cells reduces lifespan in *Drosophila melanogaster*: evidence in support of the somatic mutation theory of aging. *Mutation Research*, 338, 35–42.

Wright, S. (1932). The roles of mutation, inbreeding, crossbreeding and selection in evolution. *Proceedings of the Sixth International Congress of Genetics*, 1, 356–366.

Zera, A. J., & Harshman, L. G. (2001). The physiology of life history trade-offs in animals. *Annual Review of Ecology and Systematics*, 32, 95–126.

Zuk, M., & Stoehr, A. M. (2002). Immune defense and host life history. *American Naturalist*, 160, S9–S22.

Zuk, M., Simmons, L. W., Rotenberry, J. T., & Stoehr, A. M. (2004). Sex differences in immunity in two species of field crickets. *Canadian Journal of Zoology*, 82, 627–634.

Chapter 9

Senescence in Wild Populations
of Mammals and Birds

Anja K. Brunet-Rossinni and Steven N. Austad

I. Introduction

Senescence or, synonymously in this chapter, aging can be defined as the progressive deterioration in physiological function that accompanies increasing adult age. Like the proverbial elephant described by blind men, it has many visible forms, depending on your perspective. For instance, to a geriatrician, senescence is evident as an age-related increase in frailty or vulnerability and a mounting incidence and severity of degenerative diseases. To a demographer, it is most easily measured as an age-related increase in the probability of death, and to an evolutionary biologist, senescence might describe the progressive decline in age-specific Darwinian fitness components. These are all valid embodiments of senescence; however, some will be more easily observed and measured in natural populations and less easily confounded by other phenomena than others. Also, various signs of senescence may appear at different ages.

It has long been conjectured, particularly in the biomedical community, that animals in nature do not experience senescence (Comfort, 1979; Hayflick, 2000; Medawar, 1952). Among ecologists, such a general assumption has never been advanced; however, some animal groups, particularly birds and fishes, have been identified as likely to die at a constant rate in nature, irrespective of age (Deevey, 1947). Even this more restricted statement has met with subsequent skepticism from field biologists. Botkin and Miller (1974) pointed out that if annual mortality rate were indeed independent of age, then one or more of the royal albatrosses seen by Captain Cook during his first visit to New Zealand in 1769 should still be alive today! As remarkable as avian longevity might be, that is a hard tale to swallow. The *Guinness Book of Records* lists the oldest royal albatross identified to date as 53 years old.

The notion that animals do not senesce in nature arises from an implicit belief that life in the wild is so nasty and brutish, so beset by predation, pestilence,

Handbook of the Biology of Aging, Sixth Edition

foul weather, famine, and drought that animals must inevitably die before signs of senescence appear. According to this intuition, only under the protected conditions of captivity (or civilization) does aging become manifest. No doubt such a scenario describes life for some species. For instance, multiple field studies of house mice (*Mus musculus*) indicate that median longevity in nature is only about 3 to 4 months, with 90 percent of deaths occurring by about 6 months of age (Phelan & Austad, 1989)—ages at which senescence is indeed not readily observable even in the laboratory. This is in contrast to the 2- to 3-year mean longevity under protected conditions (Turturro *et al.* 1999).

On the other hand, the *general* claim of negligible senescence in the wild, despite its persistence in the biogerontological literature, is quite clearly incorrect, as we will show. We are not suggesting that animals in nature reach the advanced state of decrepitude found in the city or the laboratory, but only that an observable age-related decline in function is not rare.

In this article, we review evidence for senescence in birds and mammals in the wild. We have limited our survey to birds and mammals not because they are uniquely senescence-prone, but to keep the size of our review manageable and also because of the availability of numerous long-term field studies in which individuals have been monitored for a number of years, sometimes throughout life, for these two animal groups. Such studies are not *required* to detect senescence, but they are the most likely to do so. Such studies also avoid many of the pitfalls of less intensive studies. We discuss the nature of these pitfalls later on.

It is important to note that detecting senescence is the primary goal of few if any field studies. Data relevant to senescence are usually adventitiously acquired while investigating other issues. Therefore, the failure to detect senescence in a study

may say more about the length, design, and intensity of the study than the probability that the population under study did, or did not, exhibit signs of senescence.

II. Evidence of Senescence in Wild Populations

A. Demographic Senescence

The majority of articles assessing senescence in natural populations have focused on detecting an age-related increase in mortality rate (actuarial or survival senescence) and/or decrease in reproductive rate (reproductive senescence). Together we call these measures of *demographic* senescence. Increasing age-specific mortality in adulthood is widely used as the gold standard of senescence, both in natural and in laboratory populations. This choice stems from the assumption that age-specific death rate is a good indicator of intrinsic physiological hardiness. As hardiness declines with age, the probability of death should rise. Such a rise has often been found in natural populations. For instance, Promislow's (1991) analysis of 56 published life tables from mammal field studies found statistically significant evidence for survival senescence in 44 percent (26) of the studies and a nonsignificant trend in the same direction in a further 34 percent (20) of the studies. Thus, there was at least some reason to suspect the existence of senescence in nearly four of five published mammal field studies. Later, Gaillard and colleagues (1994) published a slightly more conservative reanalysis of the same data but still found statistically compelling evidence for senescence in 42 percent (25 of 59) of data sets.

Sometimes, as in the previously mentioned Royal Albatross, survival senescence can be inferred by the lack of survivors above a certain age. For instance, Ian Nisbet has been studying the common tern, a small seabird, at an island off the Massachusetts coast for more than 30 years and has individually marked thousands of birds. The annual observed adult survival rate is 0.9. If survival rate were independent of age, then about 5 percent of adults (assuming adulthood begins at age 2) should survive to 30 years of age and 1 percent should survive 45 years. However, direct observation finds that the 5 percent survival age is 18 years and the longest-lived bird seen so far is only 26 years old (Nisbet, 2001).

Measurement of survival senescence has some practical difficulties when applied to wild populations, however. One such complication is seasonality. For instance, a number of small mammals develop in the spring, mature in the summer and autumn, and tend to die in the winter. Among species such as these, increasing age-related mortality rate could indicate senescence but could just as easily indicate increasing environmental harshness from summer to autumn to winter. That is, even if no physiological deterioration has occurred in the study populations, morality rate could still increase with age. Consequently, increasing mortality rate with age does not by itself unequivocally demonstrate senescence in the wild.

Another problem is environmental change with unknown effects on demography. For instance, the common tern colony studied by Nisbet and colleagues grew from about 500 breeders in 1970 to about 4,500 breeders in 1992. An early report from this colony suggested that several markers of reproductive function (clutch size, egg volume) decreased with age (Nisbet *et al.*, 1984). However a much later report found no evidence of reproductive senescence (Nisbet *et al.*, 2002). Whether this difference was due to the increased population density, some other environmental factor, or simply more and better information is not clear.

In addition to complications involving seasonality or environmental change, several other factors warrant caution in interpreting the *failure* to find increasing mortality as indicating an *absence* of senescence. First, for any given cohort, nonseasonal, stochastic environmental factors may override or mask even the very real effects of age on physical state. As one example, a classic study of house sparrows found that a New England winter storm preferentially killed birds that were particularly large or small relative to the mean size in the population (Bumpus, 1898). Body size is not related to age in birds, therefore the storm likely killed birds with little if any relation to their age. However the mortality from that single event might have overwhelmed any underlying age-related pattern. Stochastic climatic events can also depress food availability, which is likely to lead to more risk-taking by foragers and thus a generally higher mortality rate. Environmental events of this type can confound detection of survival senescence or its absence.

Significantly, dead animals are seldom recovered in field studies. Death is typically assumed when marked animals disappear from a study area, but they could also have emigrated. As a result, mortality and emigration can easily be conflated. In addition, if individual identification is by tags or bands, these markers can fall off. If so, a death will be mistakenly recorded. Third, even if death can be unambiguously detected, mortality rates can easily be affected by behavior as well as by intrinsic deterioration. For instance, animals engaging in high-risk behaviors will obviously die at higher rates than their more cautious peers. If animals in certain age classes are particularly prone to risky behavior, underlying physical senescence patterns again may be masked (see Figure 9.1). Are there particular ages at which animals in nature are prone to engage in high-risk behaviors? Indeed, as in humans, adolescent and newly maturing animals frequently take exceptional risks. Typically, birds and mammals disperse from their birth site around the time

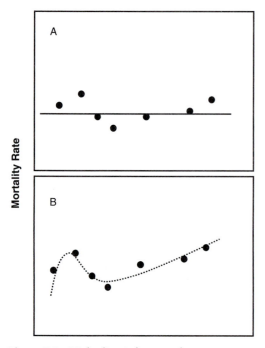

Figure 9.1 Misleading inference of no senescence caused by elevated risk-taking during dispersal or territory acquisition. A. Regression from points sampled. B. Underlying mortality pattern. •Ages sampled. Dashed line = actual adult mortality trajectory, solid line = inferred mortality trajectory from 5 sampled ages.

of sexual maturity to seek and compete for new territories and/or mates. Venturing through unknown areas and competing for territories or mates can be very dangerous. In one of the few studies in which this "dispersal risk" could be quantified, female water-voles (*Arvicola terrestris*) died at at least an 86-fold higher rate during dispersal than when remaining in their natal home range (Leuze, 1980). Any such behavior-mediated elevation of mortality rate in early life will require that statistical analyses be sensitive to the possibility that temporary, early life mortality spikes might make a simple Gompertzian analysis of the entire adult life somewhat misleading (see Figure 9.1).

Survival is only part of demography. An age-related decline in reproductive performance can also be a sensitive indicator

of physical senescence. For instance, among human females, fertility declines are detectable by about age 30, an age of minimal senescence by other measures (Dunson *et al.*, 2004; Shock, 1983). One main difficulty with using reproductive function as a measure of senescence is that, like age-specific mortality, environmental events can mask underlying patterns. Hard times—food shortages, temperature extremes, exceptional predator abundance—rather than aging may depress reproduction in a study population. Reproductive performance also has the disadvantage that it is generally much easier to monitor in one sex (females) relative to the other. So, too, there are subtleties of reproductive senescence that will be difficult to detect in either field or laboratory. For instance, reproductive senescence may manifest itself as a decline in the phenotypic quality of offspring from older females rather than a straightforward reduction in number of eggs or newborns (Saino *et al.*, 2002). As another example, slow growth of unweaned pups rather than reduced litter size marked reproductive senescence in Virginia opossums (Austad, 1993).

Both reproductive and survival senescence can also be difficult to detect in the presence of infectious disease. The relationship between senescence and disease is complex (see Masoro, Chapter 2). Decreased reproductive performance near the very end of life might as easily reflect infectious status as senescence *per se*. For instance, in a long-term study of an oceanic bird species, the black-legged kittiwake, Coulson and Fairweather (2001) observed depressed reproductive performance in the final breeding period prior to death in birds of all ages. Because this was observed in young as well as old birds, the authors interpreted this pattern as a sign of terminal illness, not senescence, although these are clearly not mutually exclusive.

Such difficulties aside, an extensive but not exhaustive survey of the literature turned up evidence for demographic senescence (either survival or reproductive) in natural populations of 42 species of mammals and 35 species of birds (summarized in Tables 9.1 and 9.2). Included in this list are the 26 species for which Promislow (1991) found statistically significant (P < 0.1) evidence of senescence. We excluded from this list data on captive or semi-wild populations and claims of senescence based only on secondary sources. However, we included any article in which the authors claimed evidence of senescence in natural populations or in which we could easily detect such evidence from the published data even if the author(s) failed to note it.

In addition to the studies we cite, of course, a number of studies have failed to find demographic senescence. However, because these studies varied in their intensity and evidentiary methodology, it

Table 9.1

Literature presenting evidence of senescence in wild populations of mammals. Survival senescence refers to an increasing age-specific mortality rate. Measures used as evidence of reproductive senescence are listed for each species and symbol in parenthesis indicates which sex was studied. Arrows indicate direction of change in variable with increasing age. Column labeled as "other" contains information regarding changes in behavior or morphology associated with increasing age.

Species	Survival senescence	Reproductive senescence	Other
Didelphis virginiana **Virginia opossum**	Austad, 1993	↑ infertility, ↓ pouch young growth rate (♀) Austad, 1993	
Pipistrellus pipistrellus **Pipistrelle bat**	Promislow 1991		
Macaca mulatta **Rhesus macaque**	Promislow 1991		
Macaca fuscata **Japanese macaque**		↓ birth rate (♀) Wolfe & Noyes 1981	
Papio hamadryas **Baboon**	Bronikowski *et al.* 2002 Packer *et al.* 1998	↓ maternity rate, ↓ fertility (♀) Packer *et al.* 1998	
Lutra canadensis **River otter**	Promislow 1991		
Martes zibellina **Sable marten**	Promislow 1991		
Panthera leo **African Lion**	Packer *et al.* 1998 Promislow 1991	↓ maternity rate (♀) Packer *et al.* 1998 ↓ surviving cubs/male (♂) Packer *et al.* 1988	
Ursus arctos **Brown bear**	Promislow 1991		
Ursus maritimus **Polar bear**		↓ litter size and mass (♂) Derocher & Stirling 1994	↓ body mass (♀) Derocher & Stirling 1994
Alces alces **Moose**	Ericsson *et al.* 2001	↓ litter size, ↑ offspring mortality (♀) Ericsson *et al.* 2001 ↓ fertility Heard *et al.* 1997	

(continues)

Table 9.1 *(Cont'd)*

Species	Survival senescence	Reproductive senescence	Other
Dama dama **Fallow deer**	McElligott *et al.* 2002	↓ reproduction probability (♂) McElligott *et al.* 2002	
Aepyceros melampus **Impala**	Promislow 1991		
Hemitragus jemlahicus **Himalayan tahr**	Promislow 1991		
Ovis dalli **Dall's sheep**	Promislow 1991		
Kobus kob **Kob**	Promislow 1991		
Rupicapra rupicapra **Chamois**	Promislow 1991		
Cervus elaphus **Red deer**	Clutton-Brock *et al.* 1988	↓ fecundity, ↑ calf mortality (♀) Clutton-Brock 1984 ↓ reproduction probability (♂) Clutton-Brock *et al.* 1979	↓ body mass Mysterud *et al.* 2001 ↓ control of harems (♂) Clutton-Brock *et al.* 1979
Tragelaphus strepsicerus **Greater kudu**	Owen-Smith 1993		
Syncerus caffer **African buffalo**	Sinclair, 1977 Promislow 1991	↓ pregnancy rate (♀) Sinclair, 1977, Grimsdell, 1969	
Ovis musimon **Mouflon**			↓ parental care (♀) Réale & Boussès 1995
Hippopotamus amphibious **Hippopotamus**	Promislow 1991		
Phacochoerus aethiopicus **Desert warthog**	Promislow 1991		
Lutra canadensis **River otter**	Promislow 1991		
Martes zibellina **Sable marten**	Promislow 1991		
Panthera leo **African Lion**	Packer *et al.* 1998 Promislow 1991	↓ maternity rate (♀) Packer *et al.* 1998 ↓ surviving cubs/male (♂) Packer *et al.* 1988	
Ursus arctos **Brown bear**	Promislow 1991		
Ursus maritimus **Polar bear**		↓ litter size and mass (♀) Derocher & Stirling 1994	↓ body mass (♀) Derocher & Stirling 1994
Lepus europaeus **European hare**	Promislow 1991		

(continues)

Table 9.1   *(Cont'd)*

Species	Survival senescence	Reproductive senescence	Other
Oryctolagus cuniculus **European rabbit**	Promislow 1991		
Sylvilagus floridanus **Eastern cottontail**	Promislow 1991		
Equus burchelli **Burchell's zebra**	Promislow 1991		
Callorhinus ursinus **Northern fur seal**	Promislow 1991		
Arctocephalus gazelle **Antarctic fur seal**		↓ reproductive rates (♀) Lunn *et al.* 1994	
Phoca hispida **Ringed seal**	Promislow 1991		
Pan troglodytes **Chimpanzee**	Promislow 1991	↓ birth rate (♀) Sugiyama 1994	
Loxodonta Africana **African elephant**	Promislow 1991		
Microtus agrestis **Field vole**	Promislow 1991		
Apodemus flavicollis **Yellow-necked mouse**	Promislow 1991		
Peromyscus maniculatus **Deer mouse**	Millar 1994 Promislow 1991		
Peromyscus leucopus **White-footed mouse**		↓ litter size of old, large females Morris 1996	
Tamiasciurus hudsonicus **Red squirrel**	Promislow 1991		
Spermophilus colombianus **Colombian ground squirrel**		↑ unsuccessful litters (♀) Broussard *et al.* 2003	

Table 9.2

Literature presenting evidence of senescence in wild populations of birds. Survival senescence refers to an increasing age-specific mortality rate. Measures used as evidence of reproductive senescence are listed for each species and arrows indicate direction of change in variable with increasing age. Column labeled as "other" contains information regarding changes in behavior or morphology associated with increasing age.

Species	Survival senescence	Reproductive senescence	Other
Aphelocoma coerulescens **Florida scrub jay**	McDonald *et al.* 1996	↓ number of fledglings, ↓ offspring survival Fitzpatrick & Woolfenden 1988	
Pica pica **Black-billed Magpie**		↓ clutch size Birkhead & Goodburn 1989	

(continues)

Table 9.2   (*Cont'd*)

Species	Survival senescence	Reproductive senescence	Other
Bucephala clangula **Common goldeneye**		↓ brood survival Milonoff *et al.* 2002 ↓ clutch and brood size Dow & Fredga 1984	
Larus glaucescens **Glaucous-winged gull**		↓ egg volume, ↓ hatching success Reid 1988	
Sula granti **Nazca booby**		↓ fledging success Anderson & Apanius, 2003	
Larus delawarensis **Ring-billed gull**		↓ hatching success Haymes & Blokpoel 1980	
Larus californicus **California gull**	Pugesek 1987 Pugesek *et al.* 1995		
Larus canus **Common gull**	Rattiste & Lilleleht 1987		
Fulmarus glacials **Northern Fulmar**	Dunnet & Ollason 1978	↓ breeding success Ollason & Dunnet 1978 ↓ fecundity, ↓ breeding success Ollason & Dunnet 1988	
Rissa tridactyla **Black-legged Kittiwake**	Aebischer & Coulson 1990 Coulson & Wooller 1976	↓ fledgling production Thomas 1983	
Somateria mollissima **Common Eider**	Coulson 1984	↓ reproductive output Bailey & Milne 1982	
Puffinus tenuirostris **Short-tailed shearwater**	Bradley *et al.* 1989	↓ reproductive performance Wooller *et al.* 1990	
Phalacrocorax aristotelis **Shag**	Aebischer 1986 Harris *et al.* 1994		
Catharacta skua **Great skua**		↓ clutch volume Hamer & Furness 1991 ↓ clutch size Ratcliffe *et al.* 1998	
Diomedea exulans **Wandering albatross**	Weimerskirch 1992	↓ egg size, ↓ breeding success and frequency Weimerskirch 1992	
Sterna hirundo **Common tern**		↓ clutch size, ↓ egg volume Nisbet *et al.* 1984	
Sterna paradisaea **Arctic tern**		↓ clutch size and volume Coulson & Horobin 1976	
Chen caerulescens **Snow goose**		↓ hatchability, ↑ brood loss Rockwell *et al.* 1993	

(*continues*)

Table 9.2   *(Cont'd)*

Species	Survival senescence	Reproductive senescence	Other
Hirundo rustica **Barn swallow**	Møller & de Lope 1999	↓ offspring quality Saino et al. 2002 ↓ number of fledglings, ↓ reproductive value Møller & de Lope 1999	↑ ectoparasite load, ↓ secondary sexual characters, ↑ fluctuating asymmetry, ↓ body mass, delayed arrival from migration Møller and de Lope 1999; ↓ humoral immunity Saino *et al.* 2003
Tachycineta bicolor **Tree swallow**		↓ breeding performance index Robertson & Rendell 2001	
Calidris temminckii **Temminck's stint**	Hilden 1978		
Parus major **Great tit**	Dhondt 1989	↓ nesting success, ↓ brood size, ↓ juvenile survival Dhondt 1989 ↓ hatching rate, ↓ fledgling survival Perrins & Moss 1974	
Parus caeruleus **Blue tit**		↓ nesting success, ↓ clutch and brood size, ↓ juvenile survival Dhondt 1989	
Parus montanus **Willow tit**	Orell & Belda 2002		
Pyrrhocorax pyrrhocorax **Red-billed chough**		↓ clutch size, ↓ fledging success Reid et al. 2003b	
Ficedula albicollis **Collared flycatcher**		↓ successful broods, ↓ number of fledglings, ↓ clutch size Gustafsson & Pärt 1990	↓ humoral immune response Cichon *et al.* 2003
Ficedula hypoleuca **Pied flycatcher**	Sternberg 1989		
Parus atricapillus **Black-capped chickadee**	Loery *et al.* 1987		
Acrocephalus sechellensis **Seycelles warbler**		↓ hatching success, ↓ number of fledglings Komdeur 1996	
Melospiza melodia **Song sparrow**		↓ number of fledglings Nol & Smith 1987	↓ Cell-mediated immune response Reid *et al.* 2003a

(continues)

Table 9.2 *(Cont'd)*

Species	Survival senescence	Reproductive senescence	Other
Anthus spinoletta **Rock pipit**		↓ second clutch size Askenmo & Unger 1986	
Geospiza conirostris **Large cactus finch**	Grant & Grant 1989		
Tetrao tetrix **Black grouse**		↓ copulation success (♂) Kruijt & de Vos 1988	
Accipiter nisus **European Sparrowhawk**	Newton & Rothery 1997	↓ reproductive output Newton *et al.* 1981 ↓ clutch size, ↓ number of young/nest, ↓ egg size Newton 1988 ↓ annual production of young, ↓ reproductive value Newton and Rothery 1997	
Aegolius funereus **Tengmalm's owl**		↓ clutch size (♂) Laaksonen *et al.* 2002	

is not possible to identify general patterns concerning species that exhibit senescence in nature relative to those that do not. For one thing, failure to observe a phenomenon of interest likely leads to reporting bias. That is, negative results often go unpublished.

This is not to say that some very thorough studies have failed to find demographic senescence. For instance, a 17-year study of Southern elephant seals tracked 1,650 individually marked pups throughout their lives. Although only 5 percent of the marked animals survived even to age 10, no statistically significant increase in age-specific mortality rate could be detected even as late as between ages 10 and 17 (Pistorius & Bester, 2002). A 30-year study of the common tern (*Sterna hirundo*) in which about 60,000 chicks have been banded has not found evidence of reproductive senescence even among the oldest 5 percent of birds in the population (Nisbet *et al.*, 2002).

Besides practical difficulties in measuring demographic senescence in nature, there are also theoretical difficulties. For instance, if animals increase reproduction with age, and there is a tradeoff between reproduction and survival, as predicted by Williams (1957) and empirically verified by many others (e.g., Koivula *et al*, 2003; Orell & Belda, 2002), then declining survival with age might reveal nothing more than increasing reproduction rather than an independently deteriorating internal state. Although evolutionary theories of senescence, such as antagonistic pleiotropy and mutation accumulation (Medawar, 1952; Williams, 1957), do not specifically predict a decline in fertility or increase in death risk alone with age, they do predict declining reproductive expectations with age. Reproductive expectations incorporate both reproduction and survival. This is why Partridge and Barton (1996) suggest Fisher's "reproductive value," which utilizes both reproduction and survival to quantify expected current and future reproduction as the best metric for assessing senescence. An interesting case illustrating the problem and how such an analytical approach may be useful is Pugesek's long-term study of California gulls (Pugesek, 1987; Pugesek & Diem, 1990; Pugesek *et al.*, 1995). Older birds in this study died at higher rates than younger birds, hence by the standard criterion of survival senescence, they aged. However, older birds also raised more chicks to fledging than did younger birds. Feeding and protecting young in the nest is energetically taxing and physically risky. That is, there is a cost to reproduction. Controlling for reproduction by comparing young (3- to 10-year-old) birds with older (11- to 17-year-old) ones that fledged the same number of young, no difference in yearly survival could be detected (Pugesek, 1987).

A potentially useful way of envisioning demographic senescence is to assess the maintenance of adaptive tradeoffs between reproduction and somatic survival as they occur in young adults. For instance, Broussard and colleagues (2003) found that the oldest Colombian ground squirrels (*Spermophilus colombianus*) in their study population were more likely than younger age classes to experience reproductive failure. Moreover, young females failing to reproduce regained healthy body mass lost during their reproductive attempt, whereas old females did not. Thus, the adaptive tradeoff between reproductive and somatic investment appears to deteriorate in old age in the Colombian ground squirrel. It is not unexpected that tradeoffs like other adaptive traits deteriorate with age and decaying physiology. This type of deterioration may provide a better indication of the effects of physiological degeneration than purely demographic parameters. Moreover, such deteriorating tradeoffs could potentially produce physiological/demographic patterns that we do not normally recognize as senescence (Blarer et al., 1995).

B. Nondemographic Measures of Senescence

The failure to find demographic evidence of senescence does not necessarily mean that animals are not experiencing it. As previously mentioned, environmental or behavioral factors may overwhelm subtle demographic indicators; therefore, physiological markers of functional decline might serve as alternative or complementary sources of information. Note that the indicators used here only need document that later life decline in function has occurred. They do not need to be useful as markers of the *rate* of functional loss. For instance, studies of three bird species have presented evidence of a decline in immune function with advancing age (Cichón et al., 2003; Reid et al., 2003a; Saino et al., 2003). Although the long-held view that aging is accompanied by a monolithic decline in immune function is gradually being supplanted by a more nuanced view that aging alters immune response in complex, potentially adaptive ways (Effros, 2001), it is probably still a safe generalization that deteriorating resistance to infectious agents is a hallmark of physiological senescence. Indeed, autopsy data on humans implicated infections in the deaths of a majority of people older than 80 years in a Japanese population (Horiuchi & Wilmoth, 1997).

Declining immunity with age seems widespread among species. It is well documented in humans and laboratory rodents of course, but it has also been reported in song sparrows (Reid et al., 2003a) and rhesus macaques (Coe & Ershler, 2001). Particularly interesting field studies combine assessment of immune competence with demographic parameters. Intriguingly, in barn swallows, humoral immunity as measured by antibody response to injection of Newcastle Disease Virus declined in females 3 years old or older relative to 1-and 2-year olds (Saino et al, 2003), but no such decline was observed in males. Survival senescence could only be detected in birds age 5 and older, whereas reproductive senescence as measured by number of fledglings produced began to decline by age 4. Thus, the decline in female immune function preceded indicators of demographic senescence. It might therefore be assumed that immune function decline is a more sensitive indicator of senescence than demographic parameters.

However, the situation is not so simple. In the collared flycatchers, a much different pattern is seen. Humoral immunity (response to injected sheep red blood cells) did not decline significantly until 5 to 6 years of age, whereas reproductive and survival performance declined after age 3 (Cichón et al., 2003; Møller & De Lope, 1999). In this case, demographic senescence preceded immunosenescence. Thus, one can't generalize about the sensitivity of immune markers of physiological senescence in wild animals. It is most useful to have both physiological and demographic measures of senescence whenever possible.

A few studies have adduced age-related declines in body mass as evidence of senescence (Berubé et al., 1999; Derocher & Stirling, 1994; Mysterud et al., 2001). The general sensitivity of body mass decline as an indicator of aging is not clear. There is substantial variability among laboratory mouse sexes and genotypes in the timing of body mass decrease relative to patterns of demographic senescence (Turturro et al., 1999). However, in the laboratory, with ad lib feeding and minimal energetic demands, body mass may decline at a more advanced age compared to the wild. Senescence in nature can affect body mass by decreasing the ability to obtain, process, and store food (Ericsson et al., 2001). For instance, tooth wear may be a significant contributor to age-related mortality in some mammals (Ericsson et al. 2001; Skogland, 1988). Tooth wear increases markedly in roe deer after the age of 7 and coincides with a decrease in survival rate (Gaillard et al., 1993). Indeed, the strongest evidence for changes in body mass relating to senescence are when simultaneous changes occur in demographic parameters. Thus, both lit-

ter size and body mass increase for female polar bears (Ursus maritimus) until ages 14 to 16, and thereafter both decline (Derocher & Stirling, 1994). However, this is not always the case, as shown by bighorn ewe body mass, which began declining at about age 11 in one study, about three years before a reduction in fertility was observed but four years after survival senescence became evident (Jorgenson et al., 1997). In sum, the meaning and reliability of age-related body mass decline as a marker of physical senescence is far from clear.

Senescence could potentially be seen as well in a reduced ability to provide nourishment to offspring. Mammary glands themselves may senesce due to a decreasing replicative capacity of mammary epithelial cells with age (Daniel, 1977). In support of this phenomenon, the lambs of old mouflon (Ovis musimon) ewes suckle less frequently, decrease total suckling time, and spend more time grazing relative to lambs of younger ewes (Réale & Boussès, 1995).

Other nondemographic indicators of senescence exist in specific instances. For instance, the ability to defend a territory or other more mobile resource such as a harem may decline with age. On the Scottish island of Rhum, the reproductive success of red deer stags declines after age 11 due to a decreased ability to fight and control harems (Clutton-Brock et al., 1979). However, this is not always true even in harem-defending species, as shown by the absence of a similar phenomenon in the American pronghorn (Byers, 1998). From the female side, calf mortality increases for red deer hinds over 12 years of age. Survival of calves depends partially on its mother's dominance rank and access to a good-quality home range, both of which decline as females age (Clutton-Brock, 1984). Therefore, change in dominance rank may serve as a marker of senescence in some species.

The ability to defend a territory declines with age in a number of species. In the small passerine bird, the great tit (*Parus major*), male territory size increases until 4 years of age and then decreases from 5 years throughout the rest of life. Some old great tits forego defending a territory altogether, although they still manage some breeding by mating with females late in the year (Dhondt, 1971). Male black grouse (*Tetrao tetrix*) defend territories that females attend only to breed. Those 6 years and older seldom occupy the highest-quality territories on display grounds, likely because they cannot defend them (Kruijt & de Vos, 1988). By contrast, young male greater white-lined bats (*Saccopteryx bilineata*) lurk on the periphery of older males' breeding territories, copulating with females opportunistically. No reports exist of males so old that they can no longer defend their territory. This may be a case where significant senescence is not seen in the wild (Heckel & Von Helversen, 2002). Hormones may serve as markers of senescence as well. Plasma testosterone level in Misaki feral horses correlates with age and harem size (Khalil et al., 1998). If senescent males no longer can mount and maintain appropriate testosterone levels during the breeding season, their ability to recruit a harem may become compromised. Thus, hormonal and reproductive aging decline synchronously.

Sometimes demographic senescence can be observed even when other well-characterized indicators of senescence cannot be detected. For instance, common terns exhibit survival senescence, yet no decline can be detected over their lifetime in immunological, endocrinological, or reproductive aging (Apanius & Nisbet, 2003).

In birds, where renewal of feathers must occur annually after molting, one might expect that the ability to produce long, healthy feathers might decrease with age. Indeed, Møller and De Lope (1999) found that both tail and wing length decreased in barn swallows 5 years old or older. In addition, these aged birds had less perfect symmetry between left and right wing and tail feathers compared with younger birds.

Finally, as biochemical markers of aging become available, studies that involve recapturing individuals can focus on directly measuring deteriorating physiology from blood or urine samples, though assays will need to be validated for the particular study organism. Regardless of the measures selected to test for senescence in natural populations, it is critical to have detailed understanding of the dynamics of the study population, the physiology of the study organism, and the life history trade-offs individuals face over their life span.

III. Patterns of Senescence

Can we glean anything about general patterns of senescence in wild populations from the information currently available? The first and most important point is that one should exercise caution when accepting and comparing published data on senescence in the wild (Nisbet, 2001). Apparent senescence can arise from short-term climatic events such as El Niño or increasing population density over the course of a study. The literature must be interpreted with sensitivity to variation among studies in the methods used to collect and analyze demographic data. Second, senescence, measured as changes in life-history traits and physical function associated with old age, is a complex phenomenon. It can defy our expectations about which species should and should not show signs of senescence and at what point during the life course indicators of senescence might become apparent. It is also critical to remember that patterns of senescence are not necessarily species-specific but may vary among populations within a species (Austad, 1993).

Generally, senescence is expected to be more apparent among species of low mortality rates and long life span because senescence reduces average life span more in such species (Ricklefs, 1998) and because high mortality rates significantly reduce the chances of any individual reaching a senescent age or remaining alive in a senescent state for long enough to be detected. However, some short-lived animals with high mortality rates have been demonstrated to experience senescence. For example, small rodents typically experience high mortality rates and small mice rarely live more than one year in the wild. Despite this, Promislow (1991) and Millar (1994) both found evidence of actuarial senescence in populations of deer mice (*Peromyscus maniculatus*), and Morris (1996) found evidence of reproductive senescence in white-footed mice (*Peromyscus leucopus*; see Table 9.1).

Is there a general age or developmental stage that is a threshold for the onset of senescence generally? Evolutionary senescence theory (Williams, 1957) suggests that aging should begin at about the time of sexual maturity. Although observations consistent with the theory have been reported for a German population of pied flycatchers (Sternberg, 1989) as well as Florida scrub jays (McDonald et al., 1996), it was not found in any of five populations of three species of ungulates (roe deer, bighorn sheep, Pyrenean chamois) (Loison et al., 1999). In a particularly thorough long-term (12 to 22 years) study, age at first reproduction in all five populations was 2 years, yet annual female survival rate high remained high (>0.9) with no statistical decline at least until age 7. Another potential stage at which senescence could conceivably begin is "social maturity," the age at which animals are capable of actively competing for reproductive

opportunities, often somewhat later than the time of sexual maturation. McElligott and colleagues (2002) evaluated such a situation in male fallow deer (*Dama dama*). They found that social maturation began at 4 to 5 years, yet annual survival rate did not begin to decrease until age 9. An even more complex situation is found in bighorn sheep (*Ovis canadensis*), in which the onset of survival senescence did not coincide with age of first reproduction in females, but did in males (i.e., rutting decreased male survival rate) (Jorgenson et al., 1997). Thus, no clear pattern about the timing of senescence's onset emerges from field data.

One point that does emerge though is that patterns of mortality dynamics in nature can be dramatically different than in captive populations. For instance, animals in captivity often exhibit Gompertzian mortality dynamics (Finch, 1990)—that is, a monotonically log-linear increase age-specific mortality rate—but many long-lived mammals and birds in nature have a more phase-specific relationship between survival, reproduction, and age. That is, survival and reproduction are relatively low and variable in young adults, both increase and remain steady in prime-aged animals, and then both decrease again in oldest individuals (Berubé et al., 1999; Caughley, 1966; Festa-Bianchet et al., 2003). Some of the difference between captive and wild populations may be explained by the greater phenotypic variability within populations in nature due to some combination of differential genetic endowment, consequent differential access to important resources, and discrete social roles. A case in point is the previously mentioned study of fallow bucks (McElligott et al., 2002). Overall, mortality dynamics fit well with a Gompertz model. However, when the population was subdivided into nonreproducers (animals that had ceased to breed later in life) and producers (animals still actively reproducing) irrespective of age, nonreproducers' survival declined after age 9 but reproducers showed no change in survival even to much later ages.

A related question concerns whether there are general patterns in the timing of the beginning of reproductive senescence *vis à vis* survival senescence? To take one well-known example, in humans, age-specific mortality increases from the age of 10 to 11 years in societies with access to modern medicine (Finch, 1990), whereas subtle evidence of reproductive senescence only becomes apparent by about age 30 (vom Saal *et al.*, 1994). Is this appearance of survival senescence prior to reproductive senescence a general phenomenon? Apparently not. Although such a pattern is seen in female bighorn sheep (Berubé *et al.*, 1999, Jorgenson *et al.*, 1997), European sparrowhawks (Newton & Rothery, 1997), European red deer (Clutton-Brock *et al.*, 1988), baboons and African lions (Packer *et al.*, 1998), the reverse—reproductive senescence preceding survival senescence—is seen in barn swallows (Møller & De Lope, 1999; Saino *et al.*, 2003) and wandering albatrosses (Weimerskirch, 1992). The difference between onset of reproductive and survival senescence can be substantial. In bighorn ewes, survival senescence appears by age 7 to 8 but reproductive senescence only after 13 years (Berubé *et al.*, 1999; Jorgenson *et al.*, 1997). Similarly, both male and female red deer (*Cervus elaphus*) experience survival senescence after 8 years of age, but reproductive senescence does not appear until age 12, as evidenced by declining female fecundity and increasing calf mortality (Clutton-Brock, 1984) and the loss of males' ability to control harems (Clutton-Brock *et al.*, 1979). In contrast, wandering albatrosses (*Diomedea exulans*) exhibit decreased egg size, breeding success, and breeding frequency after age 20 but survival decreases significantly only after age 27 (Weimerskirch, 1992).

Although the previous discussion and our summary tables have primarily focused on species patterns, it is worth recalling that not all populations of a species will necessarily exhibit the same pattern. For example, Sanz and Moreno (2000) found no evidence of declining age-specific survival rate of female pied fly-catchers (*Ficedula hypoleuca*) breeding in central Spain, the southern part of this species' breeding range, whereas Sternberg (1989), studying the same species in Germany, did observe a steady decline in annual survival after age 1. The former authors suggest that the lack of observed senescence in their population relative to Sternberg's may be due to its shorter migration route to wintering grounds in West Africa. Loison and colleagues (1999) also found marked differences in senescence patterns among different populations of roe deer and bighorn sheep.

Gaps in our knowledge of senescence patterns in wild populations stem from the limited number of field studies systematically addressing the issue. However, there are also methodological difficulties associated with assessing senescence in natural populations that may continue to make the accumulation of new knowledge slow. Reliable studies need to be based on long-term observations and/or experiments, enhanced by detailed knowledge of the mechanisms affecting age-specific mortality and fecundity, of the life-history tradeoffs at play in the population, and of the causes and dynamics of these tradeoffs (Blarer *et al.*, 1995).

IV. Methodological Difficulties in Evaluating Senescence in Wild Populations

The scarcity of studies on senescence in natural populations testifies to the logistical difficulty of observing and investigating it. Some authors urge readers to be careful when accepting published data on senescence in wild populations (Gaillard *et al.*, 1994; Nisbet, 2001) and cite a variety of methodological and interpretation problems that must be overcome before we can develop a true understanding of how, when, and why senescence occurs in the wild. Potential methodological problems include the lack of visible, anatomical markers of aging, the use of cross-sectional rather than longitudinal life tables, small sample sizes of individuals at older ages, and the assumption that an undetected individual is a dead individual. Interpretation problems include demographic heterogeneity, assumptions of temporal constancy of environmental and demographic conditions, and the choice of variables to measure senescence. We will discuss some of these problems briefly.

The first question to ask before evaluating any type of senescence in wild populations is whether you can be confident in assigning calendar age to study animals. The gold standard should continue to be unique marking of individuals as close to birth as possible. Even gold standards are not perfect, however, as individual marks such as bands or tags can be lost over time. Frequently, surrogate markers of calendar age, such as growth rings or plumage changes, are used as age estimators, sometimes without extensive validation. In fact, there are very few reliable markers of age in the wild, and even the ones that exist are often species-, population-, and even sex-specific. Thus, their uncritical use can be deceptive. Tooth wear categories, for example, are often used to estimate age in populations of ungulates. However, tooth wear changes have been shown to decelerate with age and differ between male and female Norwegian red deer (Loe *et al.*, 2003). On the other hand, the precision required of an age estimator depends on the precision necessary to answer the research question. Sometimes relative

rather than absolute age estimation is sufficient. Even when absolute age estimation is required, rough precision may suffice. For instance, if bowhead whales indeed frequently live 150 to 200 years, as one report suggests, then an age estimator such as amino acid racemization of the eye lens may be sufficiently precise for most demographic analyses, even if its margin of error is as much as a decade (George *et al.*, 1999).

Even well-established age estimators can be flawed. For example, the correlation between growth layers in dentine and age used to establish calendar age of southern elephant seals was constructed with animals only up to 8 years of age. It is known from individually marked individuals that this species can live in excess of 23 years (Hindell & Little, 1988). Whether extrapolation from known to older unknown ages is warranted will depend on the biology of the species and marker in question. Some traditional markers, such as scale rings of fishes, have failed validation tests in at least some species (Nedreaas, 1990), whereas newer techniques, such as growth rings of fish otoliths, have been extensively validated (Cailliet *et al.*, 2001).

Cross-sectional or "snapshot" studies are the easiest and quickest way to investigate senescence in the wild. That is, demographic parameters are estimated from the age distribution of a current population. Indeed, life tables used in human demography are virtually always cross-sectional. Cohort tables, in which a population of individuals born at the same time is tracked throughout life, will generally be preferred for studies of wild populations. Problems with cross-sectional life tables have to do with the assumptions required for using such life tables as surrogates for cohort tables. These include assumptions such as a stationary population age distribution and consistency of mortality patterns over time that are unlikely to be even approximately met in wild populations (Gaillard *et al.*, 1994).

If individuals in a population are not identified, even serial snapshots of a single cohort can mislead as a consequence of, say, population heterogeneity. Consider, for instance, a hypothetical cohort of five females that were born the same year (see Figure 9.2). A researcher averages the number of offspring of the females at 1 year of age and then again at 6 years in an attempt to detect reproductive senescence. Only three of the original five females make it to age 6. The results from these two snapshots appear to indicate a decline in reproduction with age—that is, reproductive senescence. However, the reproduction of individual females never changed over time. A more accurate assessment of the population would be that for some reason—a tradeoff between reproduction and survival or genetic heterogeneity or chance—females with low reproductive rates live longer. Without data on survival and number of offspring for individ-

ual females, a researcher would have an inaccurate picture concerning reproductive senescence.

Even longitudinal studies are not foolproof, of course. For instance, the length of sampling intervals must be meaningful within the context of the life of the study organism. Sampling wild mice annually would clearly be useless given that their average longevity is only 3 to 4 months (Phelan & Austad, 1989). In addition, there is the question of how long a longitudinal study should last in order to obtain accurate measures of demographic parameters and actually detect individuals that reach a senescent stage. Climatic variability and changes in population density are only two possible confounders of field demography. Consider a population of fulmars in England that has been tagged and tracked since 1950 (Dunnet & Ollason, 1978). Based on data from 1950 to 1962, researchers calculated the average adult longevity to be 15.6 ± 1.9 years (Dunnet *et al.*, 1963). Based on data from 1950 to 1970, adult longevity increased to 25.0 ± 4.3 years for males and 22.3 ± 4.2 years for females (Cormack, 1973). Finally, based on even later data (1958 to 1974), which now included only birds wearing a style of leg bands that were less likely to fall off, adult longevity was estimated at a substantially shorter 19.9 ± 1.8 years (Dunnet & Ollason, 1978). Although the analytical methods differed somewhat in each of these studies, the increasing study length combined with improved survival data from better leg bands account for at least part of the progressive changes in longevity estimates.

Although the length of a longitudinal study is important for evaluating trends in senescence, so is the number of individuals marked in the population. Needless to say, this is not a problem specific to field studies. Sample sizes limit demographic analyses in both field

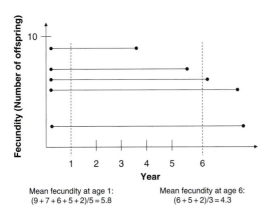

Mean fecundity at age 1:
(9 + 7 + 6 + 5 + 2)/5 = 5.8

Mean fecundity at age 6:
(6 + 5 + 2)/3 = 4.3

Figure 9.2 Misleading inference from two cross-sectional samples (year 1 and 6) of cohort from one hypothetical population. Each line represents one individual. Height of line on the y-axis represents fecundity of that individual which remains constant with age, length of the line along the x-axis represents individual longevity. An apparent decline in reproduction is caused not by individual senescence, but rather by earlier death of more fecund individuals.

and lab. For instance, if only 50 individuals are included in a study, a real 1 percent difference in mortality rate is impossible to detect (Promislow et al., 1999). Also, because fewer and fewer individuals are alive at later ages, the statistical power to determine late-life demographic trends inevitably decreases. For instance, in a typical study, only 4 percent of the willow tits (Parus montanus) reached an age at which demographic senescence could be detected (Orell & Belda, 2002).

Population heterogeneity can also obscure underlying demographic patterns (Carnes & Olshansky, 2001; Festa-Bianchet et al., 2003; McDonald et al., 1996; Service, 2000; Vaupel & Yashin, 1985), as the previous example with fallow deer indicated. This interpretation problem is not unique to field studies but may be exaggerated in nature relative to the laboratory. Such heterogeneity can arise from genotypic or phenotypic differences among individuals. Consider that it is likely that only the strongest, healthiest individuals in a population will make it to old age. As individuals of low quality are eliminated from the population, we see a resulting increase in survival rate. This increase could be interpreted as negative senescence. Yet it does not represent individuals becoming more robust as they get older. It is the result of a selection process that has changed the nature of the sample being measured and it thus may obscure a different underlying pattern if the same individuals were followed longitudinally. For instance, McDonald and colleagues (1996) found evidence of survival senescence in Florida scrub jays. The evidence was most clear when social role was controlled for and a homogenous subpopulation of high-quality individuals with the highest annual fledging rates and greatest longevity were identified. Another example in which phenotypic heterogeneity may be misleading with respect to demographic senescence may

been seen in snowshoe hares (Lepus americanus), which experience dramatic and regular population cycles. That is, periods of very high hare density are followed by population crashes to low densities, which in turn are followed by rebounds to high density again. During a 16-year breeding program, Sinclair and colleagues (2003) found that genetic lineages established from females of the high-density phase had significantly lower reproductive output and longevity than lineages established from females of the low-density phase. Furthermore, high-phase females showed declining reproductive output with age, whereas reproductive output remained constant throughout life in low-phase females.

Despite the manifold complications associated with the study of senescence in nature, an increasing number of studies are addressing the issue, with progressively more sophisticated techniques.

V. Conclusions

Studies of senescence in natural populations of mammals and birds have improved significantly in recent years with the introduction of new methodological and analytical techniques and the continuation of long-term research projects. Clearly, senescence occurs in the wild, although just as clearly it is not ubiquitous. Only by increasing the breadth of study species and focusing specifically on the question of senescence will we eventually be able to comprehensively assess interspecies patterns of senescence. Further research is also necessary to enhance our understanding of variation in senescence patterns among populations of the same species. The future of this line of research will be based on longitudinal data from large samples of marked individuals in populations that are well characterized and organisms for which we have a sound understanding of physiology, behavior, and life-history options, constraints, and tradeoffs.

Acknowledgments

We thank Ed Masoro, Daniel Promislow, Victor Apanius, and an anonymous reviewer for helpful comments on an earlier version of this manuscript. Preparation of the manuscript was supported in part by an Ellison Senior Scholar Award and NIH grant AG022873.

References

Aebischer, N. J. (1986). Retrospective investigation of an ecological disaster in the shag, *Phalacrocorax aristotelis*: a general method based on long-term marking. *Journal of Animal Ecology*, 55, 613–629.

Aebischer, N. J., & Coulson, J. C. (1990). Survival of Kittiwakes in relation to sex and position in colony. *Journal of Animal Ecology*, 59, 1063–1071.

Anderson, D. J., & Apanius, V. (2003). Actuarial and reproductive senescence in a long-lived seabird: preliminary evidence. *Experimental Gerontology*, 38, 757–760.

Apanius, V., & Nisbet, I. C. T. (2003). Serum immunoglobulin G levels in very old common terns Sterna hirundo. *Experimental Gerontology*, 38, 761–764.

Askenmo, C., & Unger, U. (1986). How to be double-brooded: trends and timing of breeding performance in the rock pipit. *Ornis Scandinavica*, 17, 237–244.

Austad, S. N. (1993). Retarded aging rate in an insular population of opossums. *Journal of Zoology*, 229, 695–708.

Bailey, S. R., & Milne, H. (1982). The influence of female age on breeding in the Eider *Somateria mollissima*. *Bird Study*, 29, 55–66.

Berubé, C. H., Festa-Bianchet, M., & Jorgenson, J. T. (1999). Individual differences, longevity and reproductive senescence in bighorn ewes. *Ecology*, 80, 2555–2565.

Birkhead, T. R., & Goodburn, S. F. (1989). Magpie. In I. Newton (Ed.), *Lifetime reproduction in birds* (pp. 173–182). London: Academic Press.

Blarer, A., Doebeli, M., & Stearns, S. C. (1995). Diagnosing senescence: inferring evolutionary causes from phenotypic patterns can be misleading. *Proceedings of the Royal Society of London B*, 262, 305–312.

Botkin, D. B., & Miller, R. S. (1974). Mortality rates and survival of birds. *American Naturalist*, 108, 181–192.

Bradley, J. S., Wooller, R. D., Skira, I. J., & Serventy, D. L. (1989). Age-dependent survival of breeding short-tailed shearwaters *Puffinus tenuirostris*. *Journal of Animal Ecology*, 58, 175–188.

Bronikowski, A. M., Alberts, S. C., Altmann, J., Packer, C., Carey, K. D., & Tatar, M. (2002). The aging baboon: comparative demography in a non-human primate. *Proceedings of the National Academy of Sciences of the USA*, 99, 9591–9595.

Broussard, D. R., Risch, T. S., Dobson, F. S., & Murie, J. O. (2003). Senescence and age-related reproduction of female Colombian ground squirrels. *Journal of Animal Ecology*, 72, 212–219.

Bumpus, H. C. (1898). The elimination of the unfit as illustrated by the introduced sparrow, *Passer domesticus*. *Biology lectures*, Marine Biological Laboratory, Woods Hole, MA.

Byers, J. (1998). *The American Pronghorn*. Chicago: University of Chicago Press.

Cailliet, G. M., Andrews, A. H., Burton, E. J., Watters, D. L., Kline, D. E., & Ferry-Graham, L. A. (2001). Age determination and validation studies of marine fishes: do deep-dwellers live longer? *Experimental Gerontology*, 36, 739–764.

Carnes, B. A., & Olshansky, S. J. (2001). Heterogeneity and its biodemographic implications for longevity and mortality. *Experimental Gerontology*, 36, 419–430.

Caughley, G. (1966). Mortality patterns in mammals. *Ecology*, 47, 906–918.

Cichón, M., Sendecka, J., & Gustafsson, L. (2003). Age-related decline in humoral immune function in collared flycatchers. *Journal of Evolutionary Biology*, 16, 1205–1210.

Clutton-Brock, T. H. (1984). Reproductive effort and terminal investment in iteroparous animals. *American Naturalist*, 123, 212–229.

Clutton-Brock, T. H., Albon, S. D., Gibson, R. M., & Guinness, F. E. (1979). The logical stag: adaptive aspects of fighting in red deer (*Cervus elaphus* L.). *Animal Behavior, 27*, 211–225.

Clutton-Brock, T. H., Albon, S. D., & Guiness, F. E. (1988). Reproductive success in male and female red deer. In T. H. Clutton-Brock (Ed.), *Reproductive success: studies of individual variation in contrasting breeding systems* (pp. 325–343). Chicago: University of Chicago Press.

Coe, C. L., & Ershler, W. D. (2001). Intrinsic and environmental influences on immune senescence in the aged monkey. *Physiology and Behavior, 73*, 379–384.

Comfort, A. 1979. *The Biology of Senescence* (3rd ed.). Edinburgh: Churchill Livingston.

Cormack, R. M. (1973). Commonsense estimates from capture-recapture studies. In M. S. Bartlett & R. W. Hiorns (Eds.), *The mathematical theory of the dynamics of biological populations* (pp. 225–234). London and New York: Academic Press.

Coulson, J. C. (1984). The population dynamics of the Eider duck *Somateria mollissima* and evidence of extensive non-breeding by adult ducks. *Ibis, 126*, 525–543.

Coulson, J. C., & Fairweather, J. A. (2001). Reduced reproductive performance prior to death in the black-legged kittiwake: senescence or terminal illness? *Journal of Avian Biology, 32*, 146–152.

Coulson, J. C., & Horobin, J. (1976). The influence of age on the breeding biology and survival of the Arctic tern (*Sterna paradisaea*). *Journal of Zoology, 178*, 247–260.

Coulson, J. C., & Wooller, R. D. (1976). Differential survival rates among breeding kittiwake gulls *Rissa tridactyla*. *Journal of Animal Ecology, 45*, 205–213.

Daniel, C. W. (1977). Cell longevity in vivo. In C. E. Finch & L. Hayflick (Eds.), *Handbook of the biology of aging* (1st ed., pp. 122–158). New York: Van Nostrand Reinhold.

Deevey, E. S. Jr. (1947). Life tables for natural populations of animals. *Quarterly Review of Biology, 22*, 238–314.

Derocher, A. E., & Stirling, I. (1994). Age-specific reproductive performance of female polar bears (*Ursus maritimus*). *Journal of Zoology (London), 234*, 527–536.

Dhondt, A. A. (1971). Some factors influencing territory in the great tit, *Parus major*. *Gerfaut, 61*, 125–135.

Dhondt, A. A. (1989). The effect of old age on the reproduction of great and blue tit. *Ibis, 131*, 268–280.

Dow, H., & Fredga, S. (1984). Factors affecting reproductive output of the Goldeneye duck *Bucephala clangula*. *Journal of Animal Ecology, 53*, 679–692.

Dunnet, G. M., & Ollason, J. C. (1978). The estimation of survival rate in the Fulmar, *Fulmarus glacialis*. *Journal of Animal Ecology, 47*, 507–520.

Dunnet, G. M., Anderson, A., & Cormack, R. M. (1963). A study of survival of adult fulmars with observations on the prelaying exodus. *British Birds, 56*, 2–18.

Dunson, D. B., Baird, D. D., & Colombo, B. (2004). Increased infertility with age in men and women. *Obstetrics and Gynecology, 103*, 51–56.

Effros, R. (2001). Immune system activity. In E. J. Masoro & S. N. Austad (Eds.), *Handbook of the biology of aging* (5th ed., pp. 324–350). San Diego: Academic Press.

Ericsson, G., Wallin, K., Ball, J., & Broberg, M. (2001). Age-related reproductive effort and senescence in free-ranging moose, *Alces alces*. *Ecology, 82*, 1613–1620.

Festa-Bianchet, M., Gaillard, J.-M., & Côté, S. D. (2003). Variable age structure and apparent density dependence in survival of adult ungulates. *Journal of Animal Ecology, 72*, 640–649.

Finch, C. E. (1990). *Longevity, senescence, and the genome*. Chicago: University of Chicago Press.

Fitzpatrick, J. W., & Woolfenden, G. E. (1988). Components of lifetime reproductive success in the Florida scrub jay. In T. H. Clutton-Brock (Ed.), *Reproductive success: studies of individual variation in contrasting breeding systems* (pp. 305–320). Chicago: University of Chicago Press.

Gaillard, J.-M., Allainé, D., Pontier, D., Yoccoz, N. G., & Promislow, D. E. L. (1994). Senescence in natural populations of mammals: a reanalysis. *Evolution, 48*, 509–516.

Gaillard, J.-M., Delorme, D., Boutin, J.-M., Van Laere, G., Boisaubert, B., & Pradel, R. (1993). Roe deer survival patterns: a comparative analysis of contrasting populations. *Journal of Animal Ecology*, 62, 778–791.

George, J. C., Bada, J., Zeh, J., Scott, L., Brown, S. E., O'Hara, T., & Suydam, R. (1999). Age and growth estimates of bowhead whales (Balaena mysticetus) via aspartic acid racemization. Canadian *Journal of Zoology*, 77, 571–580.

Grant, B. R., & Grant, P. R. (1989). *Evolutionary dynamics of a natural population: the large cactus finch of the Galapagos Islands.* Chicago: University of Chicago Press.

Gustafsson, L., & Pärt, T. (1990). Acceleration of senescence in the collared flycatcher *Ficedula albicollis* by reproductive costs. *Nature*, 347, 279–281.

Hamer, K. C., & Furness, R. W. (1991). Age-specific breeding performance and reproductive effort in great skuas, *Catharacta skua*. *Journal of Animal Ecology*, 60, 693–704.

Harris, M. P., Buckland, S. T., Russell, S. M., & Wanless, S. (1994). Year- and age-related variation in the survival of adult European shags over a 24-year period. *Condor*, 96, 600–605.

Hayflick, L. (2000). The future of ageing. *Nature*, 408, 267–269.

Haymes, G. T., & Blokpoel, H. (1980). The influence of age on the breeding biology of ring-billed gulls. *Wilson Bulletin*, 92, 221–228.

Heard, D., Barry, S., Watts, G., & Child, K. (1997). Fertility of female moose (*Alces alces*) in relation to age and body composition. *Alces*, 33, 165–176.

Heckel, G., & Von Helversen, O. (2002). Male tactics and reproductive success in the harem polygynous bat *Saccopteryx bilineata*. *Behavioral Ecology*, 13, 750–756.

Hilden, O. (1978). Population dynamics in Temminck's stint *Calidris temminckii*. *Oikos*, 30, 17–28.

Hindell, M. A., & Little, G. J. (1988). Longevity, fertility and philopatry of two female southern elephant seals (*Mirounga leonina*) at Macquarie Island. *Marine Mammal Science*, 4, 168–171.

Horiuchi, S, & Wilmoth, J. R. (1997). Age patterns of the life table aging rate for major causes of death in Japan, 1951–1990. *Journals of Gerontology. Series A, Biological Sciences and Medical Sciences*, 51, B67–B77.

Jorgenson, J. T., Festa-Bianchet, M. Gaillard, J.-M., & Wishart, W. D. (1997). Effects of age, sex, disease and density on survival of bighorn sheep. *Ecology*, 78, 1019–1032.

Khalil, A. M., Murakami, N., & Kaseda, Y. (1998). Relationship between plasma testosterone concentration and age, breeding season and harem size in Misaki feral horses. *Journal of Veterinary Medical Science*, 60, 643–645.

Koivula, M., Koskela, E., Mappes, T., & Oksanen, T. A. (2003). Cost of reproduction in the wild: manipulation of reproductive effort in the bank vole. *Ecology*, 84, 398–405.

Komdeur, J. (1996). Influence of age on reproductive performance in the Seychelles warbler. *Behavioral Ecology*, 7, 417–425.

Kruijt, J. P., & de Vos, G. J. (1988). Individual variation in reproductive success in male black grouse, *Tetrao tetrix*. In T. H. Clutton-Brock (Ed.), *Reproductive success: studies of individual variation in contrasting breeding systems* (pp. 279–290). Chicago: University of Chicago Press.

Laaksonen, T., Korpimäki, E., & Hakkarainen, H. (2002). Interactive effects of parental age and environmental variation on the breeding performance of Tengmalm's owls. *Journal of Animal Ecology*, 71, 23–31.

Leuze, C. C. C. K. (1980). The application of radio tracking and its effect on the behavioral ecology of the water vole, *Arvicola terrestris*. In C. J. Amlamer & D. W. MacDonald (Eds.), *A handbook on biotelemetry and radio tracking* (pp. 361–366). Oxford: Pergamon Press.

Loe, L. E., Mysterud, A., Langvatn, R., & Stenseth, N. C. (2003). Decelerating and sex dependent toothware in Norwegian red deer. *Oecologia*, 135, 346–353.

Loery, G., Pollock, K. H., Nichols, J. D., & Hines, J. E.(1987). Age-specificity of black-capped chickadee survival rates: analysis of capture-recapture data. *Ecology*, 68, 1038–1044.

Loison, A., Festa-Bianchet, M., Gaillard, J.-M., Jorgenson, J. T., & Jullien, J.-M. (1999). Age-specific survival in five populations of ungulates: evidence of senescence. *Ecology*, 80, 2539–2554.

Lunn, N. J., Boyd, I. L., & Croxall, J. P. (1994). Reproductive performance of male Antarctic fur seals: the influence of age, breeding experience, environmental variation and individual quality. *Journal of Animal Ecology*, 63, 827–840.

McDonald, D. B., Fitzpatrick, J. W., & Woolfenden, G. E. (1996). Actuarial senescence and demographic heterogeneity in the Florida scrub jay. *Ecology*, 77, 2373–2381.

McElligott, A. G., Altwegg, R., & Hayden, T. J. (2002). Age-specific survival and reproductive probabilities: evidence for senescence in male fallow deer (*Dama dama*). *Proceedings of the Royal Society of London B*, 269, 1129–1137.

Medawar, P. B. (1952). *An unsolved problem of biology*. London: Lewis.

Milonoff, M., Pöysä, H., & Runko, P. (2002). Reproductive performance of common goldeneye *Bucephala clangula* females in relation to age and lifespan. *Ibis*, 144, 585–592.

Millar, J. S. (1994). Senescence in a population of small mammals? *Ecoscience*, 1, 317–321.

Morris, D. W. (1996). State-dependent life history and senescence of white-footed mice. *Ecoscience*, 3, 1–6.

Møller, A. P., & De Lope, F. (1999). Senescence in a short-lived migratory bird: age-dependent morphology, migration, reproduction and parasitism. *Journal of Animal Ecology*, 68, 163–171.

Mysterud, A., Yoccoz, N. G., Stenseth, N. C., & Langvatn, R. (2001). Effects of age, sex and density on body weight of Norwegian red deer: evidence of density-dependent senescence. *Proceedings of the Royal Society of London B*, 268, 911–919.

Nedreaas, K. (1990). Age determination of Northeast Atlantic *Sebastes* species. *Journal du Conseil CIEM*, 47, 208–230.

Newton, I. (1988). Age and reproduction in the sparrowhawk. In T. H. Clutton-Brock (Ed.), *Reproductive success: studies of individual variation in contrasting breeding systems* (pp. 201–219). Chicago: University of Chicago Press.

Newton, I., & Rothery, P. (1997). Senescence and reproductive value in sparrowhawks. *Ecology*, 78, 1000–1008.

Newton, I., Marquiss, M., & Moss, D. (1981). Age and breeding in sparrowhawks *Accipiter nisus*. *Journal of Animal Ecology*, 51, 327–343.

Nisbet, I. C. T. (2001). Detecting and measuring senescence in wild birds: experience with long-lived seabirds. *Experimental Gerontology*, 36, 833–843.

Nisbet, I. C. T., Apanius, V., & Friar, M. S. (2002). Breeding performance of very old common terns. *Journal of Field Ornithology*, 73, 117–124.

Nisbet, I. C. T., Winchell, J. M., & Heise, A. E. (1984). Influence of age on the breeding biology of common terns. *Colonial Waterbirds*, 7, 117–126.

Nol, E., & Smith, J. N. M. (1987). Effects of age and breeding experience on seasonal reproductive success in the song sparrow. *Journal of Animal Ecology*, 56, 301–313.

Ollason, J. C., & Dunnet, G. M. (1978). Age, experience and other factors affecting the breeding success of the fulmar, *Fulmarus glacialis*, in Orkney. *Journal of Animal Ecology*, 47, 961–976.

Ollason, J. C., & Dunnett, G. M. (1988). Variation in breeding success in Fulmars. In T. H. Clutton-Brock (Ed.), *Reproductive success: studies of individual variation in contrasting breeding systems* (pp. 263–278). Chicago: University of Chicago Press.

Orell, M., & Belda, E. J. (2002). Delayed cost of reproduction and senescence in the willow tit *Parus montanus*. *Journal of Animal Ecology*, 71, 55–64.

Owen-Smith, N. (1993). Comparative mortality rates of male and female kudus: the costs of sexual size dimorphism. *Journal of Animal Ecology*, 62, 428–440.

Packer, C., Herbst, L., Pusey, A. E., Bygott, J. D., Hanby, J. P., Cairns, S. J., & Mulder, M. B. (1988). Reproductive success of lions. In T. H. Clutton-Brock (Ed.), *Reproductive success: studies of individual variation in contrasting breeding systems* (pp. 363–383). Chicago: University of Chicago Press.

Packer, C., Tatar, M., & Collins, A. (1998). Reproductive cessation in female mammals. *Nature*, 392, 807–810.

Partridge, L., & Barton, N. H. (1996). On measuring the rate of ageing. *Proceedings of* the *Royal Society of London B*, 263, 1365–1371.

Perrins, C. M., & Moss, D. (1974). Survival of young great tits in relation to age of female parent. *Ibis*, 116, 220–224.

Phelan, J. P., & Austad, S. N. (1989). Natural selection, dietary restriction and extended longevity. *Growth, Development, & Aging*, 53, 4–6.

Pistorius, P. A., & Bester, M. N. (2002). A longitudinal study of senescence in a pinniped. *Canadian Journal of Zoology*, 80, 395–401.

Promislow, D. E. L. (1991). Senescence in natural populations of mammals: a comparative study. *Evolution*, 45, 1869–1887.

Promislow, D. E. L., Tatar, M., Pletcher, S., & Carey, J. (1999). Below-threshold mortality: implications for studies in evolution, ecology and demography. *Journal of Evolutionary Biology*, 12, 314–328.

Pugesek, B. H. (1987). Age-specific survivorship in relation to clutch size and fledging success in California gulls. *Behavioral Ecology and Sociobiology*, 21, 217–221.

Pugesek, B. H., & Diem, K. L. (1990). The relationship between reproduction and survival in known-aged California gulls. *Ecology*, 71, 811–817.

Pugesek, B. H., Nations, C., Diem, K. L., & Pradel, R. (1995). Mark-resighting analysis of a California gull population. *Journal of Applied Statistics*, 22, 625–639.

Ratcliffe, N., Furness, R. W., & Hamer, K. C. (1998). The interactive effects of age and food supply on the breeding ecology of great skuas. *Journal of Animal Ecology*, 67, 853–862.

Rattiste, K., & Lilleleht, V. (1987). Population ecology of the common gull *Larus canus* in Estonia. *Ornis Fennica*, 64, 25–26.

Réale, D., & Boussès, P. (1995). Effect of ewe age and high population density on the early nursing behavior of mouflon. *Ethnology, Ecology and Evolution*, 7, 323–334.

Reid, J. M., Arcese, P., & Keller, L. F. (2003a). Inbreeding depresses immune response in song sparrows (*Melospiza melodia*): direct and inter-generational effects. *Proceedings of the Royal Society of London B*, 270, 2151–2157.

Reid, J. M., Bignal, E. M., Bignal, S., McCracken, D. I., & Monaghan, P. (2003b). Age-specific reproductive performance in red-billed choughs *Pyrrhocorax pyrrhocorax*: patterns and processes in a natural population. *Journal of Animal Ecology*, 72, 765–776.

Reid, W. V. (1988). Age-specific patterns of reproduction in the glaucous-winged gull: increased effort with age? *Ecology*, 69, 1454–1465.

Ricklefs, R. E. (1998). Evolutionary theories of aging: confirmation of a fundamental prediction, with implications for the genetic basis and evolution of life span. *American Naturalist*, 152, 24–44.

Robertson, R. J., & Rendell, W. B. (2001). A long-term study of reproductive performance in tree swallows: the influence of age and senescence on output. *Journal of Animal Ecology*, 70, 1014–1031.

Rockwell, R. F., Cooch, E. G., Thompson, C. B., & Cooke, F. (1993). Age and reproductive success in female lesser snow geese: experience senescence and the cost of philopatry. *Journal of Animal Ecology*, 62, 323–333.

Saino, N., Ambrosini, R., Martinelli, R., & Møller, A. P. (2002). Mate fidelity, senescence in breeding performance and reproductive trade-offs in the barn swallow. *Journal of Animal Ecology*, 71, 309–319.

Saino, N., Ferrari, R. P., Romano, M., Rubolini, D., & Møller, A. P. (2003). Humoral immune response in relation to senescence, sex and sexual ornamentation in the barn swallow (*Hirundo rustica*). *Journal of Evolutionary Biology*, 16, 1127–1134.

Sanz, J. J., & Moreno, J. (2000). Delayed senescence in a southern population of the pied flycatcher (*Ficedula hypoleuca*). *Ecoscience*, 7, 25–31.

Service, P. M. (2000). Heterogeneity in individual mortality risk and its importance for evolutionary studies of senescence. *American Naturalist*, 156, 1–13.

Shock, N (1983). Aging of physiological systems. *Journal of Chronic Diseases*, 36, 137–142.

Sinclair, A. R. E. (1977). *The Africa buffalo: a study of resource limitation of populations*. Chicago: University of Chicago Press.

Sinclair, A. R. E., Chitty, D., Stefan, C. I., & Krebs, C. J. (2003). Mammal population cycles: evidence for intrinsic differences during snowshoe hare cycles. *Canadian Journal of Zoology*, 81, 216–220.

Skogland, T. (1988). Tooth wearing by food limitation and its life history consequences in wild reindeer. *Oikos*, 51, 238–242.

Sternberg, H. (1989). Pied flycatcher. In L. Newton (Ed.), *Lifetime reproduction in birds* (pp. 55–74). London: Academic Press.

Sugiyama, Y. (1994). Age-specific birth rate and lifetime reproductive success of chimpanzees at Bossou, Guinea. *American Journal of Primatology*, 32, 311–318.

Thomas, C. S. (1983). The relationship between breeding experience, egg volume and reproductive success of the kittiwake *Rissa tridactyla*. *Ibis*, 125, 567–574.

Turturro, A., Witt, W. W., Lewis, S., Hass, B. S., Lipman, R. D., & Hart, R. W. (1999). Growth curves and survival characteristics of the animals used in the biomarkers of aging program. *Journals of Gerontology Biological Sciences*, 54A, B492–B501.

Vaupel, J. W., & Yashin, A. I. (1985). Heterogeneity's ruses: some surprising effects of selection on population dynamics. *American Statistician*, 39, 176–185.

Vom Saal, F. S., Finch, C. E., & Nelson, J. F. (1994). Natural history and mechanisms of reproductive aging in humans, laboratory rodents, and other selected vertebrates. In E. Knobil & J. D. Neill (Eds.), *The physiology of reproduction* (2nd ed., pp. 1213–1314). New York: Raven Press.

Weimerskirch, H. (1992). Reproductive effort in long-lived birds: age-specific patterns of condition, reproduction, and survival in the wandering albatross. *Oikos*, 64, 464–473.

Weladji, R. B., Mysterud, A., Holand, Ø., & Lenvik, D. (2002). Age-related reproductive effort in reindeer (*Rangifer tarandus*): evidence of senescence. *Oecologia*, 131, 79–82.

Williams, G. C. (1957). Pleiotropy, natural selection and the evolution of senescence. *Evolution*, 11, 398–411.

Wolfe, L. D., & Noyes, M. J. S. (1981). Reproductive senescence among female Japanese macaques (*Macaca fuscata fuscata*). *Journal of Mammalogy*, 62, 698–705.

Wooller, R. D., Bradley, J. S., & Croxall, J. P. (1992). Long-term population studies of seabirds. *Trends in Ecology and Evolution*, 7, 111–114.

Wooller, R. D., Bradley, J. S., Skira, I. K., & Serventy, D. L. (1990). Reproductive success of short-tailed shearwaters *Puffinus tenuirostris*: relation to their age and breeding experience. *Journal of Animal Ecology*, 59, 161–170.

Chapter 10

Biodemography of Aging and Age-Specific Mortality in *Drosophila melanogaster*

James W. Curtsinger, Natalia S. Gavrilova, and Leonid A. Gavrilov

I. Introduction

For the last 15 years there has been a high level of interest in combining the methods of biology and demography to investigate aging in experimental populations. The hybrid field of biodemography addresses a wide range of questions about aging organisms and aging populations, and also attempts to provide insights into human aging (Wachter & Finch, 1997). A handful of issues have preoccupied the nascent field: To what extent are the genetic phenomena that influence life histories age-specific in their effects? How malleable are the patterns of survival and death among the oldest organisms? Why do populations often exhibit mortality plateaus? How have observed survival patterns evolved under the influence of mutation and natural selection? To what extent do survival patterns in populations reflect underlying changes in individual organisms? All of these questions are challenging, and none fully answered yet. Addressing them requires a set of analytical techniques that are com-

monplace to demographers but foreign to most biologists. Here we review some basic analytic methods from demography and lay out essential biological methods and questions, hoping to introduce both biologists and demographers to the hybrid field.

The integration of genetic and demographic methods requires an experimental system that is genetically defined and amenable to large-scale population studies. The fruit fly *Drosophila melanogaster* is an obvious candidate, being one of the premiere experimental systems for basic research in genetics. The genome is completely sequenced, and the flies can be reared in large numbers (tens of thousands of organisms). The nematode *Caenorhabditis elegans* and some yeast species also have those desirable characteristics, but other standard experimental systems do not. The genetics of house mice (*Mus musculus*) is an important and growing area of research, but large-scale population studies with rodents are impractical. Demography of medflies

(*Cerititus capitata*) and several parasitic wasp species has been investigated in large experimental populations (Carey, 2003), but those systems are genetically undefined. An interesting feature of *Drosophila* as an experimental model is the similarity of its mortality kinetics to that of humans, first noted by Raymond Pearl (1922). Both species have a relatively short period of high initial mortality, followed by a relatively long period of mortality increase, and then deceleration at advanced ages (although the period of mortality deceleration and mortality plateau in *Drosophila* is longer than in humans).

Here we concentrate on *D. melanogaster*, a holometabolous insect. Larvae hatch from eggs about 24 hours after laying, feed voraciously for a week, and then pupate. Adults emerge from the pupal case after a few days of metamorphosis and are sexually mature within 24 hours. In the wild, *D. melanogaster* adults probably live one to two weeks. In laboratory culture, flies are normally maintained on a two-week generation schedule but can live much longer as adults. In a typical outbred population, adults survive 30 to 50 days on average, depending on temperature and other environmental conditions. Inbreeding and increased temperature reduce mean adult life spans, while artificial selection for increased life span is capable of doubling it. Maximum adult life spans observed in large experiments typically exceed 100 days. There is no precise definition of young, middle-aged, or old adult flies. At two weeks after emergence, metabolic rate and gene expression reach low levels characteristic of remaining adult life (Tahoe *et al.*, 2004; Van Voorhies *et al.*, 2003, 2004). For females, old age in flies is probably best understood as the age after egg laying has ceased, usually 40 to 60 days

after emergence, depending on genotype and environmental conditions.

A. Collection of Survival Data

Survival experiments with laboratory populations of *Drosophila* are typically longitudinal, large scale, and complete. That is, age-synchronized cohorts consisting of thousands or tens of thousands of experimental animals are established with newly emerged adults and are observed over time. As the cohorts age, dead animals are removed, counted, and recorded on a daily basis. Observations continue until the last fly dies, typically around 100 days after emergence (depending on genotype and sample size; see below). Experimental populations are maintained under controlled environmental conditions, including temperature, light cycle, and humidity. Initial population density is also controlled, at least approximately; in smaller experiments, exact numbers of flies are counted, whereas in larger experiments, density is approximated by volume or weight of anesthetized flies (one large female weighs ~ 1mg., whereas males are typically ~30 percent smaller). Experimental populations are often housed in cages of one to several liters in volume, each holding up to a thousand individuals, but half-pint milk bottles and finger-sized glass vials are sometimes used. There is always fresh fly food in the containers, which serves as both an oviposition medium and a source of nutrition for adults and larvae. Frequent replacement of the medium and changing cages prevents unwanted recruitment of new adults into experimental populations.

Populations used for survival studies typically consist of males and females in approximately equal proportions when experiments are initially set up, but because of differential survival, the sex ratio changes over time. In mixed-sex population cages, females actively reproduce and generally exhibit shorter average life spans than males (Curtsinger & Khazaeli, 2002; Curtsinger *et al.*, 1998; Fukui *et al.*, 1993, 1995, 1996; Khazaeli & Curtsinger, 2000; Khazaeli *et al.*, 1997; Pletcher, 1996; Resler *et al.*, 1998;). Because flies reach sexual maturity soon after emergence, mating behavior begins almost immediately in mixed-sex populations. It is possible to study the survival characteristics of unmated flies in single-sex populations by anesthetizing newly emerged adults and then sorting the sexes under a dissecting microscope when cohorts are initially established (Miyo & Charlesworth, 2004; Semenchenko *et al.*, 2004).

There is significant uncontrolled environmental variation that affects death rates in experimental populations of *Drosophila*. The magnitude of the variation is perhaps underappreciated. For instance, it is not unusual to see four- or five-fold variation in individual life spans among flies of the same genotype sharing the same food and population cage. This is not a peculiarity of fly life spans; biologists have long recognized that quantitative traits vary between organisms, even if they are genetically identical and reared under carefully controlled conditions (for a review, see Finch & Kirkwood, 2000; Gavrilov & Gavrilova, 1991). Because of this irreducible variation, which is not well understood, survival experiments should be highly replicated, in some cases involving hundreds of populations. Ideally, data from genotypes or treatments that are to be contrasted are collected simultaneously in order to avoid confounding uncontrolled environmental variations with treatment or genotype effects.

B. Data Analysis: Mean Life Span and Survivorship

The central problem in survival analysis is to summarize and interpret large amounts of information hidden in the survival data. Raw data consist of estimated ages at death. Mean life span, the arithmetic average survival time, has intuitive appeal as a descriptor of survival ability, but the information contained in that summary statistic is limited. The most critical limitation in the present context is that the mean gives little information about the age-specificity of survival patterns. Two cohorts could have very similar means but experience vastly different life histories. For instance, if one population suffers mortality only at middle age, whereas a second experiences mortality equally and exclusively at early and late ages, mean life spans in the two populations will be similar. Maximum observed life span is also frequently reported but is similarly uninformative about age-specific events.

The central conceptual tool for organizing and analyzing age-specific aspects of survival data in experimental populations of *Drosophila* and other species (indeed, other objects) is the cohort life table. It is interesting that *Drosophila* was the second species, after humans, for which such demographic life tables were constructed (Pearl & Parker, 1921). The essential features of the life table are that age classes are defined by sampling intervals, and for each age class (life table row) specific variables (life table columns) are estimated. The first variable is the fraction of the total population dying while in age class x, denoted d_x. The distribution of d_x, a typical example of which is shown in Figure 10.1a, is approximately bell-shaped but not symmetrical, in contrast to the normal curve. The long right-skewed tail represents the oldest survivors of the cohort and is observed even in genetically homogeneous populations. The second variable, survivorship, is represented as l_x and is defined as the probability of survival from the beginning of the experiment until the beginning age interval x. That probability is estimated by the proportion of the initial cohort that remains alive at age x. Survival curves, which show plots of l_x versus x, start at

100 percent and decline to zero at the age when the last animal in the cohort dies (see Figure 10.1b). Survival curves have built-in smoothing because they are non-increasing (the proportion of the initial cohort remaining alive at age x can only be the same or lower at age $x + \Delta x$). For this reason, even relatively small cohorts produce smoothly declining survivorship curves. Life-table values of l_x and d_x are related as follows: $l^{x+\Delta x} = l_x - d_x$, where Δx is the length of the sampling (age) interval, typically equal to one day for fly experiments. It is important to emphasize that both l_x and d_x are cumulative indicators that depend on preceding death rates. Events early in the life history, such as a temporary epizootic, can affect survivorship and the fraction dying in later age classes, even in old age. In this sense, l_x and d_x reflect the survival history of the cohort up to and including age x.

C. Data Analysis: Probability of Death and Mortality Rate

Unlike survivorship and fraction dying, which have "memory," some other life-table variables are noncumulative and better suited to detecting age-specific effects. Age-specific probability of death (q_x) is defined as the conditional probability of dying in the interval Δx for individuals that survive to the beginning of interval x. It is estimated as the number of deaths that occur in age class x, divided by the number of individuals entering class x. An example of age-specific probability of death is shown in Figure 10.1c. Note that in this particular example, the age-specific probability of death grows monotonically with age up to an advanced age and then levels off, a phenomenon discussed in detail later.

Although probability of death is useful and intuitive, it has limitations. The main problem is that the value of q_x depends on the length of the age interval Δx for which it is calculated, which hampers both analyses and interpretation. For example, one-day probabilities of death may follow the Gompertz law of mortality, but probabilities of death calculated for other age intervals with the same data may not (Gavrilov & Gavrilova, 1991; le Bras, 1976). A meaningful descriptor of the dynamics of survival should not depend on the arbitrary choice of age intervals. Another problem is that, by definition, q_x is bounded by unity, which makes it difficult to scale the variable for studies of mortality at advanced ages.

A more useful indicator of mortality is the instantaneous mortality rate, or hazard rate, μ_x, which is defined as follows:

$$\mu_x = -\frac{dN_x}{N_x dx}$$

where N_x is the number alive at age x. The hazard rate does not depend on the length of the age interval; it reflects instantaneous risk of death. It has no upper bound and has the dimension of a rate (time^{-1}). One of the first empirical estimates of hazard rate μ_x was proposed by Sacher (1956):

$$\mu_x = \frac{1}{\Delta^x}\left(ln\, l_{x-\frac{\Delta^x}{2}} - ln\, l_{x+\frac{\Delta^x}{2}}\right)$$

$$= \frac{1}{2\Delta^x}\, ln\frac{l_{x-\Delta^x}}{l_{x+\Delta^x}}$$

This estimate is unbiased for slow changes in hazard rate (Sacher, 1966). A simplified version of the Sacher estimate (for small age intervals equal to unity) is often used in biological studies of mortality: $\mu_x = -ln(1-q_x)$ (see Carey, 2003) and assumes constant hazard rate in the age interval.

The Cutler-Ederer (1958) estimate (also called the actuarial hazard rate) is based on the assumption that deaths are

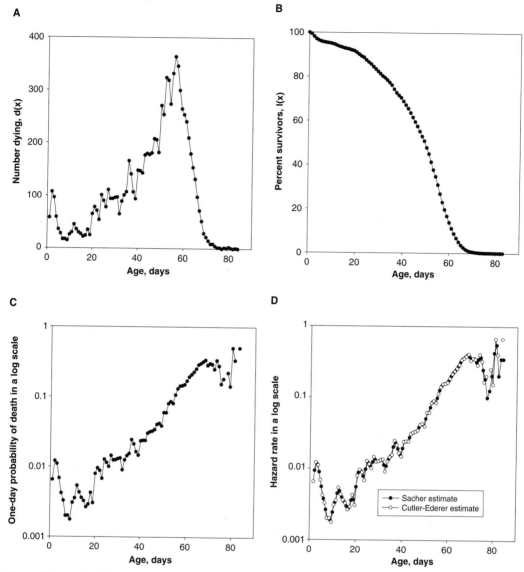

Figure 10.1   Life-table variables as a function of adult age, estimated for experimental population of 8,926 *D. melanogaster* males. (a) Number dying d_{xi} (b) survivorship l_{xi} (c) age-specific probability of death q_{xi} (d) age-specific mortality (hazard) rate μ_x. The subscript "x" indicates adult age in days since eclosion. (Unpublished data of Khazaeli, Gavrilova, Gavrilov, & Curtsinger)

uniformly distributed in the age interval and that all cases of withdrawal (censoring) occur in the middle of the age interval:

$$\mu_{x+\frac{\Delta^x}{2}} = \frac{d_x}{\Delta^x\left[l_x - \frac{c_x}{2} - \frac{d_x}{2}\right]}$$

Here, c_x is number of censored individuals during the age interval (for example, number of flies accidentally escaping the cage during food replacement). The hazard rate is measured at the midpoint of the age interval. Gehan and Siddiqui (1973) used Monte Carlo simulation to show that for samples less than 1,000, the Sacher method may produce biased results compared to the Cutler-Ederer method, whereas for larger samples, the Sacher estimate is more accurate. The advantage of the Cutler-Ederer estimate is its availability in standard statistical packages (such as SAS and *Stata*), which compute actuarial life tables. Despite the apparent differences between Cutler-Ederer and Sacher estimates, the methods produce very similar results for real data (see Figure 10.1d). Note that the mortality curve, depicting μ_x as a function of x, describes survival events in true age-specific fashion. It clearly illustrates the rate of actuarial senescence, usually defined as the slope of the mortality curve, and is particularly useful for examining details of death rates among the oldest survivors of a cohort. In contrast, the details of shape in a survivorship curve as it approaches the x-axis are generally indistinct (but see Pearl & Parker's method, described below).

The differences between survivorship and mortality are fundamental. The former depends on all previous cohort history, whereas the latter reflects risk specific solely to the age group under study. This distinction has often been misunderstood or overlooked by biologists. Rose's (1991) influential text on evolutionary biology of aging contains dozens of figures, extensive discussion of age-specific life-history phenomena, and not a single depiction of a mortality curve, either experimental or theoretical. Similarly, Kirkwood's (1999) general text on causes of aging gives considerable notice to age-specific phenomena but employs survivorship rather than mortality throughout. In an otherwise excellent paper on chromosomal mapping of genes that influence mean life spans in *Drosophila*, Nuzhdin and colleagues (1997) test an evolutionary model of senescence by examining age-specific variance in l_x, when the issue is clearly variance in μ_x.

Perhaps the most common misunderstanding among biologists about survivorship and mortality is the widespread assumption that rates of senescence can be easily seen in the slopes of survivorship curves. The apparent or actuarial rate of senescence, defined as the rate at which risk of death increases with age, is precisely reflected in the slope of the mortality curve: a steep slope indicates rapid actuarial senescence, a shallow slope indicates negligible senescence, and a zero slope indicates no senescence. Of course, the slope of the survivorship curve bears a mathematical relationship to the slope of the corresponding mortality curve, but not one that is easily grasped by visual inspection. The problem is that even populations that experience no apparent senescence (constant probability of death at all ages) will exhibit exponentially declining survivorship with increasing age. Thus, information about the rate of senescence is present in a survivorship curve only as a deviation from the exponential, a quantitative measure that is not well suited to casual inspection. Pearl and Parker (1924) addressed this problem by examining survivorship in semi-logarithmic plots. This approach may be useful in defining periods of mortality leveling-off (mortality plateaus): survivorship curves in semi-logarithmic scale should be linear if mortality is constant. Economos (1979, 1980) used this method for demonstrating non-Gompertzian mortality kinetics at advanced ages, but the technique has not been widely used in recent years.

There are probably several reasons that biologists in some fields have not, until recently, adequately appreciated the information that can be gained by estimating mortality rates. Survivorship curves have intrinsic smoothing, as mentioned above, whereas mortality curves tend to be jumpy. For a single data set plotted both ways, the mortality estimation makes the data look noisy, whereas the survivorship curve gives an appearance of orderly behavior. Accurate estimation of age-specific mortality rates requires larger sample sizes than those needed for estimating means or survivorship but provides extra sensitivity in studies of short-term response to phenomena such as heat shock (Khazaeli *et al.*, 1997) and dietary restriction (Mair *et al.*, 2003; Pletcher, 2002). The sample-size requirement is especially critical for the oldest ages; large initial cohort sizes are required in order to have adequate numbers of animals alive for estimation of death rates at the older ages.

In the 1920s, Raymond Pearl, an early advocate of biostatistics and experimental investigation of populations, published a series of papers on *Drosophila* life spans that employed relatively large sample sizes. For instance, Pearl and Parker (1924) collected survival data on about 4,000 flies from two strains. Since the 1950s, radiobiologists have routinely employed large sample sizes to estimate mortality rates in survival studies with experimental organisms. However, in spite of those pioneering efforts, up until around 1990, it was standard practice among experimental gerontologists, evolutionary biologists, and geneticists to employ small populations in studies of *Drosophila* survival, typically on the order of 50 to 100 animals per experimental treatment or genotype. Such sample sizes sufficed to give reasonably accurate estimates of mean life spans and aesthetically pleasing survivorship curves but provided virtually no information about death rates in old age.

Sample size requirements will depend on the specific question being asked. For accurate estimates of hazard rates, it is necessary to have some events (deaths) in each age interval. At younger ages, when mortality rates are low, it would be desirable to have at least one death in each observation interval. In small samples there might be no deaths during some

intervals, in which case intervals will have to be combined and the accuracy of hazard rate estimation will decline. Thus, the minimum sample size of experimental populations for hazard rate studies may be estimated on the basis of expected risk of death during younger ages, when mortality is low.

For example, if the expected risk of death is 1 per 1,000 during a one-day period, then the sample size should be at least 1,000. If mortality at younger ages is higher, then smaller sample sizes will suffice. This rule of thumb does not apply to studies of mortality deceleration and leveling-off. This phenomenon happens later in life, after a significant part of population has died and the remaining number of animals is a small fraction of the initial cohort. The empirical rule here may be to have at least 50 animals alive at the age when mortality deceleration starts so that hazard rate estimations would not be distorted by small numbers of deaths. If one is interested in short-term effects of caloric restriction or other interventions on mortality kinetics at middle ages close to the modal life span, then much smaller sample sizes may be sufficient because numbers of organisms at risk and numbers of deaths will be substantial.

D. Smoothing and Model Fitting

Two approaches are commonly used to describe trends in the (often noisy) data on age-specific mortality. One approach is to apply a non-parametric smoothing procedure. For data organized in the form of a life table, smoothing can be accomplished by widening the age intervals. If times to death for each individual in the sample are known with reasonable accuracy, and/or small sample size does not allow construction of a conventional life table, then the method of hazard rate smoothing using kernel functions may be more appropriate (Ramalu-Hansen,

1983). The latter method is more computationally complex, although special routines are available now in SAS and *Stata*. Applying methods of non-parametric smoothing decreases statistical noise and facilitates visual inspection of mortality plots but does not allow quantitative analysis of life-span data.

The second major approach for summarizing and simplifying mortality estimates is parametric model fitting, which allows researchers to describe the observed mortality kinetics using a small number of parameters of a specified mortality model. Although there are many possible models in the literature, three are widely used by biologists. The venerable model of Gompertz (1825) specifies exponentially increasing hazard rate with increasing age:

$$\mu_x = A e^{Bx}$$

where A is initial mortality rate, e is the base of the natural logarithms, and B, the slope parameter, controls the rate at which mortality increases with age. Estimates of A in laboratory populations of *D. melanogaster* are typically in the range 0.005 to 0.010 per day, whereas B often lies in the range 0.04 to 0.10 per day (Fukui *et al*, 1993). The Gompertz model produces a straight line in semi-log plots of hazard rate versus age, with the y-intercept estimating the initial mortality rate and the slope estimating the rate of senescence. The aging rate is sometimes summarized by the mortality rate doubling time (MRDT), defined as $\ln(2)/B$. However, this measure has limited applicability to *Drosophila* because of non-Gompertzian mortality dynamics at advanced ages; in particular, as B approaches zero in old age, the MRDT approaches infinity.

A second widely used model is the logistic, which is motivated by the possibility that individuals in the same population can have different frailties (age-dependent chances of death).

Differences in frailty might be innate and fixed throughout life, or modified over the life history. Strehler and Mildvan (1960) showed that when there is such heterogeneity, the observed population mortality pattern deviates from the underlying mortality for individuals. Following Beard (1963), the observed mortality in the population is

$$\mu_x = A e^{Bx}/[1 + \sigma^2 \Lambda(x)],$$

where A and B are as defined in the Gompertz model, σ^2 is the variance for frailty in the population, and $\Lambda(x) = (A/B)(e^{Bx} - 1)$. Note that when $\sigma^2 = 0$, there is no heterogeneity in the population, and the logistic reduces to the Gompertz model. However, if $\sigma^2 > 0$, then the logistic curve increases exponentially at early ages and plateaus at more advanced ages (as x becomes large, u_x approaches B/σ^2). Yashin and colleagues (1994) showed that this model applies under two biologically different circumstances: when individuals possess a fixed frailty from birth that differs from that of other individuals, and when all individuals start life with identical frailties but then randomly acquire differences in frailty during adulthood.

A third model used by biologists is also motivated by the observation that mortality data often exhibit plateaus at older ages. This approach involves fitting two curves to the mortality data. Curtsinger and colleagues (1992) proposed a two-stage Gompertz model, in which a Gompertz curve is fit to the data at young ages up to some breakpoint age, and then a second Gompertz curve with shallower slope is fit to the older ages. This model includes five parameters: two intercept and two slope parameters for two Gompertz curves, and a fifth parameter for the breakpoint. Zelterman and Curtsinger (1994, 1995) applied the method to fly data, and Vaupel and colleagues (1994) used it for nematodes.

Drapeau and colleagues (2000) employed a similar method, except older ages were fit to a linear rather than exponential curve. It should be noted that mortality trajectories following the Weibull (power) law of mortality may resemble a two-stage Gompertz model in semi-log coordinates (see Chapter 1 in this volume).

The two major methods of parameter estimation for nonlinear models are maximum likelihood and nonlinear least squares. The maximum likelihood approach is based on maximizing the likelihood function, or the probability of obtaining a particular set of data given the chosen probability model. Maximum likelihood methods provide unbiased and efficient parameter estimates for large data sets (though the estimates may be heavily biased for small samples). Another advantage is that maximum likelihood generates theoretically more accurate confidence bounds for parameter estimates. An important property of maximum likelihood for survival data is that censored observations can be readily introduced (see Filliben, 2004). The limitation of this method is the need for specifying the maximum likelihood equations for each particular function not implemented in the standard statistical software packages, which often is not trivial. Standard statistical packages provide maximum likelihood estimates for a limited number of models. For example, the *Stata* package has a procedure for maximum likelihood estimation of Gompertz and logistic models. Maximum likelihood estimation of Gompertz, Gompertz-Makeham, logistic, and logistic-Makeham models is implemented in *WinModest*, a program written and distributed by S. Pletcher (Baylor College of Medicine, Houston) specifically for calculating basic statistics, fitting mortality models to survival data, and partitioning mean longevity differences between populations (Pletcher & Curtsinger, 2000a).

The nonlinear least squares method provides an alternative to maximum likelihood. This method is implemented in most statistical software packages and allows researchers to fit a large variety of nonlinear models. The limitation of this method is its theoretically less desirable optimality properties compared to the maximum likelihood, and less applicability to censored data. Both methods are sensitive to the choice of initial parameter estimates and outliers.

There is a tradeoff between flexibility and convenience of the nonlinear least squares method and the accuracy of the maximum likelihood approach. In practice, the theoretical considerations mentioned above are apparently not crucial, and the two approaches generate similar results. For example, Gehan and Siddiqui (1973) conducted a simulation study of fitting Gompertz and some other hazard models to survival data. The authors concluded that the least squares estimates are nearly as efficient as maximum likelihood when sample size is 50 or more. They also found that the weighted least squares approach, which accounts for systematic decrease of the sample size with age, generated more efficient but less accurate parameter estimates compared to the nonweighted method. Thus, maximum likelihood is a preferred method in those cases where the statistical software is readily available or the optimization procedure can be easily implemented. Otherwise, the nonlinear least squares may be a reasonable choice.

It is important to recognize the limitations and pitfalls of model fitting. The main problem is uneven statistical power. At young ages, there are relatively few deaths; at the oldest ages, death rates are high, but there are relatively few organisms. At middle ages, there are large numbers of both organisms at risk and deaths, and so statistical power for estimation of mortality rates is concentrated in those middle age classes. Consequently, model fitting to the entire life history can give very accurate descriptions of the dynamics of middle age and can be systematically biased at early and late ages.

II. Experimental Evidence for Age-Specific Effects

If new mutations and genetic variants segregating in populations modify chances of survival by a constant factor at all ages (a situation known among demographers as "proportional hazards"), then there is no true age specificity; all is known from observations at a single age. However, if genes alter survival characteristics specifically at certain prescribed ages or stages of the life cycle, with no effect or very different effect at other ages, then the situation is more complex, and much more interesting. The evolutionary theory for the evolution of senescence requires age-specificity of genetic effects (Charlesworth, 1980; Curtsinger, 2001; Hamilton, 1966; Medawar, 1952; Williams, 1957). As we discuss below, evolutionary models currently under investigation are sensitive to the precise degree of age specificity. Proving the existence of such age-specific genetic variation is difficult, especially at the older ages, but mounting evidence suggests that there may be a substantial degree of age specificity of genetic effects in *Drosophila*. In the following sections, we describe several different types of experimental evidence that address that issue.

A. P-Element Tagging

P-elements are naturally occurring transposable genetic elements (transposons) specific to *Drosophila*. Their ability to insert into random chromosomal locations throughout the genome makes them useful tools for genetic research,

because they potentially disrupt gene expression or function at the insertion site. Screening of P-element inserts led to the discovery of life-extending "methuselah" (*mth*) and "I'm not dead yet" (*Indy*) single-gene mutations (Lin *et al.*, 1998; Rogina *et al.*, 2000). Clark & Guadalupe (1995) used P-element insertion lines to investigate the genetic basis of senescence and found that otherwise genetically identical lines differed in survivorship and mean life span under the influence of P-induced insertions. The authors claimed that some of the P-element insertions led to reduced post-reproductive survival without affecting early life history, and that P-element inserts altered the ages at which mortality curves leveled off, though few demographic details were given.

B. Mutation Accumulation Experiments

The term *mutation accumulation* refers to both a theory of the evolution of senescence (Medawar, 1952) and an experimental design pioneered in *Drosophila* (Mukai, 1964). It is the latter sense of the term that concerns us for the moment, although the former will be relevant later. The goal of a mutation accumulation experiment is to measure the rate at which new genetic variation spontaneously arises in a population, and to measure the phenotypic effects of those new mutations. General features of mutation accumulation experiments using *Drosophila* are as follows: starting with a single highly inbred line of flies, multiple sub-lines are established and maintained separately in small populations for dozens or even hundreds of generations. Spontaneous germline mutations occur independently in the various sub-lines, causing them to diverge both genetically and phenotypically. The sub-lines are kept at small census numbers so that new mutations have a reasonable chance to increase to fixation within each particular line by random genetic drift. The rate at which sub-lines diverge phenotypically provides an estimate of the rate of input of new genetic variation affecting the particular trait assayed.

The first mutation accumulation study of age-specific mortality was executed by Pletcher and colleagues (1998), who established 29 sub-lines of *D. melanogaster* from a single highly inbred progenitor pair. Sub-lines were maintained for 19 generations, and then survival data were collected on approximately 100,000 flies. Mutational effects were detected by comparing age-specific mortality rates in each sub-line with that of the progenitor stock, which was maintained in nonmutating condition by cryopreservation. Significant mutational variance for age-specific mortality was detected, but only for flies aged less than 30 days post-emergence. Most of the new mutations were highly age-specific, each affecting survival rates over a well-defined age window of one or two weeks. Mutations that affected mortality at all ages were also detected, but their contribution to overall mutational variance was small. The conclusion from this study is that most new mutations have age-specific effects, but the failure to detect mutational variance at very old ages is difficult to interpret. It is unclear whether the failure to detect late-acting mutations is due to smaller sample sizes and loss of statistical power, to inherently lower mutation rates for alleles that specifically affect old age survival, or a combination of those factors.

Pletcher and colleagues (1999) continued the mutation accumulation experiment, assaying mortality rates at 47 generations of divergence, and also jointly analyzing data at three time points (10, 19, and 47 generations). These assays involved approximately a quarter of a million flies. Further evidence for highly age-specific mutation was found, and once again there was evidence for higher levels of mutation affecting early survival than late survival. Surprisingly, there appeared to be no upward or downward bias of mutational effects on mortality rates (mutations increasing mortality are as frequent as mutations decreasing mortality), contradicting the usual assumption that almost all mutations are deleterious to carriers. One possible explanation of this paradox may be related to elimination of many deleterious mutations through selective deaths at early larval stages of *Drosophila* development.

Mack and colleagues (2000) and Yampolsky and colleagues (2001) used a different experimental design, the "middle class neighborhood" method, to accumulate mutations affecting mortality, fecundity, and male mating ability on a genetically heterogeneous background of recently collected flies. They found clear evidence of age-specific effects of new mutations after 20 generations of mutation accumulation, including many effects limited to middle and advanced ages. This result contrasts with that of Pletcher and colleagues (1998, 1999), who found mostly early age effects. In both studies, the degree of age specificity declined in later generations of the experiment.

Martorell and colleagues (1998) executed a large mutation accumulation experiment to study life history in *D. melanogaster*, maintaining 94 sub-lines for 80 generations. They found evidence for small mutational effects on mean life span, but because mortality rates were not assayed, the experiment provides no information about age specificity of genetic effects. If Pletcher and colleagues (1999) are correct about mutations decreasing mortality as often as they increase it, then Martorell and colleagues (1998) might have underestimated the rate of mutations that modify mean life spans. Similar remarks apply to studies of life span and related characters in flies exposed to mutagenic chemicals (Keightley & Ohnishi, 1998). Mutation accumulation experiments on life-history traits have also been executed using the nematode *C. elegans* (Keightley et al., 2000).

C. Neurogenetics and Gene Expression

Adult *Drosophila* are entirely post-mitotic organisms; that is, all cell division is completed when the animal metamorphoses from larval to adult stage. This contrasts sharply with other organisms, such as humans, in which cell division continues throughout the adult life span. It has been suggested that the lack of cell division in adult flies precludes late-onset genetic effects in *Drosophila*. However, recent evidence from several areas of biology that are not normally part of the discourse of demography suggests otherwise.

Neurodegenerative diseases in human, including Alzheimer's, Huntington, and Parkinson's disease, are characterized by late onset of pathology. Because *Drosophila* and humans share many functionally and structurally related genes, it is possible to model some of the human neurodegenerative pathologies by creating lines of flies that carry foreign or artificially modified genes (Driscoll & Gerstbrein, 2003; Fortini & Bonini, 2000; Mutsuddi & Nambu, 1998). Feany and Bender (2000) constructed transgenic flies carrying normal or mutant forms of the human gene for α-synuclein, a candidate cause of Parkinson's disease. All transgenics exhibited normal neural morphology and geotactic behavior as young adult flies, but beginning at 25 days after eclosion, mutant transgenics developed Parkinson-like neural morphology and a dramatic loss of locomotor ability, whereas nonmutant transgenics escaped the morphological and behavioral manifestations of disease. Of course, the primary importance of such research is its potential application to treating human disease, but the α-synuclein case

and others like it also demonstrate that genetic variation can produce specific late-onset phenotypes in adult *Drosophila*. Evidently, lack of cell division in adults does not preclude age-specific effects in older flies.

There is also evidence for age-specific genetic effects in modern studies of gene expression. It used to be widely assumed that the regulation of gene expression, which is capable of transforming single cells into highly differentiated and spatially structured mature organisms, becomes chaotic in old age. This view is now rejected, in part because of evidence from *Drosophila* (Helfand & Rogina, 2000, 2003; Rogina & Helfand, 1995; Rogina et al., 1998). Regulation of gene expression throughout the adult life span, including old age, sets the stage for age-specific genetic effects. DNA microarrays are powerful tools for the study of genome-wide patterns of gene expression in *Drosophila* and other organisms. Microarrays have been used to detect genes that vary in expression levels over the lifetimes of flies, and to detect genome-wide transcriptional responses to experimental treatments that modify life spans (McCarroll et al., 2004; Pletcher et al., 2002). Results from microarray studies bolster the view that gene expression is regulated throughout the adult life span and is therefore likely to be subject to genetic modification. Tahoe and colleagues (2005) demonstrated that age-specific patterns of gene expression differ between lines of *Drosophila* with very different mean life spans, and in some cases, including the genes encoding anti-microbial peptides, the line differences are manifest only in old age. Such observations do not prove that there are genetic differences between lines that alter survival specifically at advanced ages, but the observation of late-onset transcriptional differences does render the existence of such effects more likely. As more longitudinal studies of genome-wide transcription levels are published in the next few years, we can expect a more complete picture of genome function and its variability throughout the adult life span.

D. Mortality QTLs

Quantitative trait locus (QTL) mapping is a set of procedures for identifying approximate chromosomal locations of segregating genes that influence polygenic traits (Mackay, 2001, 2002; see Chapter 8, this volume). QTLs affecting mean life span in *Drosophila* have been identified in a number of studies (Curtsinger *et al.*, 1998; De Luca *et al.*, 2003; Forbes *et al.*, 2004; Leips & Mackay, 2000, 2002; Luckinbill & Golenberg, 2002; Khazaeli *et al.*, 2005; Nuzhdin *et al.*, 2005; Nuzhdin *et al.*, 1997; Pasyukova *et al.*, 2000; Resler *et al.*, 1998; Valenzuela *et al.*, 2004; Vieira *et al.*, 2000).

In principle, it is possible to apply the methods of QTL mapping to localize genes that affect age-specific mortality rates rather than just mean life spans. However, the requirements are stringent: not only is there the prerequisite for large sample sizes, as in any estimation of mortality rates, but it is also necessary that the populations be genetically highly defined and contain a high density of genetic markers for QTL localization. To date this has been accomplished in only two cases. Curtsinger and Khazaeli (2002) identified QTLs that affect age-specific mortality rates in recombinant inbred populations of *D. melanogaster*, finding evidence for several genetically variable chromosomal regions that influence survival in age-specific fashion. The authors also developed a graphical method for presenting age-specific QTL results, as follows. QTL mapping results are typically presented in two-dimensional graphs: the abscissa represents chromosomal position, measured in units of recombination from the left telomere, while the ordinate represents a statistical measure,

likelihood or LOD score indicating the probability that a QTL is present at a particular chromosomal position. A typical QTL map has peaks and valleys; genes affecting the quantitative trait are most likely to be located in chromosomal regions under the peaks, provided that the peaks exceed some likelihood threshold. Curtsinger and Khazaeli (2002) extended the usual analysis by mapping QTLs that affect mortality in each week of adult life and then adding a third dimension to the QTL map, indicating age. An example of a three-dimensional QTL map is shown in Figure 10.2. There is a QTL that affects age-specific mortality near the left end of chromosome III; the QTL has significant effects on

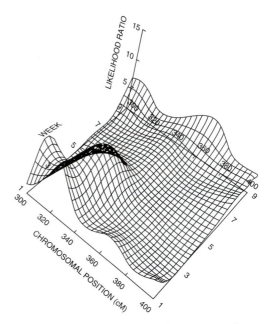

Figure 10.2 Three-dimensional QTL map of age-specific mortality rates for experimental populations of male *D. melanogaster* (Curtsinger & Khazaeli, 2002). The figure shows the chromosomal location and ontogenic timing of effects of quantitative trait loci that influence weekly mortality rates throughout the adult life span. The peak near the left telomere of chromosome III indicates genetic effects on mortality rates primarily in early adult life, with no evidence for significant effects late in adult life.

mortality in the first few weeks of adult life but has no effect on survival at later ages.

One other study of age-specific mortality rates using QTL mapping methods is that of Nuzhdin and colleagues (2005). QTLs affecting weekly mortality rates in both sexes were mapped in 144 recombinant inbred lines. Twenty-five statistically significant QTLs were found; most had positively correlated effects on mortality at several different ages, but in two cases the correlations were negative. Overall, the results suggest that the standing genetic variation in survival consists of a mixture of transient deleterious mutations that tend to increase mortality at younger ages, and a few mutations with opposing age-specific effects that are maintained by balancing selection. The latter are potentially examples of antagonistic pleiotropy, although finer genetic resolution will be required to rule out the competing linkage hypothesis.

III. Leveling-Off of Mortality Rates

In many biological species, including *Drosophila* and humans, death rates increase exponentially with age for much of the life span. However, at extreme old ages, a "mortality deceleration" occurs— the pace of mortality growth decelerates from an expected exponential curve. Sometimes this mortality deceleration progresses to the extent that mortality "leveling-off" is observed, leading to a "mortality plateau." Thus, at extreme old ages, a paradoxical situation is observed when one of the major manifestations of aging—increasing death rate—apparently fades away or even disappears.

The phenomenon of mortality deceleration has been known for a long time, although its mechanisms were not intensively studied prior to the 1990s. The first

person who noticed that the Gompertz curve is not applicable to extreme old ages was Benjamin Gompertz himself (Gompertz, 1825, 1872; see review by Olshansky, 1998). In 1867, William Makeham noted that for humans "the rapidity of the increase in the death rate decelerated beyond age 75" (p. 346). In 1919, Brownlee wondered whether it is "possible that a kind of Indian summer occurs after the age of 85 years is passed, and that conditions improve as regards length of life" (p. 385). Perks (1932) observed that "the graduated curve [of mortality] starts to decline in the neighborhood of age 84" (p. 15). Greenwood and Irwin (1939) confirmed that "the increase of mortality rate with age advances at a slackening rate, that nearly all, perhaps all, methods of graduation of the type of Gompertz's formula overstate senile mortality" (p. 14). They also suggested "the possibility that with advancing age the rate of mortality asymptotes to a finite value" (p. 14), and made the first estimates for the asymptotic value of human mortality plateau (expressed in one-year probability of death, q_x). According to their estimates of human mortality plateaus, "the limiting values of q_x are 0.439 for women and 0.544 for men" (Greenwood & Irwin, 1939, p. 21). In 1960, *Science* published an article on a "General theory of mortality and aging" that listed some "essential observations which must be taken into account in any general theory of mortality." (Strehler & Mildvan, 1960, p. 14). The first of these essential observations was the Gompertz law of mortality, while the second essential observation stated that "the Gomperzian period is followed by a gradual reduction in their rate of increase of the mortality" (Strehler & Mildvan, 1960, p.14). This observation of mortality deceleration was confirmed for several species, including *Drosophila* and *C. elegans* (Economos, 1979). The author concluded "that after a certain species-characteristic age, force of mortality and probability of death cease to increase exponentially with age . . . and remain constant at a high level on the average for the remainder of the life span." (p. 74). The author called these findings "a non-Gompertzian paradigm for mortality kinetics" (Economos, 1979, p. 74). A year later, the same author analyzed data for thoroughbred horses (mares), Dall mountain sheep, houseflies, and some other species and came to a conclusion that "Gompertz's law is only an approximation, not valid over a certain terminal part of the lifespan, during which force of mortality levels off." (Economos, 1980, p. 317). These findings failed, however, to receive attention, and the topic stagnated.

A. Recent Studies of Mortality Plateaus

Prior to 1990, the most popular explanation of mortality plateaus was based on the idea of initial population heterogeneity, suggested by British actuary Robert Eric Beard (1911–1983). Beard developed a mathematical model in which individuals were assumed to have exponential increase in their risk of death as they age, but their initial risks differed from individual to individual and followed a gamma distribution (Beard, 1959, 1963, 1971). This model produces a logistic function for mortality kinetics that is very close to the exponential function at younger ages, but then mortality rates decelerate and reach a plateau in old age. This compositional interpretation of mortality plateaus explained them as an artifact of mixture, perhaps reducing their intrinsic interest to biologists.

The situation changed in 1991, when it was found that the general theory of systems failure (known as reliability theory) predicts an inevitable mortality leveling-off as a result of redundancy exhaustion, even for initially identical individuals (Gavrilov & Gavrilova, 1991). Thus, a testable prediction from this theory was that mortality deceleration should be observed even for genetically identical individuals kept in strictly controlled laboratory conditions. Shortly thereafter, Carey and colleagues (1992) and Curtsinger and colleagues (1992) published back-to-back papers in *Science* demonstrating mortality plateaus in laboratory populations of medflies and *Drosophila*, respectively. The medfly study employed genetically heterogeneous populations, whereas the companion study in *Drosophila* used highly inbred lines that were essentially devoid of within-line genetic heterogeneity.

The medfly and *Drosophila* experimental papers generated a flurry of criticisms and responses (Carey *et al.*, 1993; Curtsinger *et al.*, 1994; Gavrilov & Gavrilova, 1993; Graves & Mueller, 1993, 1994; Kowald & Kirkwood, 1993; Nusbaum *et al.*, 1993; Robine & Ritchie, 1993; Vaupel & Carey, 1993). Within a few years, even the most ardent critics were convinced that mortality plateaus were real phenomena and not merely artifacts of contamination or declining density in population cages (Khazaeli *et al.*, 1995a, 1996). Mortality plateaus were subsequently documented on very large scales in a variety of experimental species, including yeast, nematodes, *Drosophila*, medflies, parasitic wasps, and humans (see Vaupel *et al.*, 1998, for a review).

Typical characteristics of a mortality plateau in *Drosophila* are shown in Figure 10.3 (from Pletcher & Curtsinger, 1998). In this sample of 122,000 males, age-specific mortality increases in approximately exponential fashion from emergence until 60 days. After 60 days, when 5 percent of the original cohort remains alive, mortality decelerates and remains fairly constant until 80 days of age. Thus,

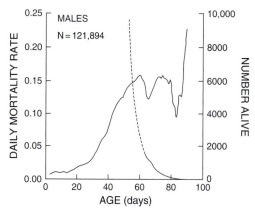

Figure 10.3 Age-specific mortality rate and survivorship in a large cohort of male *D. melanogaster* (Pletcher & Curtsinger, 1998). Age-specific mortality increases approximately exponentially until 60 days post-eclosion, and then reaches a plateau on days 60 to 80.

for a period of 20 days, or about 20 percent of the maximum life span in this particular experiment, there is no trend toward increasing mortality with increasing age. After 80 days the mortality curve shoots up, as the last few survivors die. The latter behavior is of no particular significance, and is best understood as an artifact of finite sample size, occurring when fewer than 10 flies remain alive.

The turnaround in views about applicability of the Gompertz model, which had been revered for well over a century, raises an obvious question: Why was Gompertz widely accepted until recently, and even raised to the stature of "Gompertz' law" despite various exceptions being pointed out? In addition to science's predilection for simple laws of nature, the likely explanation is that most survival experiments prior to the 1990s had been too small to detect plateaus. Mortality plateaus are late-life phenomena. Small experiments fail to detect them because there are few survivors to the age at which mortality rates begin to level off. It is also possible that biologists' habit of examining survivorship curves rather than mortality rates contributed to ignorance about

plateaus; it is difficult to see a plateau in the tail of a survivorship curve, even if sample sizes are relatively large.

B. Explaining Mortality Plateaus

Although the existence of mortality plateaus is now universally accepted, explaining why plateaus exist is controversial. It is convenient to define two general, non-exclusive classes of explanations: population heterogeneity and individual aging. Heterogeneity refers to the idea that individuals in a cohort differ in frailty, which is most conveniently parameterized as a multiplicative factor of the Gompertz hazard model. The hazard rate of an individual of age x and frailty Z is

$$\mu_{x,z} = ZAe^{Bx},$$

where Z is a gamma-distributed random variable with mean 1 and variance σ^2. Under those circumstances, the mean age-specific mortality in the population is given by the logistic equation. Individual differences in frailty can be genetic or environmental in origin and tend to produce mortality deceleration. This occurs because weaker organisms die first, leaving preferentially more robust members of the population alive for later survival measurements. The process of sorting weaker and stronger individuals by death within a generation is often referred to as "demographic selection," the first part of the term being necessary to distinguish it from selection of the Darwinian sort.

Frailty may be fixed at birth, or acquired and modified through life experience, as mentioned above. For instance, for the fixed frailty situation, we might imagine that a population of flies contains different genotypes, each with its characteristic hazard rate. Or, in a genetically homogeneous population such as an inbred line or F_1 cross between two inbred lines, differences in frailty between organisms could arise from micro-environmental effects, such as slight uncontrolled spatial variation in temperature or quality of food experienced at pupation sites. In either case, the essential feature of the fixed frailty models is that the organisms carry a certain frailty factor Z with them throughout their lives. In contrast, flies could acquire different frailty factors during their adult lifetimes as a result of exposure to infectious organisms, or differential rates of reproduction. In either case, the logistic model predicts the expected population mortality dynamics (Yashin *et al.*, 1994), and the magnitude of population variance for frailty has a strong influence on mortality dynamics.

Gavrilov and Gavrilova (1991, 2001; see Chapter 1, this volume) developed several classes of aging models based on reliability theory. Interestingly, all these models predict a mortality deceleration, no matter what assumptions are made regarding initial population heterogeneity or its complete initial homogeneity. Moreover, these reliability models of aging produce mortality plateaus as inevitable outcome for any values of considered parameters. The only constraint is that the elementary steps of the multistage destruction process of a system should occur by chance only, independent of age. The models also predict that an initially homogeneous population will become highly heterogeneous for risk of death over time (acquired heterogeneity).

Another class of explanations for mortality plateaus depends not on differences between individuals, but on changes within individuals as they age. If the hazard rates for individual organisms decelerate at older ages, then so, too, will the observed population mortality. One can imagine various biological reasons that individual hazard rates might decelerate. Older flies might incur less physiological and metabolic cost from mating behavior and reproduction, or lower activity levels in old age might entail

less exposure to infectious agents and less generation of harmful oxygen radicals. For humans, a similar hypothesis was proposed by Greenwood and Irwin (1939), who suggested that lower-than-expected mortality of centenarians could be explained by their less risky behavior.

There is a growing body of evolutionary theory that addresses ultimate causes of mortality plateaus. The basic problem to be solved by theoreticians is that evolutionary models of age-specific mortality tend to generate very high mortality rates ("walls of death") at post-reproductive ages (Charlesworth, 1980; Curtsinger, 1995a,b; Partridge & Barton, 1993; Pletcher & Curtsinger, 1998). Imagine a population in which there is initially no senescence—that is, the hazard rate is the same for all age classes. Over time, new mutations occur, some of which have age-specific effects on survival. Many of the new mutations are deleterious at all ages and are quickly eliminated from the population by natural selection. Some mutations, presumably very few, improve survival of carriers at early ages, are positively selected, and increase in frequency in the population; this causes an evolutionary lowering of the population mortality curve at juvenile and reproductive ages. Some mutations increase or decrease mortality specifically at post-reproductive ages, but because post-reproductive survival is irrelevant to Darwinian fitness, natural selection does not discriminate. The net result is that there is no evolutionary force "pushing down" on the late-life part of the mortality curve. If the majority of mutations that affect old-age survival cause a deterioration of vitality, then post-reproductive survival will erode under mutation pressure, with nothing to stop it from eventually producing a wall of death. This scenario presumes the existence of exclusively late-acting mutations, as originally postulated by Medawar (1952), and is known as the mutation accumulation model of the evolution of senescence. The central problem for evolutionists trying to understand mortality trajectories is to discover some means of counteracting the tendency of recurrent mutation to drive post-reproductive hazard rate to infinity.

One possibility, not widely considered, is that mutations that affect only the old might improve survival as often as they erode it. This might seem at first glance to be nonbiological, violating the widely held view that the vast majority of mutations are deleterious to their carriers. However, reasonable scenarios can be imagined; for instance, a mutation that reduces mobility in old age might increase survival by causing carriers to generate fewer damaging oxygen radicals. There is some suggestion in the results of mutation accumulation experiments described above that mutations increase survival as often as they decrease it, but it must be admitted that the distribution of mutational effects for old-age-specific mutations is not known in detail.

Abrams and Ludwig (1995) addressed the mortality plateau problem in an evolutionary context by analyzing an optimality model in which organisms are presumed to allocate resources to either somatic repair or reproduction. The optimal allocation was presumed to be that which maximizes lifetime reproductive output. Abrams and Ludwig (1995) found that an optimal allocation involves declining investment in repair with increasing age, which, the authors suggest, could lead to late-life mortality plateaus. However, Charlesworth and Partridge (1997) re-examined the optimality model and found that the death rate tends to infinity with increasing age. We also note that the optimality approach does not specifically incorporate deleterious mutations with age-specific effects, an important omission.

Mueller and Rose (1996) used numerical simulations to study the evolution of mortality under antagonistic pleiotropy—that

is, the assumption that mutations have negatively correlated effects on survival at young and old ages. They argued that such models easily explain mortality plateaus, but their results have been widely criticized. Mueller and Rose (1996) assumed that every mutation increases survival in one randomly chosen age class, and reduces it in another; there are no unconditionally deleterious mutations in the model. Charlesworth and Partridge (1997) noted that the Mueller-Rose model was not iterated to equilibrium, and suggested that late-life survival rates would approach zero in this model as more evolutionary time elapsed. In general, the evolutionary equilibrium state is difficult to define in numerical simulations of finite populations. Pletcher and Curtsinger (1998) argued that the Mueller-Rose model includes a strange feature that biases the results: there is an assumption that when the population mortality rate is low, new mutations tend to increase mortality, but when the mortality rate is high, new mutations tend to make it decrease. The net effect is that mortality rates are forced toward an intermediate value. Pletcher and Curtsinger (1998) showed that removing that assumption leads to a late-life wall of mortality. The most telling critique is by Wachter (1999), who obtained analytical results for a generalized class of Mueller-Rose–type models and concluded that mortality plateaus cannot be accounted for by their equilibrium behavior. Wachter (1999) states unequivocally that the Mueller-Rose model fails in this respect. Thus, it seems likely that the simulation of Mueller and Rose (1996) produced transient mortality plateaus that were erroneously interpreted as equilibrium evolutionary states.

Given strong criticisms of the Mueller-Rose simulation model and analytical invalidation of its results, it is surprising that Drapeau and colleagues (2000), Rose and Mueller (2000), and Rose and colleagues (2002) have continued to promote it. All three of those papers failed to cite the analytical results of Wachter (1999). Mueller and colleagues (2003) address the various criticisms, including Wachter's (1999) analytical results, but the responses are unconvincing (de Grey, 2003a, 2004; Service, 2004). Technical details aside, the broader point is that Rose, Mueller, and their associates endorse individual aging over population heterogeneity as a general explanation for mortality plateaus, a position that could ultimately prove to be correct. They refer to their argument as "the evolutionary theory" (Rose & Mueller, 2000, p. 1,660), implying that heterogeneity explanations are "un-evolutionary" or "anti-evolutionary." The nomenclature is unfortunate. Phenotypic variability between organisms, including genetically identical ones, is an essential feature of quantitative genetic variability and micro-evolutionary change (Falconer & Mackay, 1996). Labeling the argument "evolutionary" is just a rhetorical device, with few constraints on its use: Graves and Mueller (1993, 1994; see also Curtsinger, 1995a,b) raised the "evolutionary" flag when they argued *against the existence* of mortality plateaus in *Drosophila*, a stance that was eventually abandoned.

Pletcher and Curtsinger (1998) presented simulation results for the evolution of mortality plateaus, focusing on positive pleiotropy, in which mutations exert positively correlated effects on mortality rates at different ages. In these simulations, positive pleiotropy seemed to produce mortality plateaus, but, as in any simulation of finite populations, the definition of stable evolutionary state is difficult, and the outcomes were probably transient. Charlesworth (2001) used analytical techniques to study a similar situation by assuming that all deleterious mutations have deleterious effects at reproductive ages. This assumption prevents mutation frequencies from exploding at older ages and, thus, preserves mortality plateaus.

Service (2000a) simulated mortality dynamics under the assumption of population heterogeneity in individual age-specific risk of death. Heterogeneity was modeled by assigning each individual a unique Gompertz mortality function, with means and variances of Gompertz parameters based on the published literature for *Drosophila*. He found that the heterogeneity generated by variation in Gompertz parameters was sufficient to explain late-life mortality plateaus and could also account for late-life declines in genetic variance of mortality rates. Similar conclusions were reported by Pletcher and Curtsinger (2000b).

The reliability models of multistage destruction (Gavrilov & Gavrilova, 1991, 2001) were recently reformulated in mathematical terms of a stochastic Markov process (Steinsaltz & Evans, 2004). The authors define a Markov mortality model as a stochastic process, which is "killed" at random stopping times according to the behavior of a Markov process. A general feature of such multistage models is that they usually produce mortality plateaus, as it was demonstrated earlier with a more simple approach (Gavrilov & Gavrilova, 1991, 2001). As Steinsaltz and Evans (2004) put it, "the mortality rate stops increasing [with increasing age], not because we have selected out an exceptional subset of the population, but because the condition of the survivors is reflective of their being survivors, even though they started out the same as everyone else." Thus, the Markov mortality models explain mortality plateaus by a type of heterogeneity in acquired frailty because the underlying assumptions are similar to the earlier reliability models.

In evaluating the various theories, it is important to remember that the fact that a particular mathematical model or simulation can fit or "predict" an experimental outcome is not proof that the assumptions of the model are correct. For example, the venerable Hardy-Weinberg model of population genetics predicts certain genotypic frequencies, but observation of those frequencies in real populations does not validate the underlying assumptions of the model (random mating, absence of natural selection, etc.). Theory guides our thinking, but critical tests must come from well-designed experiments, efforts at which are described in the next section.

C. Testing the Theories

Designing critical experiments to address the causes of mortality plateaus has proven to be exceptionally difficult; in fact, all experimental tests in this area are flawed in one way or another. Thus, no final answers can be given at present, but it is instructive to review the relevant experiments and consider the pitfalls.

The first experiment specifically designed to test heterogeneity theory used lethal stress to manipulate the magnitude of population heterogeneity (Khazaeli et al., 1995b) and was inspired by demographic studies of human populations after a catastrophe (Vaupel et al., 1987). Using a single highly inbred line of flies, multiple age-synchronized cohorts were established. In control populations, flies were maintained under the usual conditions, whereas in experimental populations, flies were subjected to 24 hours of desiccation at a young age. About 20 percent of the flies died during and immediately after the desiccation stress. Post-stress mortality rates are informative about population heterogeneity; in particular, in the absence of population heterogeneity, post-stress mortality in experimental and control populations is expected to be identical. However, if there is significant population heterogeneity at the time of the stress, then post-stress mortality in the experimental populations is expected to drop below that of the control populations,

at least temporarily, because the more frail individuals will have been eliminated. The latter pattern was observed, and was interpreted by Khazaeli and colleagues (1995b) as evidence for significant levels of heterogeneity. However, the authors retracted that result when it was realized that there was a flaw in the interpretation (Curtsinger & Khazaeli, 1997). The problem is that exposure to an external stress does more than kill the more frail flies; it also induces a stress response in the survivors. This phenomenon, known as hormesis, is well documented in a variety of species and involves a rapid genomic response to severe stress. The stress response is an interesting phenomenon, but it creates difficult problems in the interpretation of the stress experiment. In particular, the post-stress decline in mortality among experimentals compared to controls could be due to reduced heterogeneity through elimination of weaker flies, hormesis induced among survivors, or both factors. The experimental design of Khazaeli and colleagues (1995b) does not permit separation of the heterogeneity and hormetic effects, and so the result is inconclusive regarding heterogeneity. Recently, the stress experiment was redesigned to correct the confounding flaw, and data have been collected in the Curtsinger lab on 100,000 male flies of one inbred genotype. Five intensities of stress were applied, including one sufficient to induce a stress response but not severe enough to cause immediate deaths. The mild stress will allow estimation of the hormesis effect independent of the heterogeneity effect, unconfounding the variables. Data analysis by the authors of this chapter and Dr. A. Khazaeli is underway.

A different and more benign experimental design was used by Khazaeli and colleagues (1998), who attempted to manipulate population heterogeneity by fractionating genetically homogeneous populations. Working with two highly inbred lines, experimental populations were subjected to the most stringent environmental controls possible, far beyond what is normally employed in fly husbandry. Eggs were collected over a seven-hour period, instead of the usual 24 hours. First instar larvae were collected from that sample for only three hours, and emerging adults were collected in three-hour windows. The result of all this careful timing of development is that within a cohort, adult flies experienced larval and pupal environmental conditions that are as similar as possible. The question then is whether the environmentally "homogeneous" populations exhibit mortality plateaus to a lesser extent than normal environmentally "heterogeneous" control populations. Khazaeli and colleagues (1998) found that 93 percent of experimental populations and 100 percent of control populations exhibited statistically significant mortality deceleration late in life. The authors concluded that reducing environmental heterogeneity during larval and pupal stages has negligible effect on adult mortality trajectories. Drapeau and colleagues (2000, p. 72) overstated this experimental result when they wrote that "Khazaeli *et al.* (1998) found no evidence to support the hypothesis that environmental heterogeneity among individual flies is a primary factor in determining late-life mortality rates." The experiment actually gives information only about larval and pupal stages, and is in the strictest sense relevant only to the "fixed-heterogeneity" model. The results are not informative about heterogeneity acquired in adulthood, which may be substantial. Perhaps a broader lesson from this study is that there is a substantial and intrinsic environmental heterogeneity in experimental populations that cannot be removed experimentally, even by Herculean efforts.

The most widely discussed experimental test of heterogeneity theory is that of Drapeau and colleagues (2000), who argued that there is a close connection between frailty and sensitivity to environmental stresses in experimental populations of *Drosophila*. They further suggested that, according to heterogeneity theory, populations differing in tolerance to stress should have different late-life mortality characteristics, though the nature of the expected differences was not spelled out. They compared mortality trajectories in fly populations that had been selected for resistance to starvation with those of unselected controls. No statistically significant differences were found, which the authors interpreted as evidence against the heterogeneity theory. Service (2000b) questioned the assertion that the populations are expected to differ in late-life mortality, noting that for the logistic model the plateau occurs at B/σ^2. Consequently, populations could differ in the intercept parameter A and have the same levels of late-life mortality. As noted by Mueller and colleagues (2000) in their response to Service (2000b), the force of this criticism is blunted by the generally accepted theoretical observation that large and biologically unrealistic amounts of variation in the intercept parameter would be required to produce mortality plateaus, if that were all that varied between individuals. Service (2000b) also noted that if σ^2 is lower in the selected population, then it is expected to have higher mortality rate than controls (when all other parameters are fixed), especially at early ages, as observed. Service concludes that the results of Drapeau and colleagues (2000) are entirely consistent with the predictions of the heterogeneity model. de Grey (2003b) criticized the use of maximum likelihood methods by Drapeau and colleagues (2000) and argued that heterogeneous Gompertz parameters could explain the experimental results. Steinsaltz (2005) reanalyzed the experimental results of Drapeau and colleagues (2000) and questioned the claim that there is no difference in late-life mortality schedules between populations. The original claim was based on comparisons of means averaged over populations. Steinsaltz (2005) noted that the data are bimodal, and means are therefore misleading. He reanalyzed the data and found that populations were actually quite different, the mortality plateau being lower in the selected populations. He concluded that the experimental results lend mild support to the heterogeneity theory, although the expected differences in timing of the plateau were not observed. In sum, the critiques of Drapeau and colleagues (2000) are varied and instructive, and illustrate some of the difficulties of the experimental task and complexities of the analysis.

Rose and colleagues (2002) studied mortality trajectories in populations of *Drosophila* that had been artificially selected for long life and compared them to unselected control populations. Mortality trajectories had previously been studied in the same populations by Service and colleagues (1998), who invoked a heterogeneity explanation. Rose and colleagues (2002) showed that control populations consistently exhibited earlier onset of mortality plateaus than selected populations. This result was interpreted as being consistent with an "evolutionary" (i.e., individual aging) model. The result is suggestive, but not critical; it is not clear that the observations are inconsistent with predictions of any particular heterogeneity model. In general, we consider it very unlikely that critical tests of heterogeneity and individual aging models can be executed with outbred experimental populations. The problem is that the variance parameter plays a central role in the predictions of heterogeneity models but is generally unknown in either relative or absolute terms for outbred, genetically uncharacterized populations. It is widely assumed that selected populations are less heterogeneous than unselected controls because

some genotypes have been eliminated by selection. However, several factors could cause selected populations to be *more* heterogeneous, both in genetic and environmental variance. If the selection response entails an increase in frequencies of initially rare alleles, genetic variance is expected to increase under selection, a prediction that has been verified experimentally (Curtsinger & Ming, 1997). This counterintuitive result occurs because the contribution to total genetic variance by any particular locus depends on $2pq$, where p and q are allelic frequencies (Falconer & Mackay, 1996); rare and common alleles contribute little to population genetic variance, but alleles at intermediate frequencies potentially contribute much. The same effect occurs if new mutations increase to appreciable frequencies during the selection process. Another factor that complicates matters is genetic homeostasis. It is well known that homozygous genotypes generally exhibit greater environmental variance than heterozygotes (see review by Phelan & Austad, 1994). If selection and/or inbreeding increase homozygosity in selected populations, then the environmental component of variance is expected to increase. In short, there are too many unknown variables in genetically uncharacterized outbred populations to allow critical tests of predictions of heterogeneity models. A better experimental design is that of Miyo and Charlesworth (2004), who studied mortality rates in hybrid progeny of crosses between inbred lines of *Drosophila*. In such populations, all individuals are genetically alike, except for recent mutations, and heterozygous at loci that differ between parental lines. Miyo and Charlesworth (2004) found that populations of both mated and unmated hybrid males exhibited mortality plateaus, and suggested that their results were consistent with underlying heterogeneity of mortality rates.

In the final analysis, evaluating the various heterogeneity models is a purely quantitative question. No reasonable person would deny that there is some heterogeneity for frailty within populations, even genetically homogeneous ones; the question is whether there is sufficient heterogeneity to produce late-life mortality plateaus. We are optimistic that large-scale, multilevel stress experiments and other designs using genetically defined populations will provide the relevant estimates. On the other hand, if the individual aging theory is correct, then there must be some important biological processes that differ between organisms at pre- and post-plateau ages and account for the change in mortality trajectory.

IV. Conclusions

The integration of biology and demography proceeded sporadically for most of the 20th century. Pearl, Sacher, Strehler, and others showed the way toward integration of the fields, but their efforts were not always widely appreciated. Now we are in a period of widespread dissemination of demographic techniques among experimental biologists. The new field of biodemography is flourishing and has rich conceptual bases to draw on in demography, evolutionary biology, reliability theory, and even theoretical physics (Pletcher & Neuhauser, 2000). Its first major conceptual challenge is to explain mortality plateaus. We are optimistic that consensus will emerge in this area as experimental designs and methods of data analysis become more sophisticated. Other important challenges include defining the nature of age-specific genetic variation and explaining the high degree of environmental variation in demographic parameters.

Acknowledgements

Research is supported by grants from the National Institute of Aging at the National Institutes of Health. We thank Dr. A. Khazaeli for comments.

References

Abrams, P. A., & Ludwig, D. (1995). Optimality theory, Gompertz' law, and the disposable soma theory of senescence. *Evolution, 49,* 1056–1066.

Beard, R. E. (1959). Note on some mathematical mortality models. In G. E. W. Wolstenholme & M. O'Connor (Eds.), *The lifespan of animals.* Boston: Little, Brown.

Beard, R. E. (1963). A theory of mortality based on actuarial, biological, and medical considerations. *Proceedings of the International Population Conference, New York,* 1, 611–625.

Beard, R. E. (1971). Some aspects of theories of mortality, cause of death analysis, forecasting and stochastic processes. In W. Brass (Ed.), *Biological aspects of demography* (pp. 57–68). London: Taylor & Francis.

Brownlee, J. (1919). Notes on the biology of a life-table. *Journal of the Royal Statistical Society, 82,* 34–77.

Carey, J. R. (2003). *Longevity: the biology and demography of life span.* Princeton, NJ: Princeton University Press.

Carey, J. R., Curtsinger, J. W., & Vaupel, J. W. (1993). Response to letters. *Science, 260,* 1567–1569.

Carey, J. R., Liedo, P., Orozco, D., & Vaupel, J. W. (1992). Slowing of mortality rates at older ages in large medfly cohorts. *Science, 258,* 457–461.

Charlesworth, B. (1980). *Evolution in age-structured populations.* New York: Cambridge University Press.

Charlesworth, B. (2001). Patterns of age-specific means and genetic variances of mortality rates predicted by mutation-accumulation theory of ageing. *Journal of Theoretical Biology, 210,* 47–65.

Charlesworth, B., & Partridge, L. (1997). Ageing: leveling of the grim reaper. *Current Biology, 7,* R440–R442.

Clark, A. G., & Guadalupe, R. N. (1995). Probing the evolution of senescence in *Drosophila melanogaster* with P-element tagging. *Genetica, 96,* 225–234.

Curtsinger, J. W. (1995a). Density and age-specific mortality. *Genetica, 96,* 179–82.

Curtsinger, J. W. (1995b). Density, mortality, and the narrow view. *Genetica, 96*, 187–89.

Curtsinger, J. W. (2001). Genetic theories of senescence. *International encyclopedia of social and behavioral sciences.* Oxford: Pergamon Press.

Curtsinger, J. W., & Khazaeli, A. (1997). A reconsideration of stress experiments and population heterogeneity. *Experimental Gerontology, 32*, 727–729.

Curtsinger, J. W., & Khazaeli, A. A. (2002). Lifespan, QTLs, age-specificity, and pleiotropy in *Drosophila. Mechanisms of Ageing and Development, 123*, 81–93.

Curtsinger, J. W., Fukui, H. H., Resler, A. S., Kelly, K., & Khazaeli, A. A. (1998). Genetic analysis of extended lifespan in *Drosophila melanogaster.* I. RAPD screen for genetic divergence between selected and control lines. *Genetica, 104*, 21–32.

Curtsinger, J. W., Fukui, H., Townsend, D., & Vaupel, J. W. (1992). Demography of genotypes: failure of the limited life-span paradigm in *Drosophila melanogaster. Science, 258*, 461–463.

Curtsinger, J. W., & Ming, R. (1997). Non-linear selection response in Drosophila: A strategy for testing the rare-alleles model of quantitative genetic variability. *Genetica, 99*, 59–56.

Curtsinger, J. W., Service, P., & Prout, T. (1994). Antagonistic pleiotropy, reversal of dominance, and genetic polymorphism. *American Naturalist, 144*, 210–228.

Cutler, S. J., & Ederer, F. (1958). Maximum utilization of the life table methodology in analyzing survival. *Journal of Chronic Disease, 8*, 699–712.

de Grey, A. D. (2003a). Overzealous maximum-likelihood fitting falsely convicts the slope heterogeneity hypothesis. *Experimental Gerontology, 38*, 921–923.

de Grey, A. D. (2003b). Critique of the demographic evidence for "late-life non-senescence." *Mathematical Society Transactions, 31*, 452–454.

de Grey, A. D. (2004). Reply to Mueller's and Rose's letter to the editor: models on trial: falsifying overstated claims of generality does not falsify correctly-stated ones. *Experimental Gerontology, 39*, 453.

De Luca, M., Roshina, N. V., Geiger-Thornsberry, G. L., Lyman, R. F., Pasyukova,

E. G., & Mackay, T. F. C. (2003). Dopa-decarboxylase affects variation in *Drosophila* longevity. *Nature Genetics, 34*, 429–433.

Drapeau, M. D., Gass, E. K., Simison, M. D., Mueller, L. D., & Rose, M. R. (2000). Testing the heterogeneity theory of late-life mortality plateaus by using cohorts of *Drosophila melanogaster. Experimental Gerontology, 35*, 71–84.

Driscoll, M., & Gerstbrein, B. (2003). Dying for a cause: invertebrate genetics takes on human neurodegeneration. *Nature Reviews Genetics, 4*, 181–194.

Economos, A. C. (1979). A non-Gompertzian paradigm for mortality kinetics of metazoan animals and failure kinetics of manufactured products. *AGE, 2*, 74–76.

Economos, A. C. (1980). Kinetics of metazoan mortality. *Journal of Social and Biological Structures, 3*, 317–329.

Falconer, D. S., & Mackay, T. F. C. (1996). *Introduction to quantitative genetics* (4th ed.). Harlow, UK: Longman Science and Tech. Feany, M. B., & Bender, W. W. (2000). A *Drosophila* model of Parkinson's disease. *Nature, 404*, 394–398.

Filliben, J. J. (2004). Exploratory data analysis. In *NIST/SEMATECH e-Handbook of Statistical Methods.* Available at http://www.itl.nist.gov/div898/handbook.

Finch, C. E., & Kirkwood, T. B. L. (2000). *Chance, development, and aging.* New York: Oxford University Press.

Forbes, S. N., Valenzuela, R. K., Keim, P., & Service, P. M. (2004). Quantitative trait loci affecting life span in replicated populations of *Drosophila melanogaster.* I. Composite interval mapping. *Genetics, 168*, 301–311.

Fortini, M. E., & Bonini, N. M. (2000). Modeling human neurodegenerative diseases in *Drosophila. Trends in Genetics, 16*, 161–167.

Fukui, H. H., Ackert, L., & Curtsinger, J. W. (1996). Deceleration of age-specific mortality rates in chromosomal homozygotes and heterozygotes of *Drosophila melanogaster. Experimental Gerontology, 31*, 517–531.

Fukui, H., Pletcher, S., & Curtsinger, J. W. (1995). Selection for increased longevity in *Drosophila melanogaster*: A response to Baret and Lints. *Gerontology, 41*, 65–68.

Fukui, H, Xiu, L., & Curtsinger, J. W. (1993). Slowing of age-specific mortality rates in

Drosophila melanogaster. Experimental Gerontology, 28, 585–599.

Gavrilov, L. A., & Gavrilova, N. S. (1991). *The biology of lifespan: a quantitative approach*. New York: Harwood Academic Publishers.

Gavrilov, L. A., & Gavrilova, N. S. (1993). Fruit fly aging and mortality. *Science*, 260, 1565.

Gavrilov, L. A., & Gavrilova, N. S. (2001). The reliability theory of aging and longevity. *Journal of Theoretical Biology*, 213, 527–545.

Gehan, E. A., & Siddiqui, M. M. (1973). Simple regression methods for survival time studies. *Journal of the American Statistical Association*, 68, 848–856.

Gompertz, B. (1825). On the nature of the function expressive of the law of human mortality, and on a new mode of determining the value of life contingencies. *Philosophical Transactions of the Royal Society (London)*, 115, 513–585.

Gompertz, B. (1872). On one uniform law of mortality from birth to extreme old age, and on the law of sickness. *Journal of the Institute of Actuaries*, 16, 329–344.

Graves, J. L., & Mueller, L. D. (1993). Population density effects on longevity. *Genetica*, 91, 99–109.

Graves, J. L., & Mueller, L. D. (1994). Population density effects on longevity revisited: a note in response to 'Density and age-specific mortality' by J. W. Curtsinger. *Genetica*, 96, 183–186.

Greenwood, M., & Irwin, J. O. (1939). The biostatistics of senility. *Human Biology*, 11, 1–23.

Hamilton, W. D. (1966). The molding of senescence by natural selection. *Journal of Theoretical Biology*, 12, 12–45.

Helfand, S. L., & Rogina, B. (2000). Regulation of gene expression during aging. *Results and Problems in Cell Differentiation*, 29, 67–80.

Helfand, S. L., & Rogina, B. (2003). Molecular genetics of aging in the fly: is this the beginning of the end? *Bioessays*, 25, 134–141.

Keightley, P. D., & Ohnishi, O. (1998). EMS-induced polygenic mutation rates for nine quantitative characters in *Drosophila melanogaster. Genetics*, 148, 753–766.

Keightley, P. D., Davies, E. K., Peters, A. D., & Shaw, R. G. (2000). Properties of ethylmethane sulfonate-induced mutations affecting life-history traits in

Caenorhabditis elegans and inferences about bivariate distributions of mutation effects. *Genetics*, 156, 143–154.

Khazaeli, A. A., & Curtsinger, J. W. (2000). Genetic analysis of extended lifespan in *Drosophila melanogaster*. III. On the relationship between artificially selected lines and wild stocks. *Genetica*, 109, 245–253.

Khazaeli, A. A., Pletcher, S. D., & Curtsinger, J. W. (1998). The fractionation experiment: reducing heterogeneity to investigate age-specific mortality in *Drosophila. Mechanisms of Ageing and Development*, 105, 301–317.

Khazaeli, A. A., Tatar, M., Pletcher, S., & Curtsinger, J. W. (1997). Heat-induced longevity extension in *Drosophila melanogaster* I. Longevity, mortality, and thermotolerance. *Journal of Gerontology, Biological Sciences*, 52A, B48–B52.

Khazaeli, A. A., Van Voorhies, W., & Curtsinger, J. W. (2005). Longevity and metabolism in *Drosophila melanogaster*: positive pleiotropy between life span and age-specific metabolic rate in populations artificially selected for long life. *Genetics*, 69, 231–242.

Khazaeli, A. A., Xiu, L., & Curtsinger, J. W. (1995a). Effect of adult cohort density on age-specific mortality in *Drosophila melanogaster. Journal of Gerontology, Biological Sciences*, 50A, 262–269.

Khazaeli, A. A., Xiu, L. & Curtsinger, J. W. (1995b). Stress experiments as a means of investigating age-specific mortality in *Drosophila melanogaster. Experimental Gerontology*, 30, 177–184.

Khazaeli, A. A., Xiu, L., & Curtsinger, J. W. (1996). Effect of density on age-specific mortality in *Drosophila melanogaster*: A density supplementation experiment. *Genetica*, 98, 21–31.

Kirkwood, T. B. L. (1999). *Time of our lives: the science of human ageing*. New York: Oxford University Press.

Kowald, A., & Kirkwood, T. B. L. (1993). Explaining fruit fly longevity. *Science*, 260, 1664–1665.

le Bras, H. (1976). Lois de mortalité et age limité. *Population*, 31, 655–692.

Leips, J., & Mackay, T. F. C. (2000). Quantitative trait loci for lifespan in

Drosophila melanogaster: interactions with genetic background and larval density. *Genetics*, 155, 1773–1788.

Leips, J., & Mackay, T. F. C. (2002). The complex genetic architecture of *Drosophila* life span. *Experimental Aging Research*, 28, 361–390.

Lin, Y. J, Seroude, L., & Benzer, S. (1998). Extended life-span and stress resistance in the *Drosophila* mutant *methuselah*. *Science*, 282, 943–946.

Luckinbill, L. S., & Golenberg, E. M. (2002). Genes affecting aging: mapping quantitative trait loci in *Drosophila melanogaster* using amplified fragment length polymorphisms (AFLPs). *Genetica*, 114, 147–156.

Mack, P. D., Lester, V. K., & Promislow, D. E. L. (2000). Age-specific effects of novel mutations in *Drosophila melanogaster*. II. Fecundity and male mating ability. *Genetica*, 110, 31–41.

Mackay, T. F. C. (2001). Quantitative trait loci in *Drosophila*. *Nature Reviews, Genetics*, 2, 11–20.

Mackay, T. F. C. (2002). The nature of quantitative genetic variation for *Drosophila* longevity. *Mechanisms of Ageing and Development*, 123, 95–104.

Mair, W., Goymer, P., Pletcher, S. D., & Partridge, L. (2003). Demography of dietary restriction and death in *Drosophila*. *Science*, 301, 1731–1733.

Makeham, W. M. (1867). On the law of mortality. *Journal of the Institute of Actuaries*, 13, 325–358.

Martorell, C., Toro, M. A., & Gallego, C. (1998). Spontaneous mutation for life-history traits in *Drosophila melanogaster*. *Genetica*, 102/103, 315–324.

McCarrol, S. A., Murphy, C. T., Zou, S., Pletcher, S. D., Chin, C. S., Jan, Y. N., Kenyon, C., Bargmann, C. I., & Li, H. (2004). Comparing genomic expression patterns across species identifies shared transcriptional profiles in aging. *Nature Genetics*, 36, 197–204.

Medawar, P. B. (1952). *An unsolved problem of biology*. London: H. K. Lewis.

Miyo, T., & Charlesworth, B. (2004). Age-specific mortality rates of reproducing ad non-reproducing males of *Drosophila melanogaster*. *Proceedings of the Royal Society of London, Series B*, 271, 2517–2522.

Mueller, L. D., & Rose, M. R. (1996). Evolutionary theory predicts late-life mortality plateaus. *Proceedings of the National Academy of Sciences of the USA*, 93, 15249–15253.

Mueller, L. D., Drapeau, M. D., Adams, C. S., Hammerle, C. W., Doyal, K. M., Jazayeri, A. J., Ly, T., Beguwala, S. A., Mamidi, A. R., & Rose, M. R. (2003). Statistical tests of demographic heterogeneity theories. *Experimental Gerontology*, 38, 373–386.

Mueller, L. D., Drapeau, M. D., & Rose, M. R. (2000). Stress resistance, heterogeneity, and mortality plateaus: response by the authors. *Experimental Gerontology*, 35, 1089–1091.

Mukai, T. (1964). The genetic structure of natural populations of *Drosophila melanogaster*. I. Spontaneous mutation rate of polygenes controlling viability. *Genetics*, 50, 1–19.

Mutsuddi, M., & Nambu, J. R. (1998). *Drosophila* degenerates for a good cause. *Current Biology*, 8, R809–811.

Nusbaum, T. J., Graves, J. L., Mueller, L. D., & Rose, M. R. (1993). Fruit fly aging and mortality. *Science*, 260, 1567.

Nuzhdin, S. V., Khazaeli, A. A., & Curtsinger, J. W. (2005). Survival analysis of life span QTLs in *Drosophila melanogaster*. *Genetics*, 170, 719–731.

Nuzhdin, S. V., Pasyukova, E. G., Dilda, C., & Mackay, T. F. C. (1997). Sex-specific quantitative trait loci affecting longevity in *Drosophila melanogaster*. *Proceedings of the National Academy of Sciences of the USA*, 94, 9734–9739.

Olshansky, S. J. (1998). On the biodemography of aging: a review essay. *Population and Development Review*, 24, 381–393.

Partridge, L., & Barton, N. H. (1993). Optimality, mutation, and the evolution of aging. *Nature*, 362, 305–311.

Pasyukova, E. G., Vieira, C., & Mackay, T. F. C. (2000). Deficiency mapping of quantitative trait loci affecting longevity in *Drosophila melanogaster*. *Genetics*, 156, 1129–1146.

Pearl, R. (1922). Experimental studies on the duration of life. VI. A comparison of the laws of mortality in *Drosophila* and in man. *American Naturalist*, 56, 398–405.

Pearl, R., & Parker, S. (1921). Experimental studies on the duration of life. I.

Introductory discussion of the duration of life in *Drosophila*. *American Naturalist*, 55, 481–500.

Pearl, R., & Parker, S. (1924). Experimental studies on the duration of life. IX. New life tables for *Drosophila*. *American Naturalist*, 58, 71–82.

Perks, W. (1932). On some experiments in the graduation of mortality statistics. *Journal of the Institute of Actuaries*, 63, 12–57.

Phelan, J. P., & Austad, S. N. (1994). Selecting animal models of human aging: inbred strains often exhibit less biological uniformity than F1 hybrids. *Journal of Gerontology, Biological Science*, 49, B1–B11.

Pletcher, S. D. (1996). Age-specific mortality costs of exposure to inbred *Drosophila melanogaster* in relation to longevity selection. *Experimental Gerontology*, 31, 605–616.

Pletcher, S. D. (2002). Mitigating the tithonus error: genetic analysis of mortality phenotypes. *Science Aging Knowledge Environment*, pe14.

Pletcher, S. D., & Curtsinger, J. W. (1998). Mortality plateaus and the evolution of senescence: Why are old-age mortality rates so low? *Evolution*, 52, 454–464.

Pletcher, S. D., & Curtsinger, J. W. (2000a). Why do lifespans differ? Partitioning mean longevity differences in terms of age-specific mortality parameters. *Journal of Gerontology, Biological Sciences*, 55, B381–B389.

Pletcher, S. D., & Curtsinger, J. W. (2000b). The influence of environmentally induced heterogeneity on age-specific genetic variance for mortality rates. *Genetical Research, Cambridge*, 75, 321–329.

Pletcher, S. D., Houle, D., & Curtsinger, J. W. (1998). Age-specific properties of spontaneous mutations affecting mortality in *Drosophila melanogaster*. *Genetics*, 148, 287–303.

Pletcher, S. D., Houle, D., & Curtsinger, J. W. (1999). The evolution of age-specific mortality rates in *Drosophila melanogaster*: Genetic divergence among unselected strains. *Genetics*, 153, 813–823.

Pletcher, S. D., Macdonald, S. J., Marguerie, R., Certa, U., Stearns, S. C., Goldstein, D. B., & Partridge, L. (2002). Genome-wide transcript profiles in aging and calorically restricted *Drosophila melanogaster*. *Current Biology*, 12, 712–723.

Pletcher, S. D., & Neuhauser, C. (2000). Biological aging: criteria for modeling and a new mechanistic model. *International Journal of Modern Physics C*, 11, 525–546.

Ramalu-Hansen, H. (1983). Smoothing counting process intensities by means of kernel functions. *Annals of Statistics*, 11, 453–466.

Resler, A. S., Kelly, K., Cantor, G., Khazaeli, A. A., Tatar, M., & Curtsinger, J. W. (1998). Genetic analysis of extended lifespan in *Drosophila melanogaster*. II. Replication of the backcross test and molecular characterization of the N14 locus. *Genetica*, 104, 33–39.

Robine, J. M., & Ritchie, K. (1993). Explaining fruit fly longevity. *Science*, 260, 1665.

Rogina, B., & Helfand, S. L. (1995). Regulation of gene expression is linked to life span in adult *Drosophila*. *Genetics*, 141, 1043–1048.

Rogina, B., Reenan, R. A., Nilsen, S. P., & Helfand, S. L. (2000). Extended life-span conferred by cotransporter gene mutations in *Drosophila*. *Science*, 290, 2137–2140.

Rogina, B., Vaupel, J. W., Partridge, L., & Helfand, S. L. (1998). Regulation of gene expression is preserved in aging *Drosophila melanogaster*. *Current Biology*, 9, 475–478.

Rose, M. R. (1991). *Evolutionary biology of aging*. New York: Oxford University Press.

Rose, M. R., & Mueller, L. D. (2000). Ageing and immortality. *Philosophical Transactions of the Royal Society of London, Series B*, 355, 1637–1662.

Rose, M. R., Drapeau, M. D., Yazdi, P. G., Shah, K. H., Moise, D. B., Thakar, R. R., Rauser, C. L., and Mueller, L. D. (2002). Evolution of late-life mortality in *Drosophila melanogaster*. *Evolution*, 56, 1982–1991.

Sacher, G. A. (1956). On the statistical nature of mortality, with special reference to chronic radiation mortality. *Radiology*, 67, 250–257.

Sacher, G. A. (1966). The Gompertz transformation in the study of the injury-mortality relationship: Application to late radiation effects and ageing. In P. J. Lindop & G. A. Sacher (Eds.), *Radiation and ageing* (pp. 411–441). London: Taylor and Francis.

Semenchenko, G. V., Khazaeli, A. A., Curtsinger, J. W., & Yashin, A. L. (2004). Stress resistance declines with age: analysis of data from a survival experiment with *Drosophila melanogaster*. *Biogerontology*, 5, 17–30.

Service, P. M. (2000a). Heterogeneity in individual mortality risk and its importance for evolutionary studies of senescence. *American Naturalist*, 156, 1–13.

Service, P. M. (2000b). Stress resistance, heterogeneity, and mortality plateaus: a comment on Drapeau *et al. Experimental Gerontology*, 35, 1085–1087.

Service, P. M. (2004). Demographic heterogeneity explains age-specific patterns of genetic variance in mortality rates. *Experimental Gerontology*, 39, 25–30.

Service, P. M., Michieli, C. M., & McGill, K. (1998). Experimental evolution of senescence: An analysis using a "heterogeneity" model. *Evolution*, 52, 1844–1850.

Steinsaltz, D. (2005). Reevaluating a test of the heterogeneity explanation for mortality plateaus. *Experimental Gerontology*, 40, 101–113.

Steinsaltz, D., & Evans, S. N. (2004). Markov mortality models: implications of quasistationarity and varying initial distributions. *Theoretical Population Biology*, 65, 319–337.

Strehler, B. L., & Mildvan, A. S. (1960). General theory of mortality and aging. *Science*, 132, 14–21.

Tahoe, N. M., Lande, J., Khazaeli, A. A., & Curtsinger, J. W. (2005). Genome-wide analysis of age-specific gene expression in populations of *Drosophila melanogaster* artificially selected for long life.

Tahoe, N. M, Mokhtarzhadeh, A., & Curtsinger, J. W. (2004). Age-related RNA decline in adult *Drosophila* melanogaster. *Journal of Gerontology: Biological Sciences*, 59, B896–901.

Valenzuela, R. K., Forbes, S. N., Keim, P., & Service, P. M. (2004). Quantitative trait loci affecting life span in replicated populations of *Drosophila melanogaster*. II. Response to selection. *Genetics*, 168, 313–324.

Van Voorhies, W., Khazaeli, A. A., & Curtsinger, J. W. (2003). Selected contribution: long-lived *Drosophila melanogaster* exhibit normal metabolic rates. *Journal of Applied Physiology*, 95, 2605–2613.

Van Voorhies, W.W., Khazaeli, A. A., & Curtsinger, J. W. (2004). Testing the "rate of living" model: Further evidence that

longevity and metabolic rate are not inversely correlated in *Drosophila melanogaster. Journal of Applied Physiology*, 97, 1915–1922.

Vaupel, J. W., & Carey, J. R. (1993). Compositional interpretations of medfly mortality. *Science*, 260, 1666–1667.

Vaupel, J. W., Carey, J. R., Christiansen, K., Johnson, T. E., Yashin, A. I., Holm, N. V., Iachine, L. A., Khazaeli, A. A., Liedo, P., Longo, V. D., Yi, Z. Y., Manton, K. G., & Curtsinger, J. W. (1998). Biodemographic trajectories of longevity. *Science*, 280, 855–860.

Vaupel, J. W., Johnson, T. E., & Lithgow, G. J. (1994). Rates of mortality in populations of *Caenorhabditis elegans. Science*, 263, 668–671.

Vaupel, J. W., Yashin, A. I., & Manton, K. G. (1987). Debilitation's aftermath: stochastic process models of mortality. *Mathematical Population Studies*, 1, 21–48.

Vieira, C., Pasyukova, E. G., Zeng, S., Hackett, J. B., Lyman, R. F. & Mackay, T. F. C. (2000). Genotype-environment interaction for quantitative trait loci affecting lifespan in *Drosophila melanogaster. Genetics*, 154, 213–227.

Wachter, K. W. (1999). Evolutionary demographic models for mortality plateaus. *Proceedings of the National Academy of Sciences of the USA*, 96, 10544–10547.

Wachter, K. W., & Finch, C. E. (Eds.). (1997). *Between Zeus and the salmon*. Washington, DC: National Academy Press.

Williams, G. C. (1957). Pleiotropy, natural selection, and the evolution of senescence. *Evolution*, 11, 398–411.

Yampolsky, L. Y, Pearse, L. E., & Promislow, D. E. L. (2001). Age-specific effects of novel mutations in *Drosophila melanogaster*. I. Mortality. *Genetica*, 110, 11–29.

Yashin. A., Vaupel, J. W., & Iachine, I. A. (1994). A duality in aging: the equivalence of mortality models based on radically different concepts. *Mechanisms of Ageing and Development*, 74, 1–14.

Zelterman, D., & Curtsinger, J. W. (1995). Survival curves subjected to occasional insults. *Biometrics*, 51, 1140–1146.

Zelterman, D., Li, C., & Curtsinger, J. W. (1994). Piecewise exponential survival curves. *Mathematical Biosciences*, 120, 233–250.

Chapter 11

Microarray Analysis of Gene Expression Changes in Aging

F. Noel Hudson, Matt Kaeberlein, Nancy Linford, David Pritchard,
Richard Beyer, and Peter S. Rabinovitch

I. Introduction

The promise of genome-wide platforms for biological discovery has been received by biological scientists with great enthusiasm. Of the global discovery technologies, the increasing accessibility of microarrays for analysis of gene expression has perhaps stirred the greatest interest, certainly within the field of gerontology. As this chapter will discuss, recent literature includes applications of these arrays to studies of aging in yeast, invertebrates, rodents, and humans. However, the very nature of the technology—the measurement of thousands or tens of thousands of variables at once—presents new challenges for the analysis and interpretation of the data, requiring the development and application of new statistical and informatics tools. We have begun to see initial fruition of this work, especially in yeast and invertebrate models. Studies in mice and humans are well underway; however, the greater inter-individual heterogeneity and tissue and genomic complexity of

these organisms remain as appreciable challenges. Because global analysis of gene expression offers great potential for the elucidation of common mechanisms, pathways, and biomarkers of aging, it is safe to predict continued enthusiasm for application of this technology toward these goals.

II. Technical Issues

A. Design of Aging Studies

1. Biological Aspects of Design

One of the most important (and often neglected) considerations in the successful design of microarray experiments is the unique properties of the biological question being explored. In the case of the biology of aging, with pleiotropic and often subtle phenotypes, careful examination of the precise biological features under scrutiny is paramount. Unfortunately, important considerations, such as how to define terms like "old" and "premature aging," are often neglected. This section attempts to deal with these issues in relationship to the experimental design of microarray studies. In particular, we will address how experimental design determines the types of gene expression biomarkers obtained. Several classes of aging-related microarray experiments are considered, including analysis of gene expression at different ages, analysis of gene expression in short-and long-lived models, and analysis of individual longevity.

a. Gene Expression Studies at Different Age. Perhaps the most common application of microarray technology to the study of aging is the search for gene expression changes that correlate with organismal age. Studies of this type typically employ a design in which RNA is obtained from "young" individuals and compared against RNA obtained from "old" individuals. Microarray analysis is then carried out and a comparison is made between "young" and "old," with lists of genes presented that either increase or decrease in expression as a function of age. These types of studies have been carried out in all of the model systems commonly used to study aging, including mammals, flies, worms, and yeast, as described in subsequent sections.

In the vast majority of "young" versus "old" studies, only two timepoints have been used. This two-timepoint design is fraught with danger because no information is gained regarding the kinetics of gene expression change. In some cases, intermediate age timepoints have been collected in addition to "young" and "old." This type of design has the advantage that it may be possible to identify genes that show trends in expression correlated across multiple age groups. In addition, it may be possible to identify and classify genes based on the kinetics with which expression changes occur. This is particularly important if any inferences regarding the causality of observed changes with

respect to aging or age-associated phenotypes are to be made. Whenever possible, it is strongly recommended that multiple timepoints be used rather than only "young" and "old."

One important consideration in the design of a study comparing young and old organisms is how to define the "young" and "old" populations. For young populations, the primary criteria should be organisms that are reproductively and developmentally mature. In order to define "old" populations, the most straightforward definition is derived from statistical parameters of the life-span distribution, such as population median and maximum life span. For example, one definition of "old" could be individuals that have achieved at least 75 percent of the population maximum life span. The potential for degenerative changes present in very old animals must be considered, however, as these secondary gene expression changes may complicate the observation of those more intimately tied to the biology of aging. An alternative definition of what age constitutes "old" might be based on the appearance of one or more phenotypes associated with old age. Such a definition, however, is complicated by the fact that a majority of aging phenotypes show incomplete penetrance, with large individual variation in age of onset and severity. On the other hand, an appropriate set of phenotypic markers might reflect biological age more accurately than does chronological age (see section II.A.1.e). In some cases, the age of the "old" population is determined by the availability of donor samples. Human studies in particular are often constrained by sample availability and must make use of tissues or cells obtained from donors of a variety of different ages. For microarray studies, as with other types of analyses, there is no clear right answer as to what the definition of "old" should be. What is clear, however, is that the parameters used to define the old population should be carefully considered and explicitly presented during both the experimental design and data interpretation. In addition, the statistical analyses used should reflect the experimental design in this regard. As stated above, a multiple timepoint design in which samples are obtained at several different ages is preferred, as this provides additional information about the kinetics of gene expression change with age and a measure of flexibility in choosing appropriate donor ages.

b. Gene Expression Analysis of Long-Lived Models. In addition to studies comparing young organisms with aged organisms, microarrays can be used to compare individuals or populations of similar age but with different aging potentials. For example, many studies have examined the gene expression profile of young mice fed a control diet relative to young mice fed a calorie restricted (CR) diet (see section III.C.2). When age-matched animals are compared across the two dietary regiments, differences reflect gene expression changes associated with caloric intake rather than age. Because CR animals have a longer life span than control-fed animals, observed gene expression changes also have been correlated with increased longevity, at least within the experiment. This distinction is an important one. In "young" versus "old" experiments, the potential exists to discover gene expression changes that correlate with chronological age (biomarkers of age or aging). In experiments carried out on young control versus long-lived individuals, it is possible to identify gene expression changes that correlated with longevity (biomarkers of longevity) and/or the rate of aging. Such studies may permit the discovery of genes with the potential to extend life span that may not be altered in normal aging.

c. Studies of Both Longevity and Age. In several studies, these two types of experimental design have been combined such that microarray analysis is carried out on control and long-lived animals at

two or more ages. The primary advantage associated with this type of design is that a single experiment can be used to identify gene expression changes correlated with aging, the model of longevity and the interaction of aging and the model of longevity. Figure 11.1 shows the possible gene expression changes in a "four-way design" experiment where young and old animals are used with and without a modification that affects longevity (Mod). Biomarkers of aging (light bars in the Old WT column of Figure 11.1, rows B, D, G, and H), which are unaffected in old members of the group modified for longevity (Figure 11.1, row B), can be distinguished from biomarkers of aging, which are attenuated in old members of the group modified for longevity (Figure 11.1, row D). The latter may include age-associated gene expression changes that are functionally important for longevity; these are predicted to be attenuated in long-lived animals relative

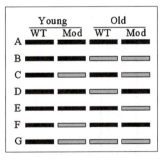

Figure 11.1 Possible expression patterns of genes regulated by aging and a modification associated with longevity (Mod). Grey bars represent expression changes relative to the black bars; black bars represent genes with unchanged expression relative to young wildtype (WT) animals. For experimental designs that include intermediate ages and so on, this basic set of possible experimental results can serve as a guideline for predicting the biological implications of potential outcomes of a gene expression study. This simplified set of results can be expanded to include experimental designs with intermediate ages, the likelihood intermediate gene expression patterns, and different interpretations depending on the direction of gene expression change relative to baseline.

to controls. The classic example of this phenomenon is the observation that many gene expression changes associated with age in control mice are reduced or absent in old mice subjected to CR (Cao *et al.*, 2001; Dhahbi *et al.*, 2004). Of note, many of the studies of CR are missing the young treated (short-term CR) control group, and this may complicate the interpretation of results. In addition, biomarkers of longevity in the modified group can be examined in the young animals (Figure 11.1, row F), old animals (Figure 11.1, row E), or both (Figure 11.1, row C), and effects of the longevity modification occurring early and late in the aging process can be distinguished. Furthermore, complex changes associated with aging and altered by the longevity modification can be identified (Figure 11.1, rows G and H). In these cases, biomarkers of aging may also be affected in the young modified group. This might represent a more complex phenomenon, such as a stress induced by the longevity modification that leads to a stress response similar to that seen in aging. A related design, typically used for dietary modification studies such as caloric restriction, is a "three-way design" in which young animals from an age prior to the start of caloric restriction are compared to older animals that have been subjected either to caloric restriction or normal feeding (Lee *et al.*, 1999). This design is effective for the study of modifications that are started after development.

d. Microarray Studies on Short-Lived Mutants. Several mutations that result in shortened life span have been suggested as models of premature aging in mammals (Warner and Sierra, 2003). Microarray analysis of tissues or cells derived from short-lived mutants offers the opportunity to identify gene expression changes correlated with short life span and, potentially, accelerated aging. In principle, such studies are identical in design to those examining gene expression changes in

models of increased longevity. It should be noted, however, that none of the "premature aging" models proposed to date recapitulate all of the phenotypic changes associated with aging in normal animals, and most have additional pathologies that do not occur during the normal aging process. Differentiating gene expression changes associated with accelerated aging (if present at all) from those associated with non-aging related pathologies is a daunting task. The most effective approach would most likely be a comparative analysis of gene expression profiles across multiple long-and short-lived mutants. In this way, gene expression biomarkers that reflect the rate of aging could potentially be identified with higher confidence.

e. Biomarkers that Predict Individual Longevity. Another potential use of microarrays applied to aging research is the large-scale identification of gene expression biomarkers that predict individual longevity. Among humans, it is clear that different individuals age at different rates, due to both genetic and environmental factors. For a particular person, chronological age may not be an accurate predictor of remaining life expectancy. In fact, several phenotypes have already been suggested as potential biomarkers of biological age in humans, including body temperature (Roth *et al.*, 2002), serum insulin levels, age-related rate of decline in serum dehydroepiandrosterone sulfate (DHEAS) (Roth *et al.*, 2002), and telomere length in blood cells (Cawthon *et al.*, 2003). To date, however, it has not been demonstrated that these biomarkers can be accurately used to predict survival.

Microarrays offer the opportunity to detect a group of gene expression biomarkers that more accurately reflect biological age (and hence life expectancy) than currently possible. Hundreds of potential biomarkers can be assayed simultaneously in a single array experiment. Appropriate experimental design for the identification of individual biomarkers of longevity using microarrays, however, is nontrivial.

One approach might be to compare gene expression profiles from a specific tissue type using samples from centenarians versus samples from the general population. A problem with studies of this type, however, is the confounding effect of gene expression changes due to age-associated disease and degenerative changes that are likely to be present in the centenarian population simply due to the extreme chronological age of these individuals. One way to get around this complication would be to compare samples from age-matched siblings or offspring of centenarians versus age-matched individuals from the general population. Because the probability of achieving extreme longevity is quantifiably higher in close relatives of centenarians (Perls *et al.*, 2000; Perls *et al.*, 2002), it might be possible to extract the genetic component of gene expression changes associated with a predisposition for longevity in this manner.

Alternatively, a mammalian model system, such as mice, could be used to identify gene expression biomarkers predictive of individual longevity. Similar to the human study mentioned above (Roth *et al.*, 2002), reduced body temperature and serum insulin are associated with longevity in mice (Weindruch and Walford, 1988). Recent work has also suggested that body weight and levels of T-cell subsets and thyroxin can be used to predict individual longevity in animals as young as 8 months old (Harper *et al.*, 2004). One approach for using microarrays to identify these types of biomarkers would involve analysis of global gene expression in particular tissue, such as blood, from individual animals at multiple age points (e.g., every 6 months). Following the death of all animals in the cohort, it should be possible to identify gene expression patterns that correlate with individual longevity relative to the population. A computational algorithm could then be generated to predict

life expectancy based on these gene expression markers.

From a clinical perspective, the use of microarrays has even greater promise than just identifying candidate genes for potential therapeutic intervention. Microarray analysis to identify biomarkers of aging and longevity could strongly influence preventative care and risk management–based decisions about screening for diseases of the elderly. It is possible that a specialized version of a microarray analysis for potential biomarkers of aging could be used in routine assessment of aging adults.

2. Sources of Variability in Microarray Experiments

When considering the design of a microarray experiment, the sources of biological and technical variability must be considered, as they affect the ability to detect true gene expression changes. Microarray experiments can most clearly detect gene expression changes with low biological variability. However, changes in genes with high biological variability may be of interest to the researcher for several reasons. Some of the sources of biological and technical variability as well as methods for addressing them are discussed below.

a. Cellular Heterogeneity. One important factor to consider in the analysis of variability in microarray experiments is the cellular heterogeneity of the samples being analyzed. In most experiments conducted on multicellular species, a single sample is derived from whole animals or organs. Therefore, changes in gene expression due to changes in underlying cell type distribution are indistinguishable from gene expression changes due to transcriptional events within a cell. This is a particularly important cautionary note when considering aging experiments where the time-dependent structural changes associated with atrophy or hypertrophy are well known and when tissues are rarely cleared of blood before RNA preparation. Gene expression differences arising from a population of cells may still provide insight into changes in the function of an organ or organism with age and are certainly interesting. However, when attempting to infer the cause of gene expression changes, it is important to consider that cell type differences may be at the root of the observed differences and that assumptions about alterations in intracellular signaling pathways may be unfounded when whole tissues are analyzed.

Techniques for measuring gene expression from single cells in an organism are being actively developed in order to address this concern. Amplification procedures allow for the labeling of RNA from samples as small as 50 nanograms (ng). Most of these amplification procedures are based on the methods developed by Van Gelder and colleagues (1990). Concerns about bias introduced by amplification appear to differ depending on the microarray platform. For Affymetrix arrays, a systematic bias introduced by amplification has been noted (Wilson *et al.*, 2004). However, this bias does not affect the genes identified as differentially expressed when data is only compared directly between samples that have undergone the same amplification procedures. For cDNA arrays, Feldman and colleagues (2002) reported that the bias introduced by amplification is negligible. Additionally, there are several reports suggesting that amplification may reduce the noise inherent in rare transcripts for cDNA arrays and produce data that is more likely to be verified by reverse transcriptase polymerase chain reaction (RT-PCR) (Feldman *et al.*, 2002; Gomes *et al.*, 2003). In addition to potential bias due to amplification, analysis of RNA from single cells may introduce stochastic and micro-environmental variability that would normally be averaged out in a sample composed of thousands of cells. The magnitude of gene expression differences between neighboring cells in a tissue

due to these effects has not been sufficiently characterized to date.

b. Temporal Heterogeneity. In addition to cellular heterogeneity, effects of temporal differences may also introduce variability into a data set. Gene expression differences can be associated with time of day or level of activity, and because a typical gene expression study is a temporal cross-section, it is difficult to determine whether the differences seen between individuals are due to a true stable heterogeneity or are the result of transient gene expression in certain animals. Care should be taken when preparing for a microarray experiment to minimize temporal factors that may affect apparent gene expression.

c. Age-Associated Biological Variability. There are several potential sources of biological variability inherent in the aging process that can affect the outcome of a microarray experiment. For example, age-associated dysregulation at the level of the genes (e.g., alterations in gene silencing), at the level of cellular signaling (e.g., alterations in functionality of signaling pathways), at the level of tissue (e.g., alterations in cell type composition), or at the level of the organism (e.g., alterations in circulating hormone levels) may cause an increase in the variability of gene expression with age. These changes are clearly associated with the aging process but may not affect the same genes in each individual to the same extent, thus appearing as an increase in the variance of samples from older individuals. Similarly, discarding as uninteresting genes that show significant expression changes in only a subset of individuals may overlook biologically important candidates. One positive aspect to the increase in gene expression variance with age is that it should be possible to obtain information regarding the pathways most affected by age-associated transcriptional dysregulation. A thorough study looking at the gene-specific variation as a function of age would be of interest.

d. Sources of Technical Variability. There are multiple sources of variability in measurements of gene expression that can mask biologically relevant signals (Parmigiani *et al.*, 2003). These sources of variability can be grouped into two main categories: systematic and stochastic (Huber, 2004). Systematic sources include the amount and quality of the labeled RNA in the sample, dye-specific effects, and proper calibration of the instrumentation used for array manufacture, hybridization, and scanning. Stochastic sources include variability in the quality of the arrays themselves, particularly the DNA on the arrays, nonspecific hybridization, stray signals, inherent variability in labeling and extraction of RNA, and day-specific effects. For spotted arrays, spotting efficiency and spot size and shape contribute to stochastic variability, and for arrays built *in situ*, efficiency of incorporation of each base is included in stochastic variability. Systematic errors can be greatly reduced by careful methodology and appropriate instrument calibration. However, stochastic errors are inherent to the microarray system being used and are handled by an experimental design that is balanced across the sources of error and the use of an appropriate statistical error model that factors in the multiple sources of variation.

The most important and correctable source of systematic variability in any microarray experiment derives from the quality of the input RNA. Differences in RNA degradation between two samples can lead to false positives upon comparison of the gene expression profiles that are indistinguishable from true positives even after statistical analysis. Use of a fluidics system such as the Agilent Bioanalyzer for determination of RNA quality is recommended. This system uses nanogram amounts of the total RNA preparation and can quantify degradation in the extracted mRNA or in the 18s and 28s rRNA bands of total RNA (a 28s:18s ratio of 1.3–2:1 is typically considered intact). Although measuring bulk degradation in total RNA does not directly address mRNA quality, intact total RNA profiles are consistently associated with measurements of RNA quality on the arrays, such as the similarity of the signal intensity histogram across samples. Affymetrix arrays, for example, provide indicators of 3' to 5' ratio for two genes using probes that hybridize along the sequence. Additionally, contaminant-free preparation, proper storage at $-70\,°C$, and minimization of freeze-thaw cycles all contribute to RNA quality. Microarray applications are highly sensitive to RNA quality and require extreme attention at this step.

Another important and correctable source of systematic variability is in the methods used for RNA labeling. Direct comparison of array results obtained through different labeling protocols should not be attempted, although differential expression (ratios) may be compared. Because even small deviations in a protocol can produce differences in the resulting signal intensities, simultaneous labeling of all samples compared in a study is preferred. When this is not possible, simultaneous labeling of samples that are balanced across the experimental conditions will minimize the bias introduced by labeling. For experiments where two or more samples are labeled with different dyes and compared directly on the same chip, systematic differences in the incorporation of dyes during RNA labeling can also lead to large artifacts. One method to control for this variability is to implement a dye flip control for each sample (see section II.A.3.c).

3. Managing Variability in Microarray Experiments

a. Replication and Sample Size Considerations. Like any other scientific experiment, the need for replication in microarray gene expression studies is well established (Lee *et al.*, 2000b). Broadly speaking, there are two types of replication: biological replicates and technical replicates. In addition, there are two main types of technical replicates: independent oligonucleotides or cDNA products representing the same gene present in multiple locations on the array, and the use of multiple RNA samples from the same source to hybridize onto multiple arrays. Only the biological replicates allow for making some inference about the population from which the individuals are drawn. Technical replicates, on the other hand, allow for the determination of measurement error or "noise." When measuring technical variability in a platform, it is common to measure the same labeled RNA sample on multiple arrays. However, there is a stochastic component to the RNA extraction and labeling, even when systematic variability is minimized, and use of independently prepared RNA samples will incorporate this aspect of

technical variability. Even so, estimates of the technical variability will always under-represent the true variability of the system, which includes large biological components.

Because the goal of a microarray experiment is to identify differentially expressed genes, it is important to have enough replicates to keep the probability of having false positives as low as possible. Having sufficient replicates to examine the probability of random variability accounting of "positive" results is an intrinsic aspect of algorithms for estimating false discovery rates (see below). There are several standard approaches for calculating how many replicates are needed when the variances of differential gene expression are known. For example, see Cui and Churchill (2004), Lee and Whitmore (2002), or Parmigiani and colleagues (2003). Figure 11.2, from Cui and

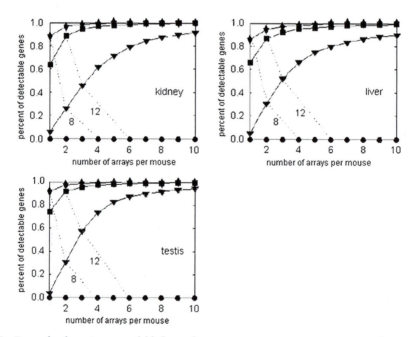

Figure 11.2 Power for detecting a two-fold change between two treatments at various combinations of number of mice per treatment (biological replicates) and number of arrays per mouse (technical replicates). Circles, triangles, squares, and diamonds represent 2, 4, 6, and 8 mice per treatment, respectively. Dotted lines represent the same number of array pairs (8 or 12) for each treatment. Significance level is 0.05 after Bonferroni correction. Biological and technical variance components are estimated from Project Normal data http://www.camda.duke.edu/camda02/datasets. The plotted data is derived from Cui and Churchill (2004).

Churchill (2004), shows the power for detecting a two-fold change for various combinations of biological and technical variations.

Sample size considerations are especially important in aging studies because the variability between individuals and between tissues can be many times larger than the changes due to aging; that is, individual variability may overwhelm changes due to aging alone. In general, biological variability is greater in higher eukaryotes, and greater in outbred, rather than inbred, organisms (although it is possible that F1 hybrids may have reduced variability compared to the parental strains; Phelan & Austad, 1994). It has been suggested, for example, that a minimum of six individual mice are required to reduce sampling errors to satisfactory levels in cDNA array experiments with mice (Cui & Churchill, 2004) and seven individual mice to detect a 1.5-fold difference in 95 percent of genes at the 0.01 level of significance with 90 percent power (Han *et al.*, 2004). However, experiments examining expression differences in human tissues show that at least 36 individuals would be required to obtain similar results in human experiments due to the increased variance present in the human population (Han *et al.*, 2004).

b. Microarrays on Individuals Versus Sample Pools. While increasing the number of arrays used in a microarray experiment increases the statistical power for detecting population differences, the cost of processing a microarray, along with the need to validate results by an independent technique, has driven researchers to look for methods to achieve similar data from a smaller number of arrays.

Pooling samples has been proposed as a strategy to identify genes displaying differences in mean expression between groups. Though pooling masks underlying biological variability, a more accurate estimate of the population mean can be determined when independent pools are used in an experiment with a fixed number of arrays. This is because more individuals from the population can be assayed than if an experiment used a single individual per array. However, this technique is highly sensitive to outliers because a single outlier may skew the perceived gene expression for an entire group. Furthermore, caution must but used when pooling across animals, organs, or even a heterogeneous single organ because small changes present in a region-specific manner will be undetectable. It has been demonstrated that when using a pooling strategy, apportioning individual samples into multiple smaller independent pools (a given sample is added to only one pool) can provide useful information on the biological variability, which cannot be obtained if all samples are pooled together and only technical replicates are performed (Kendziorski *et al.*, 2004). Technical replicates also do not provide satisfactory estimates of interassay variance, which are used to determine statistical significance and false discovery rates; this challenge has not yet been addressed in pooling experiments.

Pooling is a standard strategy when samples are from very small organisms such as yeast and invertebrates (*Drosophila* and *C. elegans*), where acquisition of RNA from a single organism is difficult and leads to an extremely low yield. This is discussed further in section II.A.2.

c. Design of Two-Channel Arrays. Array platforms such as the Affymetrix GeneChip® use a single fluorescent signal, and all replicates must be hybridized to separate chips. Two-channel spotted cDNA microarrays, however, allow investigators to perform direct comparisons of two samples on the same array; these also pose more of a challenge for determining ideal experimental design.

For more than two samples, a widely used approach is the reference design, which compares all samples to a common reference. However, as pointed out by Kerr and Churchill in a series of papers, there are more sophisticated alternatives, such as the loop design, that are more efficient for certain types of experiments, such as those with fewer than 10 samples. Because there are differences in the incorporation of the two fluorophores, leading to systematic dye-specific bias, a dye flip design (replicates balanced across both fluorescent channels) is recommended. The importance of a good design cannot be overemphasized because it is a major factor in the estimation of precision as well as the power to detect differential gene expression. Reviews of two-channel design issues can be found in Churchill (2002), Kerr (2003), Kerr and Churchill (2001a), Kerr *et al.* (2000), Lee *et al.* (2000b), Parmigiani *et al.* (2003), and Yang and Speed (2002).

4. Available Technologies for Microarrays and Validation

a. Microarray Technologies. There are two main microarray technologies in current use: cDNA spotted glass arrays and oligonucleotide arrays (both *in situ* synthesized and spotted) (Holloway *et al.*, 2002). Each type has its advantages and disadvantages. Spotted cDNA arrays usually offer the advantage of lower cost, whereas oligonucleotide arrays have much higher specificity (Hughes *et al.*, 2000). There are three main factors underlying these differences: (1) cDNA products may be recombined or contaminated such that sequences from multiple genes may be present in a single spot; (2) oligonucleotide sequences can be chosen to distinguish from among related gene family members, which cDNA sequences frequently do not; and (3) cDNA products are often both variable and large in size

(close to 1 kb), leading to inconsistent hybridization. Commercial oligonucleotide microarrays have seen dramatic price reductions over the last two years, which makes them more attractive for academic research. There are three main commercial oligonucleotide platforms: Affymetrix GeneChip® microarrays, Agilent Oligo microarrays, and Amersham Biosciences (GE Healthcare) CodeLink™ Bioarrays. Excellent reviews of the issues involved in both oligonucleotide and cDNA microarray platforms can be found in Li and colleagues (2003) and Parmigiani and colleagues (2003).

b. Validation of RNA Expression Levels. In order to be convinced that changes in gene expression associated with aging are biologically relevant, validation is required. The first step is to ensure that the RNA levels measured by the microarray experiment can be validated by an independent technique. Real-time quantitative RT-PCR and northern blotting are the primary methods used to validate candidate gene expression changes. Quantitative RT-PCR is considered the "gold standard" due to its sensitivity, reproducibility, and large dynamic range. The development of high throughput technologies for quantitative RT-PCR including the Taqman Low Density Arrays by Applied Biosystems has led to the possibility of independent validation of many candidates from initial screening experiments.

c. Biological Validation. Once candidate genes and pathways have been identified and validated, it is important to determine whether the observed gene expression changes are biologically relevant. This has been accomplished to varying degrees. Confirmation of changes at the protein level is crucial, particularly in aging experiments, because of changes in RNA and protein stability and changes in translational efficiency with age (Brewer, 2002;

Ekstrom *et al.*, 1980), and thus gene expression changes may not correspond to protein levels. Furthermore, measurement of biochemical activity of any candidate genes is also extremely important because of potential alterations in post-translational modification, inactivation, and degradation of proteins with aging. These caveats suggest that microarray studies are useful for the generation of hypotheses, but, particularly in aging, investigators must test whether the changes observed at the RNA level result in functional changes before clear biological conclusions can be drawn. It is worth noting, however, that although biological relevance is desirable, it is not a prerequisite for the identification of biomarkers of aging or longevity. In order for a gene expression biomarker to be useful, all that is required is a high degree of correlation and reproducibility.

An additional level of biological validation is using the gene candidates identified by microarrays to test hypotheses about the aging process. This is most ideally done through genetic manipulation of the model organism. For example, genes that are upregulated in long-lived organisms should increase life span when overexpressed by genetic manipulation, if they are functionally relevant. Likewise, functionally relevant genes that are down-regulated in long-lived organisms should increase life span when expression or function is decreased (e.g., by deletion or RNAi). This type of phenotypic validation has been carried out with much success in *C. elegans* and represents the most convincing demonstration of microarrays as a tool to study the aging process to date (Murphy *et al.*, 2003). Particularly in more advanced organisms, the timing, tissue specificity, and quantitative level of upregulation and downregulation of identified key regulatory genes will likely play a

role in the extent of phenotypic validation of candidate longevity-associated genes. As biological validation of microarray results from aging experiments becomes more common in *C. elegans* and other model systems, it will be possible to more accurately assess the gene expression changes that represent important aging-related biochemical pathways conserved through evolution.

B. Informatics Approaches to Gene Expression Data in Aging

The analysis of microarray data involves several sequential and parallel steps, as shown in Figure 11.3. The first three steps have been covered in some detail in previous sections. In the following sections, we focus on the pre-processing and analysis phases.

1. Preprocessing: Diagnostics and Normalization

After a set of microarrays has been hybridized and scanned, the images from the scanner need to be preprocessed before performing any statistical analysis. The preprocessing involves visual inspection of the scanner images (often TIFF files), spot quantification, slide diagnostics and quality control, and normalization.

Spot quantification software depends on the type of microarray. For commercial oligonucleotide arrays, the manufacturers offer their own quantification software. Amersham Codelink slides require the Codelink Expression Analysis program. Agilent slides use Agilent's Feature Extractor program. Affymetrix GeneChips require using GCOS. For two-color cDNA arrays, there are a variety of open-source programs as well as commercial programs (please refer to The Institute of Genomic Research's Web site for open-source

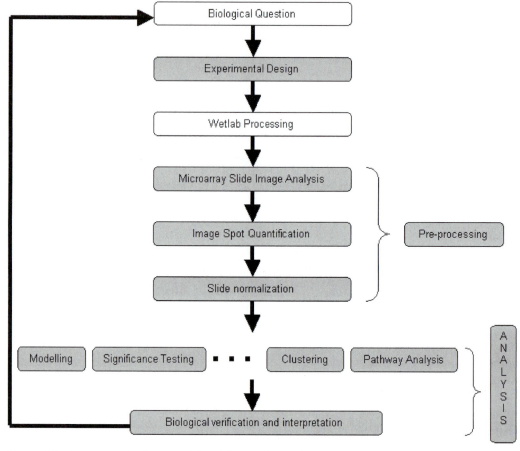

Figure 11.3 Microarray Analysis Workflow (after Dudoit *et al.*, 2002)

offerings at http://www.tigr.org). For commercial programs, choices include Axon's GenePix, BioDiscovery's Imagene, or CISRO's Spot, to name a few. Most of these programs allow visual inspection of the slide images to check for defects or damage, and many produce results of similar quality.

After the scanner images have been quantified, the next main step in preprocessing involves some type of diagnostics and/or quality control. Most of the spot quantification programs mentioned previously also perform quality control tasks, such as calculating mean signal strength, background thresholds, and control spot statistics. From these types of calculations, poor quality slides can be identified and excluded.

Normalization, the process of removing the uninteresting variability within the quantified images, also requires specialized software. There are many programs available that will take a spot quantification file as input, and perform normalization as well as other statistical tasks discussed in the next section. The specialized programs mentioned above have these statistical capabilities in addition to their image-analysis features. However, there are also open-source programs available that allow for the custom analysis of data. For example, Bioconductor (http://www.bioconductor.org)

allows the input of raw quantification data. There are many normalization routines available for any type of microarray platform, from Affymetrix to two-channel cDNA arrays. Bioconductor can also perform more sophisticated multichip normalizations, such as robust multiarray analysis, RMA, GC-RMA, variance stabilization, VSN, and dChip. Each of these methods takes a different approach to adjusting signal intensities to account for nonspecific hybridization, optical noise, and between-array variations. RMA is explained in more detail by Irizarry and colleagues (2003b), where it is shown that for Affymetrix arrays, subtracting the mismatched probes from the perfect match probes results in an exaggerated variance. Their RMA method does a background adjustment that ignores the mismatch probes. GC-RMA is explained in more detail by Wu and colleagues (2003), where it is shown that using the GC content of the mismatch probes improves the background adjustment. VSN is explained in more detail by Warner and colleagues (2002), where variance stabilizing transformations are used to normalize the microarray data. dChip is explained in more detail by Li and colleagues (2003), where a model-based expression analysis is used that normalizes Affymetrix array data based on an invariant set of genes. Each of these methods performs well on a variety of performance metrics. For further comparisons, see http://affycomp.biostat.jhsph.edu for details about a list of benchmarks for Affymetrix GeneChip expression measures.

Preprocessing of microarrays is discussed in more detail in publications by Parmigiani (2003) and Yang and Speed (2002). For the normalization of Affymetrix arrays, RMA has been demonstrated to be more robust than other available programs for identification of spike-in RNA samples of known concentrations

(Irizarry et al., 2003a). GC-RMA, which uses information about the GC content of the oligonucleotide sequences, is able to improve on the RMA algorithm to maintain precision while improving accuracy (Wu and Irizarry, 2004).

2. Statistical Methods for Identifying Differential Gene Expression

Generally speaking, there are four steps in the identification of differentially expressed genes. First is the choice of the appropriate statistical model, which is used to calculate the average intensities of gene expression for each gene across replicates and the sample variance for each gene. Appropriate models will be suggested by the experimental design and can include mixed effects models if higher-order structure is present in the data, such as groupings of covariates (Churchill, 2002). Second is the calculation of the test statistic. If only two groups are to be compared, then t-tests are useful. For more groups, some type of analysis of variance approach is more appropriate. See for example Churchill (2002), Kerr and Churchill (2001a,b), Kerr and colleagues (2000), Lee and colleagues (2000b), Parmigiani and colleagues (2003), and Yang and Speed (2002).

For data with more structure, such as balanced and unbalanced data, or when the within-group correlation is important in grouped data, mixed effects models are important (see Pinheiro and Bates, 2000). Several investigators prefer a modified version of the standard t statistic that uses information borrowed from all the genes on the array to estimate the individual gene variance (Efron and Tibshirani, 2002; Smyth, 2004; Storey and Tibshirani, 2003a). This modified test statistic approach is useful for prevention of calculating spuriously significant genes. As previously reported (Qin and Kerr, 2004), in the analysis of spike-in experiments on two-color cDNA arrays, it has been found that *t*-tests performed the worst among test statistics for correctly identifying the rankings of the spike-in genes, whereas modified versions of the *t* test were much more robust. Furthermore, it was found that for some data sets, the simple median of the log ratio across arrays performed best at correctly ranking the spike-in genes (Qin and Kerr, 2004).

The calculation of unadjusted p-values is the third step. This involves the calculation of the null distribution for the test statistics and the selection of rejection regions (symmetric or one-sided). The fourth step requires some reasonable approach to controlling the number of falsely positive genes. When testing a hypothesis, one can make either a Type I error (calling the gene significant when it is not, a false positive) or a Type II error (calling the gene not significant when it is, a false negative). However, in microarray analysis, multiple hypotheses are being tested, so it is not clear how best to specify the overall error rate. As pointed out by Storey and Tibshirani (2003b), there are a spectrum of choices. At one end are unadjusted p-values, which result in far too many false positives (if you have an array with 50,000 genes and a p-value cutoff of 0. 01, there are possibly 500 genes that are false positives). At the other end is the standard Bonferroni correction to control the family-wise error rate, which is far too conservative and results in large numbers of false negatives. What has been found to be most useful in the microarray context is the False Discovery Rate (FDR), or the positive False Discovery Rate (pFDR) or q-value. With this approach, the investigator can control the number of false positives in the number of genes called significant, rather than controlling the number of false positives out of all the genes present, by examining the distribution of p values. A detailed discussion of

these issues can be found in Storey and Tibshirani (2003a).

Software programs that do most or all of the steps described above are now present in many commercial analysis programs. One popular program is SAM (Statistical Analysis of Microarrays; see Storey and Tibshirani, 2003a,b). However, identification of differential gene expression is a very active research field. To stay most current with rapid changes in the field, we also recommend using the microarray statistical research tool Bioconductor, where many new algorithms first appear.

3. Data Visualization

The visualization of large data sets in order to discovery underlying patterns is an important aspect of microarray analysis. The goal is to use a dimension reduction algorithm such as Principle Component Analysis, Singular Value Decomposition, or multidimensional scaling to capture the essential variations in the data set in just two or three dimensions. However, an inherent danger is present in such a reduction of dimensionality, as valuable information may be lost (Slonim, 2002).

Another important goal in microarray analysis is the assignment of biological samples into groups based on their expression patterns. This process of assignment is broken out into two approaches: unsupervised and supervised learning. In unsupervised learning, also known as clustering, the groups or classes are discovered from the data, as they are not known beforehand. In supervised learning, also known as classification, the groups or classes are already known or are predefined. The task is then to predict the class of a new set of experiments.

Classification methods fall into three main groups: class comparison, class prediction, and class discovery. A discussion of statistical issues of classifiers such as types of classifiers, usefulness and limitations, classifier accuracy improvement, and performance of five main classifiers (k-nearest neighbor, naïve Bayes, logitBoost, random forests, and support vector machines) is given by Dudoit and Fridlyand (2003a,b). In Dudoit and Fridlyand (2003a), these classifiers are applied to several real data sets, and their performance is assessed. They showed that the simpler methods, such as k-nearest neighbor and naïve Bayes, were competitive with the more complex methods and are advisable for the more inexperienced user. However, they also showed that for larger data sets, the more complex methods performed best.

Clustering methods, which can be more difficult than classification, are used to group genes into clusters with similar behaviors, and usually begin with not knowing how many groupings there are in the data. Methods include hierarchical clustering, k-means clustering, self-organizing maps, and model-based approaches. Often it is useful to filter the data so as to cluster only a useful subset of genes. Such filtering can include simple nonspecific filtering such as removing low-intensity genes or more sophisticated Principle Component Analysis that is used to reduce the high-dimensionality of the data set to generate gene lists that account for most the differential changes. (Reviews of relevant clustering issues, algorithms, and software can be found in Chipman et al., 2003, Do et al., 2003, and Sebastiani et al., 2003). When repeated measurements are taken into account, it is possible to achieve more accurate and stable clusters (Yeung et al., 2003). Keep in mind that clusters will always be found by the algorithm, even if there are no true clusters in the underlying data. Choosing the most appropriate clustering method will depend on the data, design, and goals of the research (Slonim, 2002). A useful way to think about clustering methods is that they are different ways of looking at a data set. Each one gives a somewhat different view of a complex problem, and, therefore, each is useful in its own way.

Many open-source software packages such as Bioconductor, TIGR MultiExperiment Viewer, Eisen Lab's Cluster (Eisen et al., 1998), as well as commercial programs such as Silicon Genetics GeneSpring®, Iobion's GeneTraffic®, SAS® Microarray, Insightful's S + ArrayAnalyzer™, Rosetta Resolver®, and VizX Lab's GeneSifter™, to name a few, have a wide variety of clustering capabilities.

4. Gene Ontology Mining, Pathways Analysis, and Systems Biology

It is now possible to use microarray gene expression data to identify groups of genes in common gene ontology categories and thereby uncover biological processes and pathways. This visualization and analysis ability requires specialized software, such as the open-source programs GoMiner and GenMAPP (see Dahlquist et al., 2002, and Zeeberg et al., 2003). The Gene Ontology (GO) consortium (http://www.geneontology.org) has attempted to construct a standardized structure for functional categorization of genes. While there is a strong need for such a standardized categorization, the assignments are still changing as more research is conducted on gene function.

In addition to the open-source software, there are also commercial software programs that allow for the visualization of biological pathways, gene regulation networks, and protein–protein interactions, such as Iobion's Pathway Assist and Ingenuity System's Pathways Analysis. These programs are based on scans of the biomedical literature, and this is a changeable, active area of current research.

At the systems biology level of analysis, there is the open-source software program Cytoscape, which is used in conjunction with protein–protein, protein–DNA, and genetic interactions databases for investigating biomolecular interaction networks (see Shannon *et al.*, 2003, for more details).

5. Expression Databases and Meta-Analyses

High-throughput technologies such as DNA microarrays generate enormous amounts of data. This necessitates the use of data management systems for the storage and retrieval of experiments. Both open-source programs as well as commercial products are available. Most, if not all, of these data management systems also have a data analysis capability. These data management and data analysis systems come in client/server form or as standalone, Web-based, Windows, Macintosh, or various flavors of Unix/Linux. Of particular importance in choosing data management and data analysis systems is the overall cost of the software. Open-source systems have low to zero initial cost, but maintenance and support usually require more experienced bioinformatics and/or programming staff. Commercial systems usually have a much higher initial cost, but that cost usually covers user training and a support help desk. Furthermore, commercial vendors can also customize their products for some additional cost, whereas customization of open-source software is a job for your programming staff. Commercial products tend to be much more user friendly, coming equipped with easy-to-use graphical user interfaces. Open-source products, especially ones such as Bioconductor, have a much larger availability of statistical algorithms for use on complex experimental designs.

Open-source systems include BASE (http://base.thep.lu.se/) (Saal *et al.*, 2002), The National Center for Genome Resources' GeneX-Lite (http://www.ncgr.org/ genex/), The Institute for Genomic Research's TM4 suite

(http://www.tigr.org/ software/ tm4/), as well as others.

Commercial systems include Silicon Genetics' SpringCore™, Iobion's GeneTraffic®, SAS® Microarray, Insightful's S + ArrayAnalyzer™, Rosetta Resolver®, BioDiscovery's GeneDirector™ and VizX Lab's GeneSifter™, to name a few.

Public databases for the storage and retrieval of microarray data are available. These include the NIH's Gene Expression Omnibus GEO at http://www.ncbi.nlm.nih.gov/geo/ and the European Bioinformatics Institute's ArrayExpress at http://www.ebi.ac.uk/ arrayexpress/. These public repositories are becoming more widely used as more scientific journals require microarray data to be deposited in publicly accessible databases.

A new area of opportunity for microarray data analysis is the integration of microarray data generated by different research groups on different array platforms (Moreau *et al.*, 2003). Furthermore, access to microarray databases also affords opportunities for meta-analyses of cross-species comparisons of expression profiles that allows the study of biological processes and global properties of expression networks (Shah *et al.*, 2004). An ongoing effort at the NIA DNA Array Unit is the development of a Web-based database of biological pathways (http:// bbid.grc.nia.nih.gov), which is used to relate gene expression studies to complex biological processes. In addition, a second project includes a Web-based database of the genetics of common complex diseases.

III. Biological Studies

A. Gene Expression in Yeast

The budding yeast *Saccharomyces cerevisiae* has been used as a model system to investigate two fundamentally different types of cellular aging processes

(Bitterman *et al.*, 2003; Kaeberlein *et al.*, 2001). The study of chronological aging involves maintaining cells in a meta-bolically active, nondividing state and monitoring the decrease in viability with time, perhaps akin to the aging of post-mitotic cells in mammals (Fabrizio and Longo, 2003; MacLean *et al.*, 2001). Replicative aging, in contrast, is defined by the number of mitotic cycles com-pleted by a mother cell prior to senes-cence (Mortimer and Johnston, 1959). Several genes have been identified that determine chronological or replicative life span; however, the relationship, if any, between these two aging processes remains unclear.

Yeast represents an attractive model for using microarrays to study the aging process. With a doubling time of less than two hours, yeast is amenable to both classical genetic as well as high-throughput approaches. Much of the microarray technology development was carried out in studies of this organism (e.g., by Chu *et al.*, 1998; DeRisi *et al.*, 1997; Eisen *et al.*, 1998; Lashkari *et al.*, 1997; Shalon *et al.*, 1996; Spellman *et al.*, 1998), resulting in a large body of knowledge regarding appropriate design and an abundance of publicly available expression data (Horak and Snyder, 2002). In addition, metabolic and protein interaction pathways are relatively well characterized compared to other model systems (Barr, 2003). Also, unlike the case in multicellular eukaryotes, the potential complications arising from tis-sue heterogeneity and cell specificity do not apply to studies in yeast (see section II.A.2).

It is worth noting that one significant difference between microarray studies of aging in yeast compared to other sys-tems is that almost all have been carried out using spotted cDNA arrays. The rel-ative advantages and disadvantages of this type of platform are discussed in section II.A.4.a.

1. Gene Expression Changes Associated with Replicative Age in Yeast

As in other model systems, microarray analysis has been used as a tool to identify gene expression changes associated with old age in yeast. In theory, the design of such an experiment is identical to similar studies in worms, flies, and mice: RNA is obtained from old organisms and com-pared against RNA obtained from young organisms. Attempting to obtain a pure population of replicatively aged yeast, however, presents a unique challenge not present in other models. The median life span of a typical lab strain is approxi-mately 25 generations (Jazwinski, 1993). Thus, in order to obtain a single mother cell aged to the population median, that cell must be physically separated away from her ~2^{25} "progeny" cells. For life-span analysis, micromanipulation is used to separate daughter cells from 40 to 50 mother cells per strain; however, it is not feasible to use micromanipulation as a method to obtain enough cells for even one microarray experiment without extensive, and possibly biased, RNA amplification. Two technologies are cur-rently available to obtain large populations of aged cells: magnetic sorting and elutria-tion. In the magnetic sorting procedure, an unsorted population of cells is treated with biotin then allowed to grow for several generations prior to addition of streptavidin-coated magnetic beads (Park *et al.*, 2002; Smeal *et al.*, 1996). Subsequent magnetic separation allows enrichment of aged mother cells, which specifically retain biotin on their cell walls. Elutriation is a centrifugal tech-nique that separates cells based on cell size (Helmstetter, 1991). Generally, G_0 daughter cells are the smallest cells in a population, and older cells are the biggest. Thus, a population enriched for bigger cells by elutriation also tends to be enriched for aged cells (Woldringh *et al.*, 1995). Both magnetic sorting and elutriation, however, suffer from the drawback of significant contamination by daughter cells, a potential source of experimental noise that must be considered in any gene expression study of "old" versus "young" yeast.

Two studies have described the transcriptome of replicatively aged yeast. In one study, microarray analysis was carried out on "young" (0–1 generation) or "old" (7–8 generation) wildtype cells obtained by magnetic sorting (Lin *et al.*, 2001). In addition, young and old cells from a 20 percent shorter-lived *sip2Δ* mutant or a 15 percent longer-lived *snf4Δ* mutant (Ashrafi *et al.*, 2000) were examined. From this analysis, it was concluded that gluconeogenesis and glucose storage increase as cells age, suggesting a metabolic shift away from glycolysis and toward gluconeogenesis. Microanalytic biochemical assays were used to verify changes in enzyme activity consistent with the microarray results. In addition to questions regarding the purity of the aged cell population, however, the validity of defining 7–8 generation cells as "old" must be questioned. The median and maximum life spans of the strain background used in this study (S288C) are approximately 25 and 50 generations, respectively (Kaeberlein *et al.*, 2004). Thus, the use of 7–8–generation mother cells to identify gene expression changes associated with aging in yeast is analogous to using 7-month mice or 20-year-old humans as the aged population for similar studies in these organisms.

In the second study of this type, elutriation was used to obtain an aged population in which 75 percent of the cells were at least 15 generations old and 90 percent of the cells were more than 8 generations old (Lesur and Campbell, 2004). Microarray analysis of aged cells relative to young cells suggested an increase in expression of enzymes associated with glucose storage and gluconeogenesis, consistent with the previous study (Lin *et al.*, 2001). In addition, certain stress- and damage-responsive genes were also reported to

be elevated in aged cells (Lesur and Campbell, 2004). Although the average age of the "old" cells is a significant improvement over the first study of this type, it is still well below the population median. Further, both studies use an arbitrary two-fold cutoff to identify differentially expressed genes and suffer from a lack of rigorous statistical analysis. Future studies of this type should attempt to address both of these weaknesses. The fact that both studies suggest an age-associated shift toward glucose storage at ages below the median life span of the population, however, is suggestive that major metabolic changes occur early in the yeast life span. It will be of interest to determine whether these changes are retained, or perhaps enhanced, at later replicative ages.

2. Gene Expression Profiles of Long-Lived Yeast Strains

In addition to age-associated gene expression studies, microarrays have also been used to examine gene expression changes that correlate with extreme longevity in yeast. These types of experiments are simpler to perform than those described above. Because the proportion of aged cells present in a logarithmically growing yeast culture is exceedingly small (less than 1 per 2^n cells, where n equals replicative age), RNA can be harvested from an unsorted population of long-lived cells and compared against RNA from an unsorted population of wildtype cells. In theory, this approach provides an opportunity to identify molecular mechanisms of enhanced longevity in individual long-lived mutants. In addition, comparison of multiple long-lived mutants has the potential to identify gene expression biomarkers of longevity.

This type of analysis has been successfully performed using genetic models of longevity as well as environmental models of longevity, such as CR by growth on low glucose. In one study, microarray analysis was carried out on two models of CR in yeast: growth on low glucose and deletion of the gene coding for hexokinase, *HXK2* (Lin *et al.*, 2002). Based on the observed gene expression changes, it was suggested that CR of yeast cells results in a transcriptional shift from fermentation to respiration. These findings were verified by follow-up experiments showing that oxygen consumption is elevated by CR. In addition, based on the overlap between gene expression changes observed in cells lacking *HXK2* and cells grown on low glucose, 124 putative gene expression biomarkers of CR were reported. It should be noted, however, that no evidence has been presented to suggest that the observed gene expression changes play a causal role in CR-mediated life-span extension.

To date, a large-scale comparative microarray analysis of multiple long-lived mutants is lacking. At least two additional studies have compared individual gene expression data sets from cells with enhanced life span against the CR data sets described above. In one case, the transcriptional changes associated with high external osmolarity showed significant overlap with the CR data set (Kaeberlein and Guarente, 2002). In the other study, gene expression changes associated with addition of *SSD1-V*, which increases mean replicative life span by approximately 75 percent, showed no significant overlap with CR (Kaeberlein and Guarente, 2002). These results were interpreted to suggest that osmotic stress response, but not *SSD1-V*, is likely to promote longevity by a mechanism similar to CR. In both of these studies, as well as the CR study described above, only two data sets for each genotype were obtained, and an arbitrary two-fold cutoff was used to classify genes with significantly altered expression. Rigorous statistical analysis and additional data sets would improve confidence in the individual genes reported. The use of gene expression changes across a subset of genes to place long-lived mutants into genetic pathways, however, is an approach with the potential for broad applicability as additional data sets are obtained.

3. Chronological Aging in Yeast

To date, the use of microarrays to investigate yeast aging has been largely confined to studies of replicative aging. The reasons for this dichotomy are unclear, as chronological aging would seem to present a system amenable to microarray technology. Chronological life span is determined by culturing cells into stationary phase and monitoring the percentage of cells that retain viability over time (Fabrizio and Longo, 2003; MacLean *et al.*, 2001). Unlike the case with replicative age, studies examining gene expression changes associated with increased chronological age are trivial in design. In fact, one of the pioneering microarray studies examined the gene expression changes associated with the yeast diauxic shift, a transition from logarithmic growth to stationary phase (DeRisi *et al.*, 1997). A similar design, but with timepoints spaced over several weeks, could be used to identify gene expression biomarkers of chronological age. As with replicative aging, microarray studies comparing chronologically long-lived mutants to wildtype cells could also be used to potentially identify gene expression biomarkers of chronological longevity. In this regard, it would be of particular interest to determine whether there are significant similarities between the transcriptional changes associated with enhanced chronological life span and those associated with enhanced replicative life span.

4. Mutation of Orthologous Genes in Yeast

In addition to directly studying the function of genes that regulate chronological or replicative life span, an alternative approach is to use microarrays to study the function of yeast orthologs of proteins that affect aging in higher eukaryotes. For example, increased expression of the heat shock transcription factor Hsf1 has been found to increase life span in worms (Hsu *et al.*, 2003; Morley and Morimoto, 2004). Although, no chronological or replicative life span phenotype has been reported in response to Hsf1 overexpression in yeast, a recent study employed microarray technology to identify a majority of the direct transcriptional targets of yeast Hsf1 (Hahn *et al.*, 2004). Analysis of this data to determine which Hsf1 targets have worm orthologs is likely to provide information regarding potential downstream effectors of the enhanced longevity conferred by HSF-1 overexpression. This type of approach would be particularly amenable to highly conserved pathways or genes that are likely to behave similarly in higher eukaryotes.

5. Conclusions from Yeast Studies

Microarray analysis has provided valuable insight into certain aspects of the aging process in yeast, particularly the identification of global metabolic changes associated with calorie restriction and replicative age. However, this technology has not been used to its fullest potential. The use of arbitrary fold cutoffs and lack of rigorous statistical analysis, in particular, have been limitations of studies to date. Future studies should strive to improve in these areas. Given the relative ease with which a compendium of gene expression data sets could be generated for all of the mutants reported to increase yeast life span, this should become a priority for future work. In this way, it will be possible to rapidly identify gene expression changes correlated with longevity on a genome-wide scale, something for which yeast is uniquely suited.

B. Gene Expression in Invertebrate Models

A number of studies have employed microarrays to study aging in the invertebrate model systems *Drosophila melanogaster* and *Caenorhabditis elegans*. As is the case with yeast and mammalian model systems, two general strategies have been employed to identify genes important for the aging process. In the first, microarrays have been used to look for genes that are differentially expressed in aged animals relative to young animals. In the second type of study, microarrays have been used to identify genes differentially expressed in long-lived versus short-lived animals. The merit of each of these approaches is discussed in detail in section II.A.1.

Although there is still substantial disagreement as to which specific genes are differentially expressed, and even how many genes are differentially expressed, there is an emerging consensus that certain types of genes show specific changes in gene expression with age. In particular, several studies have suggested that expression of stress-response genes is elevated in old animals, and that these types of genes are also upregulated in long-lived mutants. There is also evidence that metabolic genes are downregulated during aging. In this section, we review selected microarray studies to demonstrate these themes. We also highlight discrepancies between various studies to demonstrate the limitations of current technology.

1. Overexpression of Stress Response Genes During Aging in Drosophila

Several studies in *Drosophila* have reached the conclusion that stress-response genes are overexpressed during aging (Zou *et al.*, 2000). Zou and colleagues used dual-channel cDNA arrays and probes prepared from pooled male *Drosophila* samples of diverse ages to identify genes differentially expressed during aging. The data analysis for this early study was nonstatistical and based on ratio-dependent selection of genes followed by hierarchical clustering. From this analysis, it was reported that expression of certain key metabolic genes, including glucose-3-phosphate dehydrogenase and cytochrome c, are decreased with age. An age-associated upregulation of some stress-related genes, including glutathione-s-transferase 1, was also observed. To test whether this represented a general response to oxidative stress, the gene expression profile of young animals treated with the superoxide-generating drug paraquat was obtained and compared to that of aged flies. Intriguingly, approximately one-third of genes differentially expressed in response to the oxidative challenge were also differentially expressed with normal aging.

More recently, several other studies have reached similar conclusions. Pletcher and colleagues (2002) used Affymetrix arrays containing the majority of *Drosophila* open reading frames to look for differentially expressed genes. For this study, RNA was collected only from female flies and analyzed in a pooled fashion. Samples from both control-fed and calorically restricted animals were collected at multiple time points. A sophisticated statistical analysis with false discovery rate adjustment was used to identify differentially expressed genes. Nine percent of genes on the array were differentially expressed at one or more timepoints during aging. Differentially expressed genes were then mapped against the GO gene functional ontology (http://www.geneontology.org/). Based on this analysis, stress response, antibacterial, and serine protease inhibitor functional categories were upregulated during aging, and oogenesis genes were downregulated during aging. In calorically restricted flies, genes involved in the cell cycle, DNA repair, DNA replication,

protein metabolism, and protein degradation were downregulated. Fifty percent of age-dependent changes in gene expression were ameliorated by long-term CR.

Landis and colleagues (2004) performed a microarray study with the aim of identifying gene expression biomarkers of aging in *Drosophila*. As with Pletcher and colleagues (2002), Landis and colleagues (2004) used Affymetrix arrays coupled with a sophisticated statistical analysis to identify differentially expressed genes. RNA was obtained from male flies and pooled at a variety of aging timepoints between 10 and 61 days (at the 61-day timepoint, 50 percent of the cohort was surviving). Using Significance Analysis of Microarrays (SAM), 7 percent of genes on the array were differentially expressed at one or more timepoints, in good agreement with the Pletcher study. They also observed upregulation during aging of stress-response genes, including antioxidant genes, antibacterial genes, and some heat shock proteins (hsp 22). In addition, genes coding for enzymes in the purine biosynthetic pathway were upregulated, whereas protease, proteasome, and metabolic genes were downregulated.

Landis and colleagues (2004) also exposed young flies to 100 percent oxygen to induce antioxidant genes. They observed that there was a 33 percent overlap between genes differentially expressed in response to oxygen and aging. In agreement with the fact that *Drosophila* life span scales with the temperature at which they are raised, the age-associated upregulation of antibacterial genes also scaled with temperature, suggesting that these genes may be good aging biomarkers in *Drosophila*.

2. Overexpression of Stress Response Genes in Long-Lived Invertebrates

The studies described thus far indicate that stress-response genes, such as antioxidant genes and antibacterial genes, are induced during aging in flies. Kang and colleagues (2002) observed that treating flies with the histone deacetylase inhibitor PBA increased both mean and maximum life span in two strain backgrounds. They used EST spotted nylon membrane microarrays to identify genes upregulated in PBA-treated flies. Genes upregulated in the long-lived animals included stress-response genes such as MnSOD, glutathione-s-transferase, and several chaperonins.

Several important studies using *C. elegans* have also tried to identify genes differentially expressed in short- versus long-lived animals (McElwee *et al.*, 2003; Murphy *et al.*, 2003). These studies are based on the observation that an IGF/insulin-like signaling pathway functions in early adult *C. elegans* to regulate life span.

Hypomorphic mutations in the DAF-2 insulin-like receptor double life span and increase the stress resistance of mutant worms. Mutations in the downstream DAF-16 FOXO transcription factor block the effects of DAF-2 mutations. McElwee and colleagues (2003) used cDNA microarrays, spotted with the majority of *C. elegans* genes, to identify genes differentially expressed between young (1 day) DAF-2 and DAF-2/DAF-16 pooled worm samples. In both cases, the worms had additional mutations to render them sterile. In the long-lived DAF-2 worms, upregulation of mitochondrial superoxide dismutase sod-3, as well as several heat shock proteins, was observed. In addition, substantial overlap between the differentially expressed genes and genes with DAF-16 binding sites in their promoters was reported. In order to verify the relevance of observed gene expression changes for increased life span in DAF-2 animals, RNAi was used to knock down the activities of the differentially expressed ins-7 gene, and this lengthened life span.

A similar strategy was employed by Murphy and colleagues (2003). In this study, they collected pooled samples of sterile worms from a variety of aging timepoints as well as day 1 DAF-2 versus DAF-2/DAF-16 worms. These samples were hybridized to spotted cDNA arrays containing the majority of the *C. elegans* genome. A nonstatistical analysis plus hierarchical clustering was used to identify genes that showed differential patterns of expression. In particular, genes upregulated in DAF-2 versus DAF-2/DAF-16 were selected as potential longevity-enhancing genes. Such genes included stress-response genes such as gst-4, sod-3, catalase genes, small heat shock proteins, and antibacterial defense genes. Importantly, using RNAi to inhibit the activity of these genes in DAF-2 mutants resulted in a *decrease* in life span, suggesting that their upregulation is functionally related to enhanced longevity.

These studies also identified the ins-7 gene product as the likely ligand of the IGF/insulin-signaling pathway. ins-7 expression is decreased in the long-lived DAF-2 mutant but increased in DAF-2/DAF-16 double mutants. RNAi against ins-7 in a DAF-2/DAF-16 background resulted in an increase in life span.

The study of Murphy and colleagues marks an important advance in the field, as it demonstrated convincingly that gene expression changes observed by microarray can lead to the identification of functionally relevant regulators of longevity. In addition, this study enhanced a biological model for the mechanism by which hormonal signals produced in specific cells can act globally to regulate life span in *C. elegans*.

3. Bioinformatic Analysis of Cross-Species Gene Expression Changes During Aging

Collectively, these microarray studies argue that, in general, stress-response genes are upregulated in old animals and that long-lived animals have elevated expression of stress-response genes. Also, in several of these studies, metabolic genes were noted to be downregulated during aging. In an attempt to synthesize the data from flies and worms, McCarroll and colleagues (2004) used a bioinformatic approach to compare genes differentially expressed during aging in both organisms. McCarroll first identified orthologous gene pairs across the two species and then used microarrays to analyze gene expression during aging in pooled *Drosophila* heads and in pooled worms at various ages. Orthologous gene pairs showed a limited (r = .144), but highly statistically significant (P < 10^{-11}), correlation during aging. Perhaps more importantly, McCarroll then mapped the orthologous gene pairs to GO functional categories. GO term mapping of age-associated gene expression changes in worms and flies also demonstrated a significant overlap in functional categories. Although it is important to note that the majority of differentially expressed aging genes were unique to each species, statistically significant enrichment for 14 GO categories was observed. This is many more significant GO categories than would be expected by chance, as permuting the underlying data and redoing the GO analysis showed a false positive rate of 1.4 +/− .91 GO categories. Many of these GO categories were involved in general metabolism and showed a coordinate repression in early adulthood when the IGF/insulin pathway is known to begin regulating life span in *C. elegans*. This study was the first to attempt to demonstrate the existence of broad phylogenetically conserved similarity in the types of genes showing altered transcription with age as well as specific orthologous gene pairs with similar age-associated profiles.

4. To Pool or Not to Pool Invertebrates?

Due to the small size of the experimental animal, both *Drosophila* and *C. elegans* microarray studies have generally pooled a large number of whole animals to study gene expression at each timepoint. This has advantages and disadvantages, as described in section II.A.3.b. A major disadvantage of this approach in invertebrate systems is that changes in gene expression in individual tissues are averaged out over all of the tissues in the body. For example, if a gene were strongly differentially expressed in one small organ but not differentially expressed in other tissues, it is likely that this gene would be missed in current studies.

Another disadvantage of pooling animals is that gene expression differences in individual animals are lost. To eliminate this problem, Golden and Melov (2004) analyzed gene expression changes during aging in individual *C. elegans*.

5. How Many Genes Are Differentially Expressed During Aging in Invertebrate Model Systems?

We have cited evidence that there are broad similarities in the gene expression changes associated with aging in *Drosophila* and *C. elegans*, as well as multiple conserved gene expression changes among orthologous gene pairs. However, there are still substantial disagreements between studies, even within the same species. For example, there is relatively poor agreement on which genes are differentially expressed during aging. There is also disagreement on the magnitude of differential gene expression during aging. For example, using modern Affymetrix arrays and sophisticated statistical analysis, Landis and colleagues (2004) and Pletcher and colleagues (2002) observed 7 to 9 percent of genes as being differentially expressed during aging across multiple timepoints. In contrast, rigorous statistical analysis of the data from Jin and colleagues (2001) suggests that the majority of variance in their expression data was due first to strain differences, then to sex differences, and only last to age-specific differences. This observation implies that the magnitude of gene expression changes during aging is relatively modest. Only 1 percent (1.0 percent) of genes in the Jin study showed age-dependent statistically significant differences in expression, compared to 7 to 9 percent in the other studies.

Some of the differences between the studies can be attributed to the differences in experimental design. However, by plotting P-value versus ratio change for the genes using a volcano plot, Jin and colleagues (2001) demonstrated an important aspect of their result: none of the genes identified as showing a statistically significant change in gene expression during aging showed even a two-fold ratio change, and many ratio changes were as little as 1.2-fold.

It is important to note that modern statistical array analysis tools identify genes with very modest ratio changes as differentially expressed. Furthermore, many of the studies we have reviewed do not even show the distribution of observed ratios for their data. This is unfortunate, as the biological significance of, for example, a 1.2-fold ratio change in gene expression is presently unclear. Furthermore, many array data normalization procedures can cause small consistent shifts in the ratio data. This could lead to affected genes being falsely identified as differentially expressed. Thus, the significance of statistically significant but tiny changes in gene expression must be questioned.

It can also be asked whether microarrays are missing key aspects of changes in gene function during aging in both *D. melanogaster* and *C. elegans*. As noted above, in most studies, relatively small gene expression changes have been observed in aging. However, biosynthetic activity in both invertebrate and vertebrate models plunges during aging, with decreases in both synthesis and degradation of mRNA and protein. For example, protein synthesis decreases by as much as 60 to 90 percent during aging in *Drosophila* (Arking, 1998). Such large changes may be highly significant for the aging phenotype and yet are not detected by microarrays, at least in part because current microarray studies examine only relative, not absolute, changes in gene expression.

C. Gene Expression in Rodent Models

Although studies of yeast, nematodes, and fruit flies yield important insight into evolutionarily conserved pathways of aging, the rodent model better represents aging in a complex mammalian system, and still offers time, space, and economic benefits compared to larger mammals. Additionally, the availability of long-lived genetic mouse models (such as dwarf mice deficient in growth hormone signaling), CR, and transgenic and allele replacement mice have allowed for comparisons of gene expression patterns associated with life-span extension in the mammal.

Use of a mammalian model, however, does present additional concerns. Unlike studies of lower eukaryotes, mammalian studies of gene expression changes with age are intrinsically linked to tissue type, as gene expression variability between tissues overwhelms the changes observed with aging. For most laboratories, it is not economically feasible to pursue microarray studies on all tissues, or even several tissues of interest, and, thus, most of the reported studies focus on transcriptional profiles in one or two tissues that may or may not be representative of global gene expression changes. Tissues examined to date include brain (Blalock *et al.*, 2003; Lee *et al.*, 2000a; Preisser *et al.*, 2004; Prolla, 2002; Prolla and Mattson, 2001; Weindruch and Prolla, 2002; Weindruch *et al.*, 2002), skeletal muscle (Lee et al., 1999; Tollet-Egnell et al., 2004; Weindruch et al., 2001, 2002; Welle et al., 2001), liver (Cao et al., 2001; Dozmorov et al., 2001; Dozmorov et al., 2002; Meydani et al., 1998; Miller et al., 2002; Tollet-Egnell et al., 2004; Tsuchiya et al., 2004), heart (Bronikowski et al., 2003; Csiszar et al., 2003; Edwards et al., 2003, 2004; Lee et al., 2002; Meydani et al., 1998), kidney (Preisser et al., 2004), duodenum and colon (Lee et al., 2001), adipose tissue (Higami et al., 2004; Tollet-Egnell et al., 2004), and submandibular gland (Hiratsuka et al., 2002).

The current body of literature employing microarrays to examine gene expression associated with aging in mammals is relatively young and largely descriptive. However, Helmberg (2001) and Weindruch and colleagues (2002) discuss the enormous potential utility of this approach. The possible outcomes from this work include: (1) insights into the fundamental causes of aging by, for example, the identification of biochemical pathways altered with age; (2) development of tools and biomarkers useful in the evaluation of aging interventions; and (3) perhaps even to define "individual genomic risk constellations" useful in the treatment and management of aging-associated conditions. This review highlights some of the seminal papers to date that employ microarray technology to advance our understanding of aging in mammals.

1. Gene Expression Changes Associated with Age

Lee and associates were among the first to report changes in gene expression profiles with age in mouse tissues, using microarrays to study gene expression patterns in brain (neocortex and cerebellum) and skeletal muscle from adult (5-month) and old (30-month) C57Bl/6NHsd mice (average life span 30 months), as described in a series of papers (Lee et al., 1999; Lee et al., 2000a; Weindruch et al., 2001, 2002; Prolla, 2002). (The CR component of these studies will be discussed later.) For these studies, the authors compared three animals per group using 6347-gene oligonucleotide arrays. The data were analyzed using pairwise comparisons (nine total comparisons) with Pearson correlation coefficients calculated for individual animals and a fold-change cutoff was used to classify genes as significantly upregulated or downregulated.

The principal finding of these studies is that only a small percentage of genes in each tissue (approximately 1 percent) were upregulated or downregulated by at least two-fold (1.7 fold in the neocortex), indicating that aging is unlikely to result from widespread gene expression changes of large magnitude. Furthermore, the authors observed little overlap among the individual genes altered in the tissues examined, although they did observe coordinate induction of complement cascade members and cathepsins in the neocortex and cerebellum with age. Cathepsins may be of particular interest as they are involved in the processing of amyloid precursor protein and are upregulated in Alzheimer's diseased brains. Of the genes reported to be upregulated with age in the tissues examined, the greatest proportion fell into the functional categories of inflammation and stress response, whereas decreased expression was observed for genes involved in metabolism and biosynthesis.

Although these early studies are somewhat limited by their lack of rigorous statistical analyses and validation, they were among the first to illuminate trends that seem to be recurrent in subsequent microarray studies—namely, that relatively few transcriptional changes are of great magnitude, and that transcriptional profiles across tissues and even across subregions of a particular tissue are markedly different. Furthermore, the initial findings in these studies, that genes involved in stress response and inflammation seem to increase with age while genes involved in protein turnover and structural maintenance decline, are also echoed in later studies.

Other studies have also analyzed age-associated gene expression changes (young versus old) in conjunction with gene expression changes associated with enhanced longevity. For example, Dozmorov and colleagues (2001) measured gene expression changes with age in livers of 5-, 13-, and 22-month-old mice (n = 3 to 4 mice per group). This study utilized both control and Ames *dw/dw* dwarf mice, but presently this discussion will focus on the analysis of the subset of genes altered with age. The authors measured gene expression levels using Atlas 588-gene cDNA membranes, 323 genes of which were removed from analysis due to low levels of expression or proximity on the array to highly expressed genes. Although the authors did observe large changes in the expression ratios of many of the remaining 265 genes, a closer examination revealed that high fold-change values were correlated with high variability and were likely to be false positives. Thus, of the 265 remaining genes, the authors report only four genes altered in the wildtype mice between 5 and 22 months, and only three genes altered between 5 and 13 months. Two of these seven genes, however, were directly involved in insulin signaling, IGFBP1 and IGF receptor 2, notable in particular due to the repeated implication of insulin signaling in longevity studies of lower invertebrates.

Edwards and colleagues compared cardiac gene expression profiles in young (5-month), middle-aged (15-month) and old (25-month) mice at 0, 1, 3, 5, and 7 hours after a single intraperitoneal injection of paraquat (N = 3 for each age and timepoint) (Edwards *et al.*, 2003, 2004). These authors measured expression levels of 9,977 genes using high-density oligonucleotide arrays and found an age-dependent decrease in the cardiac transcriptional response to the paraquat challenge, particularly a decrease in the stress-response pathways signaling through MAPKKK and JNK, and a decreased induction of the DNA damage-induced gene GADD45. The authors also note a shift in the spectrum of oxidative stress genes induced at different ages, with induction of glutathione-S-transferase A3 specific to young mice, glutathione peroxidase 1 and peroxiredoxin 4 specific to middle-aged mice, and superoxide dismutase 1 specific to old mice.

A recent study by Blalock and colleagues (2003) has attempted to link age-dependent expression changes with measurable functional consequences. They describe age-dependent transcriptional profiles associated with cognitive impairment in the rat hippocampus, in particular the hippocampal CA1 region. The authors trained young (4-month), middle-aged (14-month), and old (24-month) male rats on two memory tasks, the Morris spatial water maze and the object memory task, and the hippocampal CA1 region of each animal was subsequently harvested for expression analysis on individual Affymetrix oligonucleotide arrays (one chip per animal, N = 10 animals per group). The expression data were analyzed for both aging effects (ANOVA) and for cognition effects (Pearson's test), and although most of the gene expression changes were initially evident in the middle-aged group, impaired cognition was not clearly manifest until late life. The aging- and cognition-related genes identified represent familiar categories such as oxidative stress, inflammation, decreased mitochondrial function, and altered protein processing, but also include genes involved in downregulated early response signaling, cholesterol synthesis, lipid and monoamine metabolism, and other likely brain-specific categories such as activity-regulated synaptogenesis, upregulated myelin turnover, and structural reorganization genes. This study clearly benefits from the statistical power of a relatively large number of samples (N = 10 for each group), but more importantly, the inclusion of an intermediate timepoint and the correlation with a functional outcome in the study design allow the authors to put forth an integrative model of brain aging in which gene expression changes observed in early adulthood trigger subtle changes resulting in cumulative cognitive deficits not evident until a much later date.

2. Attenuation of Age-Related Expression Changes by Caloric Restriction in Rodents

The early studies by Lee and coworkers comparing genomic expression profiles in young and old brain (Lee *et al.*, 1999; Prolla, 2002) and skeletal muscle (Lee *et al.*, 1999; Weindruch *et al.*, 2001) also examined the effect of CR on the expression profiles of tissues from old (30-month) animals. In general, the authors noted that CR (initiated at 2 months) selectively prevented many of the age-related increases in inflammatory and stress-response genes while having little effect on expression of genes involved in neuronal growth and plasticity in the neocortex and cerebellum. In skeletal muscle, CR shifted the expression profile toward increased energy metabolism, increased biosynthesis, and increased protein turnover, more similar to that of younger animals.

The reversal of age-dependent expression changes by CR seems to occur whether the CR is of short or long duration. The same group (Lee *et al.*, 2002) reported in a separate paper that CR initiated at middle-age (14 months) resulted in a 19 percent global inhibition

of the age-related gene expression changes observed in 30-month-old mouse hearts (Lee *et al.*, 2002). Cao and colleagues employed a long-lived F1 hybrid strain of mice, comparing liver gene expression profiles of young (7-month) versus old (27-month) animals fed *ad libidum* or on a CR diet, and also included a short-term CR cohort consisting of 34-month-old control mice placed on a CR regimen for 4 weeks (Cao *et al.*, 2001). Gene expression changes observed with age were consistent with previous studies, reflecting increased inflammation, stress, and fibrosis with reduced expression of genes involved in apoptosis, xenobiotic metabolism, and DNA replication and cell-cycle. However, the observed changes in gene expression were attenuated by both long-term CR and 4-week short-term CR in old mice. These results imply that CR begun late in life and instituted for a short time can shift gene expression patterns for a subset of genes to a more youthful profile.

However, it may be that the short-term effects of CR on gene expression are tissue and/or age-dependent. Higami and colleagues (2004) investigated the influences of short-term and long-term CR on gene expression in white adipose tissue and report gene expression changes associated only with long-term CR. The authors compared four groups of 10- to 11-month-old male C57Bl6 mice (N = 5 per group): non-fasted controls, fasted for 18 hours before death, short-term caloric restriction for 23 days, or long-term caloric restriction for 9 months. For this study, the authors employed high-density oligonucleotide arrays with over 11,000 genes. Compared to the control mice, only a few transcripts were differentially expressed in the fasted and short-term CR groups, whereas 345 transcripts were found to be significantly altered by long-term CR, the majority of which were directly involved in metabolism or insulin signaling. The discrepancy between results of the Higami study and the Cao study likely reflects the different tissues investigated as well as the timing of the short-term CR—in the Cao study, the short-term CR was initiated in much older mice than in the Higami study (34 months versus 9 months).

Indeed, Dhahbi and colleagues (2004) demonstrate that CR begun relatively late in life (at 19 months) begins to increase the mean time to death as well as mean and maximum life spans within 2 months of initiation and is accompanied by a rapid and progressive shift toward a hepatic transcriptional profile associated with long-term CR. (Other studies, however, have failed to demonstrate a beneficial effect of late-onset CR, for example, Lipman *et al.*, 1995, 1998). For the Dhahbi study, the authors used high-density oligonucleotide arrays to compare hepatic gene expression in control mice with that of mice on a CR regimen for 2, 4, or 8 weeks (N = 3 to 4 animals per group). Additionally, a cohort of long-term CR mice was returned to a control diet for 8 weeks. Microarray analysis of livers from 19-month-old control mice switched to CR for 2, 4, or 8 weeks revealed a pattern of early and sustained gene expression changes in response to CR, with early gene expression changes occurring within 2 weeks, intermediate gene expression changes occurring between 4 and 8 weeks, and late gene expression changes occurring after 8 weeks of CR. Furthermore, analysis of the hepatic gene expression profile of mice shifted from long-term CR to a control diet demonstrated that 90 percent of the gene expression effects of long-term CR were reversed within 8 weeks. Thus, the authors' findings imply a temporal and phenotypic link between CR-induced longevity and genomic expression changes, but these changes may be limited to late onset CR.

The impact of other late-onset dietary interventions on global gene expression has also been evaluated. In particular, the effects on cardiac gene expression profiles in mice given dietary supplementation with alpha-lipoic acid (LA) or coenzyme Q(10) (CQ) started at middle age (14 months) has been examined and compared to CR as a positive control (Lee *et al.*, 2004). In contrast to CR, supplementation with LA or CQ had no impact on longevity or on the spectrum of observed tumors when compared with control mice on an isocaloric diet. Global analysis of 9977 genes demonstrated that LA, CQ, and CR mitigated age-dependent gene expression changes related to cellular and extracellular structure and protein turnover, but CR was the only intervention to affect gene expression related to energy metabolism. The authors conclude that, although supplementation with alpha-lipoic acid or coenzyme Q(10) induces a gene expression profile indicative of reduced cardiac oxidative stress, CR is much more effective at inhibiting the aging process in the heart, likely due to the observed changes in energy metabolism.

3. Gene Expression Changes in Long-Lived Dwarf Mouse Models

Genetic mutations in the growth hormone signaling pathway and targeted disruption of the growth hormone receptor in the mouse have given rise to various dwarf mice that display remarkable increases in life span. As the primary effector of growth hormone signaling is insulin growth factor 1 (IGF-1), there is considerable interest in whether the longevity observed in these mice results from a mechanism fundamentally similar to that of CR. If true, similar gene expression patterns associated with CR and dwarf models may reveal a transcriptional profile of longevity.

Miller and colleagues (2002) examined the influence of CR on gene expression in the livers of both 9-month-old control and growth-hormone receptor knockout mice (GHR-KO) (n = 8 per group) using 2352-gene cDNA arrays. In this analysis,

CR was reported to significantly alter mRNA levels for 352 genes. Although the GHR-KO genotype had little impact on gene expression in control-fed animals, the gene expression changes associated with CR were significantly diminished in the GHR-KO mice, pointing toward an interaction between the GHR-KO genotype and CR. The genes with altered expression patterns in this study were compared to those identified in a study of another long-lived dwarf mouse model, the Snell dwarf, and expression of 29 genes was found to be similarly altered in both studies. These findings lend strength to the hypothesis that various models of increased longevity share similar underlying mechanisms.

As previously mentioned, Dozmorov and colleagues (2001) conducted an aging study of hepatic gene expression in control and Ames dwarf mice, comparing 5-, 13-, and 22-month-old animals using the 588-gene Atlas cDNA arrays . Although very few genes (7) survived the statistical significance testing to demonstrate an age-dependent change, of these, none were found to be attenuated by the Ames dwarf genotype between 5 and 13 months or between 13 and 22 months of age. A separate study by the same group investigated hepatic gene expression in 6-month-old Snell dwarf mice using the Atlas 2352-gene cDNA array set (Dozmorov et al., 2002). From this analysis, the authors report several gene expression changes associated with the dwarf genotype; however, it remains to be seen which of these early-age (6-month) changes are functionally associated with longevity.

In summary, microarray analyses of gene expression changes in aging rodent tissues have revealed a trend of increased expression of genes involved in inflammation and stress response with age with a corresponding decrease in expression of genes involved in protein turnover and structural maintenance. Several

studies suggest that these observed gene expression changes are modulated to some extent by interventions that retard aging, such as CR and/or dwarf phenotype, and thus may provide insight into the molecular mechanisms associated with aging. Furthermore, that the gene expression changes are similar in nature to those observed in nonmammalian models potentially reflects a universal aging process at the transcriptional level, and the availability of long-lived rodent models will prove essential for elucidating these mechanisms in complex mammalian systems.

D. Primates

1. Primate Literature—In Vivo

To date there are few microarray studies reporting gene expression changes with age in primates, particularly in vivo studies. This undoubtedly is due to the relatively recent advent of this technology coupled with the time and logistical requirements in obtaining primate or human tissue samples for analysis, especially for longitudinal aging studies. There are, however, several studies in primates of note, with more recent studies reflecting an increased sophistication in the use of microarray profiling to derive and test hypotheses in the study of aging.

An early attempt to detect age-related gene expression changes in human samples made use of a previously existing database of gene expression profiles from colon adenocarcinoma and normal colon samples (Kirschner et al., 2002). Although the original data were not part of an aging study, the samples (n = 16) were derived from donors ranging in age from 35 to 85 years. The samples had been hybridized onto Affymetrix high-density oligonucleotide arrays, with approximately 6,800 genes represented, and initial data assessment was conducted using Affymetrix software before loading into the public database. To determine the effect of age—if any—on gene expression, the authors calculated a correlation coefficient between mRNA expression and age of donor for each gene, the significance of which was computed using a t-test. In this manner, only nine genes were found to be significantly altered with age in the normal tissue samples, of which one-third were likely to be false positives as determined by random permutation. In the tumor samples, 12 genes were found to be altered with age, again with one-third likely false, and the overlap between the normal and tumor samples was only three genes.

Another early study measured gene expression in young (age 13 and 14, n = 2) versus old (age 62 to 74, n = 3) human retinas (Yoshida *et al.*, 2002). The RNA extracted from these samples were hybridized to glass cDNA microarray slides with 2,400 genes, 80 percent of which were of neuronal origin. Most genes were unchanged with age; only a small number of (24) genes displayed differential expression, with these representing energy metabolism, stress response, cell growth, and neuronal transmission/signaling. Although this study is limited by a very small and unequal sample size as well as by the small number of genes on the slide, it does represent one of the earliest microarray studies to investigate aging in human tissues.

The National Primate Research Center at the University of Wisconsin, Madison, has maintained a colony of rhesus monkeys (*Macaca mulatta*) for conducting longitudinal studies of aging in primates, and a cohort of these monkeys are part of a long-term CR study in primates. Kayo and colleagues (2001) reported an expression analysis of 7,070 genes from the vastus lateralis muscle of these rhesus monkeys, analyzing the data by pairwise comparisons between young and old, AL

and CR . In a comparison of young (7- to 11-year-old) and old (25- to 27-year-old) monkeys (N = 3 each group), aging resulted in a selective induction of transcripts involved in inflammation, stress response and neuronal factors, with a downregulation of genes involved in mitochondrial electron transport and oxidative phosphorylation. The CR component of the study examined gene expression in middle-aged monkeys (age 19 to 21 years, N = 3 each), fed normally or on a CR regimen for 9 years at the time of biopsy. CR induced an upregulation of genes largely representing structural components and growth regulation, and the authors also observed a downregulation of genes involved in mitochondrial bioenergetics. Interestingly, the authors found little or no evidence for an inhibitory effect of adult-onset CR on the age-dependent changes in gene expression; of the 34 genes upregulated or downregulated with age in the middle-age and old monkeys, only three were found to be significantly altered by CR. Thus, it may be that, in primates, the benefit of late-onset CR is limited. The full impact of adult-onset CR on the life span of these animals is as yet unknown.

A recent study focusing on gene expression in Alzheimer's diseased brains is nevertheless noteworthy to the aging field, not only because of the increased incidence of Alzheimer's disease (AD) with age, but also due to findings of a correlation of genomic profiles with disease severity, particularly with early or incipient AD (Blalock *et al.*, 2004). The authors correlated hippocampal gene expression with severity of AD based on ante-mortem MiniMental Stage Exam (MMSE) score and post-mortem measurements of neurofibrillary tangles (NFTs) and Braak stage scoring. Subjects were assigned to four groups: control (N = 9), incipient AD (N = 7), moderate AD (N = 8), and severe AD (N = 7). Extracted RNA samples were analyzed using high-density oligonucleotide arrays (>14,000 genes), and after initial data analysis identifying AD-related genes by Pearson's correlation with MMSE and NFT, the authors employed expression analysis systematic explorer (EASE, a modified Fisher's test) to test statistically for co-regulation of genes in a common pathway or process. In this manner, the authors identified 3,413 genes as AD-related genes across all 31 subjects, with genes correlating more strongly with MMSE than with NFT. The authors then examined expression of these genes in only the control and incipient AD groups to identify early markers of AD disease, or incipient AD-related genes, and these genes were analyzed with EASE to determine over- or under-represented categories. Using this approach, the authors report that early or incipient AD is characterized by transcriptional reprogramming and cell growth in the hippocampus, with an unexpected upregulation of tumor-suppressor genes, and also by a downregulation of bioenergetic pathways. Although these findings, possible only with a global analysis of gene expression, lead to a better understanding of the early etiology of AD, they also reflect the powerful utility of microarrays in gaining information on fundamental changes associated with any age-related or progressive disease, which in turn directs research efforts toward better-targeted therapeutics and interventions.

Lastly, a study illustrating the power of microarray profiling to generate testable hypotheses is reported by Lu and colleagues in a survey of human brain gene expression profiles from individuals ranging in age from 26 to 106 years (Lu et al., 2004). The authors analyzed RNA transcripts of post-mortem prefrontal cortex samples (N = 30) using high-density oligonucleotide arrays (~11,000 genes), and age-related genes were determined by Spearman rank correlation. Hierarchical clustering of these age-related genes and pairwise comparisons of all the samples

(by Pearson correlation) reveal clusters of relatively homogenous expression in individuals under 42 and over 73 years of age, with genes upregulated in young (<42) being downregulated in old (>73) and vice versa. The data also clearly reflect considerable heterogeneity of gene expression in the middle years. The greatest number of genes upregulated with age were stress-response and DNA repair genes, whereas downregulated genes included synaptic transmission and vesicular transport. This coordinated downregulation of a defined cluster of genes and subsequent induction of antioxidant and repair genes led the authors to hypothesize that the observed downregulation results from oxidative damage to the promoters of certain genes that are prone to such damage. To test this hypothesis, the authors developed a real-time PCR assay measuring DNA damage in specific DNA sequences based on the resistance of DNA cleaved at apurinic sites to amplification, thereby allowing quantitation of DNA damage from a ratio of PCR products in cleaved versus uncleaved DNA templates. The authors assayed the promoters of 30 selected genes in individual brain samples and demonstrated an age-dependent increase in damage to the promoters of downregulated genes such as mitochondrial ATP synthase alpha, calmodulin 1, sortilin, and calbindins 1 and 2. As proof of principal, the authors demonstrated that oxidative damage (via $FeCl_2$ and H_2O_2 treatment) reduced expression of the *tau* gene in cultured neuronal cells, and that this damage and subsequent reduction in mRNA expression was prevented by concomitant overexpression of a human base-repair excision enzyme. Furthermore, the genes downregulated with age in the human brain samples displayed an increased vulnerability to oxidative DNA damage in cultured cells when compared to genes which are stable or upregulated with age, as determined by quantification of promoter damage and luciferase reporter assays. Taken together, these data support the authors' model that DNA damage in the promoters of certain susceptible genes precipitate their downregulation with age, with the hypothesis formulated by clever interpretation by the authors of the global expression profiles generated with microarray technology.

2. Primate Literature—In Vitro

Cell culture systems offer several advantages in studies of the cellular physiology aging process, while also being subject to the well-known controversy as to the relatedness of *in vitro* to *in vivo* senescence. Although cellular senescence, which is highly correlated with telomere shortening, has not been directly linked to mammalian aging, it has been argued that cellular senescence may underlie the functional decrements present in aging tissues (Bird *et al.*, 2003). Gene expression in cellular senescence has primarily been addressed using cDNA arrays. The cell culture system has the great advantage that gene expression changes can be assayed on a relatively homogeneous cellular population. Therefore, it is notable that a high degree of heterogeneity has been identified in the senescence-associated gene expression patterns between cell types even assayed on the same array platform (Bortoli *et al.*, 2003; Shelton *et al.*, 1999). Differences between platforms further complicate the comparison of results across experimental systems. Additionally, there has been little statistical analysis and almost no validation of candidate genes with a quantitative independent technique to determine exact genes involved in senescence. However, despite these problems, some patterns are emerging. Genes associated with the extracellular matrix, cell–cell signaling are reported as categories of changed genes (Minagawa *et al.*, 2004; Shelton *et al.*, 1999), and these are remarkably close to

the gene expression changes observed in organismal aging. However, these associations have all been established without quantitative methods for identifying relative appearance of functional categories as compared to the gene expression platform used. As methods for categorizing genes and identifying over- or under-represented categories are refined, we will be able to determine whether these patterns hold true across heterogeneous cultured cell populations.

In addition to seeking candidate genes associated with cellular senescence that may be biomarkers of aging, chromosomal position of gene expression changes has also been investigated. It has been hypothesized that the genes associated with replicative senescence may localize to telomere-proximal regions. However, a lack of preferential expression or repression of telomere-proximal genes has been reported (Allen *et al.*, 2004; Chen *et al.*, 2004; Minagawa *et al.*, 2004). This result suggests that *in vitro* senescence is not due to dysregulation of gene expression genes caused by proximity to shortened telomeres.

IV. Conclusions, Future Directions, and Challenges

The technologies and tools to support the use of microarrays for global analysis of gene expression have perhaps matured from infancy, but clearly remain in rapid development. Especially in applications to yeast and invertebrate models, we have begun to see the promise of this approach for elucidating expression profiles associated with aging. More importantly, studies such as those of McCarroll and colleagues (2004) have demonstrated that inter-species comparisons of gene expression can discover common ("public") transcriptional changes in aging, if only at the level of functional classification. Similarly, inter-comparisons between different models of life-span extension, such as caloric restriction and the growth hormone/IGF-1 axis, are likely to elucidate the differences and commonalities between mechanisms of longevity in a more comprehensive fashion than might otherwise be possible. Gene expression profiles can define sets of genes that serve as biomarkers of aging and predictors of longevity, both of which are greatly needed for characterization of aging phenotypes. As published databases of expression results increase in number and quality, the power of meta-analyses increases, so that discovery of complex transcriptional relationships, or coexpression networks, becomes ever more feasible (Stuart et al., 2003). Discovery and quantitation of these networks will be very important to increase the sophistication and reduce the complexity of gene expression data analysis, as smaller numbers of networks can substitute for long lists of individual genes. Quantitation of transcriptional pathways also brings transcriptomics to an interface with metabolomics, improving the understanding of changes in the programming of cell function. The limitations of transcriptomics must always be kept in sight, particularly that messenger expression may not reflect protein level and post-translational modification of proteins. For a more complete understanding, proteomics must be studied. Ultimately, using a full suite of tools for global analysis of "systems biology," we can look forward to a deeper and more integrated understanding of the molecular biology of aging.

References

Allen, G. C., West, J. R., Chen, W. J., & Earnest, D. J. (2004). Developmental alcohol exposure disrupts circadian regulation of BDNF in the rat suprachiasmatic nucleus. *Neurotoxicology Teratology*, 26, 353–358.

Arking, R. (1998). *The biology of aging* (p. 436). Sunderland, MA: Sinauer.

Ashrafi, K., Lin, S. S., Manchester, J. K., & Gordon, J. I. (2000). Sip2p and its partner snf1p kinase affect aging in *S. cerevisiae*. *Genes & Development*, 14, 1872–1885.

Barr, M. M. (2003). Super models. *Physiological Genomics*, 13, 15–24.

Bird, J., Ostler, E. L., & Faragher, R. G. (2003). Can we say that senescent cells cause ageing? *Experimental Gerontology*, 38, 1319–1326.

Bitterman, K. J., Medvedik, O., & Sinclair, D. A. (2003). Longevity regulation in *Saccharomyces cerevisiae*: linking metabolism, genome stability, and heterochromatin. *Microbiology and Molecular Biology Reviews*, 67, 376–399.

Blalock, E. M., Chen, K. C., Sharrow, K., Herman, J. P., Porter, N. M., Foster, T. C., & Landfield, P. W. (2003). Gene microarrays in hippocampal aging: statistical profiling identifies novel processes correlated with cognitive impairment. *Journal of Neuroscience*, 23, 3807–3819.

Blalock, E. M., Geddes, J. W., Chen, K. C., Porter, N. M., Markesbery, W. R., & Landfield, P. W. (2004). Incipient Alzheimer's disease: microarray correlation analyses reveal major transcriptional and tumor suppressor responses. *Proceedings of the National Academy of Sciences of the USA*, 101, 2173–2178.

Bortoli, S., Renault, V., Eveno, E., Auffray, C., Butler-Browne, G., & Pietu, G. (2003). Gene expression profiling of human satellite cells during muscular aging using cDNA arrays. *Gene*, 321, 145–154.

Brewer, G. (2002). Messenger RNA decay during aging and development. *Aging Research Reviews*, 1, 607–625.

Bronikowski, A. M., Carter, P. A., Morgan, T. J., Garland, T., Jr., Ung, N., Pugh, T. D., Weindruch, R., & Prolla, T. A. (2003). Lifelong voluntary exercise in the mouse prevents age-related alterations in gene expression in the heart. *Physiological Genomics*, 12, 129–138.

Cao, S. X., Dhahbi, J. M., Mote, P. L., & Spindler, S. R. (2001). Genomic profiling of short- and long-term caloric restriction effects in the liver of aging mice. *Proceedings of the National Academy of Sciences of the USA*, 98, 10630–10635.

Cawthon, R. M., Smith, K. R., O'Brien, E., Sivatchenko, A., & Kerber, R. A. (2003). Association between telomere length in blood and mortality in people aged 60 years or older. *Lancet*, 361, 393–395.

Chen, H.-L., Lu, C.-Y., Hsu, Y.-H., & Lin, J.-J. (2004). Chromosome positional effects of gene expressions after cellular senescence. *Biochemical and Biophysical Research Communications*, 313(3), 576–586.

Chipman, H., Hastie, T. J., & Tibshirani, R. (2003). Clustering microarray data. In T. Speed (Ed.), *Statistical analysis of gene expression microarray data*, pp. 159–200. Boca Raton, FL: Chapman & Hall/CRC.

Chu, S., DeRisi, J., Eisen, M., Mulholland, J., Botstein, D., Brown, P. O., & Herskowitz, I. (1998). The transcriptional program of sporulation in budding yeast. *Science*, 282, 699–705.

Churchill, G. A. (2002). Fundamentals of experimental design for cDNA microarrays. *Nature Genetics*, 32, 490–495.

Csiszar, A., Ungvari, Z., Koller, A., Edwards, J. G., & Kaley, G. (2003). Aging-induced proinflammatory shift in cytokine expression profile in coronary arteries. *FASEB Journal*, 17, 1183–1185.

Cui, X., & Churchill, G. A. (2003). How many mice and how many arrays? Replication in mouse cDNA microarray experiments. In K. F. Johnson, & S. M. Lin (Eds.), *Methods of Microarray Data Analysis III*, pp. 139–154. Kluwer Academic Publishers: Norwell, MA.

Dahlquist, K. D., Salomonis, N., Vranizan, K., Lawlor, S. C., & Conklin, B. R. (2002). GenMAPP, a new tool for viewing and analyzing microarray data on biological pathways. *Nature Genetics*, 31, 19–20.

DeRisi, J. L., Iyer, V. R., & Brown, P. O. (1997). Exploring the metabolic and genetic control of gene expression on a genomic scale. *Science*, 278, 680–686.

Dhahbi, J. M., Kim, H. J., Mote, P. L., Beaver, R. J., & Spindler, S. R. (2004). Temporal linkage between the phenotypic and genomic responses to caloric restriction. *Proceedings of the National Academy of Sciences of the USA*, 101, 5524–5529.

Do, K., Broom, B., & Wen, S. (2003). GeneClust. In G. Parmigiani, E. S. Garrett, R. A. Irizarry, & S. L. Zeger (Eds.), *The analysis of gene expression data: methods and software*, pp. 342–361. New York: Springer.

Dozmorov, I., Bartke, A., & Miller, R. A. (2001). Array-based expression analysis of mouse liver genes: effect of age and of the longevity mutant Prop1df. *Journals of Gerontology. Series A, Biological Sciences and Medical Sciences*, 56, B72–B80.

Dozmorov, I., Galecki, A., Chang, Y., Krzesicki, R., Vergara, M., & Miller, R. A. (2002). Gene expression profile of long-lived snell dwarf mice. *Journals of Gerontology. Series A, Biological Sciences and Medical Sciences*, 57, B99–B108.

Dudoit, S., & Fridlyand, J. (2003a). Bagging to improve the accuracy of a clustering procedure. *Bioinformatics*, 19, 1090–1099.

Dudoit, S., & Fridlyand, J. (2003b). Classification in microarray experiments. In T. Speed (Ed.), *Statistical analysis of gene expression microarray data*, pp. 93–158. Boca Raton, FL: Chapman & Hall/CRC.

Dudoit, S., Gentleman, R., Irizarry, R. A., & Yang, Y. H. (2002). Pre-processing DNA Microarray Data Bioconductor Short Course Winter 2002. Available at http://www.bioconductor.org/workshops/Wyeth Course101702/PreProc/PreProc4.pdf.

Edwards, M. G., Sarkar, D., Klopp, R., Morrow, J. D., Weindruch, R., & Prolla, T. A. (2003). Age-related impairment of the transcriptional responses to oxidative stress in the mouse heart. *Physiological Genomics*, 13, 119–127.

Edwards, M. G., Sarkar, D., Klopp, R., Morrow, J. D., Weindruch, R., & Prolla, T. A. (2004). Impairment of the transcriptional responses to oxidative stress in the heart of aged C57BL/6 mice. *Annals of the New York Academy of Sciences*, 1019, 85–95.

Efron, B., & Tibshirani, R. (2002). Empirical Bayes methods and false discovery rates for microarrays. *Genetic Epidemiology*, 23, 70–86.

Eisen, M. B., Spellman, P. T., Brown, P. O., & Botstein, D. (1998). Cluster analysis and display of genome-wide expression patterns. *Proceedings of the National Academy of Sciences of the USA*, 95, 14863–14868.

Ekstrom, R., Liu, D. S., & Richardson, A. (1980). Changes in brain protein synthesis during the life span of male Fischer rats. *Gerontology*, 26, 121–128.

Fabrizio, P., & Longo, V. D. (2003). The chronological life span of *Saccharomyces cerevisiae*. *Aging Cell*, 2, 73–81.

Feldman, A. L., Costouros, N. G., Wang, E., Qian, M., Marincola, F. M., Alexander, H. R., & Libutti, S. K. (2002). Advantages of mRNA amplification for microarray analysis. *Biotechniques*, 33, 906–912, 914.

Golden, T. R., & Melov, S. (2004). Microarray analysis of gene expression with age in individual nematodes. *Aging Cell*, 3, 111–124.

Gomes, L. I., Silva, R. L., Stolf, B. S., Cristo, E. B., Hirata, R., Soares, F. A., Reis, L. F., Neves, E. J., & Carvalho, A. F. (2003). Comparative analysis of amplified and nonamplified RNA for hybridization in cDNA microarray. *Analytical Biochemistry*, 321, 244–251.

Hahn, J. S., Hu, Z., Thiele, D. J., & Iyer, V. R. (2004). Genome-wide analysis of the biology of stress responses through heat shock transcription factor. *Molecular and Cellular Biology*, 24, 5249–5256.

Han, E. S., Wu, Y., McCarter, R., Nelson, J. F., Richardson, A., & Hilsenbeck, S. G. (2004). Reproducibility, sources of variability, pooling, and sample size: important considerations for the design of high-density oligonucleotide array experiments. *Journals of Gerontology. Series A, Biological Sciences and Medical Sciences*, 59, 306–315.

Harper, J. M., Galecki, A. T., Burke, D. T., & Miller, R. A. (2004). Body weight, hormones and T cell subsets as predictors of life span in genetically heterogeneous mice. *Mechanisms of Ageing and Development*, 125, 381–390.

Helmberg, A. (2001). DNA-microarrays: novel techniques to study aging and guide gerontologic medicine. *Experimental Gerontology*, 36, 1189–1198.

Helmstetter, C. E. (1991). Description of a baby machine for *Saccharomyces cerevisiae*. *New Biologist*, 3, 1089–1096.

Higami, Y., Pugh, T. D., Page, G. P., Allison, D. B., Prolla, T. A., & Weindruch, R. (2004). Adipose tissue energy metabolism: altered gene expression profile of mice subjected to long-term caloric restriction. *FASEB Journal*, 18, 415–417.

Hiratsuka, K., Kamino, Y., Nagata, T., Takahashi, Y., Asai, S., Ishikawa, K., & Abiko, Y. (2002). Microarray analysis of gene expression changes in aging in mouse submandibular gland. *Journal of Dental Research*, 81, 679–682.

Holloway, A. J., van Laar, R. K., Tothill, R. W., & Bowtell, D. D. L. (2002). Options available— from start to finish—for obtaining data from DNA microarrays. *Nature Genetics*, 32, 481–489.

Horak, C. E., & Snyder, M. (2002). Global analysis of gene expression in yeast. *Functional & Integrative Genomics*, 2, 171–180.

Hsu, A. L., Murphy, C. T., & Kenyon, C. (2003). Regulation of aging and age-related disease by DAF-16 and heat-shock factor. *Science*, 300, 1142–1145.

Huber, W. (2004). Courses in Practical DNA Microarray Analysis 2004, Error Models and Normalization: The Bioconductor Project. Available at http://www.bioconductor.org/workshops/Bressanone/Monday/L2/L2.pdf.

Hughes, T. R., Roberts, C. J., Dai, H. Y., Jones, A. R., Meyer, M. R., Slade, D., Burchard, J., Dow, S., Ward, T. R., Kidd, M. J., Friend, S. H., & Marton, M. J. (2000). Widespread aneuploidy revealed by DNA microarray expression profiling. *Nature Genetics*, 25, 333–337.

Irizarry, R. A., Bolstad, B. M., Collin, F., Cope, L. M., Hobbs, B., & Speed, T. P. (2003a). Summaries of Affymetrix GeneChip probe level data. *Nucleic Acids Research*, 31, E15.

Irizarry, R. A., Hobbs, B., Collin, F., Beazer-Barclay, Y. D., Antonellis, K. J., Scherf, U., & Speed, T. P. (2003b). Exploration, normalization, and summaries of high density oligonucleotide array probe level data. *Biostatistics*, 4, 249–264.

Jazwinski, S. M. (1993). The genetics of aging in the yeast *Saccharomyces cerevisiae*. *Genetica*, 91, 35–51.

Jin, W., Riley, R. M., Wolfinger, R. D., White, K. P., Passador-Gurgel, G., & Gibson, G. (2001). The contributions of sex, genotype and age to transcriptional variance in *Drosophila melanogaster*. *Nature Genetics*, 29, 389–395.

Kaeberlein, M., & Guarente, L. (2002). *Saccharomyces cerevisiae* MPT5 and SSD1 function in parallel pathways to promote cell wall integrity. *Genetics*, 160, 83–95.

Kaeberlein, M., Kirkland, K. T., Fields, S., & Kennedy, B. K. (2004). Sir2-independent life span extension by calorie restriction in yeast. *Public Library of Science Biology*, 9, E296.

Kaeberlein, M., McVey, M., & Guarente, L. (2001). Using yeast to discover the fountain of youth. *Science of Aging Knowledge Environment* [SAGE KE] 2001[1], e1.

Kang, H. L., Benzer, S., & Min, K. T. (2002). Life extension in *Drosophila* by feeding a drug. *Proceedings of the National Academy of Sciences of the USA*, 99, 838–843.

Kayo, T., Allison, D. B., Weindruch, R., & Prolla, T. A. (2001). Influences of aging and caloric restriction on the transcriptional profile of skeletal muscle from rhesus monkeys. *Proceedings of the National Academy of Sciences of the USA*, 98, 5093–5098.

Kendziorski, C. M., Irizarry, R. A., Chen, K, Haag, J. D., & Gould, M. N. (2004). To pool or not to pool: a question of microarray experimental design. Johns Hopkins University, Dept. of Biostatistics Working Papers [46]: BE Press. Available at http://www.bepress.com/jhubiostat/paper46.

Kerr, M. K. (2003). Design considerations for efficient and effective microarray studies. *Biometrics*, 59, 822–828.

Kerr, M. K., & Churchill, G. A. (2001a). Statistical design and the analysis of gene expression microarray data. *Genetical Research*, 77, 123–128.

Kerr, M. K., & Churchill, G. A. (2001b). Bootstrapping cluster analysis: assessing the reliability of conclusions from microarray experiments. *Proceedings of the National Academy of Sciences of the USA*, 98, 8961–8965.

Kerr, M. K., Martin, M., & Churchill, G. A. (2000). Analysis of variance for gene expression microarray data. *Journal of Computational Biology*, 7, 819–837.

Kirschner, M., Pujol, G., & Radu, A. (2002). Oligonucleotide microarray data mining: search for age-dependent gene expression. *Biochemical and Biophysical Research Communications*, 298, 772–778.

Landis, G. N., Abdueva, D., Skvortsov, D., Yang, J., Rabin, B. E., Carrick, J., Tavare, S., & Tower, J. (2004). Similar gene expression patterns characterize aging and oxidative stress in *Drosophila melanogaster*.

Proceedings of the National Academy of Sciences of the USA, 101, 7663–7668.

Lashkari, D. A., DeRisi, J. L., McCusker, J. H., Namath, A. F., Gentile, C., Hwang, S. Y., Brown, P. O., & Davis, R. W. (1997). Yeast microarrays for genome wide parallel genetic and gene expression analysis. *Proceedings of the National Academy of Sciences of the USA*, 94, 13057–62.

Lee, C. K., Allison, D. B., Brand, J., Weindruch, R., & Prolla, T. A. (2002). Transcriptional profiles associated with aging and middle age-onset caloric restriction in mouse hearts. *Proceedings of the National Academy of Sciences of the USA*, 99, 14988–14993.

Lee, C. K., Klopp, R. G., Weindruch, R., & Prolla, T. A. (1999). Gene expression profile of aging and its retardation by caloric restriction. *Science*, 285, 1390–1393.

Lee, C. K., Pugh, T. D., Klopp, R. G., Edwards, J., Allison, D. B., Weindruch, R., & Prolla, T. A. (2004). The impact of alpha-lipoic acid, coenzyme Q10 and caloric restriction on life span and gene expression patterns in mice. *Free Radical Biology & Medicine*, 36, 1043–1057.

Lee, C. K., Weindruch, R., & Prolla, T. A. (2000a). Gene-expression profile of the ageing brain in mice. *Nature Genetics*, 25, 294–297.

Lee, H. M., Greeley, G. H. Jr., & Englander, E. W. (2001). Age-associated changes in gene expression patterns in the duodenum and colon of rats. *Mechanisms of Ageing and Development*, 122, 355–371.

Lee, M. L. T., Kuo, F. C., Whitmore, G. A., & Sklar, J. (2000b). Importance of replication in microarray gene expression studies: Statistical methods and evidence from repetitive cDNA hybridizations. *Proceedings of the National Academy of Sciences of the USA*, 97, 9834–9839.

Lee, M. L. T., & Whitmore, G. A. (2002). Power and sample size for DNA microarray studies. *Statistics in Medicine*, 21, 3543–3570.

Lesur, I., & Campbell, J. L. (2004). The transcriptome of prematurely aging yeast cells is similar to that of telomerase-deficient cells. *Molecular Biology of the Cell*, 15, 1297–1312.

Li, C., Tseng, G. C., & Wong, W. H. (2003). Model-based analysis of oligonucleotide arrays and issues in cDNA microarray analysis. In T. Speed (Ed.), *Statistical analysis of gene expression microarray data*, pp. 1–34. Boca Raton, FL: Chapman & Hall/CRC.

Lin, S. J., Kaeberlein, M., Andalis, A. A., Sturtz, L. A., Defossez, P. A., Culotta, V. C., Fink, G., & Guarente, L. (2002). Calorie restriction extends *Saccharomyces cerevisiae* life span by increasing respiration. *Nature*, 418, 344–348.

Lin, S. S., Manchester, J. K., & Gordon, J. I. (2001). Enhanced gluconeogenesis and increased energy storage as hallmarks of aging in *Saccharomyces cerevisiae*. *Journal of Biological Chemistry*, 276, 36000–36007.

Lipman, R. D., Smith D. E., Bronson, R. T., & Blumberg, J. B. (1995). Is late-life caloric restriction beneficial? *Aging: Clinical and Experimental Research*, 7, 136–139.

Lipman, R. D., Smith D. E., Blumberg, J. B., & Bronson, R. T. (1998). Effects of caloric restriction or augmentation in adult rats: longevity and lesion biomarkers of aging. *Aging: Clinical and Experimental Research*, 10, 463–470.

Lu, T., Pan, Y., Kao, S. Y., Li, C., Kohane, I., Chan, J., & Yankner, B. A. (2004). Gene regulation and DNA damage in the ageing human brain. *Nature*, 429, 883–891.

MacLean, M., Harris, N., & Piper, P. W. (2001). Chronological lifespan of stationary phase yeast cells: a model for investigating the factors that might influence the ageing of postmitotic tissues in higher organisms. *Yeast*, 18, 499–509.

McCarroll, S. A., Murphy, C. T., Zou, S. G., Pletcher, S. D., Chin, C. S., Jan, Y. N., Kenyon, C., Bargmann, C. I., & Li, H. (2004). Comparing genomic expression patterns across species identifies shared transcriptional profile in aging. *Nature Genetics*, 36, 197–204.

McElwee, J., Bubb, K., & Thomas, J. H. (2003). Transcriptional outputs of the *Caenorhabditis elegans* forkhead protein DAF-16. *Aging Cell*, 2, 111–121.

Meydani, M., Lipman, R. D., Han, S. N., Wu, D., Beharka, A., Martin, K. R., Bronson, R., Cao, G., Smith, D., & Meydani, S. N. (1998). The effect of long-term dietary supplementation with antioxidants. *Annals of the New York Academy of Sciences*, 854, 352–360.

Miller, R. A., Chang, Y., Galecki, A. T., Al Regaiey, K., Kopchick, J. J., & Bartke, A. (2002). Gene expression patterns in calorically restricted mice: partial overlap with long-lived mutant mice. *Molecular Endocrinology (Baltimore, Md.)*, 16, 2657–2666.

Minagawa, S., Nakabayashi, K., Fujii, M., Scherer, S. W., & Ayusawa, D. (2004). Functional and chromosomal clustering of genes responsive to 5-bromodeoxyuridine in human cells. *Experimental Gerontology*, 39, 1069–1078.

Moreau, Y., Aerts, S., De Moor, B., De Strooper, B., & Dabrowski, M. (2003). Comparison and meta-analysis of microarray data: from the bench to the computer desk. *Trends in Genetics*, 19, 570–577.

Morley, J. F., & Morimoto, R. I. (2004). Regulation of longevity in *Caenorhabditis elegans* by heat shock factor and molecular chaperones. *Molecular Biology of the Cell*, 15, 657–664.

Mortimer, R. K., & Johnston, J. R. (1959). Life span of individual yeast cells. *Nature*, 183, 1751–1752.

Murphy, C. T., McCarroll, S. A., Bargmann, C. I., Fraser, A., Kamath, R. S., Ahringer, J., Li, H., & Kenyon, C. (2003). Genes that act downstream of DAF-16 to influence the lifespan of *Caenorhabditis elegans*. *Nature*, 424, 277–283.

Park, P. U., McVey, M., & Guarente, L. (2002). Separation of mother and daughter cells. *Methods in Enzymology*, 351, 468–477.

Parmigiani, G., Garrett, E. S., Irizarry, R. A., & Zeger, S. L. (2003). The analysis of gene expression data: an overview of methods and software. In G. Parmigiani, E. S. Garrett, R. A. Irizarry, & S. L. Zeger (Eds.), *The analysis of gene expression data: methods and software*, pp. 1–45. New York: Springer.

Perls, T., Shea-Drinkwater, M., Bowen-Flynn, J., Ridge, S. B., Kang, S., Joyce, E., Daly, M., Brewster, S. J., Kunkel, L., & Puca, A. A. (2000). Exceptional familial clustering for extreme longevity in humans. *Journal of the American Geriatrics Society*, 48, 1483–1485.

Perls, T. T., Wilmoth, J., Levenson, R., Drinkwater, M., Cohen, M., Bogan, H., Joyce, E., Brewster, S., Kunkel, L., & Puca, A. (2002). Life-long sustained mortality advantage of siblings of centenarians. *Proceedings of the National Academy of Sciences of the USA*, 99, 8442–8447.

Phelan, J. P., & Austad, S. N. (1994). Selecting animal models of human aging: inbred strains often exhibit less biological uniformity than F1 hybrids. *Journal of Gerontology*, 49, B1–B11.

Pinheiro, J. C., & Bates, D. M. (2000). *Mixed-effects models in S and S-PLUS*. New York: Springer.

Pletcher, S. D., Macdonald, S. J., Marguerie, R., Certa, U., Stearns, S. C., Goldstein, D. B., & Partridge, L. (2002). Genome-wide transcript profiles in aging and calorically restricted *Drosophila melanogaster*. *Current Biology*, 12, 712–723.

Preisser, L., Houot, L., Teillet, L., Kortulewski, T., Morel, A., Tronik-Le Roux, D., & Corman, B. (2004). Gene expression in aging kidney and pituitary. *Biogerontology*, 5, 39–47.

Prolla, T. A. (2002). DNA microarray analysis of the aging brain. *Chemical Senses*, 27, 299–306.

Prolla, T. A., & Mattson, M. P. (2001). Molecular mechanisms of brain aging and neurodegenerative disorders: lessons from dietary restriction. *Trends in Neurosciences*, 24, S21–S31.

Qin, L. X., & Kerr, K. F. (2004). Contributing Members of the Toxicogenomics Research Consortium. Empirical evaluation of data transformations and ranking statistics for microarray analysis. *Nucleic Acids Research*, 32(18), 5471–9

Roth, G. S., Lane, M. A., Ingram, D. K., Mattison, J. A., Elahi, D., Tobin, J. D., Muller, D., & Metter, E. J. (2002). Biomarkers of caloric restriction may predict longevity in humans. *Science*, 297, 811.

Saal, L. H., Troein, C., Vallon-Christersson, J., Gruvberger, S., Borg, A., & Peterson, C. (2002). BioArray Software Environment (BASE): a platform for comprehensive management and analysis of microarray data. *Genome Biology*, 3, SOFTWARE0003.

Sebastiani, P., Ramoni, M., & Kohane, I. S. (2003). Bayesian clustering of gene expression dynamics. In G. Parmigiani, E. S. Garrett, R. A. Irizarry, & S. L. Zeger (Eds.), *The analysis of gene expression data: methods and software*, pp. 409–427. New York: Springer.

Shah, G., Azizian, M., Bruch, D., Mehta, R., & Kittur, D. (2004). Cross-species comparison of gene expression between human and porcine tissue, using single microarray platform—preliminary results. *Clinical Transplantation*, 18 Suppl 12, 76–80.

Shalon, D., Smith, S. J., & Brown, P. O. (1996). A DNA microarray system for analyzing complex DNA samples using two-color fluorescent probe hybridization. *Genome Research*, 6, 639–45.

Shannon, P., Markiel, A., Ozier, O., Baliga, N. S., Wang, J. T., Ramage, D., Amin, N., Schwikowski, B., & Ideker, T. (2003). Cytoscape: a software environment for integrated models of biomolecular interaction networks. *Genome Research*, 13, 2498–2504.

Shelton, D. N., Chang, E., Whittier, P. S., Choi, D., & Funk, W. D. (1999). Microarray analysis of replicative senescence. *Current Biology*, 9, 939–945.

Slonim, D. K. (2002). From patterns to pathways: gene expression data analysis comes of age. *Nature Genetics*, 32 Suppl, 502–508.

Smeal, T., Claus, J., Kennedy, B., Cole, F., & Guarente, L. (1996). Loss of transcriptional silencing causes sterility in old mother cells of *S. cerevisiae*. *Cell*, 84, 633–642.

Smyth, G. K. (2004). Linear models and empirical Bayes methods for assessing differential expression in microarray experiments. *Statistical Applications in Genetics and Molecular Biology*, 3(3), 1.

Spellman, P. T., Sherlock, G., Zhang, M. Q., Iyer, V. R., Anders, K., Eisen, M. B., Brown, P. O., Botstein, D., & Futcher, B. (1998). Comprehensive identification of cell cycle-regulated genes of the yeast *Saccharomyces cerevisiae* by microarray hybridization. *Molecular Biology of the Cell*, 9, 3273–3297.

Storey, J. D., & Tibshirani, R. (2003a). Statistical significance for genomewide studies. *Proceedings of the National Academy of Sciences of the USA*, 100, 9440–9445.

Storey, J. D., & Tibshirani, R. (2003b). SAM thresholding and false discovery rates for detecting differential gene expression in DNA microarrays. In G. Parmigiani, E. S. Garrett, R. A. Irizarry, & S. L. Zeger (Eds.), *The analysis of gene expression data: methods and software*, pp. 272–290. New York: Springer.

Stuart, J. M., Segal, E., Koller, D., & Kim, S. K. (2003). A gene-coexpression network for global discovery of conserved genetic modules. *Science*, 302, 249–255.

Tollet-Egnell, P., Parini, P., Stahlberg, N., Lonnstedt, I., Lee, N. H., Rudling, M., Flores-Morales, A., & Norstedt, G. (2004). Growth hormone-mediated alteration of fuel metabolism in the aged rat as determined from transcript profiles. *Physiological Genomics*, 16, 261–267.

Tsuchiya, T., Dhahbi, J. M., Cui, X., Mote, P. L., Bartke, A., & Spindler, S. R. (2004). Additive regulation of hepatic gene expression by dwarfism and caloric restriction. *Physiological Genomics*, 17, 307–315.

Van Gelder, R. N., von Zastrow, M. E., Yool, A., Dement, W. C., Barchas, J. D., & Eberwine, J. H. (1990). Amplified RNA synthesized from limited quantities of heterogeneous cDNA. *Proceedings of the National Academy of Sciences of the USA*, 87, 1663–1667.

Warner, H. R., & Sierra, F. (2003). Models of accelerated ageing can be informative about the molecular mechanisms of ageing and/or age-related pathology. *Mechanisms of Ageing and Development*, 124, 581–587.

Warner, H. R., von Heydebreck, A., Sultmann, H., Poustka, A., & Vingron, M. (2002). Variance stabilization applied to microarray data calibration and to quantification of differential expression. *Bioinformatics*, 18, S96–S104.

Weindruch, R., Kayo, T., Lee, C. K., & Prolla, T. A. (2001). Microarray profiling of gene expression in aging and its alteration by caloric restriction in mice. *Journal of Nutrition*, 131, 918S–923S.

Weindruch, R., Kayo, T., Lee, C. K., & Prolla, T. A. (2002). Gene expression profiling of aging using DNA microarrays. *Mechanisms of Ageing and Development*, 123, 177–193.

Weindruch, R., & Prolla, T. A. (2002). Gene expression profile of the aging brain. *Archives of Neurology*, 59, 1712–1714.

Weindruch, R. H., & Walford, R. L. (1988). *The retardation of aging and disease by dietary restriction*. Springfield, IL: Thomas.

Welle, S., Brooks, A., & Thornton, C. A. (2001). Senescence-related changes in gene expression in muscle: similarities and differences between mice and men. *Physiological Genomics*, 5, 67–73.

Wilson, C. L., Pepper, S. D., Hey, Y., & Miller, C. J. (2004). Amplification protocols introduce systematic but reproducible errors into gene expression studies. *Biotechniques*, 36, 498–506.

Woldringh, C. L., Fluiter, K., & Huls, P. G. (1995). Production of senescent cells of *Saccharomyces cerevisiae* by centrifugal elutriation. *Yeast*, 11, 361–369.

Wu, Z., & Irizarry, R. A. (2004). Preprocessing of oligonucleotide array data. *Nature Biotechnology*, 22, 656–658.

Wu, Z., Irizarry, R. A., Gentleman, R., Martinez Murillo, F., & Spencer, F. A. (2003). Model based background adjustment for oligonucleotide expression arrays.

Yang, Y. H., & Speed, T. (2002). Design issues for cDNA microarray experiments. *Nature Reviews Genetics*, 3, 579–588.

Yeung, K. Y., Medvedovic, M., & Bumgarner, R. E. (2003). Clustering gene-expression data with repeated measurements. *Genome Biology*, 4(5), R34.

Yoshida, S., Yashar, B. M., Hiriyanna, S., & Swaroop, A. (2002). Microarray analysis of gene expression in the aging human retina. *Investigative Ophthalmology & Visual Science*, 43, 2554–2560.

Zeeberg, B. R., Feng, W. M., Wang, G., Wang, M. D., Fojo, A. T., Sunshine, M., Narasimhan, S., Kane, D. W., Reinhold, W. C., Lababidi, S., Bussey, K. J., Riss, J., Barrett, J. C., & Weinstein, J. N. (2003). GoMiner: a resource for biological interpretation of genomic and proteomic data. *Genome Biology*, 4(4), R28.

Zou, S., Meadows, S., Sharp, L., Jan, L. Y., & Jan, Y. N. (2000). Genome-wide study of aging and oxidative stress response in *Drosophila melanogaster*. *Proceedings of the National Academy of Sciences of the USA*, 97, 13726–13731.

Chapter 12

Computer Modeling in the Study of Aging

Thomas B. L. Kirkwood, Richard J. Boys, Colin S. Gillespie, Carole J. Procter,
Daryl P. Shanley, and Darren J. Wilkenson

I. Introduction

A. The Why, What, and How of Biological Modeling

Three intersecting processes are making the application of mathematical and computer modeling increasingly important in the biological sciences. First, biology itself has become much more of an informational science, as a result primarily of the development of genomic (based on advances in gene sequence and expression data) and post-genomic (based on advances in proteomic and functional data) sciences. Our capacity to answer questions ranging from cell and molecular function through to evolutionary genetics requires an increasing ability to acquire, store, and manipulate large volumes of raw data. This requirement has called upon biologists to develop the necessary computational skills and understanding.

Second, there is a realization that complex biological processes cannot be understood through the application of ever-more reductionist experimental programs alone. There needs to be some integration of the mass of data and insight from study of the detailed mechanisms at the level of the physiological "system."

Third, the sophistication and power of desktop computer hardware has increased to a point where the kind of model that two decades ago might have required an overnight run on a large mainframe computer can now be done in the individual scientist's lab or office with a response time that makes possible a much more interactive way of working.

Alongside these changes is the development of a different perception of the role and value of computer modeling in biomedical research. To many scientists who have trained and worked in environments where modeling has not been a part of the scientific toolkit, the nature and scope of computer modeling is still unclear. Many see models as essentially descriptive, begging the question "Why bother?" when the real answer will be revealed in time by experiment. Others have been indoctrinated with the widespread—but largely false—idea that as soon as a model has more than two or three parameters, it can "explain" anything, resulting in a suspension of belief that models, particularly of complex systems, can be of any real use at all. Fortunately, the increasing dialog between modelers and experimentalists is beginning to break down these barriers of misunderstanding and giving rise to new interactions that are likely to change the way a great deal of science will be done in the coming decades. This new approach is commonly being described as *systems biology*. This chapter reviews how computer modeling is developing within the context of the biology of aging.

The distinctive advantages of modeling a biological process with the rigor that is needed to build a computer model are as follows:

1. Model building requires that verbal hypotheses be made specific and conceptually rigorous. Before a mathematical model can be formulated, the investigator must specify each element of the model and how it interacts with other elements.

2. Starting to build a computer model may help to highlight gaps in current knowledge. The process of specifying a mathematical model will highlight any important unknowns. Sometimes these can be represented as variables yet to be estimated or determined.

3. The process of model development might lead to the recognition of a gap that needs to be filled by further experimental investigation, which may be fundamental to understanding a complex system. Thus, modeling can be useful even if the gap means that a model cannot yet be completed.

4. Computer models yield quantitative as well as qualitative predictions. A hypothesis can be tested much more rigorously by a model that permits quantitative predictions to be made. In aging, where multiple mechanisms might be at work, it often happens that data are

broadly consistent with a hypothesized mechanism, but modeling can show that the magnitude of the effect is too small to explain aging on its own.

5. Modeling can result in improved experimental design, especially where the system embodies the potential for complex interactions. Complexity is very hard to deal with experimentally but is relatively straightforward in a computer model. Models are thus ideal for analyzing complex interactions prior to experimental tests. In extreme cases, modeling may actually reveal that because of interactions within complex systems, a proposed experiment would be inconclusive.

6. Modeling can provide a low-cost, rapid test bed for candidate interventions, thereby enabling a more predictive approach and effecting significant savings in time and money.

To the non-modeler, the science of biological modeling can easily appear to involve the application of the same set of skills to a very diverse range of problems, and in much the same kind of way. A facility with numbers, knowledge of computer programming, and some understanding of the biological system seem all that is required. In reality, the range of approaches and skills in computer modeling is broad, involving a significant diversity of skills and research subdisciplines. Later sections of this chapter examine the different kinds of computer modeling, how they are performed, and what they can achieve. If the integration between theoretical and experimental science is to take place as fast and as effectively as is needed, researchers from both communities will need to learn more about each other's methods of working. Curiously, there is more similarity between the methods of working of experimenters and modelers than is usually recognized. The experimenter has to (1) decide which factors to include and vary in the study in order to address the hypothesis most efficiently and directly; (2) spend a large amount of the total effort of the study on controls in order to reduce the possibility of artifact; (3) be careful in framing the conclusions from the study so as not to extrapolate beyond what the results support; and (4) be conscious of planning the study within a constrained budget of time, money, and human resources. So does the modeler. A number of texts expand on some of the issues raised here (e.g., Hilborn & Mangel, 1997).

In parts of this chapter, we describe the mathematical, statistical, and computational approaches that have been brought to bear on understanding the aging process. Because these approaches will be unfamiliar to some readers, we have explained the terms and basic concepts as clearly as possible. It is not feasible, however, to include all of the explanation that would be necessary to equip the reader new to these approaches with a complete knowledge base. We have therefore had to find a balance between explanation and concision. At all relevant points within the text, we give references to texts where the reader can find more detailed explanation.

B. How Computer Models Have Been Instrumental in Solving Biological Problems

In many biological domains, it is difficult to see how a clear understanding of key processes could be gained without mathematical modeling. This includes, for example, the study of population dynamics in ecology, disease transmission in epidemiology, and population genetics and life history theory in evolutionary biology. In other domains, single examples exemplify the insights that mathematical investigation can provide, such as in the study of cardiac fibrillation in physiology. Modeling is making an increasingly important contribution in the relatively new field of systems biology, which aims, in part, to bridge molecular biology and physiology by capitalizing on the large amount of postgenomic data currently being generated. Many biochemical networks involve nonlinear components, which means that relying on intuition is not reliable. In a recent essay, Lander (2004) provides an excellent example of how modeling has helped reveal the details of a molecular mechanism that was proving difficult to understand from a purely experimental approach: the role of the segmentation polarity genes in maintaining the segmentation pattern during *Drosophila* development (von Dassow *et al.*, 2000). Although details differ, a similar process is shared by all insects, and to a lesser degree in vertebrates.

Drosophila embryonic development can be described as a three-stage process. In the first stage, maternally expressed mRNA enters the *Drosophila* oocyte within the ovary, and following translation, a polarized protein gradient is established. In the second stage, gap and coordinate genes are expressed in response to the protein gradient, which in turn govern the periodic expression of pair-rule genes. The final stage involves the segment polarity genes. A repetitive pattern of *engrailed* (*en*) and *wingless* (*wg*) expression is established based on the pair-rule genes. The embryo then undergoes cellularization, and the pattern of *en* and *wg* expression is transferred to an intracellular context involving signals between morphologically distinct bands. The gap and pair-rule gene products fade, *en* and *wg* expression is maintained via a complex network of transcription factors and intracellular signals, and the segmented structure is retained during substantial morphological change.

Von Dassow and colleagues (2000) constructed a mathematical model based on current information about the segment polarity gene network to test whether it could maintain a stable segmented structure. The structure was represented as a series of connected cells, each cell populated with the focal mRNAs, proteins, and protein complexes. The known intracellular and intercellular relationship between interacting molecules was then represented as a series of differential equations, with simulation used to provide information on the temporal variation in concentration of all the molecules. Although a substantial body of information existed to construct the network, it was insufficient to fully quantify the model—50 parameters were unknown. The approach taken was to run simulations with many randomly chosen parameter sets, with each parameter bounded within realistic limits. Interestingly, no solution could be found that satisfactorily reproduced the observed stable segmented pattern.

Attention was then turned to the network structure, and it was realized that modifications were needed to capture the known biology, namely the asymmetry in signaling to neighboring cells anterior and posterior. With appropriate modifications in place, the differential equations were updated and the process of simulation with randomly chosen sets of parameters was repeated. The observed segmented structure was now reproduced with surprising ease. The important result was that it was the fine detail of the network structure that was key in determining the system behavior and not exact parameter values. Interestingly, this may reflect an evolutionary adaptation as minor variations, such as mutations in components of the network or environmental fluctuations affecting levels of signals, would not unduly affect the segment structure and subsequent development. The major message was that the segment polarity genes represent a "robust developmental module" that ensures the formation of an appropriate pattern even across distantly related insect species in which earlier stages of development differ.

II. Why Aging Particularly Needs Models

Recent years have seen rapid progress in the science of aging. A key factor in this progress has been the interaction between evolutionary (why?) and mechanistic (how?) lines of research, which gives shape to the likely genetic basis of aging and to the mechanisms that may be involved (Kirkwood & Austad, 2000). This has helped overcome a situation where the field was dominated by a plethora of rival theories, with little effective dialog between them. In particular, the disposable soma theory (Kirkwood, 1977; Kirkwood & Austad, 2000) suggests that aging is caused ultimately by evolved limitations in organisms' investments in somatic maintenance and repair rather than by active gene programming. This predicts that aging is due to the gradual accumulation of unrepaired random molecular faults, leading to an increasing fraction of damaged cells and eventually to functional impairment of older tissues and organs. Genetic effects on the rate of aging are, in this view, mediated primarily through genes that influence somatic maintenance and repair.

Although the idea of aging as a buildup of damage is straightforward in principle and supported by a growing range of data, it presents a number of distinctive challenges (Kirkwood et al., 2003). First, it predicts that there are multiple mechanisms that cause aging, instead of just one or a few. Second, it predicts that aging is inherently stochastic—that is, it is modulated to an important degree by chance. Extensive evidence points to an important contribution in aging that arises from chance variations, which are not explained by genetic or environmental factors (Finch &

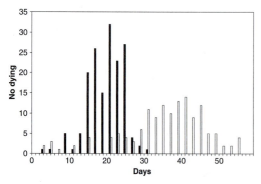

Figure 12.1 Life-span distributions for individual *Caenorhabditis elegans* nematodes in isogenic populations of wildtype (filled bars) and *age-1* (open bars) strains. Redrawn from Kirkwood and Finch (2002); original data from Johnson (1990).

Kirkwood, 2000). A particularly clear example of the role of chance in aging is the threefold range in life span (see Figure 12.1) and the apparently stochastic age-related cell degeneration of individual worms in isogenic populations of *Caenorhabditis elegans* reared under uniform laboratory conditions (Herndon *et al.*, 2002; Kirkwood & Finch, 2002). Third, since multiple mechanisms contribute to aging, a high level of complexity is to be expected. For all of these reasons, there is exceptional need in aging research for the use of computer models to help integrate findings from different lines of experimental work.

Although the multiplicity of aging mechanisms is now widely acknowledged, the reductionist nature of experimental techniques means that, in practice, most research is still narrowly focused on single mechanisms. This is where computer modeling can make a major contribution. By allowing for interaction and synergism between different processes, models reveal that the predicted effects on the system are often much greater than when mechanisms are considered one at a time. Furthermore, models can highlight important differences between the

upstream mechanisms that set a process in train and the end-stage mechanisms that dominate the cellular phenotype at the end of its life. For example, a gradual accumulation of mitochondrial (mt)DNA mutations, occurring over years, might lead to a steady increase in the production of reactive oxygen species (ROS) and a gradual decline in energy production (Kowald & Kirkwood, 1996). However, although the buildup of mtDNA mutations initiates the process, what ultimately destroys the cell is that eventually a threshold is reached where homeostatic mechanisms collapse. The end-stage of the cell's life span is dominated by dramatic biochemical changes, such as an accumulation of damaged protein. Experimental study of the latter effect, or even of the former cause, in the absence of a quantitative model to link the two would find it hard to establish the connection.

Another benefit of integrative model building is that it is well suited to take account of the fact that many of the key reactions involved in normal cell maintenance and metabolism do not act in isolation—rather, they belong to a network of activity. When the activity of one enzyme changes, all connected metabolite pools and enzyme activities may be altered. In some cases, there may be redundancy in pathways, which provides buffering against damage, whereas in other cases, the effect of damage may be propagated.

Another important area for modeling is to understand the actions of genes that affect the rate of aging. Over the past decade, scores of genes have been identified that affect aging in yeast, nematodes, fruit flies, and mice, and there is growing interest in genes affecting human longevity (Gems & Partridge, 2001; Jazwinski, 2000; Larsen, 2001; Lithgow, 1998; Tan *et al.*, 2004). Experimental data are beginning to reveal the interactions of these genes within pathways that control the aging rate, and there is evidence that several of the most important genes are those that affect basic cellular processes, such as insulin and insulin-like growth factor (IGF) signaling, which are strongly conserved across the species range (Gems & Partridge, 2001; Rincon *et al.*, 2004). Nevertheless, we are a long way from understanding the interactions between these effects. These studies need also to take account of the intrinsic stochastic nature of gene regulatory networks.

III. Different Approaches to Modeling Biological Systems

A. Descriptive Versus Predictive

A descriptive model describes a process or behavior that has already been observed. A predictive model predicts the behavior of a system not previously observed. A valid descriptive model is often easier to develop but it has less value than a model with predictive power. However, descriptive models are useful for highlighting gaps in our current knowledge. A model may start out as being descriptive but can then be used to predict outcomes when parts of the system are perturbed. For example, a descriptive model of a metabolic pathway of proteins under known conditions can be used to predict protein functions under different circumstances or in different species.

A predictive model provides quantifiable as well as qualitative predictions. The value of quantifiable predictions is that a hypothesis can be tested much more rigorously. In aging, where numerous mechanisms might be at work, data are often broadly consistent with a hypothesized mechanism, but modeling can show that the magnitude of the effect is too small to explain aging on its own. Another advantage of predictive models is that they can provide a low-cost, rapid test bed for candidate interventions.

B. Simple Versus Complex

Biological systems are complex and involve the interrelationships of many different "species," where species can refer to molecules, cells, tissues, or organisms. A model is a description of the system. The "art" in building a good model is to capture the essential details of the biology, without burdening the model with nonessential details. Every model is to some extent a simplification of the biology, but it is valuable in taking an idea that might have been expressed purely verbally and making it more explicit. Nevertheless, the question still remains: what level of complexity should be incorporated in the model?

At the most basic level, a model must be able to capture the desired inputs and outputs of a system. This is where a clear, prior specification of the problem to be addressed is as essential in modeling as it is in experimentation. For instance, if we wish to investigate how an increase of ATP will affect the production of ROS by mitochondria, then obviously these elements must be included into the model. Other elements, such as the dynamics of a cell cycle, are likely to be excluded. However, it is at this point that the modeler needs to exercise caution and to bear in mind the opportunities that are available to include further factors in the model than could easily be added to an experiment. The choice of which reactions should be left out of the model—since the activity of one enzyme may conceivably affect all connected metabolite pools—has no easy or universal answer. Some modelers prefer to start simple and add further detail as required; others prefer to recognize greater complexity from the outset. Either way, a modeler should always develop a model with as much direct biological input as possible.

Another key factor in the modelers' decision-making process is the time scale of processes involved. Molecular processes often need to be modeled on a time scale of seconds or less; outcomes affecting aging develop in months or years; evolutionary changes occur over generations. Models that seek to integrate across levels present particularly challenging problems that need to be addressed in defining the aims and scope of the project.

When modeling a process as complex as aging, an unfortunate side-effect is that very quickly, the mathematical representation can become exceedingly complex. Although the modeler may be comfortable with each and every detail of the model, the reader may be presented with an indecipherable collection of symbols. Conversely, an oversimplification of the systems may lead to the justified claim that the model does not represent the structure under consideration. Thankfully, part of this problem is being overcome with the introduction of standard methods for describing models used throughout the biological community, such as the Systems Biology Markup Language (SBML, described in more detail later). When a standard has been decided, this enables generic tools to be developed that aid the understanding of models. For instance, an SBML-aware visualization tool should accept any SBML-encoded model and return a graphical representation of it.

A barrier that limits the amount of complexity that can be included in a model is computational power. Put simply, do we have a computer powerful enough to calculate a solution to our model? It is relatively easy to construct a simple model that when simulated could take weeks to finish. With the yearly increase in processor power, models that would have taken weeks of computational time 5 years ago can now be solved in a matter of minutes. Other exciting avenues include the emergence of the GRID—the new generation of hardware/ software computer networking that is designed to facilitate the sharing of data and compute resources over a network. A benefit of the GRID is the harnessing of idle computer power. For instance, whereas a model may take weeks on a single 500-MHz processor, if 50 machines, say in a university computer laboratory, which are idle for 12 hours per day were set to the task, a properly formulated model could take hours.

C. Discrete Versus Continuous

When modeling biological processes, it is often helpful to treat time as a discrete quantity divided into a number of intervals. For instance, when dealing with the cell cycle of the budding yeast *Saccharomyces cerevisiae*, it may natural to deal in terms of generations (Gillespie *et al.*, 2004; Sinclair, 2002).

Although some types of system naturally lend themselves to discrete-time modeling, it is important to consider any distortion that may be introduced. In the yeast cell cycle example, a mother cell produces on average 24 daughter cells; however, the time taken to form a daughter cell gradually increases. So if the events being modeled were directly affected by the interbudding interval, the model may be of limited validity if only discrete generations were considered.

D. Deterministic Versus Stochastic

A model can be generally classed as deterministic or stochastic. A deterministic model is one that takes no account of random variation and therefore gives a fixed and precisely reproducible result. It can be solved by numerical analysis or computer simulation. Deterministic models are often mathematically described by sets of differential equations. Deterministic models are appropriate when large numbers of individuals of a species are involved and the importance of statistical variations in the average behavior of the system is relatively unimportant. However for many biological systems, this assumption may not be valid.

To illustrate the concepts, let us consider perhaps the simplest of molecular reactions, spontaneous degradation. The ordinary differentiation equation for the degradation of a species X at rate k_1 is given by

$$\frac{dx}{dt} = -k_1 X . \qquad (1)$$

Because this is a simple equation, it can be solved exactly to give the deterministic solution

$$X(t) = X(0)e^{-k_1 t} \qquad (2)$$

where $X(0)$ is the initial amount of species X.

A stochastic model should be used when either the number of a particular species is small or when there is reason to expect random events to have an important influence on the behavior of the system. Often, a stochastic model will be more appropriate when we need to take account of species as discrete units rather than as continuous variables, and particularly when the numbers of a particular species may become small. It may also be necessary to take account of events occurring at random times. The essential difference between a stochastic and deterministic model is that in a stochastic model, different outcomes can result from the same initial conditions.

A stochastic model is formulated in terms of probabilities and is constructed by considering the probability that an event occurs during a small time period. Formulating the model in this manner enables us to calculate the probability that the population is of size X at time t, $p_x(t)$. Because the model is reasonably simple, the exact stochastic solution can be obtained.

A stochastic model is formulated in terms of probabilities, so at each time interval, the degradation of species X has an associated probability. Again, since the model is reasonably simple, the exact stochastic solution can be obtained:

$$P_x(t) = \binom{X(0)}{X} e^{-k_1 Xt} (1 - e^{-k_1 t})^{X(0)-X} \qquad (3)$$

where X takes the values between 0 and its initial amount $X(0)$.

In most biological systems, the number of species involved and the interactions between them mean that for stochastic models, an analytical solution—that is, one that can be obtained by purely algebraic formulae without using a computer—will not be feasible. In these cases, computer simulations of the stochastic kinetics are used. A simulation keeps track of the number and state of each species over time. Therefore, it is necessary to carry out repeated simulations and then look at the distribution of results to get a picture of the central tendency, the dispersion, and outliers. This process is called *Monte Carlo simulation*.

Figure 12.2 shows a stochastic realization of a spontaneous degradation

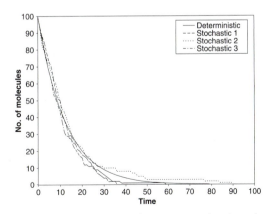

Figure 12.2 Comparison between a stochastic realization and the deterministic solution for a simple degradation reaction. In this stochastic realization, the molecules are degraded quicker than predicted by the deterministic solution.

reaction and its deterministic counterpart. For a given starting condition, a single stochastic realization may differ considerably from its deterministic counterpart. This is particularly important in models when the number of a particular species becomes low and the species may or may not become extinct. Figure 12.2 shows a clear example of a species reaching a very low concentration but never becoming totally extinct in the deterministic model, whereas in the stochastic model, the species becomes extinct and the time of extinction varies in different realizations. In the modeling of epidemic diseases within a host population, where it may matter greatly whether and when the first or last infective individual dies or recovers, the difference between stochastic and deterministic models can be very marked. Similar considerations can arise in gene regulatory networks with respect to the random association of transcription factor complexes.

Both the deterministic and stochastic methods have their respective advantages and disadvantages. The modeler should determine which method is more suitable to the task at hand (it may sometimes be both) and use that which is appropriate.

E. Software Tools

There are many ways to develop a model, from using traditional programming languages such as C, Fortran, and Java to mathematical packages such as Mathematica, Matlab, and R. Conventional publication of computer models is generally restricted to the presentation of a few key predictions, although it is common to allow the reader to download the computer program, or source. In order to replicate the same predictions as were published, the program must first be downloaded and any necessary algorithm libraries installed. To actually use the

model for further investigation generally requires a significant degree of computing skill.

As noted above (in section IIIB), there has recently been an increasing effort to agree on a standard method for representing mathematical models. One standard that has been widely adopted is the Systems Biology Markup Language (SBML). SBML provides a computer-readable format for representing models of biochemical reaction networks. Although SBML is human-readable, it is intended that it will usually be other software that would both read and write any models. This is analogous with the now widespread use of HTML for Web documents. Although a human can read HTML source documents, these are intended primarily for reading by a browser, such as Internet Explorer, that transforms the HTML code into a more easily read document on screen.

Currently there are over 60 groups using the SBML standard (see Hucka *et al.*, 2003). Some tools, such as CellDesigner, have been created that enable models to be constructed using a drag-and-drop approach. Using this approach, a user creates species that are assigned to graphical nodes. The nodes are then connected up using arrows to denote reactions (see for example Funahashi *et al.*, 2003).

Other tools, such as JigCell, allow the user to construct a model using chemical equations combined with a spreadsheet approach (Allen *et al.*, 2003). Using this approach is perhaps more useful when dealing with large and complex models, whereas the graphical approach is particularly useful when constructing a model for the first time.

SBML is not the only standard that has emerged. For example, the Petri Net Markup Language (PNML) and CellML are similar efforts in creating standards (see Lloyd *et al.*, 2004; Weber & Kindler, 2003). Although each standard focuses on different aspects of the model, they are not mutually exclusive. Hence, an effort is being made to create tools that allow the transformation from one language to another.

F. Validation of Models

Once we have constructed a model and are satisfied with its behavior, we need to test the model against observations from the biological system that it represents. This process is called *validation*. First, it is necessary to test the model to see whether it fits the data that we already have. Any discrepancies here need to be addressed. Once the model has been validated in this way, we should then test the model against data that were not used to estimate parameters for our model. If the model predictions and the observed data are not in close agreement, then the modeler needs to study the model to try and find where the discrepancies arise. This could mean modifying the model or adding further detail to the model. This is an important step as it may highlight that the current knowledge of the system is insufficient and that further experimental work should be carried out. Once modifications to the model have been made, the model is tested again, as shown in Figure 12.3.

Another aspect of validation is sensitivity analysis to assess how varying model parameters affect the model outcomes. There are two reasons why this is useful. First, we may be interested in some particular parameters—for example, the rate of degradation of a protein and how this might affect the buildup of damaged protein. Second, some of the parameter rates might not have been accurately determined and so it is important to see how sensitive the model is to small changes in these. The size of changes to make for each parameter depends on how well the parameter was determined initially. In the case of parameters that have been estimated

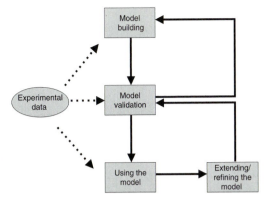

Figure 12.3 Flow diagram to show the steps in building a model. Once a model has been built, it is tested against experimental data. If the model does not agree well, then the modeler goes back to the model-building stage. Otherwise, the model can be used and then extended further as more knowledge becomes available.

from data, a multiple of the standard error is appropriate. For parameter values that have been guessed, a guess at the percentage reliability is also required. Caution needs to be taken when parameter estimates are correlated because if one parameter estimate is changed, some of the others might have to be changed too.

IV. Currently Available Models of Aging

Existing work reflects the variety of current models in aging research, which range from detailed modeling of individual intracellular mechanisms to higher-level modeling required to address the fundamental problem of why aging should occur. We will not attempt to be wholly comprehensive in this review but will illustrate the breadth of coverage and the different methodologies employed.

A. Intracellular Mechanisms

There are a large number of models currently available that focus on individual intracellular mechanisms. Currently, the models that relate directly to aging have been mainly concerned with telomere shortening, the accumulation of somatic mutations, and the accumulation of defective mitochondria.

1. Telomere Models

Telomeres are repetitive DNA sequences found at both ends of linear chromosomes. In telomerase-negative cells, telomeres shorten with each cell division, and this process eventually causes cells to enter a state of replicative senescence. One cause of telomere shortening is the end-replication problem caused by the inability of DNA polymerases to replicate a linear DNA molecule to its very end. In the 1990s, models were developed to try to explain replicative senescence in human fibroblasts based solely on the end-replication problem (Arino *et al.*, 1995; Levy *et al.*, 1992). Later models included additional mechanisms of telomere shortening. Rubelj and Vondracek (1999) modeled abrupt telomere shortening due to DNA recombination or nuclease digestion. It has been found that an increase in oxidative stress accelerates the rate of telomere shortening due to an accumulation of single-strand breaks in telomeric DNA (von Zglinicki *et al.*, 1995; von Zglinicki *et al.*, 2000). More recent models have included this additional mechanism and found that the models predict that oxidative stress plays an important role (Proctor & Kirkwood, 2002, 2003). For example, simulations showed that increasing the level of ROS led to fewer cell divisions on average. Space does not permit detail of all of the current models of telomere shortening, but the interested reader may refer to the references for further models (Aviv *et al.*, 2003; den Buijs *et al.*, 2004; Golubev *et al.*, 2003; Hao & Tan, 2002; Olofsson & Kimmel, 1999; Sidorov *et al.*, 2004; Tan, 1999a,b, 2001).

2. Somatic Mutations

The role of somatic mutations in aging is an area of particularly active research, following new methods for measuring DNA modification and repair. The somatic mutation theory was first proposed several decades ago after experiments showed that irradiation shortened life span in animal models and induced features of premature aging (Henshaw *et al.*, 1947; Lindop & Rotblat, 1961).

Szilard (1959) proposed a mathematical model that assumed that recessive mutational "hits" in diploid organisms would accumulate so that a cell could continue to function until one pair of genes had both received a "hit." Holliday and Kirkwood (1981) developed a deterministic model of the accumulation of recessive mutations in human fibroblast populations. A stochastic model of the same processes was later developed (Kirkwood & Proctor, 2003), which also considered the possibility that there may be synergistic interactions between mutations.

3. Mitochondria Models

The free-radical theory of aging proposes that ROS, which are constantly generated through normal cell metabolism in the mitochondria, cause aging by damaging membranes, proteins, and DNA (Harman, 1956). The mitochondrial theory of aging proposes that an accumulation of defective mitochondria is a major contributor to the cellular deterioration that underlies the aging process (Harman, 1972). Studies have shown that defective mitochondria accumulate with age to a greater extent in post-mitotic tissues (Cortopassi *et al.*, 1992; Lee *et al.*, 1994), although it has recently been reported that high levels of mitochondrial defects are observed in aged human colon (Taylor *et al.*, 2003). In addition, several studies have shown that muscle fibers are taken over by a single form of mutant mtDNA (Brierley *et al.*, 1998; Müller-Höcker *et al.*, 1993).

Hypotheses to explain the apparent "clonal expansion" of mutant mtDNA are a replication advantage for the mutant mtDNA; slower degradation of mutant mitochondria (de Grey, 1997); and random intracellular drift. Mathematical models have been developed to explore quantitative predictions from these ideas. Kowald and Kirkwood (2000) developed a deterministic model based on de Grey's hypothesis. Other models are based on the idea of random intracellular drift (Chinnery & Samuels, 1999; Elson *et al.*, 2001).

4. Chaperone Models

Molecular chaperones have an important role in helping to maintain protein homeostasis within cells. It has been observed that the induction of heat shock proteins, a major class of chaperones, is impaired with age and that there is also a decline in chaperone function. Although there are a few mathematical models on the role of heat shock proteins in the cell, to date only one model has looked at the role of chaperones in the aging process (Proctor *et al.*, 2005). This model describes how heat shock proteins are upregulated after an increase in intracellular stress and can be used to investigate the effect of stress on protein homeostasis.

5. Network Models

A few models exist that show how different mechanisms interact synergistically (Kowald & Kirkwood, 1994, 1996; Sozou & Kirkwood, 2001), examples being the interactions of defective mitochondria, aberrant proteins, free radicals, and scavengers in the aging process (Kowald & Kirkwood, 1996); and the interactions of telomere shortening, oxidative stress,

and somatic mutations in nuclear and mitochondrial DNA (Sozou & Kirkwood, 2001). We are currently engaged in a major effort, the Biology of Ageing e-Science Integration and Simulation (BASIS) project, to develop interactive models that can network a variety of individual processes together in a flexible, user-friendly manner (Kirkwood *et al.*, 2003). One of the aims of the BASIS project is to allow models of individual mechanisms to be linked together to form a "Virtual Aging Cell" (Proctor & Kirkwood, 2003).

B. Tissue Models

The functional properties of an aging organ or tissue can become compromised, even if most of the cells are in good working order. Mathematical models are required to help us try to understand how a fraction of damaged cells can lead to altered tissue function. Early models were motivated by the fact that cultured human diploid fibroblasts cannot be grown indefinitely in culture (Hayflick, 1972). These models were based on the commitment theory, the idea that cells become irreversibly committed to senescence while still outwardly healthy (Holliday *et al.*, 1977; Kirkwood & Holliday, 1975).

Recently, extensive experimental data has been generated on intrinsic age changes that affect the function of intestinal stem cells in aging mice (Loeffler *et al.*, 1993; Martin *et al.*, 1998a,b). This has led to a number of mathematical models (e.g., Gerike *et al.*, 1998; Loeffler *et al.*, 1993; Meineke *et al.*, 2001). Another model based on data from muscle-derived stem cells has also been developed (Deasy *et al.*, 2003).

Another tissue system that has been extensively studied and modeled is the population of T cells and their role in immunosenescence (Luciani *et al.*, 2001; Romanyukha & Yashin, 2003).

C. Organism Models

There are only a very limited number of models dealing with whole-organism aging, and these are limited to unicellular organisms. Budding yeast, *Saccharomyces cerevisiae*, is commonly used to study cellular aging. Accumulation of extrachromosomal ribosomal DNA circles (ERCs) appears to be an important contributor to aging in yeast, and a mathematical model has been developed to examine this process (Gillespie *et al.*, 2004). Another interesting model contrasts regulatory with stochastic processes in genetic segregation during division as a mechanism for the aging observed in the asexually reproducing ciliate *Styloncychia* (Duerr *et al.*, 2004).

D. Population Models

An area of research that has contributed to a fundamental understanding of why aging occurs is life-history theory—a theory that essentially deals with schedules of growth, survival, and reproduction maximizing Darwinian fitness (Kirkwood & Austad, 2000; Kirkwood & Rose, 1991; Partridge & Barton, 1993). Many classic life-history papers included an investigation of senescence (Cole, 1954; Fisher, 1930; Hamilton, 1966; Williams, 1957). Another modeling approach is represented by the disposable soma theory (Kirkwood, 1977; Kirkwood & Rose, 1991), founded on the principles of optimality theory (Parker & Maynard Smith, 1990). The disposable soma theory suggests that aging arises as part of an optimal life history due to tradeoffs in resource allocation between investment in reproduction and maintenance affecting long-term survival. There is much data in general support of the existence of such tradeoffs, including in humans (Lycett *et al.*, 2000; Westendorp & Kirkwood, 1998). More complex general life-history models that have incorporated measures of an organism's state such as size in addi-

tion to age have been analyzed using techniques such as dynamic programming, simulated annealing, and Pontryagin's maximization principle (Abrams & Ludwig, 1995; Blarer & Doebeli, 1996; Cichon, 1997; Clark & Mangel, 2000; Houston & McNamara 1999; Schaffer, 1983; Teriokhin, 1998; Vaupel *et al.*, 2004).

The following specific issues have attracted attention using approaches and modeling techniques drawn from the domains of life-history theory, demography, and population genetics.

1. Dietary Restriction

Dietary restriction is observed to cause slowing of aging and extension of life in many species. One hypothesis is that animals have evolved a response to temporary fluctuations in resource availability, in which energy is diverted from reproduction to maintenance functions in periods of food shortage, thereby enhancing survival and retaining reproductive potential for when conditions improve. A detailed quantitative development of this hypothesis using a dynamic resource allocation model revealed that the effect could be the result of the suggested evolutionary process provided that the following conditions were satisfied: (1) there is a substantial initial cost to reproduction, and (2) juveniles are at a disadvantage during periods of food shortage (Shanley & Kirkwood, 2000). An alternative approach is presented using a dynamic energy budget (van Leeuwen *et al.*, 2002). Recently, metabolic control analysis has been used to help identify an increased proton leak in the mitochondrial inner membrane as one possible mechanism whereby ROS production is reduced (Lambert & Merry, 2004).

2. Negligible Senescence

Species that exhibit negligible senescence are of particular interest (Finch, 1998) and are well represented in species that continue to grow after maturation, so-called indeterminate growth. A dynamic model that explicitly included size as a state variable predicts that this should be the case, and indeed predicts that some species should show negative senescence (Vaupel et al., 2004). Interestingly, conditions for non-aging can be found in a general life-history model in an analysis of vitality: a term that combines the declining fecundity and increasing mortality characteristic of senescence (Sozou & Seymour, 2004).

3. Gompertz, Mortality Plateaus, and Heterogeneity

Most species exhibit an exponential increase in mortality with age that can be described by the Gompertz model or by the Gompertz-Makeham model that has an extension to include extrinsic sources of mortality (Golubev, 2004). One problem in the acceptance of this model is the observation that in large laboratory populations, mortality rates appear to plateau at later ages (Vaupel et al., 1998). A number of models have been proposed to account for this pattern, such as an evolutionary trade-off (Mueller & Rose, 1996; Mueller et al., 2003), a combination of mutation accumulation and pleiotropy (Charlesworth, 2001), a state-based approach (Mangel & Bonsall, 2004), and individual heterogeneity within the population (Pletcher & Curtsinger, 1998).

4. Human Menopause

The rapid reproductive senescence associated with menopause in human females occurs well in advance of general somatic senescence and poses an interesting evolutionary problem. The reproductive life span of human females is limited, as in almost all other mammals, by a finite pool of oocytes established in the developing fetus. Menopause is manifest when this pool is near to exhaustion, and mechanistic models have focused on the follicular dynamics (Faddy et al., 1992) and problems of fetal loss that increase in frequency as the oocyte pool is depleted (O'Connor et al., 1998). Other modeling has focused on determining whether at some age mothers may increase their fitness by diverting investment from continued reproduction to existing offspring and grand-offspring (Hawkes et al., 1998; Lee, 2003; Peccei, 1995; Rogers, 1993; Shanley & Kirkwood, 2001). To date the results have not been conclusive, but given the importance of intergenerational assistance—for example, as seen in the two-fold improvement in mortality for infants with a living grandmother (Sear et al., 2002) combined with the particularly high risk of mortality in childbirth for human females—an evolutionary explanation remains a clear possibility and the development and testing of further models appears likely.

V. Models, Data Collection, and Experimental Design

Models are developed based on the collective understanding of the scientific community regarding the underlying mechanisms driving the processes of interest. The related activity of designing experiments to provide data to falsify or refine the models is essentially just a formalization of "the scientific method." However, there are a number of issues that arise in the context of complex dynamic models that make this procedure far from straightforward in practice. Models are typically concerned with underlying *mechanisms* that are difficult or impossible to measure directly through conventional experimental procedures. Consequently, they often contain *parameters* (such as various kinds of rate constants) whose values are not known.

If a model cannot make predictions regarding quantities that can (at least in principle) be measured experimentally, then it is not falsifiable, and in an important sense is not "scientific." There is therefore a requirement to develop models that are *predictive*, as this then affords an opportunity to compare the model predictions with experimentally determined *reality*. As well as providing the opportunity for falsification, this predictive behavior also potentially allows "calibration" of model parameters by finding combinations of parameters that reduce the discrepancy between the model predictions and reality.

These kinds of "inverse" problems have long been recognized in the physical and engineering sciences, and there is a large literature concerned with attempts to solve them. The problem can be understood generally as follows: a complex system has a range of inputs, and based on these, produces a range of outputs. The inverse problem is to find a set of inputs to the system that closely matches a given set of outputs (desired target or experimental observation). In the context of an attempt to match an experimentally observed history of a physical system, attempts to solve the inverse problem are often referred to as *history matching* or *calibration*, of which more is presented in the next section. Such calibration techniques are generally applied *post hoc*, after the experimental data have been collected. However, in the context of biological modeling, there is often an opportunity to go back to the lab to collect appropriate data for model validation and calibration.

A question then naturally arises as to exactly what data should be collected, and how much. In the context of complex biological models, such *experimental design* questions are difficult to tackle within a formal statistical framework, but it is relatively straightforward to justify some guiding principles. First,

it is necessary to collect data that are (or can be) predicted by the model. This may require model refinement but is necessary; otherwise, there is nothing to link the model and the data that is collected. Second, one must collect data corresponding to model predictions that are sensitive to underlying model assumptions (structural and otherwise). This is necessary on the grounds of falsifiability. Third, it is necessary to gather measurements that help to answer questions of key scientific interest. For example, if a key model parameter of interest is the degradation rate of a particular protein, then measurements should be taken on data that are sensitive to the choice of rate rather than data that are relatively robust to this choice. This will ensure that the data collected provide useful information. Fourth, enough data should be gathered to ensure that an adequate assessment can be made of inter- and intra-experimental variation; otherwise, there is no way to be sure that the data are representative and that the model is not being calibrated to fit an atypical data set. If the model being calibrated is stochastic, more data are probably required, as it is likely to be necessary to reliably determine a good approximation to the full probability distribution of key observables. These basic principles are fairly self-evident, but effectively operationalizing them for a complex dynamic simulation model is not necessarily easy. However, there are many excellent texts on experimental design that can provide further guidance (see for example Clarke & Kempson, 1997; Cochran & Cox, 1992; and Mead, 1988).

VI. Parameter Inference

A. The Calibration Problem

Many approaches have been applied to the calibration problem within the traditional engineering context. First, a (deterministic) computer simulator (model) of the physical (or biological) system under study is built, so that for a given set of inputs, a corresponding set of outputs may be computed. Next, a simple measure of "distance" for how far the output is from the desired match is defined. The input space is then searched for a set that minimizes the distance measure. This *optimization* problem can be approached using a variety of techniques for multivariate function minimization—for example, steepest descent, Newton methods, conjugate gradients, simulated annealing, genetic programming, and so on (Koza *et al.*, 2001). Such minimization techniques can work well if the computer simulator is very fast, but for a simulator of a large, complex system, which may take hours or days for a single run, such naïve approaches generally fail.

Simple search methods are very wasteful of information. Typically, a very small number of runs are used to decide on a new "best guess" for the target input parameters, and then all existing information is discarded as the search continues from this new input set. In contrast, statistical approaches to the calibration problem attempt to use all available runs from the simulator in order to infer a model for the relationship between the inputs to and outputs from the simulator. In this context, it is not necessarily optimal to always evaluate the simulator at the current "best guess" at the optimal input set, but instead to evaluate at an input set that gives the most information regarding the relationship between the inputs and outputs in the vicinity of the predicted optimal set. Thus, such statistical approaches to calibration need to combine both non-parametric statistical inference techniques and experimental design algorithms in order to effectively solve the problem (Sacks *et al.*, 1989).

A range of different approaches can be taken to carrying out statistical inference

for model parameters given data, and these correspond to different schools of statistical thought. Classical frequentist approaches seek to construct estimators that are a function of the data and have desirable properties (such as consistency and lack of bias) under repeated sampling. However, even leaving aside the serious philosophical objections many people have to the repeated sampling framework at the heart of frequentist inference, there are many practical difficulties associated with applying such techniques in the context of complex dynamic models. Consequently, few statisticians would consider a frequentist framework in this scenario.

Approaches based on the likelihood function of the data provide a more powerful and natural way of addressing the simulation model parameter inference problem. These can be divided into two main camps. The first is the maximum likelihood school, which attempts to be "objective" by using only the likelihood function of the data and seeks combinations of parameters, which makes the data as likely as possible conditional on those parameters. The likelihood (or log-likelihood) function is used as a way of "scoring" the goodness of fit, which can then be optimized. Although this sounds straightforward in principle, the likelihood function is typically not analytically tractable for complex models, and this introduces a variety of complications.

The second camp is the Bayesian school, which corrects the conditioning from data on parameters to parameters on data, and thereby seeks parameters that are likely given the data. This is done at the expense of introducing prior distributions into the problem but has a range of benefits as a result. These include the fact that the resulting framework is fully probabilistic, and that probabilistic information regarding all parameters can be obtained from the posterior distribution. The use of priors is also valuable, as they help regularize the problem and allow the modeler to incorporate information regarding realistic parameter ranges into the inference algorithm. A further benefit of the Bayesian framework is that because it is probabilistic, powerful computational algorithms may be naturally applied to problems where the likelihood is analytically intractable. Markov chain Monte Carlo (MCMC) algorithms (Gamerman, 1997) use stochastic simulation techniques to obtained realizations from the (complex) posterior distribution, which are then used to draw inferences about model parameters. For more information about Bayesian inference, see Bernardo and Smith (2000), O'Hagan and Forster (2004), and references therein.

B. Statistical Approaches to Simulation Model Calibration

Although non-Bayesian approaches to the calibration problem are possible, the complexity and dimensionality of the problem, together with the need to incorporate available expert prior information regarding, *inter alia*, plausible ranges for rate constants and information on data quality, mean that a Bayesian approach is particularly attractive. Typically, (in the context of deterministic processes), a model is specified in the following form:

$$z_i = \zeta(x_i) + \varepsilon_i, \quad \zeta(x_i) = \rho\eta(x_i, \theta) + \delta(x_i) \quad (4)$$

Here $z = (z_1, z_2, \ldots, z_n)$ represents the available experimental data, obtained from n different experimental conditions $x_1, x_2, \ldots x_n$; $\zeta(x_i)$ is the real behavior of the biological system under experimental condition x_i; ε_i is the measurement error associated with the ith experiment; ρ is a bias associated with the computer simulator of the biochemical system; $\eta(x_i, \theta)$ is the result of running the computer simulator under experimental condition x_i with the "perfect" set of calibration parameters θ; and $\delta(x_i)$ represents model inadequacy

that is independent of the calibration issue. In addition to the experimental data, there will be data $y = (y_1, y_2, \ldots, y_N)$ obtained from N runs of the computer simulator (where N will typically be larger than n, even in the case of an expensive simulator), where

$$y_j = \eta(x_j^\star, t_j) \quad (5)$$

is the result of the jth computer experiment, $x_j^\star$ is the experimental condition associated with the jth computer experiment and t_j is the set of calibration parameters associated with the jth computer experiment (Kennedy & O'Hagan, 2001).

Note that within this framework, the computer simulator of the biological model is represented by a (deterministic) function $\eta(\cdot, \cdot)$, which can be evaluated at any combination of experimental conditions and calibration parameters by running the simulator with the specified input. If the simulator were very fast, so that evaluating $\eta(\cdot, \cdot)$ were cheap, then standard Bayesian inference techniques could be used in order to make direct inferences for θ using (1), generating data of the form (2) as and when required. However, due to the expense of evaluating $\eta(\cdot, \cdot)$ for large complex models, $\eta(\cdot, \cdot)$ is often regarded as an unknown function, modeled using a Gaussian process. Thus inference may proceed for θ using only the N computer simulator runs available. Bayesian inference is typically carried out using a mixture of analytic direct matrix computations related to Gaussian processes together with computationally intensive techniques, using Markov chain Monte Carlo (MCMC) methods.

Note that in the context of biological modeling, choice of the experimental conditions for the n "wet lab" experiments will often (though not always) be predetermined. However, the choice of conditions for the N computer simulator runs will be at least partly under the calibrator's control and will be of key importance to the over-all effectiveness of the procedure. This is a nontrivial (sequential) experimental design problem, but limited literature already exists that will provide guidance in this area (Craig *et al.*, 1996; Currin *et al.*, 1991; Kennedy & O'Hagan, 2001; Sacks *et al.*, 1989).

Many complex computer codes have the facility to be run at different levels of sophistication, and hence accuracy. The BASIS simulator, for example, may be run in "exact" mode, where the simulation of the stochastic process used to model a given biochemical system is "perfect," based on a discrete event simulation strat-egy similar to the Gillespie algorithm. Such exact simulation procedures are desirable but are typically very expensive to carry out. On the other hand, the sys-tem may also be run in an approximate mode, based on a time-discretization of the process, where both the accuracy of the procedure and the time taken for a run depend on the size of time-step adopted. In this case, it can often be optimal to combine a large number of fast (but less accurate) runs with a small num-ber of slow (but accurate) runs in order to make most efficient use of computer time. There is already a sizable literature in this area; see for example Higdon and colleagues (2003), Kennedy and O'Hagan (2001), and references therein.

C. Direct Statistical Parameter Inference

The calibration techniques alluded to above work well in the deterministic con-text but are not completely straightfor-ward to extend to the case of stochastic simulation models. For a stochastic model of relatively low dimension, it may be pos-sible to make a direct attempt to carry out statistical inference for the parameters of the system given (for example, time course) experimental data on the system dynamics. Here, rather than regarding the simulator as an "unknown function," the

stochastic process corresponding to the simulator is modeled directly, and all aspects of the process that are not observed are "filled-in" probabilistically using appropriate MCMC techniques. Conditional on complete knowledge of the stochastic process, inference for any rate parameters driving the system dynamics is straightforward. The difficulty of such methods is in the construction of the MCMC algorithms to fill in the missing aspects of the stochastic process. This is very problem-specific and generally requires a fairly detailed understanding of the underlying dynamics, including the likelihood function, as well as experience in the use of MCMC algorithms. The use of these techniques for identification of biological models is still in its infancy, but see Boys and colleagues (2004), Gibson & Renshaw (2001), Golightly & Wilkinson (2005), and O'Neill (2002) for some suc-cessful examples.

VII. Conclusions

This chapter has examined the rationale for the use of computer models in study-ing the aging process and has reviewed the range of models that have been developed. It has also described some of the generic issues that need to be addressed in terms of the methodology of modeling. In com-ing years, it is likely to be essential, if aging research is to realize its potential, that modeling studies are greatly extended and that models are increasingly used to link together the pieces of the picture that are revealed by reductionist experimental techniques. These developments are an inherent part of the "new" ways of doing science that are commonly described as "systems biology." Whether systems biol-ogy is really new or not is a matter for debate, and a spectrum of opinion can be found. What is unquestionably new is the mass of detailed information emerging at accelerating pace from functional genomic technologies, the rapid expansion of raw computing power, the developing connectivity offered by advances in Internet (soon to be GRID-enabled) Web services, and the recruitment of increasing numbers of mathematicians, statisticians, and computer scientists into the life sciences.

Not all areas of biology need to be taken over by the systems approach, but few are likely to remain untouched by it. The biology of aging is one area where it is hard to envisage the necessary progress being made without embracing the systems approach. There are just too many mechanisms, levels of action, and experimental models for it to be realistic to anticipate integration without the use of computer models. Effecting the building of the cross-disciplinary research programs to bring this about is going to be a challenge, but it should also prove to be intellectually stimulating and fun.

References

Abrams, P. A., & Ludwig, D. (1995). Optimality theory, Gompertz' law, and the disposable soma theory of senescence. *Evolution*, 49, 1055–1066.

Allen, N. A., Calzone, L., Chen, K. C., Ciliberto, A., Ramakrishman, N., Shaffer, C. A., Sible, J. C., Tyson, J. J., Vass, M. T., Watson, L. T., & Zwolak, J. W. (2003). Modeling regulatory networks at Virginia Tech. *OMICS, A Journal of Integrative Biology*, 7, 285–299.

Arino, O., Kimmel, M., & Webb, G. F. (1995). Mathematical modelling of the loss of telomere sequences. *Journal of Theoretical Biology*, 177, 45–57.

Aviv, A., Levy, D., & Mangel, M. (2003). Growth, telomere dynamics and successful and unsuccessful human aging. *Mechanisms of Ageing & Development*, 124, 829–837.

Bernardo, J. M., & Smith, A. F. M. (2000). *Bayesian theory*. Chichester, NY: Wiley.

Blarer, A., & Doebeli, M. (1996). Heuristic optimization of the general life history problem: a novel approach. *Evolutionary Ecology*, 10, 81–96.

Boys, R. J., Wilkinson, D. J., & Kirkwood, T. B. L. (2004). Bayesian inference for a stochastic kinetic model. Submitted.

Brierley, E. J., Johnson, M. A., Lightowlers, R. N., James, O. F. W., & Turnbull, D. M. (1998). Role of mitochondrial DNA mutations in human aging: implications for the central nervous system and muscle. *Annals of Neurology*, 43, 217–223.

Charlesworth, B. (2001). Patterns of age-specific means and genetic variances of mortality rates predicted by the mutation-accumulation theory of ageing. *Journal of Theoretical Biology*, 210, 47–65.

Chinnery, P. F., & Samuels, D. C. (1999). Relaxed replication of mtDNA: a model with implications for the expression of disease. *American Journal of Human Genetics*, 64, 1158–1165.

Cichon, M. (1997). Evolution of longevity through optimal resource allocation. *Proceedings of the Royal Society of London Series B*, 264, 1383–1388.

Clark, C. W., & Mangel, M. (2000). *Dynamic state variable models in ecology: methods and applications*. England: Oxford University Press.

Clarke, G. M., & Kempson, R. E. (1997). Introduction to the Design and Analysis of Experiments. London: Arnold.

Cochran, W., & Cox, G. (1992). *Experimental designs*. Chichester, NY: Wiley.

Cole, L. C. (1954). The population consequences of life history phenomena. *Quarterly Review of Biology*, 29, 103–137.

Cortopassi, G. A., Shibata, D., Soong, N. W., & Arnheim, N. (1992). A pattern of accumulation of a somatic deletion of mitochondrial-DNA in aging human tissues. *Proceedings of the National Academy of Sciences of the USA*, 89, 7370–7374.

Craig, P. S., Goldstein, M., Seheult, A. H., & Smith, J. A. (1996). Bayes linear strategies for matching hydrocarbon reservoir history. In A. F. M. Smith (Ed.), *Bayesian statistics 5*. (pp. 69–95). Oxford: Oxford Science Publications.

Currin, C., Mitchell, T., Morris, M., & Ylvisaker, D. (1991). Bayesian prediction of deterministic functions, with applications to the design and analysis of computer experiments. *Journal of the American Statistical Association*, 86, 953–963.

de Grey, A. D. N. J. (1997). A proposed refinement of the mitochondrial free radical theory of aging. *BioEssays*, 19, 161–166.

Deasy, B. M., Jankowski, R. J., Payne, T. R., Cao, B., Goff, J. P., Greenberger, J. S., & Huard, J. (2003). Modeling stem cell population growth: incorporating terms for proliferative heterogeneity. *Stem Cells*, 21, 536–545.

den Buijs, J. O., van den Bosch, P. P. J., Musters, M., & van Riel, N. A. W. (2004). Mathematical modeling confirms the length-dependency of telomere shortening. *Mechanisms of Ageing & Development*, 125, 437–444.

Duerr, H. P., Eichner, M., & Ammermann, D. (2004). Modeling senescence in hypotrichous ciliates. *Protist*, 155, 45–52.

Elson, J. L., Samuels, D. C., Turnbull, D. M., & Chinnery, P. F. (2001). Random intracellular drift explains the clonal expansion of mitochondrial DNA mutations with age. *American Journal of Human Genetics*, 68, 802–806.

Faddy, M. J., Gosden, R. G., Gougeon, A., Richardson, S. J., & Nelson, J. F. (1992). Accelerated disappearance of ovarian follicles in midlife: implications for forecasting menopause. *Human Reproduction*, 7, 1342–1346.

Finch, C. E. (1998). Variations in senescence and longevity include the possibility of negligible senescence. *Journals of Gerontology A: Biological Sciences*, 53, B235–B239.

Finch, C. E., & Kirkwood, T. B. L. (2000). *Chance, development & aging.* New York: Oxford University Press.

Fisher, R. A. (1930). *The genetical theory of natural selection.* Oxford: Clarendon Press.

Funahashi, A., Tanimura, N., Morohashi, M., & Kitano, H. (2003). CellDesigner: a process diagram editor for gene-regulatory and biochemical networks. *Biosilico*, 1, 159–162.

Gamerman, D. (1997). *Markov chain Monte Carlo: stochastic simulation of Bayesian inference.* London: Chapman & Hall.

Gems, D., & Partridge, L. (2001). Insulin/IGF signalling and ageing: seeing the bigger picture. *Current Opinions in Genetics & Development*, 11, 287–292.

Gerike, T. G., Paulus, U., Potten, C. S., & Loeffler, M. (1998). A dynamic model of proliferation and differentiation in the intestinal crypt based on a hypothetical intraepithelial growth factor. *Cell Proliferation*, 31, 93–110.

Gibson, G. J., & Renshaw, E. (2001). Likelihood estimation for stochastic compartmental models using Markov chain methods. *Statistics & Computing*, 11, 347–358.

Gillespie, C. S., Proctor, C. J., Boys, R. J., Shanley, D. P., Wilkinson, D. J., & Kirkwood, T. B. L. (2004). A mathematical model of ageing in yeast. *Journal of Theoretical Biology*, 229, 189–196.

Golightly, A., & Wilkinson, D. J. (2005). Bayesian inference for stochastic kinetic models using a diffusion approximation. *Biometrics*, 61, 781–788

Golubev, A. (2004). Does Makeham make sense? *Biogerontology*, 5, 159–167.

Golubev, A., Khrustalev, S., & Butov, A. (2003). An in silico investigation into the causes of telomere length heterogeneity and its implications for the Hayflick limit. *Journal of Theoretical Biology*, 225, 153–170.

Hamilton, W. D. (1966). The moulding of senescence by natural selection. *Journal of Theoretical Biology*, 12, 12–45.

Hao, Y. H., & Tan, Z. (2002). The generation of long telomere overhangs in human cells: a model and its implication. *Bioinformatics*, 18, 666–671.

Harman, D. (1956). A theory based on free radical and radiation chemistry. *Journal of Gerontology*, 11, 298–300.

Harman, D. (1972). The biologic clock: the mitochondria? *Journal of American Geriatics Society*, 20, 145–147.

Hawkes, K., O'Connell, J. F., Jones, N. G. B., Alvarez, H., & Charnov, E. L. (1998). Grandmothering, menopause, and the evolution of human life histories. *Proceedings of the National Academy of Sciences of the USA*, 95, 1336–1339.

Hayflick, L. (1972). In H. Bredt, & J. W. Rohen, (Eds.), *Ageing and Development*, Vol. 4, pp. 1–15. Stuttgart: Schattaner Verlag.

Henshaw, P. S., Riley, E. F., & Stapleton, G. E. (1947). The biologic effects of pile radiation. *Radiology*, 49, 349–364.

Herndon, L. A., Schmeissner, P. J., Dudaronek, J. M., Brown, P. A., Listner, K. M., Sakano, Y., Paupard, M. C., Hall, D. H., & Driscoll, M. (2002). Stochastic and genetic factors influence tissue-specific decline in ageing *C. elegans*. *Nature*, 419, 808–814.

Higdon, D., Lee, H., & Holloman, C. (2003). Markov chain Monte Carlo-based approaches for inference in computationally intensive inverse problems. In M. West (Ed.), *Bayesian Statistics 7* (pp. 181–197). Oxford: Oxford Science Publications.

Hilborn, R., & Mangel, M. (1997). *The ecological detective. Confronting models with data*. Princeton, NJ: Princeton University Press.

Holliday, R., & Kirkwood, T. B. L. (1981). Predictions of the somatic mutation and mortalization theories of cellular aging are contrary to experimental-observations. *Journal of Theoretical Biology*, 93, 627–642.

Holliday, R., Huschtscha, L. I., Tarrant, G. M., & Kirkwood, T. B. L. (1977). Testing the commitment theory of cellular aging. *Science*, 198, 366–372.

Houston, A. I., & McNamara, J. M. (1999). *Models of adaptive behaviour: an approach based on state*. Cambridge: Cambridge University Press.

Hucka, M., Finney, A., Sauro, H. M., Bolouri, H., Doyle, J. C., & Kitano, H. (2003). The Systems Biology Markup Language (SBML): a medium for representation and exchange of biochemical network models. *Bioinformatics*, 19, 524–531.

Jazwinski, S. M. (2000). Metabolic mechanisms of yeast ageing. *Experimental Gerontology*, 35, 671–676.

Jahnson, T. E. (1990). Increased life span of age-1 mutants in caenorhabditis elegans and lower Gompertz rate of aging. *Science* 249, 908–912.

Kennedy, M. C., & O'Hagan, A. (2001). Bayesian calibration of computer models. *Journal of the Royal Statistical Society Series B-Statistical Methodology*, 63, 425–450.

Kirkwood, T. B. L. (1977). Evolution of ageing. *Nature*, 270, 301–304.

Kirkwood, T. B. L., & Austad, S. N. (2000). Why do we age? *Nature*, 408, 233–238.

Kirkwood, T. B. L., & Finch, C. E. (2002). The old worm turns more slowly. *Nature*, 419, 794–795.

Kirkwood, T. B. L., & Holliday, R. (1975). Commitment to senescence: a model for the finite and infinite growth of diploid and transformed human fibroblasts in culture. *Journal of Theoretical Biology*, 53, 481–496.

Kirkwood, T. B. L., & Proctor, C. J. (2003). Somatic mutations and ageing in silico. *Mechanisms of Ageing & Development*, 124, 85–92.

Kirkwood, T. B. L., & Rose, M. R. (1991). Evolution of senescence—late survival sacrificed for reproduction. *Philosophical Transactions of the Royal Society of London Series B-Biological Sciences*, 332, 15–24.

Kirkwood, T. B. L., Boys, R. J., Gillespie, C. S., Proctor, C. J., Shanley, D. P., & Wilkinson, D. J. (2003). Towards an e-biology of ageing: integrating theory and data. *Nature Reviews Molecular Cell Biology*, 4, 243–249.

Kowald, A., & Kirkwood, T. B. L. (1994). Towards a network theory of ageing: a model combining the free radical theory and the protein error theory. *Journal of Theoretical Biology*, 168, 75–94.

Kowald, A., & Kirkwood, T. B. L. (1996). A network theory of ageing: the interactions of defective mitochondria, aberrant proteins, free radicals and scavengers in the ageing process. *Mutation Research – DNAging Genetic Instability and Aging*, 316, 209–236.

Kowald, A., & Kirkwood, T. B. L. (2000). Accumulation of defective mitochondria through delayed degradation of damaged organelles and its possible role in the ageing of post-mitotic and dividing cells. *Journal of Theoretical Biology*, 202, 145–160.

Koza, J. R., Mydlowec, W., Lanza, G., Yu, J., & Keane, M. A. (2001). Automated reverse engineering of metabolic pathways from observed data by means of genetic programming. In H. Kitano (Ed.), *Foundations of systems biology* (pp. 95–121). Cambridge, MA: MIT Press.

Lambert, A. J., & Merry, B. J. (2004). Effect of caloric restriction on mitochondrial reactive oxygen species production and bioenergetics: reversal by insulin. *American Journal of Physiology-Regulatory, Integrative & Comparative Physiology*, 286, 71–79.

Lander, A. D. (2004). A calculus of purpose. *Plos Biology*, 2, 712–714.

Larsen, P. L. (2001). Asking the age-old questions. *Nature Genetics*, 28, 102–104.

Lee, C. M., Pang, C. Y., Hsu, H. S., & Wei, Y. H. (1994). Differential accumulation of 4977 bp deletion in mitochondrial DNA of various tissues in human ageing. *Biochemica Et Biophysica Acta*, 1226, 37–43.

Lee, R. D. (2003). Rethinking the evolutionary theory of aging: transfers, not births, shape social species. *Proceedings of the National Academy of Sciences of the USA*, 100, 9637–9642.

Levy, M. Z., Allsopp, R. C., Futcher, A. B., Greider, C. W., & Harley, C. B. (1992). Telomere end-replication problem and cell aging. *Journal of Molecular Biology*, 225, 951–960.

Lindop, P. J., & Rotblat, J. (1961). Shortening of life and causes of death in mice exposed to single whole-body dose of radiation. *Nature*, 189, 645–648.

Lithgow, G. J. (1998). Aging mechanisms from nematodes to mammals. *Nutrition*, 14, 522–524.

Lloyd, C. M., Halstead, M. D. B., & Nielsen, P. F. (2004). CellML: its future, present and past. *Progress in Biophysics & Molecular Biology*, 85, 433–450.

Loeffler, M., Birke, A., Winton, D., & Potten, C. (1993). Somatic mutation, monoclonality and stochastic-models of stem-cell organization in the intestinal crypt. *Journal of Theoretical Biology*, 160, 471–491.

Luciani, F., Valensin, S., Vescovini, R., Sansoni, P., Fagnoni, F., Franceschi, C., Bonafe, M., & Turchetti, G. (2001). A stochastic model for CD8(+) T cell dynamics in human immunosenescence: Implications for survival and longevity. *Journal of Theoretical Biology*, 213, 587–597.

Lycett, J. E., Dunbar, R. I. M., & Voland, E. (2000). Longevity and the costs of reproduction in a historical human population. *Proceedings of the Royal Society of London Series B-Biological Sciences*, 267, 31–35.

Mangel, M., & Bonsall, M. B. (2004). The shape of things to come: using models with physiological structure to predict mortality trajectories. *Theoretical Population Biology*, 65, 353–359.

Martin, K., Kirkwood, T. B. L., & Potten, C. S. (1998a). Age changes in stem cells of murine small intestinal crypts. *Experimental Cell Research*, 241, 316–323.

Martin, K., Potten, C. S., Roberts, S. A., & Kirkwood, T. B. L. (1998b). Altered stem cell regeneration in irradiated intestinal crypts of senescent mice. *Journal of Cell Science*, 111, 2297–2303.

Mead, R. (1988). *The design of experiments*. England: Cambridge University Press.

Meineke, F. A., Potten, C. S., & Loeffler, M. (2001). Cell migration and organization in the intestinal crypt using a lattice-free model. *Cell Proliferation*, 34, 253–266.

Mueller, L. D., & Rose, M. R. (1996). Evolutionary theory predicts late-life mortality plateaus. *Proceedings of the National Academy of Sciences of the USA*, 93, 15249–15253.

Mueller, L. D., Drapeau, M. D., Adams, C. S., Hammerle, C. W., Doyal, K. M., Jazayeri, A. J., Ly, T., Beguwala, S. A., Mamidi, A. R., & Rose, M. R. (2003). Statistical tests of demographic heterogeneity theories. *Experimental Gerontology*, 38, 373–386.

Müller-Höcker, J., Seibel, P., Schneiderbanger, K., & Kadenbach, B. (1993). Different *in situ* hybridization patterns of mitochondrial DNA in cytochrome c oxidase-deficient extraocular muscle fibres in the elderly. *Virchows Arch (A)*, 422, 7–15.

O'Connor, K. A., Holman, D. J., & Wood, J. W. (1998). Declining fecundity and ovarian ageing in natural fertility populations. *Maturitas*, 30, 127–136.

O'Hagan, A., & Forster, J. J. (2004). *Bayesian inference*. London: Hodder Arnold.

Olofsson, P., & Kimmel, M. (1999). Stochastic models of telomere shortening. *Mathematical Biosciences*, 158, 75–92.

O'Neill, P. D. (2002). A tutorial introduction to Bayesian inference for stochastic epidemic models using Markov chain Monte Carlo methods. *Mathematical Biosciences*, 180, 103–114.

Parker, G. A., & Smith, J. M. (1990). Optimality Theory in Evolutionary Biology. *Nature*, 348, 27–33.

Peccei, J. S. (1995). A hypothesis for the origin and evolution of menopause. *Maturitas*, 21, 83–89.

Pletcher, S. D., & Curtsinger, J. W. (1998). Mortality plateaus and the evolution of senescence: Why are old-age mortality rates so low? *Evolution*, 52, 454–464.

Proctor, C. J., & Kirkwood, T. B. L. (2002). Modelling telomere shortening and the role of oxidative stress. *Mechanisms of Ageing & Development*, 123, 351–363.

Proctor, C. J., & Kirkwood, T. B. L. (2003). Modelling cellular senescence as a result of telomere state. *Aging Cell*, 2, 151–157.

Proctor, C. J., Söti, C., Boys, R. J., Gillespie, C. S., Shanley, D. P., Wilkinson, D. J., & Kirkwood, T. B. L. (2005). Modelling the actions of chaperones and their role in ageing. *Mechanisms of Ageing & Development*, 126, 119–131.

Rincon, M., Muzumdar, R., Atzmon, G., & Barzilai, N. (2004). The paradox of the insulin/IGF-1 signaling pathway in longevity. *Mechanisms of Ageing & Development*, 125, 397–403.

Rogers, A. R. (1993). Why menopause. *Evolutionary Ecology*, 7, 406–420.

Romanyukha, A. A., & Yashin, A. I. (2003). Age related changes in population of peripheral T cells: towards a model of immunosenescence. *Mechanisms of Ageing & Development*, 124, 433–443.

Rubelj, I., & Vondracek, Z. (1999). Stochastic mechanism of cellular aging: abrupt telomere shortening as a model for stochastic nature of cellular aging. *Journal of Theoretical Biology*, 197, 425–438.

Sacks, J., Welch, W., Mitchell, T., & Wynn, H. (1989). Design and analysis of computer experiments. *Statistical Science*, 4, 409–435.

Schaffer, W. M. (1983). The application of optimal control theory to the general life history problem. *American Naturalist*, 121, 418–431.

Sear, R., Steele, F., McGregor, A. A., & Mace, R. (2002). The effects of kin on child mortality in rural Gambia. *Demography*, 39, 43–63.

Shanley, D. P., & Kirkwood, T. B. L. (2000). Calorie restriction and aging: a life-history analysis. *Evolution*, 54, 740–750.

Shanley, D. P., & Kirkwood, T. B. L. (2001). Evolution of the human menopause. *Bioessays*, 23, 282–287.

Sidorov, I. A., Gee, D., & Dimitrov, D. S. (2004). A kinetic model of telomere shortening in infants and adults. *Journal of Theoretical Biology*, 226, 169–175.

Sinclair, D. A. (2002). Paradigms and pitfalls of yeast longevity research. *Mechanisms of Ageing & Development*, 123, 857–867.

Sozou, P. D., & Kirkwood, T. B. L. (2001). A stochastic model of cell replicative senescence based on telomere shortening, oxidative stress, and somatic mutations in nuclear and mitochondrial DNA. *Journal of Theoretical Biology*, 213, 573–586.

Sozou, P. D., & Seymour, R. M. (2004). To age or not to age. *Proceedings of the Royal Society of London Series B-Biological Sciences*, 271, 457–463.

Szilard, L. (1959). On the nature of the aging process. *Proceedings of the National Academy of Sciences of the USA*, 45, 35–45.

Tan, Q., Yashin, A. I., Christensen, K., Jeune, B., De Benedictis, G., Kruse, T. A., & Vaupel, J. W. (2004). Multidisciplinary approaches in genetic studies of human aging and longevity. *Current Genomics*, 5, 409–416.

Tan, Z. (1999a). Intramitotic and intraclonal variation in proliferative potential of human diploid cells: Explained by telomere shortening. *Journal of Theoretical Biology*, 198, 259–268.

Tan, Z. (1999b). Telomere shortening and the population size-dependency of life span of human cell culture: further implication for two proliferation-restricting telomeres. *Experimental Gerontology*, 34, 831–842.

Tan, Z. (2001). Simulated shortening of proliferation-restricting telomeres during clonal proliferation and senescence of human cells. *Experimental Gerontology*, 36, 89–97.

Taylor, R. W., Barron, M. J., Borthwick, G. M., Gospel, A., Chinnery, P. F., Samuels, D. C., Taylor, G. A., Plusa, S. M., Needham, S. J., Greaves, L. C., Kirkwood, T. B. L., Turnbull, D. M. (2003). Mitochondrial DNA mutations in human colonic crypt stem cells. *Journal of Clinical Investigation*, 112(9), 1351–1360.

Teriokhin, A. T. (1998). Evolutionary optimal age schedule of repair: computer modelling of energy partition between current and future survival and reproduction. *Evolutionary Ecology*, 12, 291–307.

van Leeuwen, I. M. M., Kelpin, F. D. L., & Kooijman, S. (2002). A mathematical model that accounts for the effects of caloric restriction on body weight and longevity. *Biogerontology*, 3, 373–381.

Vaupel, J. W., Baudisch, A., Dolling, M., Roach, D. A., & Gampe, J. (2004). The case for negative senescence. *Theoretical Population Biology*, 65, 339–351.

Vaupel, J. W., Carey, J. R., Christensen, K., Johnson, T. E., Yashin, A. I., Holm, N. V., Iachine, I. A., Kannisto, V., Khazaeli, A. A., Liedo, P., Longo, V. D., Zeng, Y., Manton, K. G., & Curtsinger, J. W. (1998). Biodemographic trajectories of longevity. *Science*, 280, 855–860.

von Dassow, G., Meir, E., Munro, E. M., & Odell, G. M. (2000). The segment polarity network is a robust developmental module. *Nature*, 406, 188–192.

von Zglinicki, T., Pilger, R., & Sitte, N. (2000). Accumulation of single-strand breaks is the major cause of telomere shortening in human fibroblasts. *Free Radical Biology & Medicine*, 28, 64–74.

von Zglinicki, T., Saretzki, G., Docke, W., & Lotze, C. (1995). Mild hyperoxia shortens telomeres and inhibits proliferation of fibroblasts: a model for senescence. *Experimental Cell Research*, 220, 186–193.

Weber, M., & Kindler, E. (2003). Petri net technology for communication-based systems: Advances in Petri nets. In H. Weber (Ed.), *The Petri Net Markup Language* (pp. 124–144). Heidelberg: Springer-Verlag.

Westendorp, R. G. J., & Kirkwood, T. B. L. (1998). Human longevity at the cost of reproductive success. *Nature*, 396, 743–746.

Williams, G. C. (1957). Pleiotropy, natural selection, and the evolution of senescence. *Evolution*, 11.

Section II:

Non-Mammalian Models

Chapter 13

Dissecting the Processes of Aging Using the Nematode *Caenorhabditis elegans*

Samuel T. Henderson, Shane L. Rea, and Thomas E. Johnson

Genetic variants that live longer than parental strains seem more likely than shorter-lived variants to be altered in primary rate-limiting processes that determine life-span.

—Johnson & Wood, 1982

I. Introduction

A. *Caenorhabditis elegans* as a Model System for the Analysis of Biological Function

Genetic analysis of *C. elegans* was initiated by the epic paper of Sydney Brenner (Brenner, 1974) in which the entire genetic map of "the worm" was first published. This paper also set the "style" for *C. elegans* research and described about 30 years of work, much of it from the hands of the author himself. Similar seminal papers described the cell lineage of all 959 cells making up the soma and reproductive system (Kimble & Hirsh, 1979; Sulston & Horvitz, 1977), the systematic cloning of the genome (Coulson *et al.*, 1988), the entire DNA sequence (*C. elegans* Sequencing Consortium, 1998), a description of a gene expression "map" using microarrays (Kim *et al.*, 2001), and

an analysis of gene function using whole-genome RNAi libraries (Kamath & Ahringer, 2003). In little more than 30 years, this lowly round worm has become, arguably, the best genetic model system among metazoa, and certainly the best species in which to study the genetics of aging. Soon after the founding of the National Institute on Aging in 1974, a Request for Applications (RFA) was issued stating that "Applications for work on genetic analyses of aging in *C. elegans* . . . . are welcome." This RFA was a harbinger of the future impact of this species on the understanding of the processes of aging, the subject of this chapter. Throughout its relatively brief history, the study of *C. elegans* has relied on current methodology in both molecular genetics and in computer sciences, the first allowing the breakthroughs and the second allowing the wide dissemination of the results and rapid access to biological materials and information. These resources continue to be developed with centralized bioinformatics resources (http://www.wormbase.org) and genetic stocks maintained by the *C. elegans* Genetics Center.

B. *C. elegans* as a Model for Aging

C. elegans represents a relative newcomer among model genetic systems used in the study of aging. In fact, the species was not even listed in the Index in the first edition of the *Handbook of the Biology of Aging* in 1977. However, a full chapter appeared in the next three editions (Johnson, 1990a; Lithgow, 1996; Russell & Jacobson, 1985); but the absence of a chapter in the fifth edition, during a time of massive discoveries, leaves a huge amount of work to be described and integrated by the authors of this chapter. Prior to 1982, the worm was used as a model for only a few aging studies, especially into altered rates of protein synthesis during aging and effects of drug interventions on longevity (Epstein & Gershon, 1972; Rothstein, 1980). Undoubtedly, the main reason for the prevalence of aging research on *C. elegans* ("the worm") in recent years has been the ability to use increased longevity as a gold standard for detecting genetic alterations that change the aging process, as highlighted by the excerpt serving as the frontispiece of this chapter. The tremendous success of the genetic approach to dissecting aging processes is noted by the fact that some 200 or more genes have now been found to extend life as a result of hypomorphic (reduced function) mutations in the worm. These results are now commonplace, a far cry from the way that the first gerontogene in the worm was greeted in 1983 (Klass, 1983). (We will use the term *gerontogene* [Rattan, 1985] to refer to genes in which one or more alleles extend life over that of the wildtype strain, N2 Bristol.) This definition is necessarily broad in that it encompasses both gain-and loss-of-function mutations. An alternate term, *longevity assurance gene* (Lag), coined by Jazwinski (D'Mello *et al.*, 1994), wrongly implies that hypomorphic mutants should be life shortening, and thus is an incorrect approbation for these genes, which lead to life extension and slowed aging when hypomorphic. We will also refer to the long-life phenotype associated with any gerontogene as "Age." A word of caution: the success of *C. elegans* research and the many highly cited publications in journals such as *Science* and *Nature* have resulted in an oversell of the worm (and perhaps invertebrate models in general), and many results stemming from this research have yet to be shown to be relevant to human aging. Such problems have been highlighted elsewhere (Austad, 2005; Johnson, 2003).

In the present review we have attempted to cover most topics relevant to *C. elegans* aging research that have occurred within the last eight years. Due to space restrictions, we could not be exhaustive, and so we apologize to our colleagues if their work has not received mention. Although the vast majority of researchers in *C. elegans* are geneticists, we anticipate that the readers of this chapter are not, so we have attempted to define specialized genetic terms wherever used. More than 50 reviews of *C. elegans* aging studies have been published, focusing especially on the identification and interpretation of mutants that lead to life extension (Braeckman *et al.*, 2002; Finkel & Holbrook, 2000; Gershon & Gershon, 2001; Guarente & Kenyon, 2000; Hekimi & Guarente, 2003; Johnson, 2003; Johnson *et al.*, 2000; Johnson *et al.*, 2001; Kirkwood & Austad, 2000; Lithgow, 2001; Longo & Finch, 2003; Martin *et al.*, 1996; Murakami *et al.*, 2000; Rea & Johnson, 2003; Tatar *et al.*, 2003; Tavernarakis & Driscoll, 2002; Van Voorhies, 2001b). Other areas studied in such reviews include resistance to stress, particularly reactive oxidants, and metabolic alterations leading to increased longevity. Moreover, automated resources such as PubMed allow ready identification of papers over all of this period.

II. Biology of *C. elegans*

In the laboratory, *C. elegans* is typically raised at 20 °C on a simple *Escheriscia coli* diet, where an average wildtype hermaphrodite will develop from egg to adult (by way of four larval stages, termed L1 to L4) in 3 days, produce 250 to 300 eggs over the next 3 to 4 days, and live another 10 to 30 days. Timing of these life-history traits is dependent on temperature, since the worm can be grown and maintained over the range of 10 to 25.5 °C (Klass, 1977; Figures 13.1A and B). When growth conditions become limiting, an alternative third-larval stage, known as a *dauer*, serves as a migratory form, allowing worms to find new sites of bacteria in their native soil environment. The dauer stage provides a "timeout" from normal reproduction and aging and can enhance the survival of an individual by months (Klass & Hirsh, 1976).

There are two sexes in the worm—males and self-fertilizing hermaphrodites—and they age differently (Gems & Riddle, 2000; Johnson & Hutchinson, 1993; Johnson & Wood, 1982). As expected, due to its self-fertilizing nature, *C. elegans* does not show hybrid vigor (Johnson & Hutchinson, 1993; Johnson & Wood, 1982). Aging worms display many behavioral, morphological, and molecular signs of senescence (Johnson, 1990a; Lithgow, 1996; Russell & Jacobson, 1985). Behavioral signs of aging are first evident as decreases in spontaneous or stimulated movement, eating, and defecation rates. Eventually, animals stop moving and defecating altogether (Bolanowski *et al.*, 1981). Although old animals may not move, they still respond to gentle prodding, and they can persist in this state for several days. Death is identified by a lack of spontaneous movement, a lack of response to touch, loss of turgor pressure, and visible tissue degeneration due to bacterial invasion (Johnson & Wood, 1982). Movement has been considered as a marker for robustness and for age or aging itself; indeed the rate of decline in movement is a predictor of life expectancy (see Figure 13.1B, Johnson, 1987; Figure 13.1C, Herndon *et al.*, 2002).

Morphological changes also become evident as worms age. Old worms look old. Old animals take on a mottled, less-defined look and begin to accumulate dark pigments and lipofuscin (Bolanowski *et al.*, 1981; Klass, 1977). Closer examination reveals tissue degeneration, cell vacuoles, and tissue borders of uncertain distinction (see Figure 13.2) (Garigan *et al.*, 2002; Herndon *et al.*, 2002). Section VII.C will discuss these changes in more detail. More extensive reviews of the general biology of *C. elegans* are available in book form (Riddle *et al.*, 1997; Wood, 1988).

III. The *age-1* Pathway

A. Historical Background

Molecular genetic analysis of aging in *C. elegans* began with the startling discovery of the first gerontogene. Michael Klass (1983) identified long-lived mutants using a brute-force approach that few have utilized since (Duhon *et al.*, 1996). The mutants he found all were in a single genetic locus, subsequently named *age-1*, and were mapped and characterized by the Johnson and Ruvkun laboratories (Friedman & Johnson, 1988a,b; Johnson, 1990b; Morris *et al.*, 1996). Key to the rapid expansion of interest in these Age mutants was the demonstration that *age-1* and another Age mutant, called *daf-2* (DAuer Formation), both lengthened the life of adult worms and, in addition, affected the differentiation of the long-lived dauer

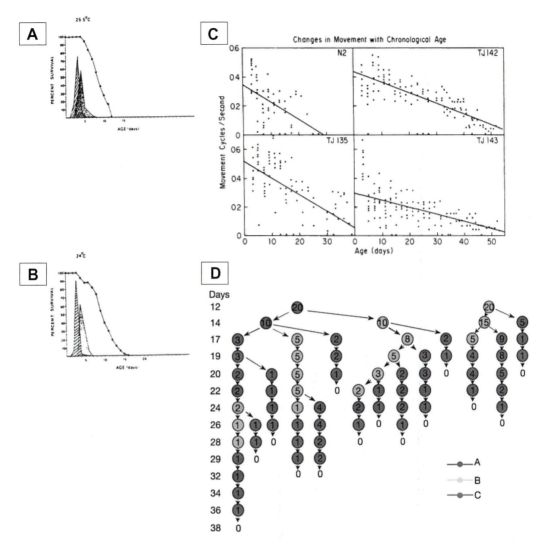

Figure 13.1 Aging in *C. elegans*. Panels A and B depict survival curves for wildtype *C. elegans* hermaphrodites raised at 25.5 °C (panel A) or 24 °C (panel B). Lines represent fraction surviving at given interval after hatching (time 0). Note extension of life span by lowered temperature. Hatched regions represent fertilized eggs laid during each time interval. Shaded regions represent unfertilized eggs (oocytes) laid during each time interval. Life span quickly declines once reproduction has ceased. Reprinted from *Mechanisms of Ageing and Development*, Volume 6, M. R. Klass, "Aging in the nematode Caenorhabditis elegans: major biological and environmental factors influencing life span," pp. 413–429, Copyright 1977, with permission from Elsevier. Panel C depicts how decline in movement correlates with increasing chronological age. Long-lived strains of *C. elegans* not only show a slowed rate of aging but also a slowed rate of movement decline that predicts the life expectancy and maximum life span of each strain. Reprinted from *Proceedings of the National Academy of Sciences of the USA*, 84(11), T. E. Johnson, "Aging can be genetically dissected into component processes using long-lived lines of Caenorhabditis elegans," pp. 3777–3781, Copyright 1987, with permission from author.Panel D shows classification of wildtype *C. elegans* based on movement at 12 days of age and older (described in text). Class A animals move spontaneously, class B animals move only when prodded, class C animals are alive but move only the head when gently prodded. Individual animals typically transit through each class before death. Entry into class C is a redictor of death. Reprinted from *Nature*, Volume 419, L. A. Herndon, P. J. Schmeissner, J. M. Dudaronek, P. A. Brown, K. M. Listner, Y. Sakano, M. C. Paupard, D. H. Hall, &M. Driscoll, "Stochastic and genetic factors influence tissue-specific decline in ageing C. elegans," pp. 808–814, Copyright 2002, with permission from Nature Publishing Group.

larva (Kenyon *et al.*, 1993; Malone *et al.*, 1996).

B. Brief Overview of the Insulin/IGF-Like Signaling (IIS) Pathway

The insulin/insulin-like growth factor (IGF) signaling (IIS) pathway is evolutionarily ancient and is found in species ranging from worms and flies to humans. Central to this pathway is a plasma membrane–bound tyrosine kinase (DAF-2 in worms [capital letters signify the protein]) that acts to transduce signals to responsive tissue following activation by insulin or insulin-like ligands. In the worm, there are 37 genes that encode putative insulin-like (*ins*) molecules (Pierce *et al.*, 2001). The IIS pathway is also comprised of several sequentially acting components, all of which are present

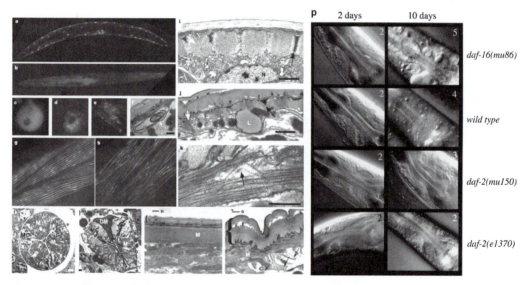

Figure 13.2 Old worms look old. Panels **a-o** depict tissue deterioration in aging *C. elegans*. Reprinted from *Nature*, Volume 419, L. A. Herndon, P. J. Schmeissner, J. M. Dudaronek, P. A. Brown, K. M. Listner, Y. Sakano, M. C. Paupard, D. H. Hall, & M. Driscoll, "Stochastic and genetic factors influence tissue-specific decline in ageing C. elegans," pp. 808–814, Copyright 2002, with permission from Nature Publishing Group. Panels **a-e** depict animals carrying a p_{myo}-3::GFP/NLS transgene, which expresses nuclear localized green fluorescent protein (GFP) in body-wall muscle cells. (**a**) Whole worm at day 8. (**b**) Whole worm at day 14. Note loss of nuclear GFP signal due to fragmentation of nuclear structure over time. (**c-e**) Individual muscle nuclei at days 7, 12, and 18, respectively. (**f**) A rare muscle nucleus (arrow) undergoing autophagy at day 18. (**g**, **h**) Body wall muscle sarcomeres as detected by a p_{myo-3}MYO-3/GFP translational fusion, highlighting myosin heavy chain A. Sarcomeres are shown at days 4 and 18, respectively. Note extensive deterioration. (**i–k**) Electron micrograph (EM) cross-sections of body wall muscle (M = muscle, MC = marginal cells, DM = deteriorated muscle, L = lipid inclusion). (**i**) Day 4, white arrow indicates sarcomere. (**j**) Day 18, note loss of sarcomere volume. (**k**) Frayed sarcomere from a day 18 animal. (**l**, **m**) EM cross-section of pharynx of day 4 and 18 animals, respectively. Note extensive disorganization. (**n**, **o**) EM cross-section of cuticle, day 4 and 18, respectively. (**p**) Reprinted from *Genetics*, 161(3), D. Garigan, A. L. Hsu, A. G. Fraser, R. S. Kamath, J. Ahringer, & C. Kenyon, "Genetic analysis of tissue aging in Caenorhabditis elegans: a role for heat-shock factor and bacterial proliferation," pp. 1101–1112, Copyright 2002, The Gerontological Society of America, reproduced by permission of the publisher. Panels depict tissue deterioration over time in different mutant backgrounds. Left panels show animals at 2 days of adulthood; right panels show animals at 10 days of adulthood. Note extensive tissue degeneration in the absence of *daf-16*, whereas conversely, decreasing *daf-2* function preserves tissue integrity. Numbers in upper right corner represent score of tissue deterioration on a scale of 1 to 5.

in the worm: an insulin receptor substrate (IRS-1), a phosphatidylinositol-3-kinase (AGE-1), a phosphoinosotide dependent kinase (PDK-1), a serum glucocorticoid kinase (SGK-1), two protein kinase B homologs (also known as akt) (AKT-1/2), and a forkhead transcription factor (DAF-16) (see Figure 13.3C). A phosphatase (DAF-18 in worms and homologous to the human tumor suppressor PTEN) also acts to counter the activity of AGE-1. The role of this pathway in nematode aging has been extensively reviewed (Guarente & Kenyon, 2000). Most importantly, reducing the function of many components of this signaling module invokes prolonged life span and/or dauer formation. In *C. elegans*, bioinformatics and molecular analyses have predicted most of the functions of this signaling module in the absence of any biochemical experiments. Molecular studies in *C. elegans* have focused largely on the downstream target of this pathway—namely, DAF-16.

C. Details on the IIS Module

Inhibition of *daf-2* by mutation or RNA interference can dramatically increase mean life span up to 150 percent (Gems *et al.*, 1998). DAF-2 is the sole member of the insulin/IGF receptor tyrosine kinase family in *C. elegans* (Rikke *et al.*, 2000). Although other putative insulin-like receptors have been identified, they lack a tyrosine kinase domain and have no known functions (Dlakic, 2002). Like the mammalian insulin receptor, DAF-2 is a single-pass transmembrane receptor with an extracellular ligand binding domain and an intracellular tyrosine kinase domain. The tyrosine kinase domain is well conserved between human and worm, sharing six out of eight critical catalytic residues and containing conservative substitutions at the remaining two sites. Mutations have also been identified within the kinase domain that increase

life span. For example, the commonly used *daf-2(e1370)* allele is a P1465S mutation within the kinase domain (Kimura *et al.*, 1997). The temperature-sensitive alleles of *daf-2* have been separated into two classes (I and II) based on the severity of their associated phenotype (Gems *et al.*, 1998). All class I alleles are dauer formation-constitutive (Daf-c), Age, intrinsically thermo-tolerant (Itt), and exhibit low levels of L1 larval arrest at 25.5°C. Class 2 mutants exhibit the class 1 defects as well as some or all of the following: reduced adult motility, abnormal adult body and gonad morphology, high levels of embryonic and L1 arrest, production of progeny late in life, and reduced brood size (Gems *et al.*, 1998).

Mutation of any one of several downstream components in the IIS pathway also slows the rate of aging and increases mean life span. *age-1* (PI3Kinase) mutants live 65 percent longer (Johnson, 1990b). Similarly, alteration of *pdk-1* increases mean life span by 60 percent (Paradis *et al.*, 1999). *C. elegans* contains two homologues of mammalian akt, called *akt-1* and *akt-2*, that appear to be functionally redundant (Paradis & Ruvkun, 1998). It is possible to inactivate both genes by either co-injecting double-stranded RNA (dsRNA) into adult animals and examining the resulting progeny, which form dauers constitutively (Daf-c) and localize DAF-16 to the nucleus (Henderson & Johnson, 2001), or by feeding *akt-2(ok393)* (a knockout allele of *akt-2*) bacteria expressing dsRNA to *akt-1*, which increases life expectancy about 20 percent (Hertweck *et al.*, 2004). (This method of inhibiting gene function is called RNAi and is described in more detail in section IV.B). The dauer observation illustrates the important point that most IIS pathway mutations are hypomorphic so that growth at 25.5 °C results in a Daf-c phenotype because dauer formation is intrinsically temperature sensitive (Riddle & Albert, 1997).

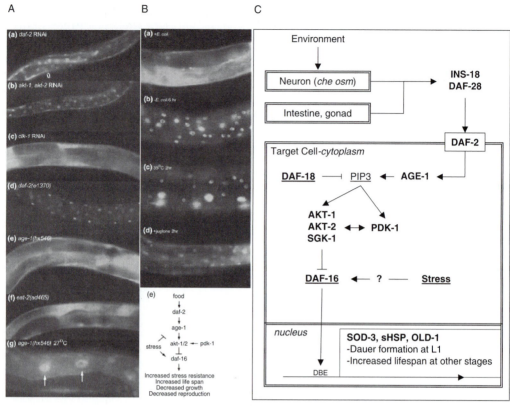

Figure 13.3   Insulin/IGF-like signaling (IIS) in *C. elegans*. Panels A and B are reprinted from *Current Biology*, Volume 11, No 24, S. T. Henderson and T. E. Johnson, "Daf-16 integrates developmental and environmental inputs to mediate aging in the nematode *Caenorhabditis elegans*," pp. 1975–1980, Copyright 2001, with permission from Elsevier. Panels A (a)–(g) depict animals carrying a DAF-16::GFP fusion transgene in the presence of the listed RNAi or mutant genetic background. Note nuclear localization of DAF-16::GFP following reduction of the IIS components DAF-2 and AKT-1/2. Panel B (a)–(d) depicts strong nuclear localization of DAF-16::GFP fusion protein in response to indicated stressors. Panel B(e) depicts model of DAF-16 as "gerontostat." Panel C gives an overview of the IIS pathway. IIS influences both dauer entry at the L1 stage and life span at other stages. Environmental conditions, such as food availability, are sensed primarily through ciliated sensory neurons located in the head and tail. These sensory neurons secrete insulin-like peptides (for example, INS-18 and DAF-28) in response to environmental cues. Other tissues, such as intestinal or gonadal cells, may also secrete insulin-like peptides acting either as agonists or antagonists to the single insulin/IGF-like receptor, DAF-2. Positive signaling through DAF-2 activates a conserved series of kinases (AKT-1/2, PDK-1, and SGK-1), which phosphorylate and negatively regulate the DAF-16 transcription factor. The mechanism of inhibition is sequestration in the cytoplasm and the result is shortened life span. Inhibition of IIS allows DAF-16 to accumulate in the nucleus, thereby activating or repressing a series of target genes, resulting in life-span extension. Genes upregulated by DAF-16 include *sod-3* (a mitochondrial superoxide dismutase), several members of the small heat shock genes (sHSP), and OLD-1, a tyrosine kinase. Inhibition of IIS may occur at many points, from improper sensory neuron development (for example, mutations in *che* and *osm* genes) to mutations directly in components of the IIS pathway, such as *daf-2, age-1, sgk-1*, and *pdk-1* mutations. DAF-16 may also be directly activated by stress by an unknown mechanism. **DAF-2,** insulin/IGF-1 receptor-like tyrosine kinase; **AGE-1,** phosphaditylinositol-3-kinase; **DAF-18,** PTEN homolog; **PDK-1,** phosphoinsotide dependent kinase; **SGK-1,** serum glucocorticoid kinase; **AKT-1/2,** protein kinase B homologs 1 and 2 (also known as PKB); **DAF-16,** FOXO-like forkhead transcription factor; PIP3, phosphoinositide-3-phosphate.

As mentioned, *C. elegans* contains a large family of insulin-like sequences. The genes frequently are found in clusters and were likely derived from recent duplication events. The gene family shares roughly 25 to 40 percent amino acid identity, yet they all contain signatures of insulin-like molecules: A and B chains and the potential to form at least three disulfide bonds. Consistent with a role of integrating environmental cues, many of the *ins* genes are expressed in sensory neurons or other neuronal cells (Pierce *et al.*, 2001) (see also section III.D). Given the large number of insulins, some may function as agonists, whereas others function as antagonists of the DAF-2 receptor. Therefore, some are predicted to shorten life span, whereas others may increase life span. This appears to be the case. For example, increased dosage of *ins-1* has been shown to promote dauer formation and increase life span, suggesting it acts as an antagonist (Pierce *et al.*, 2001). Conversely, *ins-18* may function as an agonist. Inhibition of *ins-18* results in an approximately 30 to 40 percent increase in mean life span (Kawano *et al.*, 2000).

Another possible DAF-2 agonist is encoded by *daf-28*. *daf-28* was first isolated as a mutant, causing transient dauer arrest and a modest increase in life span (10 percent) (Malone & Thomas, 1994). Li and colleagues later identified DAF-28 as an insulin-like protein that was expressed in two pairs of sensory neurons (ASI and ASJ) (Li *et al.*, 2003). Importantly, the expression of a *daf-28*::GFP fusion was found to be downregulated by dauer-inducing environmental cues—that is, starvation and exposure to crude dauer pheromone extracts dramatically decreased its expression. These findings draw a parallel between *daf-28* and mammalian insulin signaling, where in both instances conditions suitable for reproductive development are biochemically announced. The modest effects of *daf-28*

mutation on increasing nematode life span may be related to the redundancy and complex expression pattern of the *ins* genes in *C. elegans* (Li *et al.*, 2003; Pierce *et al.*, 2001).

Recently, a homolog of mammalian serum- and glucocorticoid-inducible kinase (SGK) was identified in *C. elegans*. SGK kinases are similar in sequence to AKT kinases, and in mammals they are thought to function in IIS through direct regulation of the mammalian homologs of DAF-16 (Brunet *et al.*, 2001). Analogously, in *C. elegans*, SGK-1 may act in a complex with AKT-1/2 and function to directly phosphorylate DAF-16, thereby preventing the latter's nuclear entry and shortening life span. Inhibition of *sgk-1* by RNA interference increased life span by approximately 70 percent (Hertweck *et al.*, 2004).

A major function of active IIS is to phosphorylate DAF-16, thereby excluding it from the nucleus (see Figure 13.3A a–g). Conversely, inhibition of IIS causes nuclear localization of DAF-16, leading to increased stress resistance and life span (Henderson & Johnson, 2001; Lee *et al.*, 2001; Lin *et al.*, 2001). As indicated above, inhibition of *daf-2* by mutation or RNA interference can more than double mean life span; the precise degree depends on the site of mutation and/or other manipulations. Increases in both stress resistance and longevity are, however, lost in *daf-16;daf-2* double mutants (Arantes-Oliveira *et al.*, 2003; Kenyon *et al.*, 1993). This epistasis of *daf-16* logically means that DAF-16 functions later in the pathway than does DAF-2 (i.e., DAF-16 is downstream of DAF-2), and it illustrates the fundamental role this transcription factor has in specifying life span.

D. Upstream Input into the IIS Pathway

Soil is the natural habitat of the free-living nematode *C. elegans*, and when a food source is exhausted, or in response to other adverse conditions (such as high temperature or overcrowding), an alternative developmental program called the *dauer pathway* is activated. The decision to suspend reproductive development and instead become a long-lived, growth-arrested dauer is made at the first larval stage (L1). Adverse conditions are sensed by chemosensory and thermosensitive mechanisms, whereas overcrowding is detected by the local concentration of a lipid soluble pheromone secreted by L1 animals (see Riddle & Albert, 1997). All this information is integrated into the decision to form a dauer. The dauer larvae functions as a dispersal form and exhibits behaviors that are adaptive to this end, such as nictation, in which dauers move to the surface and stand on end, extending themselves into the air sometimes as far as a few inches by making long ropes of multiple dauers. Dauers do not feed, are stress resistant, and can live six to nine times longer than adults. If dauer larvae are dispersed to a new, more favorable environment, they will resume development and become fertile adult animals with normal life spans. Therefore, dauers are often considered to be a non-aging, or at the most, a very slow-aging form (Klass & Hirsh, 1976).

The decision to enter the dauer larval stage has been extensively studied (for an overview see Riddle & Albert, 1997). It consists of multiple parallel pathways that integrate sensory input into the final decision. Genetic and molecular analyses have revealed that the dauer pathway consists of two main arms, corresponding to the IIS pathway and a transforming growth factor beta (TGFβ) pathway. Formation of the dauer can be considered the default pathway since active signaling by the IIS and TGFβ modules are required to prevent dauer formation. Therefore, mutations in many dauer genes, such as *daf-28*, result in constitutive dauer formation (Daf-c). Other genes are required to form and maintain the dauer, and mutations in these genes

result in a dauer-defective phenotype (Daf-d).

C. elegans senses its outside environment primarily through ciliated sensory neurons located in the head and tail. The major sensory neurons in the head are contained within paired structures called *amphids*. Each amphid contains the ciliated endings of 12 sensory neurons, a sheath cell and a socket cell, which together form a pore to the exterior. Phasmids are minor sensory organs located in the tail and have a similar structure to the amphids (Chalfie & White, 1988). These sensory neurons are used to monitor the environment, and they function toward both aversive stimuli and attractants, such as bacteria (food) and chemical messengers like pheromones.

Many genes have been identified that affect the function and development of sensory neurons. These include classes of genes that affect the animal's ability to detect a variety of chemical stimuli (*che*) and changes in osmolarity (*osm*). Mutations in these genes give rise to animals that are impaired in their ability to detect their environment. These animals frequently demonstrate a Daf-c phenotype at elevated temperature (27 °C) (Vowels & Thomas, 1992). For example, mutations in any of a number of *che* and *osm* genes, such as *che-2*, *che-11*, *che-13*, *osm-1*, *osm-5*, and *osm-6*, result in greater than 90 percent dauer formation at 27 °C (Apfeld & Kenyon, 1999). If these animals are raised at lower temperatures, they do not form dauers, but are long-lived. For example, *che-2(e1033)* animals live approximately 43 percent longer than wildtype at 20 °C. Other *che* and *osm* mutants behave similarly, with some exhibiting more than a doubling of life span, such as *che-3(p801)* 100 percent, *che-11(e1810)* 45 percent, *osm-1(p808)* 37 percent, and *osm-5(p813)* 120 percent. In addition, several mutants are known in which the amphids do not develop properly, such as *mec-8(e398)*, which exhibits a ~59 percent increase in life span. In nematodes, it is possible to directly test the role of amphids in life span by ablating the structures with a laser. Such sensory-deprived worms live approximately 33 percent longer than non-ablated animals (Apfeld & Kenyon, 1999).

The Daf-c phenotype of many Che and Osm mutants suggests that their increased life span may be regulated by one of the dauer genes. In fact, all of the increases in dauer formation and longevity in the *che* and *osm* mutants were found to be suppressed by mutations in *daf-16*, the paragon Daf-d gene (Apfeld & Kenyon, 1999). The dependence of *daf-16* on life-span extension suggests that sensory cues are transmitted through insulin-like signaling to influence life span (see Figure 13.3C).

E. DAF-16

Modulating DAF-16 transcriptional activity is a major function of insulin signaling in *C. elegans* and, as described above, nuclear localized DAF-16 plays a necessary role in increased longevity. A key role for *daf-16* in regulating changes to environmental inputs was demonstrated by Henderson and Johnson (2001), who found that several different environmental stressors caused nuclear localization of DAF-16 (see Figure 13.3B a–d). Additionally, the authors demonstrated that simply increasing the dosage of *daf-16* resulted in increased stress resistance and life span, while at the same time slowed growth and reproduction (Henderson & Johnson, 2001). Both of these outcomes are consistent with DAF-16 functioning as a "gerontostat," a regulator of aging. DAF-16 has exactly the right properties for regulating response to hard times, as predicted by evolutionary theories of aging. Under conditions conducive to growth and

reproduction. DAF-16 is phosphorylated by the action of the upstream IIS elements and is consequently found in the cytoplasm. The result is reproduction, normal levels of stress resistance, and a normal life span. Under difficult conditions, especially reduced food concentration, DAF-16 instead moves to the nucleus, where it stimulates the synthesis of many transcripts leading to stress resistance and increased longevity (see Table 13.1). If these signals occur early enough in life, then DAF-16 stimulates dauer formation in response to environmental stress. Kenyon has postulated multiple downstream targets for the IIS pathway at various stages of life in her models of an active death program causing aging (Alcedo & Kenyon, 2004) but, using Occam's razor, it seems more likely that the genomic response to DAF-16 activation is merely dependent on the development stage of the worm when environmental stress is encountered. We suggest that the primary role of IIS and DAF-16 is not to cause aging but to regulate the worm's response to stress and its metabolic reserves.

Given the importance of DAF-16 in increasing mean life span, gene targets of DAF-16 are likely to be highly informative about the aging process. Several authors have attempted to identify targets of DAF-16 by use of DNA microarrays and computational methods. Murphy and colleagues (2003) used both mutant animals and RNA interference to look at *daf-16*-dependent changes in expression that occur when IIS is inhibited. The authors classify the genes into either Class 1 genes that are upregulated (induced) in *daf-2*, partial loss-of-function (lf) animals, or Class 2 genes that were downregulated (repressed) under the same conditions. Interestingly, among the Class 1 genes were several members of the small heat shock genes, such as *hsp-16.1*, *hsp-12.6*, *hsp-16.11*, *sip-1*, and *hsp-16.2*. Some of

Table 13.1
Genes Regulated by DAF-16

Gene (Size Amino Acids)	Closest Match in Human	% Identity/% Homology Size (Amino Acids)	E Value	Function in C. elegans	Function in Humans
ctl-1 (497)[a]	catalase (527)	63%/76% (489)	0.0	Cytoplasmic catalase	Peroxisomal[a]
ctl-2 (500)[a]	catalase (527)	63%/79% (494)	0.0	Peroxisomal catalase	Peroxisomal[b]
mtl-1 (75)	metallothionein 3 (68)	40%/47% (59)	2e-06	Metallothionein, metal detoxification/ homeostasis	Antioxidant protective against various ROS
sod-3 (218)[c]	SOD2 (222)	61%/76% (217)	1e-77	Mitochondrial Mn SOD	Mitochondrial Mn SOD
vit-2 (1613)[d]	APOB (4563***)	19%/36% (935)	4e-06	Yolk protein	Main apolipoprotein of chylomicrons and low-density lipoproteins
vit-5 (1603)[d]	MNS1 **(495)	22%/45% (306)	1e-07	Yolk protein	Meiosis-specific nuclear structural protein

[a]There are three catalase genes in *C. elegans*: Y54G11A.6 (*ctl-1*), Y54G11A.5 (*ctl-2*), and Y54G11.13. *ctl-2* is differentially spliced. There is a single catalase gene present in the human genome.

[b]Most organisms use either a PST1 or PST2 type signal for targeting proteins to peroxisomes (PEX). *C. elegans* only contains machinery that accommodates the former. In line with this observation, *ctl-1* (and Y54G11.13) lack a PST1 type, C terminal PEX targeting signal.

[c]*C. elegans* contains two MnSODs (*sod-2* and *sod-3*) and three Cu/ZnSODs (*sod-1*, *sod-4* and *sod-5*). Humans contain three SODs (SOD1, Cu/Zn cytoplasmic; SOD2 mitochondrial MnSOD; and SOD3 Cu/Zn extracellular). *sod-2* of *C. elegans* is the best match with SOD2 in humans (63 percent identity, E: 9e-82). *sod-2* and *sod-3* of *C. elegans* share 86 percent identity. Note that there are three types of SODs: the Cu/Zn, Mn, and Fe SODs. Only the latter two are evolutionarily related.

[d]There are six vitellogenin genes in *C. elegans* (*vit-1–6*). (K09F5.2, C42D8.2, F59D8.1, F59D8.2, C04F6.1, and K07H8.6). Probably all are APOB related molecules, despite proteins such as MNS1 having higher domain homologies in the case of *vit-5* that skew BLAST results. *vit-1*, *vit-2*, and *vit-6* are most related to APOB.

these same small heat shock genes are upregulated by the hormetic treatments that increase nematode life span that are described below (section IV.A) (Cypser & Johnson, 2002; Link et al., 1999). Additionally, several other stress-related genes, including antioxidant genes, were upregulated, and these included *ctl-1* and *ctl-2* (catalases) (see Table 13.1), *mtl-1* (metallothionein-related cadmium binding protein), and *sod-3* (superoxide dismutase) (Murphy et al., 2003). Class 2 (repressed) genes included some genes with obvious roles in reproduction, such as *vit-2* and *vit-5*, two vitellogenin (yolk protein) genes. In addition, many other genes were identified as upregulated or downregulated, but speculation about what role such genes could play in *C. elegans* lifespan extension, and how they might fit into any simple aging framework, is difficult without further study.

In a separate analysis, McElwee and colleagues used microarrays to compare RNA profiles of *daf-2(e1370);glp-4(bn2)* to *daf-16(m27);daf-2(e1370);glp-4(bn2)* animals (McElwee et al., 2003). Mutations in *glp-4* were included to sterilize the animals and prevent contamination with progeny. Unfortunately, there was not a large overlap of regulated genes between the Murphy and McElwee data, a frequent problem with microarray studies. Some common genes were present. For example, McElwee and colleagues found that some classes of heat shock genes were upregulated, in particular *hsp-70* and several members of the *hsp-16* family. In addition, *sod-3* was similarly found to be upregulated. Here, both sets of results confirmed earlier work implicating *sod-3* as a DAF-16 target (Honda & Honda, 1999). Both groups used RNAi to test the role of genes identified in the microarray studies to see whether they were required for increased longevity. Murphy and colleagues generally found that many genes had small effects; typically, knocking out single genes reduced life span of *daf-2(e1370)* 10 to 15 percent, and few of the genes had strong effects. Surprisingly, in the case of *sod-3* inhibition, Murphy and colleagues found a 5 to 15 percent decrease in life span, whereas McElwee and colleagues actually observed a slight increase in life span.

From these studies it has been difficult to identify a single factor that may be leading to increased life span. Nonetheless, several candidate genes have been proposed. McElwee identified a protease (*ZK384.3*) that when inhibited in *daf-2(e1370)* animals shortened their life span 33 percent (McElwee *et al.*, 2003). Others have found that inhibition of single genes reduces *daf-2* mutants back to wildtype. For example, Melendez and colleaguesfound that inhibition of *bec-1*, the *C. elegans* ortholog of the yeast and mammalian autophagy gene *APG6/VPS30/beclin1*, reduced *daf-2(e1370)* life span back to wildtype (Melendez *et al.*, 2003). In another experiment, Okuma and colleagues also identified *scl-1*, a gene required for long life of *daf-2* mutant animals (Ookuma *et al.*, 2003). Murakami and Johnson identified the *old-1* gene as a key downstream target of DAF-16 (section VII.B). The OLD-1 protein is predicted to encode a single-pass transmembrane protein with a short extracellular domain and cytoplasmic tyrosine kinase domain. *C. elegans* contains several members of this class of tyrosine kinase that may be unique to nematodes (Rikke *et al.*, 2000). OLD-1 expression was found to be upregulated in the long-lived strains *age-1(hx546)* and *daf-2(e1370)*. Inhibition of *old-1* by RNA interference returned *daf-2(e1370)* to wildtype life span; *age-1(hx546);old-1(mk1)* double mutants also had wild-type life spans (Murakami & Johnson, 2001). In addition, increased dosage of the *old-1* gene greatly lengthened the life span of wildtype animals (Murakami & Johnson, 1998). As a tyrosine kinase, OLD-1 may function in a signaling pathway downstream of DAF-16 to influence life span. While much progress has been made on how IIS influences life span, clearly, further experimentation is required to precisely define how DAF-16 exerts such profound effects on aging.

F. Conservation of the IIS Module in Higher Animals?

Because of the central role of the IIS pathway in transmittance of environmental cues throughout *C. elegans*, it is not surprising that this pathway appears conserved and operates in a somewhat analogous function in mammals. Although this does not necessarily mean that hypomorphic mutations in mammalian IIS homologs will be long-lived, it is true that insulin signaling in mammals not only plays a critical role in maintaining glucose homeostasis (Rea & James, 1997), but it also acts to modify metabolism throughout the body in response to nutrients. In humans, for example, insulin can generally be considered to signal that nutrients are plentiful, and it promotes glucose and fat storage. When insulin signaling is decreased or inhibited, this generally signals that nutrients are limiting, so fat stores are mobilized (for an overview see (Saltiel & Kahn, 2001). Insulin-like signaling can be considered to function in a similar manner in *C. elegans*. When resources are abundant, insulin signaling is active, the dauer pathway is suppressed, and reproduction is favored. If resources are scarce, insulin signaling is reduced and the non-reproducing, dispersal, dauer form is favored. The IIS pathway is likely to function not only in the dauer decision, but also throughout the life of the animals to adjust to a changing environment (Henderson & Johnson, 2001).

The picture that has emerged from the role of insulin signaling in *C elegans* is shown in Figure 13.3, which summarizes the various findings in the worm. Increasing IIS is thought to sequester the forkhead transcription factor DAF-16 in the cytoplasm and favor reproductive development and shorter life span, whereas inhibition of IIS increases the amount of nuclear localized DAF-16 and leads to increased life span.

IV. Mutations in Mitochondrial Components

Based on the large number of deleterious mitochondrial disorders that have been detected in humans (Wallace, 1999), it seems almost heretical to propose that reducing mitochondrial electron transport chain (ETC) activity might extend life span, but in *C. elegans*, several studies suggest this to be true. The Mit (*Mit*ochondrial) class of long-lived mutants (see Table 13.2) generally contain loss-or reduced-in-function alterations in mitochondrial proteins. Almost all of these mutations directly affect components of the canonical ETC (or their proper functioning), and most exhibit a 20 to 40 percent increase in mean adult life span (reviewed in Rea & Johnson, 2003). Genetic epistasis experiments indicate that almost all of the Mit mutants tested

act independently of the insulin-like *daf-2* signaling pathway.

A. Clk Mutants

The Clock (Clk) class of mutants (named rather fancifully for abnormal functions of biological clocks (Wong *et al.*, 1995) were found to result in a modest Age phenotype (Lakowski & Hekimi, 1996). This class of mutants is heterogeneous and classified on the basis of their slow and non-synchronous rates of development and rhythmic behaviors, and also on the basis of exhibiting "maternal-effect rescue," (i.e., homozygous *clk-1* animals born of a heterozygotic hermaphrodite are wildtype). The *clk-1* mutant, which is the best characterized of the Clk family, has a defective demethoxyubiquinone (DMQ) monoxygenase, preventing synthesis of 5-hydroxyubiquinone, the penultimate intermediate of ubiquinone (Q) (Brunet *et al.*, 2001; Jonassen *et al.*, 2001; Stenmark *et al.*, 2001), and consequently accumulates significant quantities of DMQ_9. (Note that the subscript refers to the number of isoprenyl units attached to the quinone ring head group.) Early studies suggested DMQ_9 could functionally replace Q_9 as an electron acceptor at Complexes I and II, albeit less effectively in the latter instance (Miyadera *et al.*, 2001). Although measurement of the standard midpoint potentials of Q_2 (+85 mV) and DMQ_2 (+68 mV) indicated DMQ should be a less effective antioxidant than Q, that was not the case; instead, under certain conditions, DMQ had a slower oxidation rate than Q (Miyadera *et al.*, 2002) (for potential reasons see Joela *et al.*, 1997). This led to the suggestion that the life-span increase in *clk-1* nematodes might result from a reduction in the amount of life damaging reactive oxidant species (ROS) emanating from their mitochondria (Miyadera *et al.*, 2002). Substantial evidence, however, weighs against a possible role for DMQ_9 in the longevity enhancement of *clk-1*

Table 13.2
Age Genes that Affect Mitochondrial Function in *C. elegans* (Not Exhaustive)

Gene	Mutation/ RNAi	Function	Phenotype[*]	Homolog	Notes[†]	Reference
nuo-2 (T10E9.7)	RNAi	Complex I	Emb, Gro, Etv, Lva, Age[**]	–	30 kDa Subunit, alternatively spliced – T10E9.7a & b	(Dillin *et al.*, 2002)
D2030.4	RNAi	Complex I	Gro, Age	–	B18 Subunit, L4 arrest when RNAi present in egg	(Lee *et al.*, 2003)
gas-1	fc21	Complex I	Gas, Short-Lived	T26A5.3	49kDa Subunit, Complex I activity reduced by 60%, Complex II activity increased 2 fold, T26A5.3 remained undetectable	(Kayser *et al.*, 2001)
nuo-1	ua1	Complex I	Emb, Lva (L3), Age	–	51 kDa Subunit, Gonadal development arrested at L2 stage	(Tsang *et al.*, 2001)
mev-1	kn1	Complex II	Short-lived	–	Large subunit of memb-bound Cyt b (RNAi – Stp, Emb, Gro)	(Senoo-Matsuda *et al.*, 2001)
cyc-1	RNAi	Complex III	Emb, Gro, Sle, Age	–	Cytochrome c_1	(Dillin *et al.*, 2002)
isp-1	qm150	Complex III	Gro, Age	–	Reiske Iron-Sulfur Protein, RNAi – Emb, Ste	(Feng *et al.*, 2001)
F26E4.6	RNAi	Complex IV	Ste, Age	–	Subunit VII c, Lva (L2) when RNAi present in egg	(Lee *et al.*, 2003)
cco-1 (F26E4.9)	RNAi	Complex IV	Clr, Emb, Gro, Ste, Age	–	Subunit Vb	(Dillin *et al.*, 2002; Lee *et al.*, 2003)
W09C5.8	RNAi	Complex IV	Ste, Age	–	Subunit IV, also Gro when RNAi present in egg	(Lee *et al.*, 2003)
H28O16.1	RNAi	Complex V	Emb, Gro, Etv, Lva (L2/L3)	VHA-12 (vacuolar)	F1 ATPase ??- subunit (isoform 1)	(Lee *et al.*, 2003)
atp-3 (F27C1.7)	RNAi	Complex V	Emb, Lva, Age	–	ATP synthase ? – subunit (oligomycin-sensitivity conferring protein)	(Dillin *et al.*, 2002)

(continues)

Table 13.2   (Cont'd)

Gene	Mutation/ RNAi	Function	Phenotype[*]	Homolog	Notes[†]	Reference
atp-2	ua2	Complex V	Lva (L3), Age	Y49A3A.2 (vacuolar)	F1 ATPase ??- subunit, L2 arrested gonad, RNAi – Emb,Ste	(Tsang et al., 2001)
clk-1	qm30, e2519, qm51	UQ biosynthesis	Mat, Gro, Age	–	DMQ Mono-oxygenase, Bacterial UQ$_8$ is an essential dietary supplement	(Jonassen et al., 2002)
lrs-2	mg312	Mitoch. Leucine tRNA synthetase	Gro, Ste, Age	LRS-1 (cytosolic)	Adults small (L4 size), decreased pumping and defecation rates, probable null (and ETC null)	(Lee et al., 2003)
F13G3.7	RNAi	Mitoch. Carrier	Age	Y43C5B.3	probable IMM dicarboxylate (?) exchanger, RNAi effect daf-16 dependent	(Lee et al., 2003)
B0261.4	RNAi	Mitoch. Ribosomal Protein	Bmd, Emb, Gro, Age	–	Similar to mouse L47 protein, mildly Gro when RNAi present in egg	(Lee et al., 2003)

[*]Bmd: Body morphology defect; Clr: clear; Gas: Volatile-anaesthetic sensitive; Gro: Slow growth; Emb: Embryonic lethal; Etv: Embryonic terminal-arrest, variable; Lva: Larval arrest; Mat: Maternal effect; Sle: Slow embryonic development; Ste: Sterile; Stp: Sterile progeny.
[†]Subunit designations are based on *Bos Taurus* nomenclature, IMM: Inner Mitochondrial Membrane.
[**]Animals were not long lived in Lee et al., 2003.

nematodes. First, three *clk-1* alleles (*e2519*, *qm30*, and *qm50*) have been identified that all accumulate the same amount of DMQ$_9$ (Jonassen et al., 2001) but differ in the severity of both their *clk-1* lesion and corresponding increase in life span (Wong et al., 1995). Second, mice homozygous for a *clk-1* mutation developmentally arrest at day 10.5 and later die despite the presence of DMQ$_9$ (Nakai et al., 2001). Finally, more recent studies using the yeast *Saccharomyces cerevisiae* reveal DMQ cannot functionally replace Q at either Complex I or II (Padilla et al., 2004). Indeed, it is now clear that the original *clk-1* mitochondrial studies were confounded by the presence of Q$_8$ obtained from their bacterial food source, which they retained for use in their own mitochondria (Jonassen et al., 2001). Even at levels less than 5 percent that of the endogenous Q$_9$, exogenous Q$_8$ appears sufficient for both development and fertility of *clk-1* mutants. When, however, *clk-1* animals are cultured on bacteria unable to produce Q$_8$, they arrest at the L2 larval stage—strongly implying that DMQ$_9$ cannot replace a critical requirement of Q$_9$ (Jonassen et al., 2002). More recent studies in mice have similarly shown that low levels of Q_9 can overcome fetal lethality (Nakai *et al.*, 2004). If not DMQ_9, what then might be responsible for the longevity enhancement of *clk-1* animals?

Two hypotheses have recently been proposed. Santos-Ocana and colleagues (Padilla *et al.*, 2004) showed that in the yeast *S. cerevisiae*, mutations in *coq7* that corresponded to the nematode *clk-1* alleles *e2519*, *qm30*, and *qm50* resulted in a dramatic reduction in the c-type cytochromes of the ETC. The reduction in cytochrome c levels partially correlated with the severity of the mutant *coq7* allele. These researchers found that exogenous Q was sufficient to rescue both the cytochrome c phenotype and respiration, leading them to suggest that in *clk-1* nematodes, low levels of bacterial Q_8 may begin to perform a similar function and, furthermore, that this low level of ETC activity might correlate with both survival and low levels of ROS production (see section IV.D). On the contrary, though, these researchers also discovered that the presence of DMQ_8 in yeast correlated with oxidant sensitivity, not resistance as suggested by Miyadera and colleagues (2001), but that low levels of Q_8 prevented this. To reconcile this DMQ pro-oxidant finding with low ETC ROS production, they suggested that bacterial Q_8 may function in conjunction with DMQ_9 at sites such as the Q_N site of Complex III to swap reducing equivalents from DMQ_9 to Q_8 and subsequently move electrons down the ETC, simultaneously invoking a function for DMQ_9 and countering its pro-oxidant properties.

In another study, Morgan and colleagues (Kayser *et al.*, 2004b) extensively characterized mitochondria from *clk-1* and N2 worms that had each been cultured in liquid medium and fed wildtype *E. coli*. Their key finding was that Complex I in *clk-1* mitochondria operated at ~30 percent of the activity level observed for N2 mitochondria when examined using endogenous quinone carriers only (DMQ_9,

Q_8, and rhodoquinone). Oddly, Complex II remained unaltered. This defect was found not to be due to a reduction in maximal attainable Complex I activity, nor to a reduction in the activity of Complex I substrate transporters; rather, it was shown to be specific to the types of endogenous quinones present. DMQ_9 could not functionally replace Q_9. These findings were in direct contrast to earlier studies (Felkai *et al.*, 1999; Jonassen *et al.*, 2003; Miyadera *et al.*, 2001), which reported there were no differences in Complex I (NADH oxidoreductase) activity in *clk-1* animals. As pointed out by Kayser and colleagues, these earlier studies presumably either missed the observation due to the absence of appropriate wildtype controls, or they failed to include inhibitors that discounted possible nonspecific NADH oxidation (Kayser *et al.*, 2004a). In a set of parallel studies, Kayser and colleagues (2004a) also showed that *clk-1* nematodes display a reduced level of oxidized mitochondrial proteins relative to those from wildtype animals. These findings led to the suggestion that senescence in *clk-1* animals might be delayed because of a lowered electron flux through Complex I and a consequent reduction in oxidative damage—consistent with the free-radical hypothesis of aging (Harman, 1956).

B. Screens Using RNA Inhibition (RNAi)

With the advent of genomic RNAi libraries (Kamath & Ahringer, 2003), it became feasible to screen the entire *C. elegans* genome, one gene at a time, for longevity-enhancing, loss-of-function mutations. Both the Kenyon and Ruvkun labs (Dillin *et al.*, 2002; Lee *et al.*, 2003) independently unveiled the surprising finding that the (presumed) downregulation by RNAi of many mitochondrial genes paradoxically extended worm life span (see Table 13.2). Of particular note, the Ruvkun group found that of the 5,690 genes they screened, 1.8 percent extended life span by 5 to 30 percent relative to wildtype; 15 percent of these encoded mitochondrial proteins. Interestingly, almost all affected components of the ETC, and there seemed no preference for one complex over any other. Many of the mitochondrial genes inactivated by RNAi did not have redundant genetic homologs, and almost all caused a reduction in adult size. Also, similar to *clk-1* and other Clk mutants, each RNAi led to a reduction in many physiological rates. Furthermore, many of the RNAi clones induced alterations in mitochondrial morphology, and the treated animals exhibited no obvious relationship between their relative resistance to either H_2O_2 or paraquat (Lee *et al.*, 2003) and life extension. Indeed, there was often no relationship between H_2O_2 and paraquat resistance. Perhaps the most surprising finding, however, was that the life-span enhancing effects of the RNAi clones were only observed if the RNAi was fed to animals during the larval period (Dillin *et al.*, 2002). This was despite evidence showing animals fed the same RNAi as adults caused an equivalent reduction in the total amount of whole worm ATP. These findings suggest that specific, mitochondrial-dysfunction signals have to be sensed some time during development for animals to adapt with an increased life span. Rather disappointing were the findings that there were no overlaps between the sets of mutants found in the two different laboratories. Our own studies suggest, however, that the efficacy of RNAi-mediated life extension is very dependent on subtle differences in conditions (Rea *et al.*, unpublished).

C. *isp-1, lrs-2,* and *frh-1*

Several Clk-like Mit mutants have been identified that do not exhibit maternal-effect rescue but do display slowed development and rythmicity. Two of these mutants have been characterized in detail: *isp-1* and *lrs-2* (see Table 13.2). *isp-1(qm50)* was identified in a screen for mutants that specifically displayed a Clk-like phenotype without a maternal effect, and it exhibits an ~80 percent increase in mean adult life span at both 20 and 25 °C (Feng *et al.*, 2001). *isp-1* encodes the Rieske iron-sulphur protein subunit of Complex III. The *qm50* mutant allele contains a missense point mutation, the result of which is postulated to affect the redox potential of the 2Fe-2S cluster housed in the head region of the ISP-1 protein. This region normally acts to transfer single reducing equivalents within Complex III from ubiquinone to cytochrome c1 when the former resides in the Q_P binding site of the cytochrome b subunit. It has been postulated that the *qm50* mutant allele results in fewer electrons moving down this high affinity arm of the Q-cycle (Mitchell, 1975) and hence onto cytochrome c. Consistent with this idea, oxygen consumption is reduced by 60 percent in L1 larvae (Feng *et al.*, 2001). Based on this finding, as well as the observed increase in resistance to the redox cycling molecule paraquat, it was postulated that a reduction in electron transfer may translate into a reduction of life-shortening ROS production. That is, generation of ubisemiquinone within Complex III might be reduced. Normally, ubisemiquinone is thought to be formed at two sites during the Q-cycle, first when ISP-1 oxidizes Q at the Q_P site, and again when a second molecule of fully oxidized Q essentially retrieves the second electron held at Q_P via the low affinity arm of the Q-cycle (Iwata *et al.*, 1998).

lrs-2(mg312) is perhaps the most interesting of the Mit mutants. This mutation was identified in a screen for genetic alterations that increased nematode life span in a *daf-16*-independent manner (Lee *et al.*, 2003). At 20 °C, *lrs-2(mg312)* exhibits a 200 percent increase in life span relative to wildtype animals. This reduces to only a 30 percent increase at 25 °C. *lrs-2* encodes a mitochondrial tRNA synthetase. The *mg312* allele encodes a truncated version of this protein that is predicted to be inactive. The mitochondrial genome of *C. elegans* encodes 12 polypeptides, all of which are components of the ETC—specifically, cytochrome b, subunits I–III of cytochrome c oxidase, the a-chain of the Fo ATPase, and subunits 1–6 and 4L of NADH dehydrogenase (Okimoto et al., 1992). The purported absence of these 12 subunits in *lrs-2(mg312)* suggests this mutant might have no ETC activity.

In humans, defective expression of the mitochondrial protein frataxin causes Friedreich ataxia, a hereditary neurodegenerative syndrome characterized by progressive ataxia that is associated with reduced life expectancy (Puccio & Koenig, 2002). In mice, homozygous inactivation of the frataxin gene is embryonic lethal (Cossee et al., 2000). Frataxin is required for the proper assembly of Fe-S clusters, which in turn are necessary for the proper functioning of key components of the ETC (Huynen et al., 2001). Ventura and colleagues (2005) generated a nematode model of the frataxin defect and found that reduced *frh-1* expression resulted in extended life span as well as resistance to some stressors (Ventura et al., 2005). These findings make *frh-1* the latest member of the Mit class of long-lived worm mutants and also underscore the earlier point that worms do not always replicate phenomenon seen in humans.

D. Hypotheses for Longevity Extension of the Mit Mutants

Reactive oxygen species (ROS) encompass a variety of destructive, short-lived compounds that include the likes of superoxide, the hydroxy radical, nitric oxide, lipid peroxides, and many xenobiotic intermediates. They are a likely cause of senescence (Droge, 2003; Finkel & Holbrook, 2000; Golden et al., 2002; Martin et al., 1996; Nohl, 1994; Sohal, 2002) and most of the ROS in the cell comes from the energy-generating process of oxidative phosphorylation in the mitochondrial ETC (see Chapters 5 and 6, this volume). Complexes I and III, and to a lesser extent Complex II, are the major sites of ROS production in *C. elegans* (Kristal & Krasnikov, 2003; Senoo-Matsuda et al., 2001). One simple explanation, then, for why the Mit mutants are long-lived may simply be that these animals generate fewer reactive species, either because their ETCs are not in use or, if they are, the inner mitochondrial membrane potential might be reduced. But could it really be so simple? Inhibitor studies using purified mitochondria have long shown that superoxide production becomes *elevated* when upstream ETC sites become loaded with reducing equivalents. One could easily imagine that for at least some of the Mit mutants, their mitochondria might become overt radical generators. Perhaps in this instance such signals might initiate life-long, or life-lasting, protective responses that are the equivalent of hormesis (Lithgow, 2001; Rattan, 2001; Van Voorhies, 2001a) (see section VI.A). Yet for all Mit mutants, it would seem that two problems evidently still exist: how to generate ATP in the absence of a functional mitochondrial ETC, and how to get rid of their reducing equivalents? Many helminthes are capable of employing alternate pathways for generating ATP while simultaneously maintaining redox balance (Barrett, 1984). This also appears to be the case for the nematode *C. elegans* (Foll et al., 1999), where such mechanisms seem necessary in a species that must make its living in a sometimes anoxic and/or hypoxic soil environment. Indeed, mutants in *daf-2* lead to increased survival under just such conditions (Scott et al., 2002). It is in this light it has been proposed (Rea & Johnson, 2003) that the Mit mutants could be long-lived because they are forced to use alternate mechanisms for ATP and redox balance (see Figure 13.4)—the consequence of which would be lowered ROS production and its concomitant damage. However, for now at least, the physiological basis for the long life of the Mit class of mutants remains unknown.

One of the most intriguing puzzles of the Mit mutants revolves around the finding that the life-span enhancing effects of the RNAi-mediated mutants was only observed if RNAi was fed to animals during the larval period (Dillin *et al.*, 2002). RNAi is generally a knockdown, rather than knockout, technology, suggesting there may be residual ETC activity in the long-lived Mit mutants—at least enough to get them partway through larval development and to avoid dauer formation. All

the Mit mutants are characterized by either sterility or a reduced brood size and egg-laying rate (Dillin *et al.*, 2002; Lee *et al.*, 2003; Shibata *et al.*, 2003; Wong *et al.*, 1995). Gonad development accelerates at the L4/young adult stage at the same time as the total amount of mitochondrial DNA undergoes a 30-fold expansion (Tsang & Lemire, 2002). *clk-1* mutants in which gonad expansion is blocked fail to show an extended life span (Dillin *et al.*, 2002). This observation implies that low levels of Q, per se, in somatic tissue are not enough to extend life span. Furthermore, it suggests that another signal generated elsewhere in the organism acts to alter somatic cells. Since a 30-fold increase in mitochondrial DNA accompanies germline expansion at

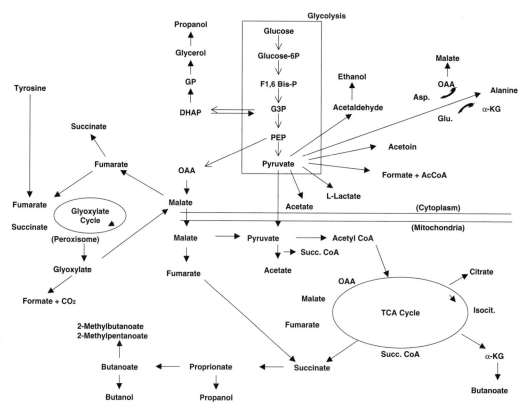

Figure 13.4 Under anaerobic conditions, energy generation in nematodes can proceed by the many pathways depicted, but not all are common to every species. Redox balance is maintained by regulating the amounts of various reduced and oxidized end-products excreted. Only terminal end-products and key metabolic intermediates are shown. Some pathways remain hypothetical.

the L4 and YA stages (Tsang & Lemire, 2002), it is reasonable to assume there must normally be a particularly intense requirement for mitochondrial oxidative metabolism at this developmental point. We suggested (Rea & Johnson, 2003) that for *clk-1* and other Mit mutants, the inability to meet this very specific and time-dependent need for mitochondrial activity is the trigger that ultimately leads to their increased longevity. Presumably, activation of the alternate energy-producing pathways just mentioned occurs at this time. This idea provides a simple explanation for why the RNAi Mit mutants have a time-dependent requirement for RNAi addition to signal a life span increase.

E. Relevance to Human Aging

If we suppose the life extension of Mit mutants results exclusively from using alternate energy-generating pathways, then we must ask, do they have any relevance to human aging? The answer is yes. First, certain tissues in the adult human, such as keratinocytes, run almost exclusively on lactate fermentation (Ronquist et al., 2003). Indeed, whole periods of human development (e.g., organogenesis, Jauniaux et al., 2003; New, 1978) require hypoxic, and possibly even anoxic, conditions. Second, the Mit mutants confirm a long-held suspicion that general aerobic mitochondrial activity (and ROS formation) contributes significantly to normal aging (Hartman et al., 2001; Kayser et al., 2004b; Nicholls, 2002). Thus, the Mit mutants may hold a key through which we can now unlock and define parameters necessary for long life.

V. Caloric Restriction

In *C. elegans*, restriction of caloric intake (CR), in three distinct ways, has been demonstrated to extend life span: by reduc-

ing food (bacteria) concentration (Klass, 1977), by growth in axenic media (De Cuyper & Vanfleteren, 1982; Houthoofd et al., 2002), and by genetically reducing feeding rate (Eat mutants) (Lakowski & Hekimi, 1998) (see Figure 13.5). The first CR studies, undertaken by Klass (1977), demonstrated that reducing the levels of food (bacterial concentration) greatly increased life span—increasing mean survival approximately 60 percent—but at the same time significantly decreased reproduction to less than 25 percent of animals fed high concentrations of food. The most dramatic increases in life span have been reported when nematodes are grown in axenic (semi-defined) media (Houthoofd et al., 2003), where about a threefold increase in life span has been observed for the wildtype strain N2. Under CR conditions, worms develop and reproduce slowly and exhibit increased stress resistance. For example, wildtype animals grown in liquid axenic cultures at 24 °C have a generation time of 5.5 days, 3 days longer than when raised on bacteria. Furthermore, animals raised in liquid axenic cultures demonstrate remarkable thermotolerance, roughly 50 percent better than bacteria-fed animals (Houthoofd et al., 2002).

A. CR and the IIS Pathway

The increase in life span that occurs by raising animals in axenic media is largely independent of the insulin/IGF-1 signaling pathway (IIS). In fact, IIS seems to work in combination with CR to extend life span even more. Because *daf-16* is required for the life span increases found in IIS mutants, Houthoofd and colleagues (2003) asked whether *daf-16* played a similar role in axenic cultures. Intriguingly, *daf-16* mutants still exhibited greatly extended mean life spans in axenic media, increasing the mean ~150 percent, about the same as that observed for wildtype animals. In addition, *daf-16 (lf)*

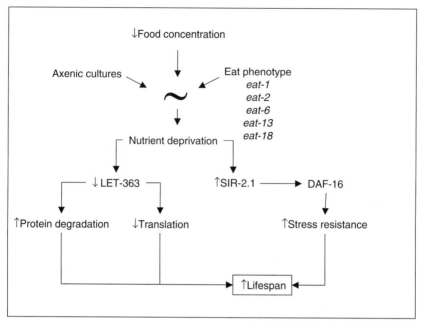

Figure 13.5 Caloric restriction in *C. elegans*. Caloric restriction (CR) can be imposed on nematodes by several mechanisms, including growth in axenic cultures, decreasing food concentrations, and by genetic mutation (e.g., Eat mutants such as *eat-1, 2, 6, 13*, and *18*, which impair the animal's ability to feed). Each of these methods results in nutrient deprivation at the cellular level and increased life span. The mechanism may work through decreased TOR (*let-363*) activity, increased SIR-2.1 activity, or both. Decreasing *let-363* activity has been shown to inhibit protein translation and increase protein degradation as well as increase life span. Similarly, increasing dosage of *sir-2.1* increases life span in *C. elegans* through a *daf-16*-dependent mechanism.

mutants also showed greatly increased thermotolerance, roughly 80 percent better than bacteria-fed controls. Growth in axenic media also seems to work synergistically with inhibition of IIS. Raising *daf-2(e1370)* animals in axenic cultures leads to dramatic increases in longevity, increasing the mean to 300 percent that of *daf-2(e1370)* and 525 percent of N2-fed live bacteria (Houthoofd *et al.*, 2003), a remarkable seven-fold increase in adult life expectancy, which is the current record (Houthoofd *et al.*, 2004).

B. Eat Mutants

Another approach to CR in *C. elegans* has been to inhibit the efficiency of the animal's ability to feed. *C. elegans* feed by pumping bacteria into the buccal cavity using a pharynx. Numerous Eat mutants have been identified that have reduced pharyngeal pumping rates and therefore a presumed reduced food intake. As a class, the Eat mutants are thin and have a mottled appearance, similar to starved worms (Avery, 1993). Many of the Eat mutants are long-lived; their percent increase of life expectancy varies with gene and allele—for example, *eat-1(ad427)* 33 percent, *eat-2(ad465)* 29 percent, *eat-3(ad426)* 11 percent, *eat-6(ad792)* 36 percent. Similar to the axenicly grown animals, the increase in life span afforded by *eat-2(ad465)* was found to be largely independent of *daf-16*, such that *daf-16(m26);eat-2(ad465)* double mutants lived ~36 percent longer then *daf-16(m26)* alone (Lakowski & Hekimi, 1998). However, not all Eat mutants were long-lived, some in fact were short-lived—

for example, *eat-5(ad464)*–6 percent, *eat-7(ad450)*–35 percent (Lakowski & Hekimi, 1998). This may be similar to decreasing caloric intake below required levels for CR, which also shortens life span in rodents (Masoro, 1998), or simply to other complications.

C. TOR

If CR works by nutrient deprivation, it might be possible to mimic the effects by inhibiting nutrient sensing or uptake mechanisms. A major nutrient-sensing mechanism across species is the Target Of Rapamycin (TOR) gene. The TOR gene encodes a large protein that is a member of the phosphatidylinositol kinase (PIK)-related kinase family. TOR acts by sensing nutrient availability and regulating transcription and translation, and exerts an overall control on cell growth and proliferation. TOR may be activated by amino acids or charged tRNAs and promotes translation while inhibiting protein degradation. Inhibition of TOR by rapamycin result in blocks in translation and increases in protein degradation (for overview see Rohde *et al.*, 2001). *C. elegans* contains a single TOR homolog called *let-363* (or ceTOR), and inhibition of the gene suggests that LET-363 plays a role in *C. elegans* similar to other species. Loss of *let-363* function results in larval arrest at the L3 stage, with severe intestinal atrophy and the appearance of refractile intestinal vesicles, which may be autophagic (Long *et al.*, 2002). Inhibition of *let-363*, either by mutation or RNA interference, also increases life span of wildtype animals about 35 percent (Meissner *et al.*, 2004; Vellai *et al.*, 2003). Similar to the effects of the *eat* mutants and growth in axenic cultures, the life-span increases conferred by inhibiting *let-363* were also independent of *daf-16* (Vellai *et al.*, 2003).

Mutations in the *Drosophila* homolog of Tor have been shown to extend life (Kapahi *et al.*, 2004).

D. SIR2

Studies in the yeast *Saccharomyces cerevisiae* identified the SIR2 and NPT1 genes as part of another metabolic sensing mechanism involved in caloric restriction. NPT1 is required for nicotinamide adenine dinucleotide (NAD) synthesis, whereas SIR2 encodes an NAD^+ dependent deacetylase (Lin *et al.*, 2000). The involvement of these genes in the longevity conferred by CR in yeast led to the model that SIR2 functions to sense the levels of NAD^+ and thereby regulate gene expression by deacetylating histones (for a review, see Lin & Guarente, 2003). This model was based on findings that revealed that overexpressing SIR2 in yeast increased life span (Lin *et al.*, 2000). The *C. elegans* genome contains four putative SIR2-like genes, *sir-2.1*, *sir-2.2*, *sir-2.3*, and *sir-2.4*. Of these genes, the one most similar to yeast SIR2 is *sir-2.1*. Tissenbaum and Gaurente (2001) showed that increased dosage of *sir-2.1* increased the life span of *C. elegans*. They constructed an extra chromosomal array and integrated lines that harbored increased dosage of the *sir-2.1* gene and found that in multiple independent lines, these strains exhibited increased life span, with the largest being a 37 percent increase (Tissenbaum & Guarente, 2001). Surprisingly, unlike CR manipulations in nematodes, the increase in life span conferred by increased dosage of *sir-2.1* was found to be dependent on *daf-16*. Furthermore, *sir-2.1* overexpression did not further increase the life span of long-lived *daf-2(e1370)* animals, both suggesting that, in *C. elegans*, *sir-2.1* acts via IIS to increase life span.

E. Summary Thoughts

The IIS independence of axenic media and Eat mutants is surprising because in mammals CR is known to reduce insulin and IGF levels, and it seemed logical to assume the benefits of mammalian CR stem from reduced IIS. Yet this may highlight a fundamental difference in the way nematodes and mammals utilize insulin and IGF. Several lines of evidence suggest that in *C. elegans*, insulin-like proteins are secreted from neurons based on direct chemosensation of the environment. First, studies on the effect of defective sensory neurons and life span demonstrate that disrupting the function of the sensory neurons results in increased dauer formation (Vowels & Thomas, 1992) and life span (Apfeld & Kenyon, 1999). Second, many of the *ins* genes are expressed in neurons (Pierce *et al.*, 2001), and in the case of *daf-28*, the level of expression is lowered during food deprivation (Li *et al.*, 2003). The secretion of insulin by sensory input would be analogous to Beta cells secreting insulin when an animal smells food. Instead, in mammals, insulin is secreted in response to nutrient availability in the bloodstream and in particular ATP levels within the Beta cells. In mammals, therefore, insulin levels more accurately reflect food consumption, whereas in worms it is relatively easy to disconnect food availability from food intake. Eat mutant animals still sense food is available and secrete normal amounts of insulin, yet do not take in as many nutrients as the wild-type, thereby disconnecting CR from IIS.

These results suggest that, in *C. elegans*, decreased nutrient intake exerts a life-span-prolonging mechanism that is independent of IIS signaling. Consistent with this interpretation is the finding that *eat-2(ad465);daf-2(e1370)* double mutants live longer than either single mutant (Lakowski & Hekimi, 1998), and that axenicly grown *daf-2(e1370)* also exhibits

large increases in life span (Houthoofd *et al.*, 2003). One possible transducer of this IIS independent signal is *let-363* (ceTOR); when inhibited, it extends life span in a *daf-16*-independent manner (Vellai *et al.*, 2003). The mechanism of action remains unknown but may be related to increased protein turnover, or perhaps decreased protein translation (Long *et al.*, 2002). Yet other CR-related interventions such as increased dosage of SIR-2.1 exhibit a *daf-16* dependent function on life span, indicating that some metabolic integration with insulin signaling is occurring. This type of metabolic signaling may measure intracellular energy levels to alter transcriptional activity. A direct role for the SIR2 class of proteins in regulating the FOXO class of transcription factors comes from studies showing that mammalian SIR2 can deacetylate FOXO1 and increase its activity (Daitoku *et al.*, 2004). Further work will elucidate the interconnectedness of these pathways.

VI. Other Non-Genetic Ways to Extend Life

A. Hormesis

A direct prediction of the link between stress resistance and aging is that increasing the level of expression of stress genes in the absence of a deleterious stressor will increase life span. Conversely, decreasing the ability to express stress genes may decrease life span. The extensive genetic and molecular tools available to nematode researchers have led *C. elegans* to become a good test of these predictions.

One method for increasing expression of stress-response genes is to expose the animals to a stressor that is not damaging to the animal yet is sufficient to induce a stress response. This has been given the general name of *hormesis*. Hormesis has been observed in response to a broad variety of harmful physical agents and environmental stressors. The common demonstration of hormesis is the observation that exposure to one type of stressor results in much greater resistance to subsequent challenges by the same stressor (for a review, see Minois, 2000). This is true in *C. elegans* (see Figure 13.5); for example, exposing adult animals to 35(C for 2 hours leads to significant increases in thermotolerance 12 hours later (Cypser & Johnson, 2002). Such treatments also lead to upregulation of stress-response genes, such as the small heat shock genes like *hsp-16.2* (Link *et al.*, 1999). Identical treatments (2 hours at 35° C) also increase mean life span ~23 percent, whereas longer treatments reduced life span. Other stressors have also resulted in increased life span in *C. elegans*. Notably, exposure to hyperbaric oxygen (95 percent, 40 psi for 8 hours) increases mean life span ~20 percent. Exposure to the latter condition has been demonstrated to increase the expression of antioxidant genes such as glutathione S-transferase 4 (*gst-4*) (Link & Johnson, 2002). Importantly, though, not all stressors result in hormesis or increased life span in *C. elegans* (e.g., treatment with ultraviolet light). This likely represents a species-specific response, as *C. elegans*, a soil dwelling nematode, may not be commonly exposed to ultraviolet light and thus may not retain the capacity to respond to such a stress.

The potential mechanism leading to an increased resistance to some later challenge by the same stressor is conceptually simple, but the increase in life span is not. Cypser and Johnson examined the role of genes in the dauer pathway known to affect life span on the hormetic response in *C. elegans* (Cypser & Johnson, 2003). They found that several dauer-defective genes (*daf-12*, *daf-16*, and *daf-18*) were required for heat-induced increased life span, whereas those same genes were only weakly required for the subsequent thermotolerance. Genes in the other arm of the dauer pathway, *daf-3* and *daf-5*, had no effect. This suggests a significant role for a subset of dauer genes in long-term

adaptation to stress. In particular, those homologous with IIS may play a prominent role. Consistent with a role for *daf-16* in hormetic life-span extension is the observation that the DAF-16 protein is nuclear localized in response to a variety of stressors and may generally function to prepare the animal for adverse conditions (Henderson & Johnson, 2001).

B. Drug Interventions that Extend Life

An elixir for life extension has been a goal of mankind for eons, probably since our species first gained self-awareness and the ability to sense our own mortality (Post & Binstock, 2004). The recent discoveries of genetic interventions that lead to life extension have obvious implications for life (and health) extension in humans. Two of the authors Samuel T. Henderson and Thomas E. Johnson have even been involved in commercial enterprises to develop interventions that might extend human life and health, as have other researchers in this field. C. Kenyon and L. Guarante, the founders of Elixir Pharmaceuticals, have most notably promoted life-extension drugs based on their fundamental discoveries in nematodes and yeast, respectively. See Johnson (2003; in press) for a more complete discussion.

Several other investigators have used *C. elegans* to screen for compounds that lead to life extension (for a review, see Sampayo *et al.*, 2003). Babar and colleagues used wortmanin and LY294002, compounds that specifically targeted the AGE-1 protein (PI3K), and found modest effects (Babar *et al.*, 1999). Worm life span was extended by about 20 percent, and both thermotolerance and the tendency to form dauers were also increased. Extracts from *Ginkgo biloba* have been reported to extend life by 8 percent (Wu *et al.*, 2002), as has tamarixetin, purified from this extract. Utilizing a few synthetic compounds developed by Eukarion that mimic SOD and catalase activity (SCMs),

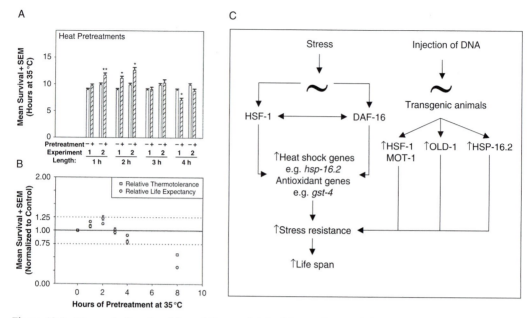

Figure 13.6 Hormesis. Reprinted from *J Gerontol A Biol Sci Med Sci*, 57(3), J. R. Cypser and T. E. Johnson, "Multiple stressors in *Caenorhabditis elegans* induce stress hormesis and extended longevity," pp. B109–B114, 2002, Copyright The Gerontological Society of America, reproduced by permission of the publisher. Panels A and B depict increased thermotolerance and life span, respectively, of wildtype *C. elegans* when pre-exposed to a modest heat challenge. Too much stress is damaging for the animal, as seen by pretreatment doses >4 hours. The right panel depicts an overview of the hormesis pathway. Mild stress may activate stress genes without causing damage. Such stressors may act through the transcription factors HSF-1 and/or DAF-16 to elevate stress genes such as small HSP and *gst-4*, resulting in increased stress resistance and life span. Similarly, stress proteins may be elevated in the absence of a stressor by increasing gene dosage through creation of transgenic lines. This has been demonstrated for *hsf-1, mot-1, old-1*, and *hsp-16.2* (see text for details).

thus reducing the levels of intracellular free-radicals, Melov and colleagues (2000) reported dramatic life extensions of about 120 percent in both mean and maximum life span in *C. elegans* (see Figure 13.7) (Melov *et al.*, 2000). Controversy exists as to replicability and generalness of the effects of these SCMs, and it may be that these compounds have limited usefulness (Sampayo *et al.*, 2003).

An interesting addition to the list of proven pro-longevity drugs (at least in the worm) appeared as this chapter was going to press. Evason and colleagues (2005) showed that ethosuximide and other anti-convulsants approved for human use also extend the life of the worm. Both mean and maximum life were extended by as much as 50 percent. These extensions

were partially dependent on *daf-16* but seemed independent of other longevity pathways and mutants. These results were dependent on activity of the drug and stimulated early egg lay in the worm as well as hyperactivity consistent with a neuromuscular target (Evason *et al.*, 2005). We speculate that a possible action of the drug is to stimulate the muscular system, which is the first system to degenerate, and thus stimulate increased longevity.

VII. Other Discoveries

A. Stress Response

Inhibition of the IIS pathway not only increases life span but also leads to large increases in resistance to a variety

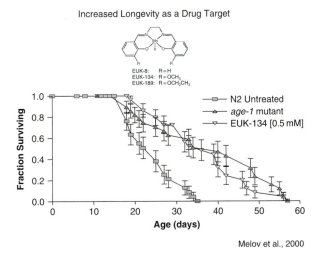

Figure 13.7 **Increased longevity as a drug target.** Several exogenously applied compounds have been shown to increase life span of *C. elegans*. LY294002, a PI3K inhibitor, increases life span 15 percent through inhibition of AGE-1 activity. EUK-134, a superoxide dismutase/catalase mimetic, increases life span by 44 percent. Survival curve reprinted with permission from *Science*, 289 (5484), S. Melov, J. Ravenscroft, S. Malik, M. S. Gill, D. W. Walker, P. E. Clayton, D. C. Wallace, B. Malfroy, S. R. Doctrow, & G. J. Lithgow, "Extension of life-span with superoxide dismutase/catalase mimetics," pp. 1567–1569, Copyright 2000, AAAS.

of stressors (Johnson *et al.*, 2000; Johnson *et al.*, 2001). This has been best studied in the *age-1* mutant. The long-lived *age-1(hx546)* allele shows resistance to a remarkable number of stressors, including hydrogen peroxide (Larsen, 1993), paraquat (Vanfleteren, 1993), ultraviolet light (Murakami & Johnson, 1996), heat (Lithgow *et al.*, 1995), the potent bacterial pathogen *Pseudomonas aeruginosa* (Mahajan-Miklos *et al.*, 1999), and to MPTP, a compound used to produce a mouse model of Parkinson's disease (Johnson *et al.*, 2002). Such strong increases in stress resistance have been reported in other components of the IIS pathway as well. Inhibition of *sgk-1* resulted in resistance to both heat and paraquat (Hertweck *et al.*, 2004). In all cases, gains in stress resistance appear to require a functional *daf-16* gene. Although correlation does not mean causality, most Age mutants of *C. elegans* (see Figure 13.8), and indeed in many other

species, also demonstrate increased stress resistance (Finkel & Holbrook, 2000). A common theme therefore appears to be that both the genetic and environmental manipulations that increase life span also increase resistance to exogenous stress (for an overview, see Johnson *et al.*, 2000). An immediate corollary presents itself—that organismal life span might be increased by either reducing the generation of endogenous damaging molecular species or by increasing the organism's ability to repair damage from them. This in many ways is similar to evolutionary theories of aging in which life span can be considered a tradeoff between devoting metabolic resources to reproduction versus cellular maintenance (Martin *et al.*, 1996).

Three groups have used the tight relationship between increased stress resistance and increased longevity to select for mutants that increase stress resistance and then ask whether these show increased life span (de Castro *et al.*, 2004;

Correlation Between Life Expectancy and Stress Resistance

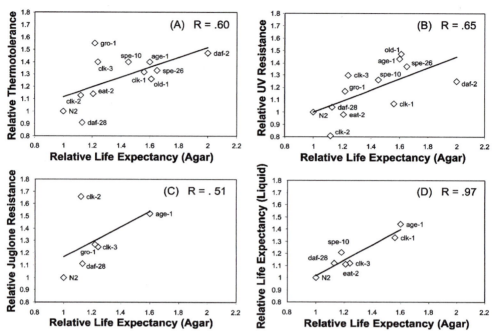

Figure 13.8 Stress resistance and life span correlate. Reprinted from *Experimental Gerontology*, Volume 35, No 6–7, T. E. Johnson, J. Cypser, E. de Castro, S. de Castro, S. Henderson, S. Murakami, B. Rikke, P. Tedesco, & C. Link, "Gerontogenes mediate health and longevity in nematodes through increasing resistance to environmental toxins and stressors," pp. 687–694, Copyright 2000, with permission from Elsevier. This figure depicts positive correlation between resistance to various stressors and life expectancy in many long-lived *C. elegans* strains. (a) Heat (35° C until death). (b) UV (2000 J/m²). (c) Juglone, a superoxide generator (240 μM) until death. (d) Food deprivation (growth in liquid media with low food, 10^9 bacteria/ml). All values are normalized against the corresponding wildtype, N2, internal control.

Munoz & Riddle, 2003; Sampayo *et al.*, 2000). Using increased stress resistance as a surrogate marker for increased longevity served as a very effective enrichment strategy. These results are consistent with a causal relationship between increased stress resistance and increased longevity but do not prove it.

Another commonly encountered stressor is low food availability. One well-studied outcome of mild food reduction is increased life span. This treatment has been extensively studied since its first report by McCay and colleagues over 60 years ago (McCay *et al.*, 1935) and has been referred to as either caloric restriction (CR) or dietary restriction (DR) and

was reviewed above. Similar to the concept of hormesis, where too great a stress is harmful, too great a restriction in calories is also deleterious to the organism, while mild 20 to 40 percent reduction in *ad lib* amounts of food intake has been shown to increase both life span and stress resistance (for a review, see Masoro, 1998). This has been extensively reported in rodent models, where CR increases life span 30 to 40 percent. CR also increases resistance to a variety of stressors, such as thermotolerance (Hall *et al.*, 2000). Importantly, CR also frequently has consequences on reproduction. Reducing calories and body fat will cause a reproductive pause in female mammals. This halting of reproduction may be regulated by neuroendocrine signaling, which slows reproduction until resources become more abundant (for a review, see Nelson *et al.*, 1995). The mechanism by which CR increases life span is not fully understood, yet the decrease in fertility and reciprocal increase in stress resistance is consistent with CR inducing a shift in the allocation of resources away from reproduction and toward somatic maintenance.

B. Overexpression Mutants, QTLs

Another method to increase expression of stress response genes is to introduce transgenes that either increase dosage or constitutively express stress response genes (see Figure 13.5C). This was first done by Murakami and Johnson, who showed that overexpression of the *old-1* tyrosine kinase (TK) gene led to life extension and increased stress resistance in a DAF-16-dependent manner (Murakami & Johnson, 1998) (see section III.E). Yokoymana and colleagues introduced a transgene into *C. elegans* carrying a muscle-specific promoter driving a member of the HSP70 family (HSP70F, also known as *mot-1*). The resultant transgenic lines showed a 43 percent increase in mean life span (Yokoyama *et al.*, 2002). In a similar set of experiments, Walker and Lithgow increased the dosage of the small heat shock genes, *hsp-16*, and found slightly increased life span (Walker & Lithgow, 2003). Furthermore, Hsu and colleagues found that increasing the dosage of heat shock factor (*hsf-1*), a key regulator of stress-response genes, also increased wildtype life span approximately 40 percent (Hsu *et al.*, 2003). Similar to the Cypser and Johnson hormesis experiments, the increased life span conferred both by increased dosage of *hsp-16* and *hsf-1* were dependent on the presence of a functional *daf-16* gene, suggesting that the transcription factor

DAF-16 may work in coordination with *hsf-1* to control the expression of small heat shock genes and other stress-response genes (Hsu *et al.*, 2003).

A corollary to hormetic increases in life span is that increasing the production of internal stressors or inhibiting the ability of the animal to respond to stress might lead to shorter life span. The *mev-1* mutant has been shown to have a defect in the large cytochrome c subunit of mitochondrial Complex II and to result in profound shortening of life (Ishii *et al.*, 1998). In a RNA interference screen for progeric phenotypes, inhibition of *hsf-1* was found to result in accelerated tissue aging and shortened life span (Garigan *et al.*, 2002). Inhibiting *hsf-1* by RNAi was also found to shorten the life span of long-lived strains of *C. elegans* such as those in the IIS pathway, for example, *daf-2(e1370)*, suggesting that HSF is required for long life. Although inhibiting *hsf-1* had the most profound effects on life span, inhibition of any one of four small heat shock genes, *hsp-16.1*, *hsp-16.49*, *hsp-12.6*, or *sip-1*, has also been reported to shorten the life spans of both wildtype and *daf-2(e1370)* animals (Hsu *et al.*, 2003). Therefore, stress-response genes may play a key role in preserving the integrity of cellular components and ultimately specifying life span. In addition, it appears that stress-response genes work together with other signaling pathways to influence aging.

The first long-lived strains to be produced in *C. elegans* were not made by inducing mutants or making transgenes but by a much more traditional quantitative genetic approach: generating recombinant inbred (RI) strains (Johnson, 1987; Johnson & Wood, 1982). Several studies have utilized these RI strains to detect and map genes (quantitative trait loci, or QTLs) specifying life span, fertility, and other life-history traits (Shook & Johnson, 1999; Shook *et al.*, 1996). Shook and colleagues (1996) and Shook and Johnson (1999) found four major QTLs; two showed genotype-by-environment interactions, and genetic epistasis and pleiotropy was also detected. Ayyadavara and colleagues (2001, 2003) have tuned this approach to even higher levels, and may be converging on the genes underlying individual QTLs for life span in *C. elegans*, which has so far proven problematic (Ayyadevara *et al.*, 2001; Ayyadevara *et al.*, 2003). In general, these QTLs specify only one trait and show little antagonistic pleiotropy or tradeoffs between different traits.

C. Biomarkers of Aging

Several studies have revealed that the behavioral declines and tissue degeneration seen in old worms can be slowed by alterations that increase life span. For example, Age mutations lead to both increased mobility and fewer morphological signs of degeneration over time (Duhon & Johnson, 1995; Garigan *et al.*, 2002; Herndon *et al.*, 2002; Hosono *et al.*, 1980; Johnson, 1987). The decrease in physical markers of aging in long-lived mutants is consistent with the hypothesis that these manipulations affect the fundamental aging process itself. A point often overlooked in the above studies is that *C. elegans* populations are typically isogenic and usually maintained in a homogenous environment. Despite this, there is a large variation in age at which animals die. The rates of decline in both behavioral and morphological signs of aging are also quite variable among individuals. This heterogeneity within identical populations reveals the stochastic nature of aging (Kirkwood & Austad, 2000).

Herndon and colleagues (2002) classified aging isogenic populations of *C. elegans* into three classes of animals: Class A, those that are highly mobile; Class B, those that do not move unless prodded; and Class C, those that do not move, even

when prodded, but do twitch their heads in response to touch (see Figure 13.1D; Herndon *et al.*, 2002). These behavioral markers are very good predictors of life span, such that progression to Class C proved to be a better marker for life expectancy than chronological age. With increasing age, tissue degeneration became more evident, particularly in muscle cells. In a related set of experiments, Herndon and colleagues utilized both a translational reporter construct, consisting of green fluorescent protein (GFP) fused to myosin heavy chain A, and electron microscopy to visualize changes in sarcomere integrity in young and old animals (see Figure 13.2). Such experiments revealed that, like mammals, *C. elegans* show signs of sarcopenia with age. Sarcomeres were found to become disorganized and contained fewer myosin thick filaments per sarcomere unit in older animals. In very old animals (18 days), muscle cells were frequently smaller and highly invaginated, especially in Class C animals. The appearance of sarcopenia is consistent with the observed decline in locomotion of old animals. Interestingly, neurons did not show gross signs of morphological disturbances with age, suggesting that different tissues may age at different rates (Herndon *et al.*, 2002).

In another effort to identify markers that change with age, Lund and colleagues analyzed gene expression using whole-genome microarrays made by the Kim lab to study changes during chronological aging of the worm (Lund *et al.*, 2002). They collected worms at six ages, providing a rich database of age-specific changes in gene expression. Using a rigorous statistical model with multiple replicates, they found only 164 genes to show statistically significant changes in transcript levels with chronological age. This represents less than 1 percent of the genes on the arrays, much less than had been found in other studies. They found that expression of heat shock proteins decrease as a class; no changes

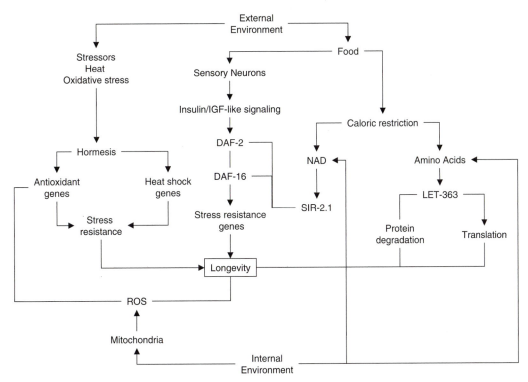

Figure 13.9   Specification of aging in *C. elegans*. Arrows indicate stimulatory action; absence of arrows indicates inhibitory action. Environmental factors that affect aging in *C. elegans* can be divided into two main types: internal and external. External factors include food and environmental stress and perhaps others still to be defined. Internal factors, at bottom, include energy supply, such as NAD+ and amino acid levels. The former may be sensed by SIR-2.1 proteins and the latter by LET-363. The production and elimination of ROS by mitochondria are major internal factors. Food availability is detected by direct chemosensation of the environment as well as by the ability to actually consume it. Environmental food abundance may be transduced to cells via the IIS pathway, whereas food consumption may be sensed by internal sensors such as LET-363. Heat exposure may be transduced through HSF-1 and DAF-16 to modulate levels of stress proteins. Developmentally unprogrammed increases in stress resistance, via inappropriate activation of stress genes, may lead to increased longevity.

were seen in genes that respond to oxidative stress, as a class. The largest changes were increased expression of certain transposases in older worms, consistent with higher mortality risk due to a failure in homeostenosis and destabilization of the genome in older animals. Interestingly, changes in mitochondrial stability had been seen (Melov *et al.*, 1994), and these alterations appeared to be reduced in the *age-1* mutant (Melov *et al.*, 1995).

VIII. Summary

Many manipulations (both genetic andenvironmental) increase life span in *C. elegans* (see Figure 13.9). For all its complexity, there does, however, appear to be a common theme. Many alterations that increase life span may be considered to "fool" the animal into signaling that resources are either scarce or damaging agents are present, when in fact they are not. This may lead the animal to invest resources into somatic maintenance and thereby minimize damage to cellular constituents. If, for example, signals are inappropriately sent that oxidants are present, the animal may then devote resources toward repair of oxidative damage, resulting in a longer life span. Such a scenario would be disadvantageous in the wild, where reproduction is more important than a longer life span and resources cannot be wasted. (The inability of *age-1* mutants to survive in a competitive experiment with wild type animals under changing environmental conditions supports this notion; Jenkins *et al.*, 2004; Walker *et al.*, 2000). With this framework in mind, interventions that increase life span in *C. elegans* can be put into three broad categories. First, non-stressful alterations to the animal lead to the activation of stress-response pathways under conditions that do not require them. These include manipulation of sensory and signaling pathways. Second are alterations that reduce the availability of resources to a point that repair pathways are activated but are not damaging to the animal. One simple example of this is caloric restriction. Third are non-lethal, stressful interventions that stimulate stress genes to a point where the beneficial effects of the stress response outweighs the harmful effects of the stressor—such interventions can be broadly defined as hormesis.

So at the end we see there is no aging program *per se*. Life is measured by what extent resources are directed from reproduction to maintenance; aging is simply a byproduct of the program we call life!

References

Alcedo, J., & Kenyon, C. (2004). Regulation of *C. elegans* longevity by specific gustatory and olfactory neurons. *Neuron*, 41(1), 45–55.

Apfeld, J., & Kenyon, C. (1999). Regulation of lifespan by sensory perception in *Caenorhabditis elegans*. *Nature*, 402(6763), 804–809.

Arantes-Oliveira, N., Berman, J. R., & Kenyon, C. (2003). Healthy animals with extreme longevity. *Science*, 302(5645), 611.

Austad, S. N. (2005). Diverse aging rates in metazoans: targets for functional genomics. *Mechanisms of Ageing and Development*, 126(1), 43–49.

Avery, L. (1993). The genetics of feeding in *Caenorhabditis elegans*. *Genetics*, 133(4), 897–917.

Ayyadevara, S., Ayyadevara, R., Hou, S., Thaden, J. J., & Shmookler Reis, R. J. (2001). Genetic mapping of quantitative trait loci governing longevity of *Caenorhabditis elegans* in recombinant-inbred progeny of a Bergerac-BO x RC301 interstrain cross. *Genetics*, 157(2), 655–666.

Ayyadevara, S., Ayyadevara, R., Vertino, A., Galecki, A., Thaden, J. J., & Shmookler Reis, R. J. (2003). Genetic loci modulating fitness and life span in *Caenorhabditis elegans*: categorical trait interval mapping in CL2a x Bergerac-BO recombinant-inbred worms. *Genetics*, 163(2), 557–570.

Babar, P., Adamson, C., Walker, G. A., Walker, D. W., & Lithgow, G. J. (1999). P13-kinase inhibition induces dauer formation, thermotolerance and longevity in *C. elegans*. *Neurobiology of Aging*, 20(5), 513–519.

Barrett, J. (1984). The anaerobic end-products of helminths. *Parasitology*, 88 (Pt 1), 179–198.

Bolanowski, M. A., Russell, R. L., & Jacobson, L. A. (1981). Quantitative measures of aging in the nematode *Caenorhabditis elegans*. I. Population and longitudinal studies of two behavioral parameters. *Mechanisms of Ageing and Development*, 15(3), 279–295.

Braeckman, B. P., Houthoofd, K., & Vanfleteren, J. R. (2002). Assessing metabolic activity in aging *Caenorhabditis elegans*: concepts and controversies. *Aging Cell*, 1(2), 82–88; discussion 102–103.

Brenner, S. (1974). The genetics of *Caenorhabditis elegans*. *Genetics*, 77(1), 71–94.

Brunet, A., Park, J., Tran, H., Hu, L. S., Hemmings, B. A., & Greenberg, M. E. (2001). Protein kinase SGK mediates survival signals by phosphorylating the forkhead transcription factor FKHRL1 (FOXO3a). *Molecular and Cellular Biology*, 21(3), 952–965.

Chalfie, M., & White, J. (1988). The nervous system. In W. B. Wood (Ed.), *The nematode Caenorhabditis elegans* (pp. 337–393). Cold Spring Harbor: Cold Spring Harbor Press.

C. elegans Sequencing Consortium. (1998). Genome sequence of the nematode *C. elegans*: a platform for investigating biology. *Science*, 282(5396), 2012–2018.

Cossee, M., Puccio, H., Gansmuller, A., Koutnikova, H., Dierich, A., LeMeur, M., Fischbeck, K., Dolle, P., & Koenig, M. (2000). Inactivation of the Friedreich ataxia mouse gene leads to early embryonic lethality without iron accumulation. *Human Molecular Genetics*, 9(8), 1219–1226.

Coulson, A., Waterston, R., Kiff, J., Sulston, J., & Kohara, Y. (1988). Genome linking with yeast artificial chromosomes. *Nature*, 335(6186), 184–186.

Cypser, J. R., & Johnson, T. E. (2002). Multiple stressors in *Caenorhabditis elegans* induce stress hormesis and extended longevity. *Journals of Gerontology Series A: Biological Sciences and Medical Sciences*, 57(3), B109–B114.

Cypser, J. R., & Johnson, T. E. (2003). Hormesis in *Caenorhabditis elegans* dauer-defective mutants. *Biogerontology*, 4(4), 203–214.

Daitoku, H., Hatta, M., Matsuzaki, H., Aratani, S., Ohshima, T., Miyagishi, M., Nakajima, T., & Fukamizu, A. (2004). Silent information regulator 2 potentiates Foxo1-mediated transcription through its deacetylase activity. *Proceedings of the National Academy of Sciences of the USA*, 101(27), 10042–10047.

de Castro, E., Hegi de Castro, S., & Johnson, T. E. (2004). Isolation of long-lived mutants in Caenorhabditis elegans using selection for resistance to juglone. *Free Radical Biology and Medicine*, 37(2), 139–145.

De Cuyper, C., & Vanfleteren, J. R. (1982). Oxygen consumption during development and aging of the nematode Caenorhabditis elegans. *Comparative Biochemistry and Physiology*, 73A, 283–289.

Dillin, A., Hsu, A. L., Arantes-Oliveira, N., Lehrer-Graiwer, J., Hsin, H., Fraser, A. G., Kamath, R. S., Ahringer, J., & Kenyon, C. (2002). Rates of behavior and aging specified by mitochondrial function during development. *Science*, 298(5602), 2398–2401.

Dlakic, M. (2002). A new family of putative insulin receptor-like proteins in *C. elegans*. *Current Biology*, 12(5), R155–R157.

D'Mello, N., P., Childress, A. M., Franklin, D. S., Kale, S. P., Pinswasdi, C., & Jazwinski, S. M. (1994). Cloning and characterization of LAG1, a longevity-assurance gene in yeast. *Journal of Biological Chemistry*, 269(22), 15451–15459.

Droge, W. (2003). Oxidative stress and aging. *Advances in Experimental Medicine and Biology*, 543, 191–200.

Duhon, S. A., & Johnson, T. E. (1995). Movement as an index of vitality: comparing wild type and the age-1 mutant of *Caenorhabditis elegans*. *Journals of Gerontology Series A: Biological Sciences and Medical Sciences*, 50(5), B254–B261.

Duhon, S. A., Murakami, S., & Johnson, T. E. (1996). Direct isolation of longevity mutants in the nematode *Caenorhabditis elegans*. *Developmental Genetics*, 18(2), 144–153.

Epstein, J., & Gershon, D. (1972). Studies on ageing in nematodes IV. The effect of antioxidants on cellular damage and life span. *Mechanisms of Ageing and Development*, 1, 257–264.

Evason, K., Huang, C., Yamben, I., Covey, D. F., & Kornfeld, K. (2005). Anticonvulsant medications extend worm life-span. *Science*, 307(5707), 258–262.

Felkai, S., Ewbank, J. J., Lemieux, J. J., Labb, C., Brown, G. G., & Hekimi, S. (1999). CLK-1 controls respiration, behavior and aging in the nematode Caenorhabditis elegans. *Embo Journal*, 18(7), 1783–1792.

Feng, J., Bussiere, F., & Hekimi, S. (2001). Mitochondrial electron transport is a key determinant of life span in *Caenorhabditis elegans*. *Developmental Cell*, 1(5), 633–644.

Finkel, T., & Holbrook, N. J. (2000). Oxidants, oxidative stress and the biology of ageing. *Nature*, 408(6809), 239–247.

Foll, R. L., Pleyers, A., Lewandovski, G. J., Wermter, C., Hegemann, V., & Paul, R. J. (1999). Anaerobiosis in the nematode *Caenorhabditis elegans*. *Comparative Biochemistry and Physiology. Part B,*

Biochemistry & Molecular Biology, 124(3), 269–280.

Friedman, D. B., & Johnson, T. E. (1988a). A mutation in the age-1 gene in *Caenorhabditis elegans* lengthens life and reduces hermaphrodite fertility. *Genetics*, 118(1), 75–86.

Friedman, D. B., & Johnson, T. E. (1988b). Three mutants that extend both mean and maximum life span of the nematode, Caenorhabditis elegans, define the age-1 gene. *Journal of Gerontology*, 43(4), B102–B109.

Garigan, D., Hsu, A. L., Fraser, A. G., Kamath, R. S., Ahringer, J., & Kenyon, C. (2002). Genetic analysis of tissue aging in Caenorhabditis elegans: a role for heat-shock factor and bacterial proliferation. *Genetics*, 161(3), 1101–1112.

Gems, D., & Riddle, D. L. (2000). Genetic, behavioral and environmental determinants of male longevity in *Caenorhabditis elegans*. *Genetics*, 154(4), 1597–1610.

Gems, D., Sutton, A. J., Sundermeyer, M. L., Albert, P. S., King, K. V., Edgley, M. L., Larsen, P. L., & Riddle, D. L. (1998). Two pleiotropic classes of daf-2 mutation affect larval arrest, adult behavior, reproduction and longevity in Caenorhabditis elegans. *Genetics*, 150(1), 129–155.

Gershon, H., & Gershon, D. (2001). Critical assessment of paradigms in aging research. *Experimental Gerontology*, 36(7), 1035–1047.

Golden, T. R., Hinerfeld, D. A., & Melov, S. (2002). Oxidative stress and aging: beyond correlation. *Aging Cell*, 1(2), 117–123.

Guarente, L., & Kenyon, C. (2000). Genetic pathways that regulate ageing in model organisms. *Nature*, 408(6809), 255–262.

Hall, D. M., Oberley, T. D., Moseley, P. M., Buettner, G. R., Oberley, L. W., Weindruch, R., & Kregel, K. C. (2000). Caloric restriction improves thermotolerance and reduces hyperthermia-induced cellular damage in old rats. *FASEB Journal*, 14(1), 78–86.

Harman, D. (1956). Aging: a theory based on free radical and radiation chemistry. *Journal of Gerontology*, 2, 298–300.

Hartman, P. S., Ishii, N., Kayser, E. B., Morgan, P. G., & Sedensky, M. M. (2001). Mitochondrial mutations differentially affect aging, mutability and anesthetic sensitivity in *Caenorhabditis elegans*.

Mechanisms of Ageing and Development, 122(11), 1187–1201.

Hekimi, S., & Guarente, L. (2003). Genetics and the specificity of the aging process. *Science*, 299(5611), 1351–1354.

Henderson, S. T., & Johnson, T. E. (2001). daf-16 integrates developmental and environmental inputs to mediate aging in the nematode *Caenorhabditis elegans*. *Current Biology*, 11(24), 1975–1980.

Herndon, L. A., Schmeissner, P. J., Dudaronek, J. M., Brown, P. A., Listner, K. M., Sakano, Y., Paupard, M. C., Hall, D. H., & Driscoll, M. (2002). Stochastic and genetic factors influence tissue-specific decline in ageing *C. elegans*. *Nature*, 419(6909), 808–814.

Hertweck, M., Gobel, C., & Baumeister, R. (2004). C. elegans SGK-1 is the critical component in the Akt/PKB kinase complex to control stress response and life span. *Developmental Cell*, 6(4), 577–588.

Honda, Y., & Honda, S. (1999). The daf-2 gene network for longevity regulates oxidative stress resistance and Mn-superoxide dismutase gene expression in *Caenorhabditis elegans*. *Faseb Journal*, 13(11), 1385–1393.

Hosono, R., Sato, Y., Aizawa, S. I., & Mitsui, Y. (1980). Age-dependent changes in mobility and separation of the nematode *Caenorhabditis elegans*. *Experimental Gerontology*, 15(4), 285–289.

Houthoofd, K., Braeckman, B. P., Johnson, T. E., & Vanfleteren, J. R. (2004). Extending life-span in *C. elegans*. *Science*, 305(5688), 1238–1239.

Houthoofd, K., Braeckman, B. P., Johnson, T. E., & Vanfleteren, J. R. (2003). Life extension via dietary restriction is independent of the Ins/IGF-1 signalling pathway in *Caenorhabditis elegans*. *Experimental Gerontology*, 38(9), 947–954.

Houthoofd, K., Braeckman, B. P., Lenaerts, I., Brys, K., De Vreese, A., Van Eygen, S., & Vanfleteren, J. R. (2002). Axenic growth up-regulates mass-specific metabolic rate, stress resistance, and extends life span in *Caenorhabditis elegans*. *Experimental Gerontology*, 37(12), 1371–1378.

Hsu, A. L., Murphy, C. T., & Kenyon, C. (2003). Regulation of aging and age-related disease by DAF-16 and heat-shock factor. *Science*, 300(5622), 1142–1145.

Huynen, M. A., Snel, B., Bork, P., & Gibson, T. J. (2001). The phylogenetic distribution of frataxin indicates a role in iron-sulfur cluster protein assembly. *Human Molecular Genetics*, 10(21), 2463–2468.

Ishii, N., Fujii, M., Hartman, P. S., Tsuda, M., Yasuda, K., Senoo-Matsuda, N., Yanase, S., Ayusawa, D., & Suzuki, K. (1998). A mutation in succinate dehydrogenase cytochrome b causes oxidative stress and ageing in nematodes. *Nature*, 394(6694), 694–697.

Iwata, S., Lee, J. W., Okada, K., Lee, J. K., Iwata, M., Rasmussen, B., Link, T. A., Ramaswamy, S., & Jap, B. K. (1998). Complete structure of the 11-subunit bovine mitochondrial cytochrome bc1 complex. *Science*, 281(5373), 64–71.

Jauniaux, E., Gulbis, B., & Burton, G. J. (2003). The human first trimester gestational sac limits rather than facilitates oxygen transfer to the foetus: a review. *Placenta*, 24 Suppl A, S86–S93.

Jenkins, N. L., McColl, G., & Lithgow, G. J. (2004). Fitness cost of extended lifespan in *Caenorhabditis elegans*. *Proceedings of the Royal Society of London Series B-Biological Sciences*, 271(1556), 2523–2526.

Joela, H., Kasa, S., Lehtovuori, P., & Bech, M. (1997). EPR, ENDOR and TRIPLE resonance and MO studies on ubiquinones (Q-n): comparison of radical anions and cations of coenzymes Q-10 and Q-6 with the model compounds Q-2 and Q-0. *Acta Chemica Scandinavica*, 51(2), 233–241.

Johnson, T. E. (1987). Aging can be genetically dissected into component processes using long-lived lines of Caenorhabditis elegans. *Proceedings of the National Academy of Sciences of the USA*, 84(11), 3777–3781.

Johnson, T. E. (1990a). *Caenorhabditis elegans* offers the potential for molecular dissection of the aging processes. In E. L. Scheider & J. W. Rowe (Eds.), *Handbook of the biology of aging* (3rd ed., pp. 45–59). New York: Academic Press.

Johnson, T. E. (1990b). Increased life-span of age-1 mutants in *Caenorhabditis elegans* and lower Gompertz rate of aging. *Science*, 249(4971), 908–912.

Johnson, T. E. (2003). Advantages and disadvantages of *Caenorhabditis elegans* for aging research. *Experimental Gerontology*, 38(11–12), 1329–1332.

Johnson, T. E., & Hutchinson, E. W. (1993). Absence of strong heterosis for life span and other life history traits in *Caenorhabditis elegans*. *Genetics*, 134(2), 465–474.

Johnson, T. E., & Wood, W. B. (1982). Genetic analysis of life-span in *Caenorhabditis elegans*. *Proceedings of the National Academy of Sciences of the USA*, 79(21), 6603–6607.

Johnson, T. E., Cypser, J., de Castro, E., de Castro, S., Henderson, S., Murakami, S., Rikke, B., Tedesco, P., & Link, C. (2000). Gerontogenes mediate health and longevity in nematodes through increasing resistance to environmental toxins and stressors. *Experimental Gerontology*, 35(6–7), 687–694.

Johnson, T. E., de Castro, E., Hegi de Castro, S., Cypser, J., Henderson, S., & Tedesco, P. (2001). Relationship between increased longevity and stress resistance as assessed through gerontogene mutations in *Caenorhabditis elegans*. *Experimental Gerontology*, 36(10), 1609–1617.

Johnson, T. E., Henderson, S., Murakami, S., de Castro, E., de Castro, S. H., Cypser, J., Rikke, B., Tedesco, P., & Link, C. (2002). Longevity genes in the nematode *Caenorhabditis elegans* also mediate increased resistance to stress and prevent disease. *Journal of Inherited Metabolic Disease*, 25(3), 197–206.

Jonassen, T., Davis, D. E., Larsen, P. L., & Clarke, C. F. (2003). Reproductive fitness and quinone content of *Caenorhabditis elegans* clk-1 mutants fed coenzyme Q isoforms of varying length. *Journal of Biological Chemistry*, 278(51), 51735–51742.

Jonassen, T., Larsen, P. L., & Clarke, C. F. (2001). A dietary source of coenzyme Q is essential for growth of long-lived *Caenorhabditis elegans* clk-1 mutants. *Proceedings of the National Academy of Sciences of the USA*, 98(2), 421–426.

Jonassen, T., Marbois, B. N., Faull, K. F., Clarke, C. F., & Larsen, P. L. (2002). Development and fertility in *Caenorhabditis elegans* clk-1 mutants depend upon transport of dietary coenzyme Q8 to mitochondria. *Journal of Biological Chemistry*, 277(47), 45020–45027.

Kamath, R. S., & Ahringer, J. (2003). Genome-wide RNAi screening in *Caenorhabditis elegans*. *Methods*, 30(4), 313–321.

Kapahi, P., Zid, B. M., Harper, T., Koslover, D., Sapin, V., & Benzer, S. (2004). Regulation of lifespan in *Drosophila* by modulation of genes in the TOR signaling pathway. *Current Biology*, 14(10), 885–890.

Kawano, T., Ito, Y., Ishiguro, M., Takuwa, K., Nakajima, T., & Kimura, Y. (2000). Molecular cloning and characterization of a new insulin/IGF-like peptide of the nematode *Caenorhabditis elegans*. *Biochemical and Biophysical Research Communications*, 273(2), 431–436.

Kayser, E. B., Morgan, P. G., Hoppel, C. L., & Sedensky, M. M. (2001). Mitochondrial expression and function of GAS-1 in *Caenorhabditis elegans*. *Journal of Biological Chemistry*, 276(23), 20551–20558.

Kayser, E. B., Sedensky, M. M., & Morgan, P. G. (2004a). The effects of complex I function and oxidative damage on lifespan and anesthetic sensitivity in *Caenorhabditis elegans*. *Mechanisms of Ageing and Development*, 125(6), 455–464.

Kayser, E. B., Sedensky, M. M., Morgan, P. G., & Hoppel, C. L. (2004b). Mitochondrial oxidative phosphorylation is defective in the long-lived mutant clk-1. *Journal of Biological Chemistry*, 279(52), 54479–54486.

Kenyon, C., Chang, J., Gensch, E., Rudner, A., & Tabtiang, R. (1993). A *C. elegans* mutant that lives twice as long as wild type. *Nature*, 366(6454), 461–464.

Kim, S. K., Lund, J., Kiraly, M., Duke, K., Jiang, M., Stuart, J. M., Eizinger, A., Wylie, B. N., & Davidson, G. S. (2001). A gene expression map for *Caenorhabditis elegans*. *Science*, 293(5537), 2087–2092.

Kimble, J., & Hirsh, D. (1979). The postembryonic cell lineages of the hermaphrodite and male gonads in *Caenorhabditis elegans*. *Developmental Biology*, 70(2), 396–417.

Kimura, K. D., Tissenbaum, H. A., Liu, Y., & Ruvkun, G. (1997). daf-2, an insulin receptor-like gene that regulates longevity and diapause in *Caenorhabditis elegans*. *Science*, 277(5328), 942–946.

Kirkwood, T. B., & Austad, S. N. (2000). Why do we age? *Nature*, 408(6809), 233–238.

Klass, M. R. (1977). Aging in the nematode *Caenorhabditis elegans*: major biological and environmental factors influencing life span. *Mechanisms of Ageing and Development*, 6(6), 413–429.

Klass, M. R. (1983). A method for the isolation of longevity mutants in the nematode *Caenorhabditis elegans* and initial results. *Mechanisms of Ageing and Development*, 22(3–4), 279–286.

Klass, M. R., & Hirsh, D. (1976). Non-ageing developmental variant of *Caenorhabditis elegans*. *Nature*, 260(5551), 523–525.

Kristal, B. S., & Krasnikov, B. F. (2003). Structure-(Dys)function relationships in mitochondrial electron transport chain complex II? *Science of Aging Knowledge Environment*, 2003(5), PE3.

Lakowski, B., & Hekimi, S. (1996). Determination of life-span in *Caenorhabditis elegans* by four clock genes. *Science*, 272(5264), 1010–1013.

Lakowski, B., & Hekimi, S. (1998). The genetics of caloric restriction in *Caenorhabditis elegans*. *Proceedings of the National Academy of Sciences of the USA*, 95(22), 13091–13096.

Larsen, P. L. (1993). Aging and resistance to oxidative damage in Caenorhabditis elegans. *Proceedings of the National Academy of Sciences of the USA*, 90(19), 8905–8909.

Lee, R. Y., Hench, J., & Ruvkun, G. (2001). Regulation of *C. elegans* DAF-16 and its human ortholog FKHRL1 by the daf-2 insulin-like signaling pathway. *Current Biology*, 11(24), 1950–1957.

Lee, S. S., Lee, R. Y., Fraser, A. G., Kamath, R. S., Ahringer, J., & Ruvkun, G. (2003). A systematic RNAi screen identifies a critical role for mitochondria in *C. elegans* longevity. *Nature Genetics*, 33(1), 40–48.

Li, W., Kennedy, S. G., & Ruvkun, G. (2003). daf-28 encodes a *C. elegans* insulin superfamily member that is regulated by environmental cues and acts in the DAF-2 signaling pathway. *Genes & Development*, 17(7), 844–858.

Lin, K., Hsin, H., Libina, N., & Kenyon, C. (2001). Regulation of the *Caenorhabditis elegans* longevity protein DAF-16 by insulin/IGF-1 and germline signaling. *Nature Genetics*, 28(2), 139–145.

Lin, S. J., & Guarente, L. (2003). Nicotinamide adenine dinucleotide, a metabolic regulator of transcription, longevity and disease. *Current Opinions in Cell Biology*, 15(2), 241–246.

Lin, S. J., Defossez, P. A., & Guarente, L. (2000). Requirement of NAD and SIR2 for life-span extension by calorie restriction in Saccharomyces cerevisiae. *Science*, 289(5487), 2126–2128.

Link, C. D., & Johnson, C. J. (2002). Reporter transgenes for study of oxidant stress in Caenorhabditis elegans. *Methods in Enzymology*, 353, 497–505.

Link, C. D., Cypser, J. R., Johnson, C. J., & Johnson, T. E. (1999). Direct observation of stress response in Caenorhabditis elegans using a reporter transgene. *Cell Stress & Chaperones*, 4(4), 235–242.

Lithgow, G. J. (1996). The molecular genetics of *Caenorhabditis elegans* aging. In J. W. Rowe & E. L. Schneider (Eds.), *Handbook of the biology of aging* (4th ed., pp. 55–73). New York: Academic Press.

Lithgow, G. J. (2001). Hormesis: a new hope for ageing studies or a poor second to genetics? *Human & Experimental Toxicology*, 20(6), 301–303; discussion 319–320.

Lithgow, G. J., White, T. M., Melov, S., & Johnson, T. E. (1995). Thermotolerance and extended life-span conferred by single-gene mutations and induced by thermal stress. *Proceedings of the National Academy of Sciences of the USA*, 92(16), 7540–7544.

Long, X., Spycher, C., Han, Z. S., Rose, A. M., Muller, F., & Avruch, J. (2002). TOR deficiency in *C. elegans* causes developmental arrest and intestinal atrophy by inhibition of mRNA translation. *Current Biology*, 12(17), 1448–1461.

Longo, V. D., & Finch, C. E. (2003). Evolutionary medicine: from dwarf model systems to healthy centenarians? *Science*, 299(5611), 1342–1346.

Lund, J., Tedesco, P., Duke, K., Wang, J., Kim, S. K., & Johnson, T. E. (2002). Transcriptional profile of aging in *C. elegans*. *Current Biology*, 12(18), 1566–1573.

Mahajan-Miklos, S., Tan, M. W., Rahme, L. G., & Ausubel, F. M. (1999). Molecular mechanisms of bacterial virulence elucidated using a Pseudomonas aeruginosa-*Caenorhabditis elegans* pathogenesis model. *Cell*, 96(1), 47–56.

Malone, E. A., & Thomas, J. H. (1994). A screen for nonconditional dauer-constitutive mutations in *Caenorhabditis elegans*. *Genetics*, 136(3), 879–886.

Malone, E. A., Inoue, T., & Thomas, J. H. (1996). Genetic analysis of the roles of daf-28 and age-1 in regulating *Caenorhabditis elegans* dauer formation. *Genetics*, 143(3), 1193–1205.

Martin, G. M., Austad, S. N., & Johnson, T. E. (1996). Genetic analysis of ageing: role of oxidative damage and environmental stresses. *Nature Genetics*, 13(1), 25–34.

Masoro, E. J. (1998). Caloric restriction. *Aging (Milano)*, 10(2), 173–174.

McCay, C. M., Crowell, M. F., & Maynard, L. A. (1935). The effects of retarded growth upon the length of life span and upon the ultimate body size. *Journal of Nutrition*, 10, 63–79.

McElwee, J., Bubb, K., & Thomas, J. H. (2003). Transcriptional outputs of the *Caenorhabditis elegans* forkhead protein DAF-16. *Aging Cell*, 2(2), 111–121.

Meissner, B., Boll, M., Daniel, H., & Baumeister, R. (2004). Deletion of the intestinal peptide transporter affects insulin and TOR signaling in *C. elegans*. *Journal of Biological Chemistry*, 279(35), 36739–36745.

Melendez, A., Talloczy, Z., Seaman, M., Eskelinen, E. L., Hall, D. H., & Levine, B. (2003). Autophagy genes are essential for dauer development and life-span extension in *C. elegans*. *Science*, 301(5638), 1387–1391.

Melov, S., Hertz, G. Z., Stormo, G. D., & Johnson, T. E. (1994). Detection of deletions in the mitochondrial genome of *Caenorhabditis elegans*. *Nucleic Acids Research*, 22(6), 1075–1078.

Melov, S., Lithgow, G. J., Fischer, D. R., Tedesco, P. M., & Johnson, T. E. (1995). Increased frequency of deletions in the mitochondrial genome with age of

Caenorhabditis elegans. Nucleic Acids Research, 23(8), 1419–1425.

Melov, S., Ravenscroft, J., Malik, S., Gill, M. S., Walker, D. W., Clayton, P. E., Wallace, D. C., Malfroy, B., Doctrow, S. R., & Lithgow, G. J. (2000). Extension of life-span with superoxide dismutase/catalase mimetics. *Science*, 289(5484), 1567–1569.

Minois, N. (2000). Longevity and aging: beneficial effects of exposure to mild stress. *Biogerontology*, 1(1), 15–29.

Mitchell, P. (1975). The protonmotive Q cycle: a general formulation. *FEBS Letters*, 59(2), 137–139.

Miyadera, H., Amino, H., Hiraishi, A., Taka, H., Murayama, K., Miyoshi, H., Sakamoto, K., Ishii, N., Hekimi, S., & Kita, K. (2001). Altered quinone biosynthesis in the long-lived clk-1 mutants of Caenorhabditis elegans. *Journal of Biological Chemistry*, 276(11), 7713–7716.

Miyadera, H., Kano, K., Miyoshi, H., Ishii, N., Hekimi, S., & Kita, K. (2002). Quinones in long-lived clk-1 mutants of *Caenorhabditis elegans. FEBS Letters*, 512(1–3), 33–37.

Morris, J. Z., Tissenbaum, H. A., & Ruvkun, G. (1996). A phosphatidylinositol-3-OH kinase family member regulating longevity and diapause in *Caenorhabditis elegans. Nature*, 382(6591), 536–539.

Munoz, M. J., & Riddle, D. L. (2003). Positive selection of *Caenorhabditis elegans* mutants with increased stress resistance and longevity. *Genetics*, 163(1), 171–180.

Murakami, S., & Johnson, T. E. (1996). A genetic pathway conferring life extension and resistance to UV stress in *Caenorhabditis elegans. Genetics*, 143(3), 1207–1218.

Murakami, S., & Johnson, T. E. (1998). Life extension and stress resistance in *Caenorhabditis elegans* modulated by the tkr-1 gene. *Current Biology*, 8(19), 1091–1094.

Murakami, S., & Johnson, T. E. (2001). The OLD-1 positive regulator of longevity and stress resistance is under DAF-16 regulation in *Caenorhabditis elegans. Current Biology*, 11(19), 1517–1523.

Murakami, S., Tedesco, P. M., Cypser, J. R., & Johnson, T. E. (2000). Molecular genetic mechanisms of life span manipulation in *Caenorhabditis elegans. Annals of*

the New York Academy of Sciences, 908, 40–49.

Murphy, C. T., McCarroll, S. A., Bargmann, C. I., Fraser, A., Kamath, R. S., Ahringer, J., Li, H., & Kenyon, C. (2003). Genes that act downstream of DAF-16 to influence the lifespan of *Caenorhabditis elegans. Nature*, 424(6946), 277–283.

Nakai, D., Shimizu, T., Nojiri, H., Uchiyama, S., Koike, H., Takahashi, M., Hirokawa, K., & Shirasawa, T. (2004). coq7/clk-1 regulates mitochondrial respiration and the generation of reactive oxygen species via coenzyme Q. *Aging Cell*, 3(5), 273–281.

Nakai, D., Yuasa, S., Takahashi, M., Shimizu, T., Asaumi, S., Isono, K., Takao, T., Suzuki, Y., Kuroyanagi, H., Hirokawa, K., Koseki, H., & Shirsawa, T. (2001). Mouse homologue of coq7/clk-1, longevity gene in *Caenorhabditis elegans*, is essential for coenzyme Q synthesis, maintenance of mitochondrial integrity, and neurogenesis. *Biochemical and Biophysical Research Communications*, 289(2), 463–471.

Nelson, J. F., Karelus, K., Bergman, M. D., & Felicio, L. S. (1995). Neuroendocrine involvement in aging: evidence from studies of reproductive aging and caloric restriction. *Neurobiology of Aging*, 16(5), 837–843; discussion 855–836.

New, D. A. (1978). Whole-embryo culture and the study of mammalian embryos during organogenesis. *Biological Reviews of the Cambridge Philosophical Society*, 53(1), 81–122.

Nicholls, D. G. (2002). Mitochondrial function and dysfunction in the cell: its relevance to aging and aging-related disease. *International Journal of Biochemistry & Cell Biology*, 34(11), 1372–1381.

Nohl, H. (1994). Generation of superoxide radicals as byproduct of cellular respiration. *Annales de Biologie Clinique (Paris)*, 52(3), 199–204.

Okimoto, R., Macfarlane, J. L., Clary, D. O., & Wolstenholme, D. R. (1992). The mitochondrial genomes of two nematodes, *Caenorhabditis elegans* and Ascaris suum. *Genetics*, 130(3), 471–498.

Ookuma, S., Fukuda, M., & Nishida, E. (2003). Identification of a DAF-16 transcriptional target gene, scl-1, that regulates longevity and stress resistance in *Caenorhabditis elegans*. *Current Biology*, 13(5), 427–431.

Padilla, S., Jonassen, T., Jimenez-Hidalgo, M. A., Fernandez-Ayala, D. J., Lopez-Lluch, G., Marbois, B., Navas, P., Clarke, C. F., & Santos-Ocana, C. (2004). Demethoxy-Q, an intermediate of coenzyme Q biosynthesis, fails to support respiration in Saccharomyces cerevisiae and lacks antioxidant activity. *Journal of Biological Chemistry*, 279(25), 25995–26004.

Paradis, S., & Ruvkun, G. (1998). *Caenorhabditis elegans* Akt/PKB transduces insulin receptor-like signals from AGE-1 PI3 kinase to the DAF-16 transcription factor. *Genes & Development*, 12(16), 2488–2498.

Paradis, S., Ailion, M., Toker, A., Thomas, J. H., & Ruvkun, G. (1999). A PDK1 homolog is necessary and sufficient to transduce AGE-1 PI3 kinase signals that regulate diapause in *Caenorhabditis elegans*. *Genes & Development*, 13(11), 1438–1452.

Pierce, S. B., Costa, M., Wisotzkey, R., Devadhar, S., Homburger, S. A., Buchman, A. R., Ferguson, K. C., Heller, J., Platt, D. M., Pasquinelli, A. A., Liu, L. X., Doberstein, S. K., & Ruvkun, G. (2001). Regulation of DAF-2 receptor signaling by human insulin and ins-1, a member of the unusually large and diverse *C. elegans* insulin gene family. *Genes & Development*, 15(6), 672–686.

Post, S. G., & Binstock, R. H. (2004). *The fountain of youth: cultural, scientific, and ethical perspectives on a biomedical goal*. Oxford: Oxford University Press.

Puccio, H., & Koenig, M. (2002). Friedreich ataxia: a paradigm for mitochondrial diseases. *Current Opinion in Genetics & Development*, 12(3), 272–277.

Rattan, S. I. (1985). Beyond the present crisis in gerontology. *Bioessays*, 2, 226–228.

Rattan, S. I. (2001). Hormesis in biogerontology. *Critical Reviews in Toxicology*, 31(4–5), 663–664.

Rea, S., & James, D. E. (1997). Moving GLUT4: the biogenesis and trafficking of GLUT4 storage vesicles. *Diabetes*, 46(11), 1667–1677.

Rea, S., & Johnson, T. E. (2003). A metabolic model for life span determination in *Caenorhabditis elegans*. *Developmental Cell*, 5(2), 197–203.

Riddle, D. L., & Albert, P. S. (1997). Genetic and environmental regulation of dauer larva development. In D. L. Riddle, T. Blumenthal, B. J. Meyer, & J. R. Priess (Eds.), *C. elegans II* (pp. 739–768). Plainview, NY: Cold Spring Harbor Press.

Riddle, D. L., Blumenthal, T., Meyer, B. J., & Priess, J. R. (Eds.). (1997). *C. elegans II*. Plainview, NY: Cold Spring Harbor Laboratory Press.

Rikke, B. A., Murakami, S., & Johnson, T. E. (2000). Paralogy and orthology of tyrosine kinases that can extend the life span of *Caenorhabditis elegans*. *Molecular and Biological Evolution*, 17(5), 671–683.

Rohde, J., Heitman, J., & Cardenas, M. E. (2001). The TOR kinases link nutrient sensing to cell growth. *Journal of Biological Chemistry*, 276(13), 9583–9586.

Ronquist, G., Andersson, A., Bendsoe, N., & Falck, B. (2003). Human epidermal energy metabolism is functionally anaerobic. *Experimental Dermatology*, 12(5), 572–579.

Rothstein, M. (1980). Nematodes as biological models. In B. M. Zuckerman (Ed.), *Aging and other model systems* (Vol. 2, pp. 29–46). New York: Academic Press.

Russell, R. L., & Jacobson, L. A. (1985). Some aspects of aging can be studied easily in nematodes. In C. E. Finch & E. L. Schneider (Eds.), *Handbook of the biology of aging* (2nd ed., pp. 128–145). New York: Van Nostrand Reinhold.

Saltiel, A. R., & Kahn, C. R. (2001). Insulin signalling and the regulation of glucose and lipid metabolism. *Nature*, 414(6865), 799–806.

Sampayo, J. N., Gill, M. S., & Lithgow, G. J. (2003). Oxidative stress and aging: the use of superoxide dismutase/catalase mimetics to extend lifespan. *Biochemical Society Transactions*, 31(Pt 6), 1305–1307.

Sampayo, J. N., Jenkins, N. L., & Lithgow, G. J. (2000). Using stress resistance to isolate novel longevity mutations in *Caenorhabditis elegans*. *Annals of the New York Academy of Sciences*, 908, 324–326.

Scott, B. A., Avidan, M. S., & Crowder, C. M. (2002). Regulation of hypoxic death in C. elegans by the insulin/IGF receptor homolog DAF-2. *Science, 296*(5577), 2388–2391.

Senoo-Matsuda, N., Yasuda, K., Tsuda, M., Ohkubo, T., Yoshimura, S., Nakazawa, H., Hartman, P. S., & Ishii, N. (2001). A defect in the cytochrome b large subunit in complex II causes both superoxide anion overproduction and abnormal energy metabolism in Caenorhabditis elegans. *Journal of Biological Chemistry, 276*(45), 41553–41558.

Shibata, Y., Branicky, R., Landaverde, I. O., & Hekimi, S. (2003). Redox regulation of germline and vulval development in *Caenorhabditis elegans. Science, 302*(5651), 1779–1782.

Shook, D. R., & Johnson, T. E. (1999). Quantitative trait loci affecting survival and fertility-related traits in *Caenorhabditis elegans* show genotype-environment interactions, pleiotropy and epistasis. *Genetics, 153*(3), 1233–1243.

Shook, D. R., Brooks, A., & Johnson, T. E. (1996). Mapping quantitative trait loci affecting life history traits in the nematode Caenorhabditis elegans. *Genetics, 142*(3), 801–817.

Sohal, R. S. (2002). Role of oxidative stress and protein oxidation in the aging process. *Free Radical Biology and Medicine, 33*(1), 37–44.

Stenmark, P., Grunler, J., Mattsson, J., Sindelar, P. J., Nordlund, P., & Berthold, D. A. (2001). A new member of the family of di-iron carboxylate proteins. Coq7 (clk-1), a membrane-bound hydroxylase involved in ubiquinone biosynthesis. *Journal of Biological Chemistry, 276*(36), 33297–33300.

Sulston, J. E., & Horvitz, H. R. (1977). Post-embryonic cell lineages of the nematode, *Caenorhabditis elegans. Developmental Biology, 56*(1), 110–156.

Tatar, M., Bartke, A., & Antebi, A. (2003). The endocrine regulation of aging by insulin-like signals. *Science, 299*(5611), 1346–1351.

Tavernarakis, N., & Driscoll, M. (2002). Caloric restriction and lifespan: a role for protein turnover? *Mechanisms of Ageing and Development, 123*(2–3), 215–229.

Tissenbaum, H. A., & Guarente, L. (2001). Increased dosage of a sir-2 gene extends lifespan in *Caenorhabditis elegans. Nature, 410*(6825), 227–230.

Tsang, W. Y., & Lemire, B. D. (2002). Mitochondrial genome content is regulated during nematode development. *Biochemical and Biophysical Research Communications, 291*(1), 8–16.

Tsang, W. Y., Sayles, L. C., Grad, L. I., Pilgrim, D. B., & Lemire, B. D. (2001). Mitochondrial respiratory chain deficiency in *Caenorhabditis elegans* results in developmental arrest and increased life span. *Journal of Biological Chemistry, 276*(34), 32240–32246.

Van Voorhies, W. A. (2001a). Hormesis and aging. *Human & Experimental Toxicology, 20*(6), 315–317; discussion 319–320.

Van Voorhies, W. A. (2001b). Metabolism and lifespan. *Experimental Gerontology, 36*(1), 55–64.

Vanfleteren, J. R. (1993). Oxidative stress and ageing in *Caenorhabditis elegans. Biochemical Journal, 292*(Pt 2), 605–608.

Vellai, T., Takacs-Vellai, K., Zhang, Y., Kovacs, A. L., Orosz, L., & Muller, F. (2003). Genetics: influence of TOR kinase on lifespan in *C. elegans. Nature, 426*(6967), 620.

Ventura, N., Rea, S., Henderson, S. T.,Condo, I., Johnson, T. E., & Testi, R. (2005). Suppression of Frataxin extends the life span of *Caenorhabditis elegans. Aging Cell, 4*(2), 109–112.

Vowels, J. J., & Thomas, J. H. (1992). Genetic analysis of chemosensory control of dauer formation in *Caenorhabditis elegans. Genetics, 130*(1), 105–123.

Walker, D. W., McColl, G., Jenkins, N. L., Harris, J., & Lithgow, G. J. (2000). Evolution of lifespan in *C. elegans. Nature, 405*(6784), 296–297.

Walker, G. A., & Lithgow, G. J. (2003). Lifespan extension in *C. elegans* by a molecular chaperone dependent upon insulin-like signals. *Aging Cell, 2*(2), 131–139.

Wallace, D. C. (1999). Mitochondrial diseases in man and mouse. *Science, 283*(5407), 1482–1488.

Wong, A., Boutis, P., & Hekimi, S. (1995). Mutations in the clk-1 gene of *Caenorhabditis elegans* affect developmental and behavioral timing. *Genetics,* 139(3), 1247–1259.

Wood, W. B. (Ed.). (1988). *The nematode Caenorhabditis elegans.* Plainview, NY: Cold Spring Harbor Press.

Wu, Z., Smith, J. V., Paramasivam, V., Butko, P., Khan, I., Cypser, J. R., & Luo, Y. (2002). Ginkgo biloba extract EGb 761 increases stress resistance and extends life span of *Caenorhabditis elegans. Cellular and Molecular Biology (Noisy-le-Grand, France),* 48(6), 725–731.

Yokoyama, K., Fukumoto, K., Murakami, T., Harada, S., Hosono, R., Wadhwa, R., Mitsui, Y., & Ohkuma, S. (2002). Extended longevity of *Caenorhabditis elegans* by knocking in extra copies of hsp70F, a homolog of mot-2 (mortalin)/ mthsp70/Grp75. *FEBS Letters,* 516(1–3), 53–57.

Chapter 14

Genetic Manipulation of Life Span in *Drosophila melanogaster*

Daniel Ford and John Tower

I. Introduction

For nine decades, *Drosophila mela-nogaster* has been an effective model system for investigating genetics. Knowledge of genetic recombination, gene regulation, and development have all benefited from experiments with *Drosophila*. Furthermore, recent research on *Drosophila* aging has led to the discovery of multiple genes and pathways that extend life span. The purpose of this chapter is to review some of the techniques available for studying aging in *Drosophila melanogaster* and to describe several experiments that have yielded a substantial increase in *Drosophila* life span. For a review of quantitative trait loci (QTL) mapping and population selection studies, see Mackay, 2002, or Chapter 7 of this volume.

II. Genetic Methods for Manipulating *Drosophila* Life Span

A. P Elements and *Drosophila* Genetics

P elements are one of the primary advantages to using *Drosophila* as a model system. They are naturally occurring transposable elements that have been isolated for use in genetic experiments (Ryder & Russell, 2002). DNA constructs can be cloned between the 5′ and 3′ P element ends. This DNA can then be injected along with DNA encoding the transposase enzyme into the germ-line cells of *Drosophila* embryos. The transposase catalyzes the transposition of the P element ends (and all sequences in between) into one of the fruit fly's four chromosomes. The injected DNA and transposase is degraded, and stable transgenic lines are derived from the progeny of the injected flies (Rubin & Spradling, 1982). However, since a P element inserts randomly into the *Drosophila* genome, it is possible that it can disrupt either a gene or regulatory region, altering the life span of the fly (Kaiser *et al.*, 1997). This is generally controlled for by generating multiple independent insertions and looking for affects that are consistent across the different lines.

B. Conditional Systems for Transgene Expression and Studying Life Span

Methods for transgene expression in *Drosophila* can be classified as either conditional (inducible) or non-conditional (non-inducible). Conditional systems require an environmental stimulus such as a heat pulse or a drug to initiate expression of the transgene. Conditional systems possess several advantages over non-conditional systems, particularly for studying a quantitative trait such as life span. First, non-conditional systems are generally implemented so that control and experimental groups are taken from two separate crosses (see Figure 14.1A). This results in slightly different environments for each group during development and the first few hours of adult life span. In contrast with conditional systems, the control and experimental flies come from the same cross (see Figure 14.1B). Second, non-conditional systems result in different genetic backgrounds for control and experimental groups. In all non-conditional *Drosophila* experiments, at least one chromosome is not identical between control and experimental groups (see Figure 14.1A). Since life span is a complex phenotype influenced by multiple genes, variations in genetic background can result in both false positives and false negatives with respect to genes modulating life span. In contrast, with conditional systems, the control and experimental animals have identical genetic backgrounds. Third, with conditional systems, expression of the transgene can be initiated at any timepoint in the life cycle. For example, an introduced gene could be expressed during development, adulthood, or both, depending on the demands of the experiment. This is important because the same gene that extends life span during adulthood may decrease life span when it is expressed during development, or vice versa.

Conditional systems have at least one minor disadvantage in that the stimulus used to initiate expression of the construct in the experimental group may itself affect life span. This problem can be addressed by assaying the effects of the stimulus in control backgrounds where no transgene is expressed.

The conditional systems currently available in *Drosophila* include tet-on, Gene Switch, and FLP-*out*. Each technique presents specific advantages and disadvantages.

C. The Tet-on Conditional System

In the tet-on system, the tetracycline derivative doxycycline (DOX) is added to fly food in order to initiate transcription of the gene of interest (Bieschke *et al.*, 1998). This system consists of two constructs. In the first construct, the powerful cytoplasmic actin (*actin5C*) promoter drives expression of the reverse tetracycline trans-activator protein (rtTA) in all tissues. The second construct consists of a synthetic promoter driving expression of the gene of interest (see Figure 14.2). The synthetic promoter in the second construct contains seven copies of the tetracycline operator linked to a core promoter (the tet-on promoter), which is the binding site for rtTA. When the tet-on system is activated in the experimental group by DOX feeding, the DOX binds to rtTA and causes a conformational change. The activated rtTA

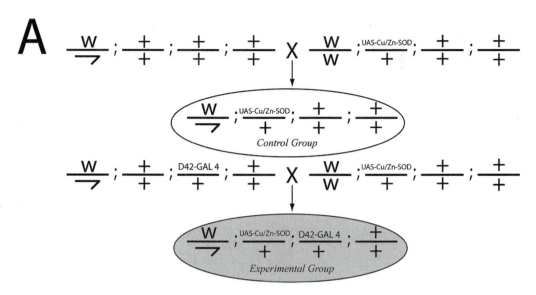

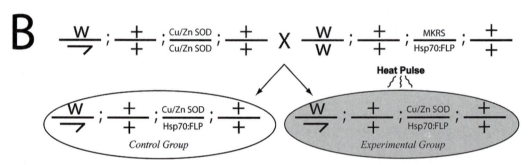

Figure 14.1 Crossing schemes for driving transgene expression in *Drosophila*. **(A)** A cross driving non-conditional expression of copper zinc superoxide dismutase (Cu/Zn-SOD) through the GAL4/UAS system. Control and experimental groups come from separate crosses, and their genetic background varies on one chromosome. **(B)** Cu/Zn-SOD is driven through the conditional FLP-*out* system. Experimental and control *Drosophila* are taken from the same pool of progeny. A heat pulse initiates expression of the gene of interest.

protein is then able to bind to the tetra-cycline operators, resulting in high-level expression of the gene of interest. The control group receives no DOX, and therefore the gene of interest is not expressed in the control group. DOX must be continuously added to fly food throughout life in order to maintain expression of the gene of interest.

One problem presented by the tet-on system is that under certain conditions, the antibiotic DOX can itself alter the life span of *Drosophila*. This can be identified by assaying the effects of the DOX in control backgrounds where no transgene is expressed. Taken together the data suggest that a 0 to 8 percent increase in life span due to the antibiotic effect of the DOX is common (Landis *et al.*, 2004). Investigators are currently trying to eliminate this small background effect of DOX by adding non-tetracycline antibiotics to both groups, as well as by other approaches.

D. The GeneSwitch Conditional System

The GeneSwitch system is directly analogous to the tet-on system. However, in this case, the progesterone antagonist RU486 is used as the stimulus (Roman

A

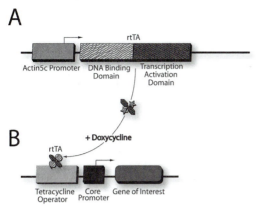

B

Figure 14.2 The tet-on conditional system. **(A)** The actin5c promoter drives expression of the reverse tetracycline trans-activator (rtTA), which changes conformation in the presence of doxycycline. **(B)** rtTA binds to the seven tet operators and initiates transcription of the gene of interest.

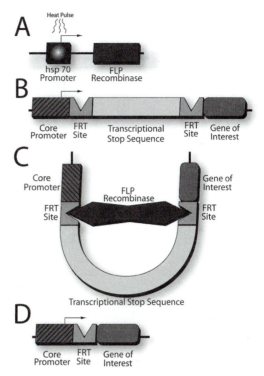

Figure 14.3 The FLP-*out* conditional system. **(A)** A heat pulse activates the *hsp70* promoter and drives the expression of the FLP recombinase. **(B)** Transcription of the gene of interest is blocked by a stop sequence, which is flanked by two FRT sites. **(C)** The FLP recombinase binds to the two FRT sites and removes the stop sequence. **(D)** With the stop sequence excised, the core promoter can drive expression of the gene of interest. The remaining FRT site is transcribed but not translated.

et al., 2001). The transcription factor (GeneSwitch) is a fusion of the yeast Gal4 DNA binding domain and transcriptional activation domain with the human progesterone receptor regulatory domain. The result is a synthetic transcription factor that binds to a upstream activating sequence (UAS) target site and activates transcription only in the presence of the artificial hormone RU486. The RU486 itself was found to have no detectable effect on life span (Giannakou *et al.*, 2004; Hwangbo *et al.*, 2004). *Drosophila* does not possess endogenous progesterone, so the impact of adding this hormone to the experimental group is expected to be minimal.

E. The FLP-*out* Conditional System

The FLP-*out* system requires a heat pulse as the trigger to cause expression of the gene of interest (Basler & Struhl, 1994; Struhl & Basler, 1993). Like the other systems, FLP-*out* consists of two constructs (see Figure 14.3). In the first construct, the promoter from the heat shock protein 70 gene (*hsp70*) is used to drive expression of yeast FLP recombinase. The second construct consists of a transcriptional

stop sequence located between the *actin5C* promoter and the gene of interest. The stop sequence is flanked by FLP recombination target (FRT) sites. When a 37-degree heat pulse is applied to the transgenic flies, the *hsp70* promoter drives high-level expression of the FLP recombinase in all tissues. Next, the FLP recombinase binds to the two FRT sites in the second construct, resulting in the excision of the transcriptional stop sequence. With the stop sequence removed, the *actin5C* promoter is free to drive high-level, tissue-general expression of the gene of interest from that point in time onward. FLP-*out* was found to work efficiently even in post-mitotic cells of the adult fly (Sun & Tower, 1999).

One advantage of FLP-*out* over the other two conditional systems is that the environmental stimulus doesn't require constant application in order to express the gene of interest. One or two heat pulses are sufficient to permanently remove the transcriptional stop sequence from the majority of the *Drosophila's* DNA.

F. Tissue-Specific Expression and the GAL4/UAS System

When P elements are introduced into fruit flies, the strength, location, and timing of their expression are often affected by where they insert into the genome. This phenomenon is referred to as *chromosomal position effect* and is caused by endogenous transcriptional regulatory sequences (enhancers) spread throughout the *Drosophila* genome. The advantage of chromosomal position effect is that useful enhancers can be discovered through "enhancer trapping" (Bellen, 1999; Bellen, et al., 1989). In enhancer trapping, a P element containing a reporter gene driven by a weak promoter is introduced into the *Drosophila* genome. Depending on where in the chromosome the construct inserts, nearby enhancers can act on the promoter, causing expression of the reporter in a constitutive, tissue-specific, and/or temporally specific manner.

Trapped enhancers are especially beneficial when combined with the GAL4/UAS system (Brand & Perrimon, 1993); which consists of two constructs (see Figure 14.4). The first construct is the enhancer trap, which is used to drive tissue-specific expression of GAL4. Such lines are commonly called *GAL4 drivers*. A large collection of GAL4 drivers exist, and there are a plethora of tissue and temporally specific expression patterns from which to choose. The second construct is a gene of interest driven by a promoter containing the upstream activating

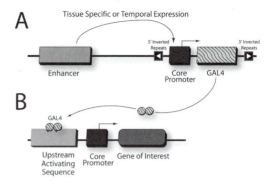

Figure 14.4 The GAL4/UAS system. **(A)** An endogenous enhancer trap drives tissue or temporal specific expression of a P-element insert containing a weak promoter and GAL4. **(B)** GAL4 is produced only in the specific circumstances designated by the enhancer trap and binds to a constitutively expressed construct containing the upstream activating sequence (UAS). The core promoter and UAS can then drive expression of the gene of interest.

sequence (UAS) binding site for GAL4. GAL4 will only be expressed in the tissues designated by the enhancer trap. Consequently, GAL4 is only able to bind to UAS and initiate transcription in the specified tissues. Because it is non-conditional, the GAL4/UAS system is subject to the variation seen in all non-conditional systems, as described above (see Figure 14.1A).

It is important to note that the GAL4/UAS system can be combined with either the tet-on or FLP-*out* systems described earlier in this chapter. Three constructs are required to combine GAL4/UAS with the tet-on system. First, an enhancer trap is used to drive GAL4. The second construct is a bridge construct where UAS drives rtTA (Stebbins *et al.*, 2001). The third construct is the tet-on promoter, driving the gene of interest.

G. dsRNA Inhibition of Gene Expression in *Drosophila*

Another way to study *Drosophila* aging is to turn off or turn down the expression of the gene in the adult fly. Antisense inhibition of gene expression has been found to work well in *Drosophila* (Ruohola-Baker *et al.*, 1993). Antisense RNA appears to mediate its effects through a double-strand RNA (dsRNA) intermediate, and dsRNA has been found to be dramatically more effective than simple antisense RNA in several systems, including *Drosophila* (Kennerdell & Carthew, 1998). dsRNA appears to function in an evolutionarily conserved pathway in which only a few dsRNA molecules per cell are sufficient to cause the destruction of most or all homologous transcripts (Fire, 1999; Fire *et al.*, 1998; Sharp, 1999). dsRNA inhibition of gene expression has also been combined with the tetracycline-conditional system to allow convenient, DOX-regulated inactivation of potentially any cloned gene in transgenic flies (Allikian *et al.*, 2002). A 0.5- to 1-kb segment of the gene coding region is cloned as an inverted repeat downstream of the tet-on promoter. The transgenes are then crossed to the rtTA trans-activator, and feeding of tetracycline causes expression of the inverted repeat RNA, which then folds into a dsRNA hairpin. The dsRNA then causes the inactivation of the corresponding endogenous gene. In addition, it is possible to include genes in *Drosophila* using inverted repeats expressed through the GAL4/UAS system (Fortier & Belote, 2000; Kennerdell & Carthew, 2000).

III. Screening for *Drosophila* Genes Affecting Life Span

A. Knockout Screens

1. Chemical Mutagenesis and Irradiation

Mutagenesis with chemicals such as EMS or irradiation with gamma or X-rays both result in a high frequency of mutations. However, it is difficult to determine where these mutations occur in the genome. Therefore, P element or other types of transposon mutagenesis is generally favored.

2. P Element Mutagenesis

In P element mutagenesis, *Drosophila* containing a P element are crossed to a strain that expresses transposase. The transposase causes the P element to excise and insert into a new location in the genome, potentially disrupting a gene. The mutation frequency is less than that resulting from chemicals or irradiation. However, inverse PCR can be employed to determine exactly where the P element inserted. Consequently, this technique is generally preferred over chemical mutagenesis or irradiation.

3. P Element Loss of Function Screens

In a loss of function screen, P element mutagenesis is used to make multiple insertions in a *Drosophila* population. DNA is then extracted from the *Drosophila*, and inverse PCR is employed to determine whether the P element inserted into a gene (Ballinger & Benzer, 1989). Finally, a life-span assay can determine whether the mutation increases the *Drosophila* life span. This method was used to identify both the *methuselah* and *indy* genes, which are discussed in detail in section III.

B. P Element-Based Mis-Expression Screens

1. EP Lines

The enhanced P-insertion (EP) system is a misexpression strategy that makes use of GAL4/UAS. The purpose of EP lines is to randomly overexpress a potential gene of interest. This is accomplished though the use of a P element that contains an upstream activating sequence. *Drosophila* that carry the UAS-containing P element are crossed to a transposase line, causing the transposon to be randomly incorporated into a new section of the genome. When the P element inserts directly before a gene, an enhancer trap containing GAL4 can be employed to overexpress it. The resulting fly can then be assayed for an alteration in life span.

One disadvantage of the EP lines system is that it is non-conditional, which prevents controlled expression of the gene.

2. The PdL System

The PdL system is also an overexpression screen; however, it uses the tet-on system instead of GAL4/UAS. In this case, the P element contains the tetracycline operator and a core promoter instead of the UAS. This strain can be crossed with *Drosophila* carrying rtTA. Then, the presence of DOX will result in the overexpression of the gene downstream of the transposon insertion.

IV. Specific Genes Used to Extend the Life Span of *Drosophila melanogaster*

A. The Insulin/Insulin-Like Pathway in *Drosophila*

Early discoveries in the insulin-like pathway were made with the model system *Caenorhabditis elegans* (Kenyon *et al.*, 1993; Klass, 1983); however, a number of key experiments have also been performed in *Drosophila*. The determination that partial knockouts of INR and CHICO increased the life span of *Drosophila melanogaster* confirmed that insulin signaling could affect life span in other species (Clancy *et al.*, 2001; Tatar *et al.*, 2001). The insulin receptor INR is analogous to the *C. elegans* receptor daf-2, and CHICO is the substrate for this receptor (see Figure 14.5). It is important to note that these mutations are more effective at increasing the life span of female *Drosophila* than male *Drosophila*. For

example, the INR mutation increased the life span of female flies by 85 percent but did not increase male life span (see Table 14.1) (Tatar *et al.*, 2001). Furthermore, homozygous CHICO mutations extended female life span by 48 percent but had no effect on male life span (Clancy *et al.*, 2001). However, male heterozygotes lived 13 percent longer than controls. Female heterozygotes still benefited from the CHICO mutation more than male heterozygotes and possessed a 36 percent increase in life span. The reason for this relative lack of effect in males is currently unknown. Both INR and CHICO activate PI3K, which in turn activates protein kinase B (PKB). Unfortunately, manipulations of these genes have not resulted in a positive effect on life span. However, overexpression of PTEN, an enzyme that inhibits PI3K, in the fat body of the head extended life span by 20 percent (Hwangbo *et al.*, 2004). Additionally, overexpression of dFOXO, the downstream forkhead transcription factor inhibited by these genes, increased life span by 56 percent (Hwangbo *et al.*, 2004). This gene only increased life span when it was expressed in the fat body of *Drosophila*. dFOXO increased life span in females, but it is not clear whether it had the same effect in males. One of the two groups working on dFOXO has reported that the forkhead transcription factor caused males to live longer, whereas the other reported no effect on male life span (Giannakou *et al.*, 2004; Hwangbo *et al.*, 2004). In summary, the upstream portion of the insulin-like pathway negatively regulates life span, whereas dFOXO positively regulates life span.

Several of the genetic interventions in the insulin-like pathway have an effect on fertility and size. Homozygotes and transheterozygotes for INR hypomorph mutations are dwarfed and have decreased fecundity, whereas INR heterozygotes are normal (Clancy *et al.*, 2001; Tatar *et al.*, 2001). The CHICO mutation resulted in a similar phenotype; heterozygous flies

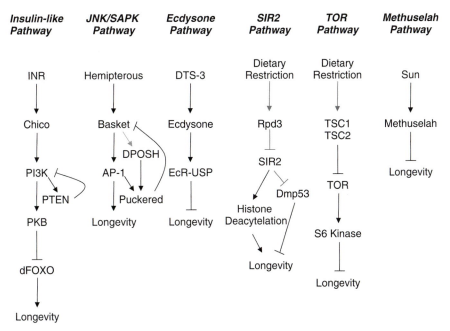

Figure 14.5 Pathways that extend *Drosophila* life span. Bold arrows denote proven pathways, whereas gray markings designate potential interactions. Inhibitory gene interactions are indicated by arrows with horizontal bars, and genes with positive interactions are denoted by normal arrows.

showed reduced fertility, and homozygous flies were dwarfed and practically sterile (Clancy *et al.*, 2001).

B. The JNK/SAPK Pathway

The JNK pathway is activated by environmental stress and offers protection against oxidative damage. Multiple genes in this pathway have been implicated in the determination of life span (see Figure 14.5). Wang and colleagues determined that overexpressing *hemipterous* in *Drosophila* neurons, and a heterozygote knockout of its downstream gene *pucker*, both increase life span (Wang *et al.*, 2003). In addition, Seong and colleagues showed that misexpression of DPOSH in the neurons extended fly life span by 14 percent (Seong *et al.*, 2001). Genes in the JNK/SAPK pathway predominantly have a positive effect on life span; however, *pucker* forms a negative feedback loop and inhibits this pathway.

C. The Ecdysone Pathway

In fruit flies, the ecdysone hormone is synthesized in part by DTS-3, and it binds to the ecdysone hormone receptor (see Figure 14.5). Heterozygote knockouts of both DTS-3 and the receptor genes extended life span (Simon *et al.*, 2003). The DTS-3 knockout extended the life span of *Drosophila* by 19 percent in females only. Simon and colleagues. have shown that feeding the DTS-3 knockout flies ecdysone reverses this increase in life span (Simon *et al.*, 2003). The heterozygote knockouts of the ecdysone receptor resulted in a life-span extension of 54 percent for both sexes, without a negative effect on fertility. Therefore, the ecdysone pathway negatively regulates life span in adult *Drosophila*. In Chapter 15, Tu and colleagues provide a more in-depth examination of the effect of ecdysone and other hormones on the life span of *Drosophila melanogaster*.

Table 14.1

Genes Reported to Extend the Life Span of *Drosophila melanogaster*. Entries marked as N/A indicate information that was not provided. In general, where there were conflicting results on a particular gene, the more positive findings were included.

Gene Name	Control Life Span	Experimental Life Span	Increase in Longevity	Increase in Maximum Life span	Genetic Manipulation	Sex	Specific Tissues	Oxygen Consumption	Mortality Rate Doubling Time	Citation
DNA Repair										
mei-41	47	58	22%	N/A	Overexpression	Male	Whole Fly	N/A	N/A	Symphorien 2003
Histone Deacetylases										
Rpd3+	N/A	N/A	47%	N/A	Heterozygote Knockout	Male/Female	Whole Fly	N/A	N/A	Rogina 2002
dSIR2‡	43	60	57%	74%	Overexpression	Male/Female	Whole Fly, Neurons	N/A	Decreased	Rogina, 2004
Hormones										
DTS-3	N/A	N/A	19%	N/A	Heterozygote Knockout	Female	Whole Fly	N/A	N/A	Simon 2003
Ecdysone Receptor	N/A	N/A	54%	N/A	Heterozygote Knockout	Male/Female	Whole Fly	N/A	N/A	Simon 2003
JNK / SAPK Pathway										
Hemipterous	N/A	N/A	N/A	N/A	Overexpression	Male	Neurons	N/A	N/A	Wang 2003
Pucker	N/A	N/A	N/A	N/A	Heterozygote Knockout	Male	Whole Fly	N/A	N/A	Wang 2003
Oxidative Defense										
Cu/Zn SOD‡	45	64	41%	48%	Overexpression	Male/Female	Whole Fly, Neurons	No Change	Constant	Parkes 1998
Mn SOD‡	41	54	33%	37%	Overexpression	Male/Female	Whole Fly	No Change	Constant	Sun 2002
MSRA	55	95	73%	N/A	Overexpression	Male/Female	Neurons	N/A	Constant	Ruan 2002

Protein Repair										
Hsp 22	60	79	30%	N/A	Overexpression	Male	Whole Fly, Neurons	N/A	N/A	Morrow 2004
Hsp26	43	57	31%	N/A	Overexpression	Male	Whole Fly	N/A	N/A	Wang 2004
Hsp 27	43	57	31%	N/A	Overexpression	Male	Whole Fly	N/A	N/A	Wang 2004
Hsp 68	N/A	N/A	N/A	N/A	Overexpression	Male	Whole Fly	N/A	N/A	Wang 2003
Hsp 70	N/A	N/A	4%	N/A	Overexpression	Male	Whole Fly	N/A	N/A	Tartar 1997
Signal Transduction										
Chico+	44	65	48%	41%	Homozygote Hypomorph*	Female**	Whole Fly	N/A	Decreased	Clancy 2001
dFOXO	32	50	56%	N/A	Overexpression	Male/Female	Fat Body	N/A	N/A	Hwangbo 2004
INR Tatar 2001	32	60	85%	N/A	Transheterozygote	Female	Female	Whole Fly	No Change	Constant
Methuselah	57	77	35%	N/A	Hypomorph Homozygote Knockout	Male	Whole Fly	N/A	Constant	Lin 1998
Sun	37	56	51%	N/A	Heterozygote Hypomorph	Female	Whole Fly	N/A	N/A	Cvejic 2004
TOR Pathway										
dS6K***	30	26	22%	N/A	Dominant Negative	Male	Whole Fly	N/A	N/A	Kapahi 2004
dTSC1***	29	26	14%	N/A	Overexpression	Male	Whole Fly, Muscle	N/A	N/A	Kapahi 2004
dTSC2	58	69	19%	N/A	Overexpression	Male	Whole Fly	N/A	N/A	Kapahi 2004
dTOR	58	72	24%	N/A	Dominant Negative	Male	Whole Fly	N/A	N/A	Kapahi 2004

(continues)

Table 14.1 (Cont'd)

Gene Name	Control Life Span	Experimental Life Span	Increase in Longevity	Increase in Maximum Life span	Genetic Manipulation	Sex	Specific Tissues	Oxygen Consumption	Mortality Rate Doubling Time	Citation
Transporter Proteins										
Indy?	37	71	92%	45%	Heterozygote Knockout	Male/Female	Whole Fly	N/A	Decreased	Rogina 2000
Sugar Baby	74	80	9%	N/A	Overexpression	Male	Whole Fly	N/A	N/A	Landis 2003
VhaSFD	69	76	11%	N/A	Overexpression	Male	Whole Fly	N/A	N/A	Landis 2003
Other										
EF1-?	38	45	18%	N/A	Overexpression	Male	Whole Fly	N/A	N/A	Shepherd 1989
fwd	59	63	7%	N/A	Overexpression	Male	Whole Fly	N/A	N/A	Landis 2003
Ovo	N/A	N/A	50%	N/A	Heterozygote Hypomorph	Female	Whole Fly	N/A	Constant	Sgro 1999
Identified Through Misexpression										
cct	60	64	8%	N/A	Overexpression	Male	Whole Fly	N/A	N/A	Landis 2003
DPOSH	43	49	14%	N/A	Overexpression	Male	Neurons	N/A	N/A	Seong 2001
Filamin	59	64	9%	N/A	Overexpression	Male	Whole Fly	N/A	N/A	Landis 2003

*Longevity is also increased in heterozygote knockouts, but to a lesser extent.

**Male life span is also increased slightly.

***Life span calculated at 29°.

+Life span values use median instead of average

pMaximum life span calculated as time to reach 90 percent mortality.

§Maximum life span calculated as time to reach 99 percent mortality.

D. The Regulation of SIR2 and Histone Deacytelation

Histone deacetylation through the SIR2 pathway may be a mechanism for life-span extension through caloric restriction (see Figure 14.5). Rogina and colleagues (2002) used partial heterozygote knockouts of *rpd3* to extend the life span of male fruit flies by 52 percent. Reduction of rpd3 resulted in the increase of dSIR2, and over-expression of dSIR2 through GAL4/UAS resulted in an increase in life span of up to 57 percent (Rogina & Helfand, 2004). Increased levels of dSIR2 increased life span in both females and males when it was expressed either ubiquitously or in pan-neuronal cells. Conditional overexpression of dSIR2 through the GeneSwitch system also increased life span; however, this increase was smaller then with non-conditional expression. Caloric restriction did not confer an additional life span increase to *Drosophila* with either the *rpd3* partial knockout or the overexpression of dSIR2.

E. The TOR Pathway

The Target Of Rapamycin (TOR) pathway is another potential candidate for the effect of caloric restriction on life span. In this pathway, the TOR gene controls growth, and overexpression of its dominant-negative form throughout all *Drosophila* tissues increased life span by 24 percent (Kapahi *et al.*, 2004). TOR is inhibited by two tuberous sclerosis complex genes (TSC1 and TSC2) (see Figure 14.5). Overexpression of TSC1 increased life span by 14 percent at 29 degrees, whereas TSC2 overexpression increased life span by 12 percent at 29 degrees and 19 percent at 25 degrees (Kapahi *et al.*, 2004). Furthermore, dominant-negative overexpression of S6 kinase, located downstream of TOR, increased life span by 22 percent when the flies were kept at 29 degrees.

F. The Methuselah Gene in *Drosophila*

Methuselah was one of the first genes found to regulate the life span of fruit flies. Homozygous partial-loss-of-function alleles of this G-protein-coupled receptor increased *Drosophila* life span and body size by 35 percent (Lin *et al.*, 1998). Interestingly, this increase in life span resulted from a decrease in initial mortality rate and did not alter mortality rate doubling time. Methuselah's ligand sun was recently discovered, and two different heterozygous *sun* mutants increased life span by 25 percent and 50 percent, respectively (Cvejic *et al.*, 2004) (see Figure 14.5). Mutants for either *methuselah* or *sun* possess an increased resistance to the chemical oxidant paraquat. In conclusion, both elements of the methuselah pathway negatively regulate *Drosophila* life span.

G. Oxidative Defense Enzymes

Copper zinc superoxide dismutase (Cu/Zn-SOD) was overexpressed in the motor neurons using the GAL4/UAS system and resulted in a 40 percent life-span increase (Parkes *et al.*, 1998). Similarly, conditional overexpression of Cu/Zn-SOD using the FLP-*out* system increases the life span of adult flies up to 40 percent (Sun & Tower, 1999). Cu/Zn-SOD is present in an active form in the cytoplasm, and in the inter-membrane space of mitochondria. This enzyme protects against oxidative stress by converting two superoxide anions to hydrogen peroxide.

Manganese superoxide dismutase (MnSOD) performs the same reaction; however, it is found only in the inner mitochondrial space. MnSOD extends the life span of flies when it is overexpressed using either the FLP-*out* or tet-on conditional systems (Sun *et al.*, 2002). Genetic manipulation of MnSOD increased the life span of *Drosophila* by up to 33 percent.

Methionine sulfoxide reductase A (MSRA) is another oxidative defense gene shown to increase *Drosophila* life span.

MSRA reduces an oxidatively damaged methionine back to normal and was reported to extend life span by up to 73 percent in flies when it was overexpressed in neurons (Ruan *et al.*, 2002). Overexpression of MSRA did not cause a decline in *Drosophila* fertility. In addition, MSRA overexpression protected against paraquat toxicity.

H. Heat Shock Proteins

Heat shock proteins are chaperones that prevent the aggregation and precipitation of misfolded proteins. Transient overexpression of hsp70 transgenes was triggered by heat stress in young adults and resulted in a significant decrease in mortality rate. However, it only increased fly life span by about 4 percent relative to controls (Tatar *et al.*, 1997). Overexpression of hsp22 using the GAL4/UAS system extended life span by up to 30 percent, whereas null mutants were found to decrease life span (Morrow *et al.*, 2000). The GAL4/UAS system was also used to overexpress hsp26 and hsp27, both of which increased life span by 30 percent (Wang *et al.*, 2004). Heat shock proteins have been implicated in both the insulin-like and JNK pathways. For example, small heat shock proteins are regulated by the forkhead transcription factor in multiple species (Longo & Finch, 2003). In addition, Wang and colleagues report that hsp68 is regulated by the JNK pathway and increases life span when it is overexpressed (Wang *et al.*, 2003).

I. Indy

The gene I'm not dead yet (*Indy*) encodes a sodium dicarboxylate transporter protein. Heterozygous *Indy* mutations increased life span by up to 92 percent and decreased the morality rate doubling time of *Drosophila melanogaster* (Rogina *et al.*, 2000). However, life span was only extended by about 15 percent when *Indy* was mutated in long-lived *Drosophila*.

V. Conclusions

It is important to note that most of the genes that extend the life span of *Drosophila melanogaster* have been tested in genetic backgrounds with short or average life spans. Only a few studies have been performed on flies with an average life span greater than 70 days (Spencer *et al.*, 2003). It is not clear if all of the transgenes and mutations mentioned above will have the same beneficial effect in the longest-lived strains. Another area of potential future work is the use of microarrays to determine whether the genes mentioned above are interacting with each other to increase life span. Microarray studies may also lead to the discovery of new genes acting downstream from those previously mentioned that also have a positive effect on life span.

References

Allikian, M. J., Deckert-Cruz, D., Rose, M. R., Landis, G. N., & Tower, J. (2002). Doxycycline-induced expression of sense and inverted-repeat constructs modulates phosphogluconate mutase (pgm) gene expression in adult *Drosophila melanogaster*. *Genome Biology*, 3(5), research0021.

Ballinger, D. G., & Benzer, S. (1989). Targeted gene mutations in *Drosophila*. *Proceedings of the National Academy of Sciences of the USA*, 86, 9402–9406.

Basler, K., & Struhl, G. (1994). Compartment boundaries and the control of *Drosophila* limb pattern by *hedgehog* protein. *Nature*, 368, 208–214.

Bellen, H. J. (1999). Ten years of enhancer detection: lessons from the fly. *Plant Cell*, 11, 2271–2282.

Bellen, H. J., O'Kane, C. J., Wilson, C., Grossniklaus, U., Perason, R. K., & Gehring, W. J. (1989). P-element-mediated enhancer detection: a versatile method to study development in *Drosophila*. *Genes and Development*, 3, 1288–1300.

Bieschke, E. T., Wheeler, J. C., & Tower, J. (1998). Doxycycline-induced transgene expression during *Drosophila* development and aging. *Molecular Genes and Genetics*, 258(6), 571–579.

Brand, A. H., & Perrimon, N. (1993). Targeted gene expression as a means of altering cell fates and generating dominant phenotypes. *Development*, 118, 401–415.

Clancy, D. J., Gems, D., Harshman, L. G., Oldham, S., Stocker, H., Hafen, E., Leevers, S. J., & Partridge, L. (2001). Extension of life-span by loss of CHICO, a *Drosophila* insulin receptor substrate protein. *Science*, 292, 104–106.

Cvejic, S., Zhu, Z., Felice, S. J., Berman, Y., & Huang, X. (2004). The endogenous ligand stunted of the CPCR methuselah extends lifespan in *Drosophila*. *Nature Cell Biology*, 6, 540–546.

Fire, A. (1999). RNA-triggered gene silencing. *Trends in Genetics*, 15, 358–363.

Fire, A., Xu, S., Montgomery, M. K., Kostas, S. A., Driver, S. E., & Mello, C. C. (1998). Potent and specific genetic interference by double-stranded RNA in *Caenorhabditis elegans*. *Nature*, 391, 806–811.

Fortier, E., & Belote, J. M. (2000). Temperature-dependent gene silencing by an expressed inverted repeat in *Drosophila*. *Genesis*, 26, 240–244.

Giannakou, M. E., Goss, M., Junger, M. A., Hafen, E., Leevers, S. J., & Partridge, L. (2004). Long-lived *Drosophila* with overexpressed dFOXO in adult fat body. *Science*, 305, 361.

Hwangbo, D. S., Gersham, B., Tu, M. P., Palmer, M., & Tatar, M. (2004). *Drosophila* dFOXO controls lifespan and regulates insulin signalling in brain and fat body. *Nature*, 429(6991), 562–566.

Kaiser, M., Gasser, M., Ackermann, R., & Stearns, S. C. (1997). P element inserts in transgenic flies: a cautionary tale. *Heredity*, 78, 1–11.

Kapahi, P., Zid, B. M., Harper, T., Koslover, D., Sapin, V., Benzer, S. (2004). Regulation of lifespan in *Drosophila* by modulation of genes in the TOR signaling pathway. *Current Biology*, 14(10), 885–890.

Kennerdell, J. R., & Carthew, R. W. (1998). Use of dsRNA-mediated genetic interference to demonstrate that *frizzled* and *frizzled 2* act in the wingless pathway. *Cell*, 95, 1017–1026.

Kennerdell, J. R., & Carthew, R. W. (2000). Heritable gene silencing in *Drosophila* using double-stranded RNA. *Nature Biotechnology*, 18, 896–898.

Kenyon, C., Chang, J., Gensch, A., Rudner, A., & Tabtiang, R. (1993). A *C. elegans* mutant that lives twice as long as wild type. *Nature*, 366, 461–464.

Klass, M. R. (1983). A method for the isolation of longevity mutants in the nematode *Caenorhabditis elegans* and initial results. *Mechanisms of Ageing and Development*, 22(3–4), 279–286.

Landis, G., Bhole, D., & Tower, J. (2003). A search for doxycyline-dependant mutations that increase *Drosophila melanogaster* life span identifies the VhaSFD, Sugar Baby, filamin, fwd, and, Cctl genes. *Genome Biology*, 4(2), R8.

Landis, G. N., Abdueva, D., Skvortsov, D., Yang, J., Rabin, B. E., Carrick, J., Tavare, S., & Tower, J. (2004). Similar gene expression patterns characterize aging and oxidative stress in *Drosophila melanogaster*. *Proceedings of the National Academy of Sciences of the USA*, 100(20), 7663–7668.

Lin, Y. J., Seroude, L., & Benzer, S. (1998). Extended life-span and stress resistance in the *Drosophila* mutant *methuselah*. *Science*, 282, 943–946.

Longo, V. D., & Finch, C. E. (2003). Evolutionary medicine: from dwarf model systems to healthy centenarians? *Science*, 299, 1342–1346.

Mackay, T. F. C. (2002). The nature of quantitative genetic variation for *Drosophila* longevity. *Mechanisms of Ageing and Development*, 123, 95–104.

Morrow, G., Samson M., Michand, S., & Tanquay R. M. (2004). Overexpression of the small mitochondrial Hsp22 extends *Drosophila* life span and increases resistance to oxidative stress. *FASEB Journal*, 18(3), 598–599.

Morrow, G., Inaguma, Y., Kato, K., & Tanguay, R. M. (2000). The small heat shock protein hsp22 of *Drosophila melanogaster* is a mitochondrial protein displaying oligomeric organization. *Journal of Biological Chemistry*, 275(40), 31204–31210.

Parkes, T. L., Elia, A. J., Dickson, D., Hilliker, A. J., Phillips, J. P., & Boulianne, G. L. (1998). Extension of *Drosophila* lifespan by overexpression of human *sod1* in motorneurons. *Nature Genetics*, 19, 171–174.

Rogina, B., Helfand, S. L., & Frankel, S. (2002). Longevity regulation by *Drosophila* rpd3 deacetylase and caloric restriction. *Science*, 294, 1745.

Rogina, B., Reenan, R. A., Nilsen, S. P., & Helfand, S. (2000). Extended life-span conferred by cotransporter gene mutations in *Drosophila*. *Science*, 290, 2137–2140.

Rogina, B., & Helfand, S. L. (2004). SIR2 mediates longevity in the fly through a pathway related to calorie restriction. *Proceedings of the National Academy of Sciences of the USA*, 101(45), 15998–16003.

Roman, G., Endo, K., Zong, L., & Davis, R. L. (2001). P[switch], a system for spatial and temporal control of gene expression in *Drosophila melanogaster*. *Proceedings of the National Academy of Sciences of the USA*, 98, 12602–12607.

Ruan, H., Tang, X. D., Chen, M. L., Joiner, M. L., Sun, G., Brot, N., Weissbach, H., Heinemann, S. H., Iverson, L., Wu, C. F., Hoshi, T. (2002). High-quality life extension by the enzyme peptide methionine sulfoxide reductase. *Proceedings of the National Academy of Sciences of the USA*, 99, 2748–2753.

Rubin, G. M., & Spradling, A. C. (1982). Genetic transformation of *Drosophila* with transposable element vectors. *Science*, 218, 348–353.

Ruohola-Baker, H., Grell, E., Chou, T.-B., Baker, D., Jan, L. Y., & Jan, Y. N. (1993). Spatially localized rhomboid is required for establishment of the dorsal-ventral axis in *Drosophila* oogenesis. *Cell*, 73, 953–965.

Ryder, E., & Russell, S. (2002). Transposable elements as tools for genomics and genetics in *Drosophila*. *Brief Functional Genomics and Proteomics*, 2, 57–71.

Seong, K. H., Matsuo, T., Fuyama, Y., & Aigaki, T. (2001). Neural-specific overexpression of *Drosophila plenty of sh3s* (*dposh*) extends the longevity of adult flies. *Biogerontology*, 2, 271–281.

Sgro, C. M., & Partridge, L. (1999). A delayed wave of death from reproduction in *Drosophila Science*, 286(5449), 2521–2524.

Sharp, P. A. (1999). RNAi and double-strand RNA. *Genes and Development*, 13, 139–141.

Shepherd, J. C., Walldorf, U., Hug, P., & Gehring, W. J. (1989). Fruit flies with additional expression of elongation factor EF-1 alpha live longer. *Proceedings of the National Academy of Sciences of the USA*, 86(19), 7520–7521.

Simphorein, S., & Woodruff, R. C. (2003). Effect of DNA repair on aging of Drosophila melanogaster: I. mei-41 locus. Journal of Gerontology A: Biological Sciences and medical Sciences. 58(9), 782–787.

Simon, A. F., Shih, C., Mack, A., & Benzer, S. (2003). Steroid control of longevity in *Drosophila melanogaster*. *Science*, 299(5611), 1407–1410.

Spencer, C. C., Howell, C. E., Wright, A. R., & Promislow, D. E. (2003). Testing an 'aging gene' in long-lived *Drosophila* strains: increased longevity depends on sex and genetic background. *Aging Cell*, 2(2), 123–130.

Stebbins, M. J., Urlinger, S., Byrne, G., Bello, B., Hillen, W., & Yin, J. C. P. (2001). Tetracycline-inducible systems for *Drosophila*. *Proceedings of the National Academy of Sciences of the USA*, 98, 10775–10780.

Struhl, G., & Basler, K. (1993). Organizing activity of wingless protein in *Drosophila*. *Cell*, 72, 527–540.

Sun, J., & Tower, J. (1999). FLP recombinase-mediated induction of Cu/Zn-superoxide dismutase transgene expression can extend the life span of adult *Drosophila melanogaster* flies. *Molecular Cell Biology*, 19(1), 216–228.

Sun, J., Folk, D., Bradley, T. J., & Tower, J. (2002). Induced overexpression of mitochondrial Mn-superoxide dismutase extends the life span of adult *Drosophila melanogaster*. *Genetics*, 161(2), 661–672.

Symphorein, S., & Woodruff, R. C. (2003). Effect of DNA repair on aging of *Drosophila melanogaster:* I. mei-41 locus. *Journal of Gerontology A: Biological Sciences and Medical Sciences.* 58(9), 782–787.

Tatar, M., Khazaeli, A. A., & Curtsinger, J. W. (1997). Chaperoning extended life. *Nature*, 390, 30.

Tatar, M., Kopelman, A., Epstein, D., Tu, M. P., Yin, C. M., & Garofalo, R. S. (2001). A mutant *Drosophila* insulin receptor homolog that extends life-span and impairs neuroendocrine function. *Science*, 292(5514), 107–110.

Wang, M. C., Bohmann, D., & Jasper, H. (2003). JNK signaling confers tolerance to oxidative stress and extends lifespan in *Drosophila*. *Developmental Cell*, 5(5), 811–816.

Wang, H. D., Kazemi-Esfarjani, P., & Benzer, S. (2004). Multiple-stress analysis for isolation of *Drosophila* longevity genes. *Proceedings of the National Academy of Sciences of the USA*, 34, 12610–12615.

Chapter 15

Juvenile and Steroid Hormones in *Drosophila melanogaster* Longevity

Meng-Ping Tu, Thomas Flatt, and Marc Tatar

I. Introduction

Hormones coordinate diverse developmental and physiological processes and regulate the allocation of metabolic resources to different organs and life-history stages (Finch & Rose, 1995). Many insects display an amazing amount of phenotypic variation in their life histories, which is mediated by the effects of hormones (Dingle & Winchell, 1997; Nijhout, 1994). Juvenile hormone (JH)[1] and the steroid hormone ecdysone (active form: 20-hydroxy-ecdysone, 20E) have fascinating physiological effects on various

aspects of development and the adult phenotype. Consequently, the endocrine effects of a single hormone on multiple traits ("hormonal pleiotropy") may offer promising insights into the mechanisms regulating complex phenotypes (Dingle & Winchell, 1997; Ketterson & Nolan, 1992; Zera & Harshman, 2001), including the aging phenotype (Bartke & Lane, 2001; Finch & Rose, 1995; Kenyon, 2001; Tatar, 2004; Tatar *et al.*, 2003).

The study of endocrine aspects of aging is not new. In 1889, Charles-Edouard Brown-Séquard, the "father" of endocrinology, was one of the first to suggest that alterations of endocrine glands or hormone metabolism may be determinants of human aging (Hayflick, 1994). For the case of insects, Meir Paul Pener showed more than 30 years ago that removal of JH extends life span in three grasshopper species (Pener, 1972). While JH and 20E are best known for their major roles in pre-adult development and adult reproduction (Kozlova & Thummel, 2000; Riddiford, 1993, 1994; Truman & Riddiford, 2002;

---

[1] Abbreviations: aa,. abnormal abdomen; CA, corpus allatum, corpora allata; CC, corpus cardiacum, corpora cardiaca; CNS, central nervous system; DAF, dauer formation; dFOXO, *Drosophila* forkhead transcription factor FOXO; DILPs, Drosophila insulin-like peptides; EcR, ecdysone receptor; 20E, 20-hydroxy-ecdysone; IGF, insulin-like growth factor; InR, insulin-like receptor; IPCs, insulin-producing cells; JH, juvenile hormone; JHA, juvenile hormone analog; JHB$_3$, juvenile hormone 3 bisepoxide; MET, methoprene-tolerant; MNCs, median neurosecretory cells; USP, ultraspiracle.

Wyatt & Davey, 1996), these hormones also show intriguing effects on insect longevity. Recent studies have shown that downregulation of JH or 20E can slow senescence (Herman & Tatar, 2001; Simon et al., 2003; Tatar et al., 2001a,b). Here we review hormonal effects on aging in *Drosophila melanogaster* (for a review of the genetics of aging in *Drosophila*, see Stearns & Partridge, 2001; also see Ford & Tower, Chapter 14, this volume). Although we will focus our discussion on *Drosophila*, a model system with both ample genetic and endocrinological data, we will also draw parallels to the endocrine control of aging in other systems (other insects, the nematode *Caenorhabditis elegans*, and vertebrates). We shall argue that studying endocrine regulation can offer promising insights into the mechanisms and the evolution of senescence.

II. JH and 20E: Two Major Insect Hormones

A. JH

The insect hormone JH is a sesquiterpenoid compound produced by the corpora allata (CA), a pair of endocrine glands with nervous connections to the brain (Nijhout, 1994; Tobe & Stay, 1985). In larval *Drosophila*, the single corpus allatum (CA) makes part of the so-called ring gland, a compound structure consisting of the CA and two other endocrine tissues, the prothoracic glands and the corpora cardiaca (CC); in adult flies, the CA is closer to the CC, whereas the prothoracic cells of the ring gland have degenerated (see Bodenstein 1950; Richard et al., 1989; Siegmund & Korge, 2001).

JH is a major insect hormone but may also exist in other arthropods and can be produced by some plant species (Tobe & Bendena, 1999). In most insects, JH regulates critical physiological processes, including metamorphosis

and reproduction (Dubrobsky, 2005; Gilbert et al., 2000; Riddiford, 1993). Insects produce at least eight different types of juvenoids (0, I, II, III, 4-Methyl-JH, JH III-bis-epoxide [JHB$_3$], and the two hydroxy-JH's 8'-OH-JH III and 12'-OH-JH III), the most common type being JH III (Darrouzet et al., 1997; Richard et al., 1989; Riddiford, 1994). *D. melanogaster* produces both JH III and JHB$_3$, both of which have endocrine function in dipterans (Riddiford, 1993; Yin et al., 1995). Whereas the effects of JH III are better known, JHB$_3$ appears to be the major product of the CA in higher dipterans (so-called cyclorrhaphan flies, including *Drosophila* and the housefly *Musca domestica*), yet its function awaits further study (Richard et al., 1989; Teal & Gomez-Simuta, 2002; Yin et al., 1995).

In pre-adult development and metamorphosis, JH functions as a "status quo" hormone, allowing continued growth after ecdysteroid-induced molting (Riddiford, 1996). Metamorphosis can only take place when the ecdysteroids act in the absence of JH. During the final larval instar, the JH titer declines due to a cessation of synthesis and increased degradation in the hemolymph and target tissues. Absence of JH triggers the release of prothoracicotropic hormone (PTTH), which in turn induces the secretion of 20E and the onset of metamorphosis (Nijhout, 1994). Although an experimental withdrawal of JH during development can lead to premature metamorphosis, an excess of JH prior to pupation results in delayed metamorphosis (Hammock et al., 1990; Nijhout, 2003; Riddiford, 1985). Unlike in some other insects, application of exogenous JH does not prevent the larval-pupal transformation in *Drosophila* (Riddiford & Ashburner, 1991). However, JH can disrupt the metamorphosis of the nervous and muscular system and disturb the normal differentiation of the abdomen in the fly (Restifo & Wilson, 1998; Riddiford &

Ashburner, 1991). Furthermore, high concentrations of exogenous JH can prolong developmental time or even inhibit eclosion without affecting the larval-pupal transformation (Riddiford & Ashburner, 1991).

In the adult fly, JH is crucial for the coordination of reproductive maturation in both sexes. In females, JH acts on oocyte maturation, including stimulation of vitellogenin synthesis and uptake of vitellogenin by the ovary (Bownes, 1982, 1989; Dubrovsky *et al.*, 2002; Gavin & Williamson, 1976; Postlethwait & Weiser, 1973; Shemshedini & Wilson, 1993), and sexual receptivity (Manning, 1966; Ringo *et al.*, 1991). In contrast, much less is known about the effects of JH on male reproduction. By analogy with other insects, JH may affect protein synthesis in the male accessory glands, sexual maturation, courtship behavior, and pheromone production (Bownes, 1982; Cook, 1973; Manning, 1967; Nijhout, 1994; Teal *et al.*, 2000; Wilson *et al.*, 2003). In other insects, JH can also affect diapause regulation, migratory behavior, wing length polyphenism, horn development in scarab beetles, seasonal form development, locomotory behavior, immune function, caste determination and division of labor in social hymenopterans and isopterans, and learning and memory (Belgacem & Martin, 2002; Hartfelder, 2000; Nijhout, 1994; Riddiford, 1994; Rolff & Siva-Jothy, 2002; Teal *et al.*, 2000; Wyatt & Davey, 1996). Thus, JH is truly a "master" hormone in insects (Hartfelder, 2000; Wheeler & Nijhout, 2003). As we shall discuss in this review, JH also has intriguing effects on insect aging.

B. 20E

Steroid hormones, such as ecdysteroids (including ecdysone and its active form 20-hydroxyecdysone, 20E), are another class of vital hormones in insects. In pre-adult flies, 20E is produced in the lar-

val prothoracic gland, which (together with the larval CA and the CC) makes part of the larval ring gland in dipterans (Bodenstein, 1950). In adult female flies, the ovary is the major 20E producing tissue (Chavez *et al.*, 2000; Gäde *et al.*, 1997; Gilbert *et al.*, 2002; Hagedorn, 1985; Kozlova & Thummel, 2000), and 20E appears to be produced in both ovarian follicle and nurse cells (Chavez *et al.*, 2000, Gilbert *et al.*, 2002; Schwartz *et al.*, 1985, 1989). Unfortunately, we know almost nothing about the production and metabolism of 20E in adult male *Drosophila* and other insects (Nijhout, 1994; Riddiford, 1993); by analogy with other insects, *Drosophila* males may produce 20E in their testes (Gäde *et al.*, 1997; Hagedorn, 1985). Together with JH, 20E is an important regulator of developmental transitions and metamorphosis (Dubrovsky, 2005; Kozlova & Thummel, 2000). In adults, 20E is well known for its effects on oogenesis, much like JH, yet other adult functions have remained elusive (Dubrovsky, 2005; Kozlova & Thummel, 2000). Similarly, the adult function of 20E in male *Drosophila* is poorly understood (Riddiford, 1993); 20E may affect *Drosophila* spermatogenesis, as it does in other insects (Nijhout, 1994).

C. Interaction Between JH and 20E

Both JH and 20E play major antagonistic or synergistic roles in regulating *Drosophila* development (Dubrovsky, 2005; Kozlova & Thummel, 2000, Riddiford, 1993; Truman & Riddiford, 2002; Zhou & Riddiford, 2002). The interaction between JH and 20E seems to take place in target tissues such as the fat body (adipose tissue), epithelium, and the ovary. For example, 20E circulating in the hemolymph appears to inhibit JH-induced production of vitellogenin in the fat body (Engelmann, 2002; Soller *et al.*, 1999; Stay *et al.*, 1980). However, in some insects, such as the silkworm

Bombyx mori, 20E can stimulate JH synthesis (Gu & Chow, 2003), and JH itself can stimulate 20E production in certain immature lepidopterans and possibly other insect species (Hiruma *et al.*, 1978). Thus, while 20E and JH appear to co-regulate reproduction, there is an intricate yet not well understood hormonal feedback between these key hormones (Dubrovsky, 2005).

III. Effects of JH and 20E on *Drosophila* Aging

A. JH and Agings

As we will discuss below, there is now increasing evidence showing that JH is a key regulator of aging in several insect species, including *Drosophila* (see also Tatar, 2004; Tatar *et al.*, 2003).

1. JH and the Abnormal Abdomen Syndrome

One of the first indications of an effect of JH on dipteran life history was found in Hawaiian *Drosophila mercatorum* (DeSalle & Templeton, 1986; Templeton, 1982, 1983; Templeton & Rankin, 1978; Thomas, 1991). In this species, the *abnormal abdomen* (*aa*) genotype has a decreased JH esterase (JHE) activity, which may lead to a high JH titer in the hemolymph (Templeton *et al.*, 1993; Thomas, 1991). The *aa* phenotype has increased developmental time, early sexual maturation, increased fecundity, and decreased longevity among females (Hollocher & Templeton, 1994; Templeton, 1982, 1983; Templeton & Rankin, 1978; but see Thomas, 1991). In males, developmental time is not affected, whereas sexual maturation is delayed, mating success decreased, and longevity increased (Hollocher & Templeton, 1994). Thus, the *aa* genotype affects male and female life history differently.

Although *aa* females seem to be long-lived (Templeton, 1982, 1983), the effects of *aa* on life span and other life-history traits may depend on nutrient conditions (Thomas, 1991). Contrary to the findings of Templeton (1982, 1983), both males and females of *aa* genotypes generally exhibited greater longevity than non-*aa* genotypes when reared on various concentrations of dry yeast in the food medium (Thomas, 1991). This life-span extension was observed for all yeast concentrations, except for the concentration used by Templeton (1982, 1983), which reduced life span. Thus, nutrition may affect *D. melanogaster* life span and other life-history traits through changes in JH signaling (see section V).

In addition, reproduction appears not to trade off with survival in these long-lived *aa* genotypes because females showed both greater fecundity and longevity than non-*aa* females (Thomas, 1991). This contradicts many experiments in *Drosophila* that show that life-span extension is typically accompanied by reduced reproduction (for a review, see Stearns & Partridge, 2001). Thus, the study by Thomas (1991) adds to a growing number of examples suggesting that the tradeoff between reproduction and life span can be uncoupled under some circumstances (Barnes & Partridge, 2003; Good & Tatar, 2001; Hwangbo *et al.*, 2004; Leroi, 2001; Marden *et al.*, 2003; Tu & Tatar, 2003).

While the various life-history effects observed in *D. mercatorum* may indeed be proximally controlled by JH, a direct proof for such an effect is lacking. Whether the *aa* genotype has an increased JH titer remains to be determined using a direct JH titer assay rather than measuring the turnover rate of degradation enzymes (Thomas, 1991). Yet, despite the uncertainty surrounding the pleiotropy of the *aa* genotype and the role of JH in the *aa* syndrome, it is interesting to note that *aa* genotypes differ remarkably from wildtype flies in *both* life span and JH metabolism, suggesting that JH may be a proximate determinant of life span.

2. JH, Reproductive Diapause, and Senescence Plasticity

Many adult insects use token cues to initiate diapause in response to seasonably predictable stressful or harsh environmental conditions. Diapause is a hormonally mediated state of reduced metabolism, developmental arrest, increased stress resistance, and altered behavior (Nijhout 1994; Tatar & Yin, 2001); the developmental arrest associated with diapause is reflected in an arrest of oogenesis, male accessory gland synthesis, and mating ("reproductive diapause"). In many insects, JH is proximately involved in regulating diapause (Nijhout, 1994; Tatar, 2004; Tatar & Yin, 2001).

JH controls reproductive diapause in insects as variable as butterflies (*Danaus plexippus*; Herman & Tatar, 2001; Tatar, 2004; Tatar & Yin, 2001), several grasshopper species (Pener, 1972; Tatar & Yin, 2001), and several species of *Drosophila* (*D. macroptera* and *D. grisea*: Kambysellis & Heed, 1974; *D. melanogaster*: Saunders *et al.*, 1989; Tatar & Yin, 2001; Tatar *et al.*, 2001a).

For example, several temperate-zone species of *Drosophila*, including *D. melanogaster*, *D. triauraria*, *D. littoralis*, and the cave-dwelling species *D. grisea* and *D. macroptera*, are known to over-winter as diapausing adults (Kambysellis & Heed, 1974; Saunders *et al.*, 1989; Tatar, 2004; Tatar & Yin, 2001). As shown by Tatar and colleagues (2001a), traits specific for diapause in *D. melanogaster* (arrest of oogenesis, resistance to exogenous stress, negligible senescence during diapause) are controlled by JH (Tatar & Yin, 2001). JH may thus be a key mediator of senescence plasticity and the tradeoff between reproduction and longevity.

Diapausing females downregulate JH synthesis in response to shorter day length and cool temperatures. Consequently, females enter ovarian arrest and show reduced age-specific mortality as compared to non-diapausing female cohorts that were started synchronously with the diapausing cohort. The diapause phenotype can be rescued by application of the synthetic JH methoprene; this treatment terminates ovarian arrest, makes flies more sensitive to oxidative stress, and reduces post-diapause longevity (Tatar *et al.*, 2001b). Methoprene is a JH analog (JHA) that is chemically more stable and much more potent than JH itself (see Wilson, 2004, and references therein). Although high doses of methoprene, a commonly used insecticide, can be toxic to insects, insect physiologists have confirmed in numerous reports that methoprene behaves as a faithful mimic of JH action in insects in general and in *Drosophila* in particular, both *in vivo* and *in vitro* (e.g., Riddiford & Ashburner, 1991; Wilson, 2004, and references therein; but also see Zera, 2004).

In *C. elegans*, larval diapause (formation of so-called dauer larvae) is under the control of the insulin signaling pathway, which signals through an insulin-like receptor encoded by the *dauerformation 2* gene (*daf-2*), the homolog of the *Drosophila insulin-like receptor* (*InR*) locus. Mutations in *daf-2* cause dramatic life-span extension (Dorman *et al.*, 1995; Kenyon *et al.*, 1993; Kenyon, 2001). Interestingly, in *D. melanogaster*, mutant *InR* genotypes live longer and exhibit small and immature ovaries, very similar to those observed in diapausing wildtype *Drosophila* (Tatar *et al.*, 2001b). This suggests that flies in reproductive diapause "phenocopy" the phenotype of *InR* mutants. Thus, there may exist an analogy between diapause and insulin signaling in *C. elegans* and *D. melanogaster*.

3. JH in Mutants of the Insulin Signaling Pathway

Several *D. melanogaster* mutant genotypes of *InR* and *chico* (encoding the insulin-receptor substrate) are long-lived (Clancy *et al.*, 2001; Tatar *et al.*, 2001b; Tu *et al.*, 2002a). For example, a heteroallelic *InR* mutant (InR^{p5545}/InR^{E19}) produces dwarf females with extended life span up to 85 percent (Tatar *et al.*, 2001b). Similarly, homozygous mutants of *chico* are sterile and very long-lived dwarfs, whereas heterozygous mutants of *chico* exhibit normal body size, reduced fecundity, and extended life span (Clancy *et al.*, 2001; Tu *et al.*, 2002a).

However, not all *InR* mutant alleles increase longevity: since *InR* gene is a highly pleiotropic locus, some alleles may have deleterious developmental effects carrying over to adults and counterbalancing the positive effects on aging (Tatar *et al.*, 2001b). Furthermore, unlike in *C. elegans*, hypomorphic insulin signaling mutants in *Drosophila* may have different effects on life span in males and females (Tu *et al.*, 2002a). While *Drosophila* mutants of *InR* and *chico* extend female longevity by 36 to 85 percent, the same alleles do not seem to produce an extension of mean longevity in males (Clancy *et al.*, 2001; Tatar *et al.*, 2001b). However, males of *InR* heteroallelic mutants have an increased life expectancy measured at age 20 days (Tatar *et al.*, 2001b), and the *chico*[1] mutation extends male longevity but has age-independent effects on adult mortality that counteract the strong impact of slow aging on life expectancy seen in *chico* mutant females (Tu *et al.*, 2002a). Similarly, reducing insulin signaling by experimental ablation of insulin-producing cells (IPCs) reduces age-dependent mortality, yet this effect is masked at young ages due to a high age-independent risk of death (Wessells *et al.*, 2004; but see Broughton *et al.*, 2005).

Interestingly, the extended life-span phenotype of some insulin signaling mutants is likely to be caused by JH deficiency. JH synthesis is negligible in *InR* dwarfs (Tatar *et al.*, 2001b), and homozygous *chico* mutants are also JH deficient (Tu *et al.*, 2005). Although *InR* mutant females are infertile with non-vitellogenic ovaries, egg development can be restored by application of methoprene. Furthermore, treatment with methoprene restores wildtype longevity to the long-lived *InR* mutants. Thus, JH deficiency, resulting from mutation in the insulin signaling pathway, may retard senescence, possibly through hormone-mediated effects on adult reproduction, physiology, and somatic maintenance. Consequently, Tatar and colleagues (2001b) suggest that infertility may not be the direct cause of slowed aging but that JH may simply control both fertility and longevity; JH may therefore be a key regulator for both traits. However, JH synthesis is also known to be reduced in a homozygous *InR* mutant genotype with normal life span; thus, the lack of JH may not be sufficient to extend life span under all circumstances (Tatar *et al.*, 2001b). Similarly, whether short-lived insulin signaling mutants have upregulated JH is currently unknown.

4. Effects of Manipulating JH on Life Span

Using mutants to examine the effects of JH on life span may be problematic because mutants can exhibit unspecific pleiotropic effects that are unrelated to changes in JH signaling. This problem may be overcome by examining the effects of applying exogenous JH or JHAs such as methoprene. Treating wildtype flies with methropene increases early fecundity but decreases longevity and stress resistance (Flatt & Kawecki, in preparation; Salmon *et al.*, 2001, Tatar *et al.*, 2001a,b). For example, methoprene treatment of diapausing *D. melanogaster* restores vitellogenesis and egg production yet increases demographic senescence (Tatar *et al.*, 2001a). Similarly, as discussed above (section III.A.3), Tatar and colleagues (2001b) found that the sterility phenotype of *InR* mutants can be rescued by methoprene treatment, which restores egg development and reduces life expectancy to that of wildtype flies, whereas methoprene treatment of *InR* wildtype controls did not increase adult mortality.

Application of commonly used JH inhibitors, such as precocene (Wilson *et al.*, 1983) or fluvastatin (Debernard *et al.*, 1994), can reduce or inhibit JH synthesis in the CA and may thus be used to study the effects of JH deficiency upon life span. However, these inhibitors also appear to have unspecific and toxic effects (e.g., Debernard *et al.*, 1994; Zera, 2004, and references therein). For example, high doses of fluvastatin kill locusts, whereas surgical removal of CA is not lethal (Debernard *et al.*, 1994). Thus, the usefulness of JH inhibitors for manipulating life span through changes in JH signaling is questionable. A different approach is to select wildtype flies for resistance to toxic doses of methoprene (T. Flatt & T. J. Kawecki, unpublished results). Flies that evolve specific insensitivity to JH, either by constitutive upregulation of JH esterases or by reduced JH binding, may exhibit increased longevity because JH deficiency is known to slow aging. Interestingly, flies selected for methoprene resistance rapidly evolved both methoprene- and JH III-resistance and showed extended life span (T. Flatt & T. J. Kawecki, unpublished results). However, the underlying mechanisms for this lifespan extension are unknown and may not be JH-related.

B. 20E and Aging

Although we know far less about the effects of steroid hormones on life span than about JH effects on aging, it now seems clear that 20E is a second candidate regulator of *Drosophila* aging (also see Simon *et al.*, 2003; Tatar, 2004; Tatar *et al.*, 2003).

1. Long-Lived Insulin Signaling Mutants Have Reduced 20E Titers

In adult insects, ecdysteroids are made in the ovaries and the testes (Chavez *et al.*, 2000; Gäde *et al.*, 1997; Gilbert *et al.*, 2002; Hagedorn, 1985). Tu and colleagues (2002b) measured ecdysteroid synthesis in isolated ovaries of *InR* mutants *in vitro* and found that ovarian ecdysteroid synthesis of mutant females was reduced as compared to wildtype. How 20E deficiency affects aging in *InR* mutants is currently not understood; 20E may affect life span by serving as a pro-aging hormonal signal or by regulating the relationship between reproduction and aging (Tatar, 2004; Tatar et al., 2004; Tu *et al.*, 2002b). Clearly, it would be interesting to see whether and how treatment of 20E-deficient *InR* mutants with 20E affects aging. In addition, because 20E is a major product of the *Drosophila* ovary and plays a pervasive role in female reproduction, we may speculate that the sex-specific effects of insulin signaling on aging seen in the fly may be related to differences in 20E signaling between males and females.

2. Mutations in the Ecdysone Receptor Extend Life Span

Simon and colleagues (2003) demonstrate that flies heterozygous for mutations of the *ecdysone receptor* (*EcR*) gene exhibit increased life span and stress resistance without decreases in reproduction or activity. Although almost nothing is known about the production, metabolism, and role of 20E in adult male *Drosophila*, it is interesting to note that mutations in *EcR* extended life span in both males and females, suggesting that 20E signaling affects aging in both sexes. Furthermore, a mutant involved in the 20E biosynthesis pathway (*DTS-3*) displays the same phenotype; this phenotype can be rescued by the application of 20E (Simon *et al.*, 2003). These results are consistent with reduced post-eclosion levels of ecdysteroids in long-lived females from a selection experiment for life-span extension (Harshman, 1999). Thus, the few examples at hand clearly suggest that 20E deficiency slows aging.

C. Interaction Effects of JH and 20E on Aging

Interactions between JH and 20E may not be restricted to pre-adult development, metamorphosis, and reproduction (Dubrovsky, 2005), but may also extend to the aging phenotype. In mosquitoes, application of bovine insulin acts directly in the ovary to regulate ecdysteroid synthesis (Riehle & Brown, 1999); insulin is also known to regulate germ-line stem cell proliferation in *D. melanogaster* ovaries (Drummond-Barbosa & Spradling, 2001). As discussed above (sections II.C and III.B.1), the ovaries of the JH-deficient *InR* mutants produce little ecdysteroids (Tu *et al.*, 2002b), and 20E can, depending on the species, inhibit or stimulate JH synthesis (Gu & Chow, 2003; Soller *et al.*, 1999). Thus, 20E may be a gonad-derived signal through which insulin and JH affect insect aging (Tatar, 2004; Tatar et al., 2003). In addition, reproductive diapause and diapause senescence may not be exclusively controlled by JH. Application of JH III or JHB$_3$ to abdomens of diapausing female flies can restore vitellogenesis (Saunders *et al.*, 1989). However, terminating diapause by warming flies from 11 °C to 25 °C results in a significant increase in the synthesis of ecdysteroids, but not JH (Saunders *et al.*, 1989). Furthermore, the injection of 20E can also elicit vitellogenesis and terminate diapause (Richard *et al.*,

1998, 2001), as has been observed with JH. This suggests that JH and 20E may interact in affecting diapause and levels of age-specific mortality during diapause. Interestingly, although JH and 20E often have antagonistic effects on the same trait or process, both hormones seem to have positive effects on female reproduction and negative effects on female life span. However, whether and how 20E interacts with JH to affect male life history remains unknown. Clearly, the interactive effects of these hormones on aging await further study.

IV. Candidate Genes Affecting Life Span Through JH and 20E Signaling

A. Insulin Signaling Affects Both JH and 20E

The insulin/IGF (insulin-like growth factor) signaling pathway has profound effects on aging in a variety of organisms, such as the nematode *C. elegans*, *Drosophila*, and rodents, and is suspected to have similar effects in humans (Kenyon, 2001; Partridge & Gems, 2002; Tatar, 2004; Tatar et al., 2003). Studies of mutants of *InR*, *chico*, and *EcR* suggest that JH and 20E may be secondary pro-aging signals downstream of insulin/IGF (see section III). As discussed above, long-lived mutants of *InR* are both JH and 20E-deficient, suggesting that insulin signaling is a major regulator of these secondary hormones. Indeed, the stimulation of ecdysteroid synthesis by insulin signaling is well known in many insects (Graf *et al.*, 1997; Hagedorn, 1985; Nagasawa, 1992; Riehle & Brown, 1999). For example, mosquitoes synthesize ovarian ecdysteroids after a blood meal, and this synthesis depends on insulin signaling. Sugar-fed mosquito females do not produce ecdysteroids, but application of exogenous bovine insulin can stimulate ovarian ecdysteroid synthesis (Riehle & Brown, 1999). But how does insulin signaling regulate JH and 20E synthesis?

In response to environmental or internal stimuli such as nutrition, insulin-producing cells (IPCs, belonging to the class of median neurosecretory cells, MNCs) located in the *pars intercerebralis* of the brain produce seven different *Drosophila* insulin-like peptides (DILPs; Brogiolo et al., 2001; Broughton et al., 2005). These DILPs are then released into the protocerebrum, at the CC, and into the hemolymph (Ikeya et al., 2002; Rulifson et al., 2002). Little is known about the effects of individual DILPs, but the expression of the genes *dilp3* and *dilp5* seems to be regulated by nutrition, and overexpression of *dilp1–7* promotes growth (Hwangbo et al., 2004; Ikeya et al., 2002; Rulifson et al., 2002). Insulin signaling may regulate JH and 20E synthesis in at least two not mutually exclusive ways (Tatar, 2004). First, circulating DILPs in the hemolymph activate insulin signaling by binding to the *InR* receptors in the target tissues and hence stimulate growth in these tissues. For example, *InR* mutants are dwarfs with both reduced JH synthesis and corpus allatum (CA) size; insulin may thus affect JH synthesis by affecting CA development and growth (Tatar et al., 2001b; Tu et al., 2005). Similarly, *InR* mutants have an approximately 50 percent reduction of wildtype ovariole number; mutants may therefore produce less 20E because of a reduced number of ovarian follicle cells synthesizing 20E (Tu & Tatar, 2003; Tu et al., 2002b;). Second, JH and 20E synthesis may be indirectly modulated by insulin signaling. For example, because JH synthesis is regulated by neuropeptides (Tobe & Bendena, 1999), DILPs may indirectly regulate the production of JH by affecting these neuropeptides. In *chico* mutants, JH synthesis relative to CA size is disproportionately reduced, suggesting that insulin signaling can regulate adult JH synthesis

independent of affecting CA development and growth (Tu et al., 2005). The insulin signaling–dependent regulation of JH and 20E may also be supported by the observation that ablation of IPCs can extend life span in *Drosophila* (Broughton et al., 2005; Wessells et al., 2004). However, it is currently unknown whether this effect occurs through the downregulation of JH or 20E. Clearly, future work needs to test whether ablation of IPCs or downregulation of DILP expression reduces JH and/or 20E. Similarly, reducing insulin signaling by transgenically overexpressing *dPTEN* (encoding a phosphatase and tensin homolog protein that antagonizes insulin signaling) and *dFOXO* (a forkhead transcription factor downstream of insulin signaling whose activity is inhibited by insulin signaling) in the head fat body of the fly can slow aging (Hwangbo et al., 2004), yet it remains to be tested whether these genes regulate longevity through effects on JH or 20E production. Figure 15.1 shows an integrated model of the endocrine regulation of *Drosophila* aging.

Although JH and 20E are not produced by *C. elegans* and rodents, the existence of secondary pro-aging hormones in these organisms has been postulated (Tatar et al., 2003; also see Gill et al., 2004). For example, in rodents, insulin signaling in the hypothalamus regulates the pituitary gland, which secretes secondary hormones such as thyroid-stimulating hormone (TSH), follicle-stimulating hormone (FSH), growth hormone (GH), and luteinizing hormone (LH); TSH in turn regulates the thyroid gland to produce the thyroid hormones T3 and T4. The pituitary may be seen as the mammalian equivalent of the CC and CA, and thyroxine (T4) has been tentatively suggested to share cellular functions with JH (Davey, 2000). Remarkably, a new study supports the idea that T4 may be a pro-aging hormone like JH (Vergara et al., 2004). Long-lived Snell dwarf mice (mice homozygous for the *Pit1*

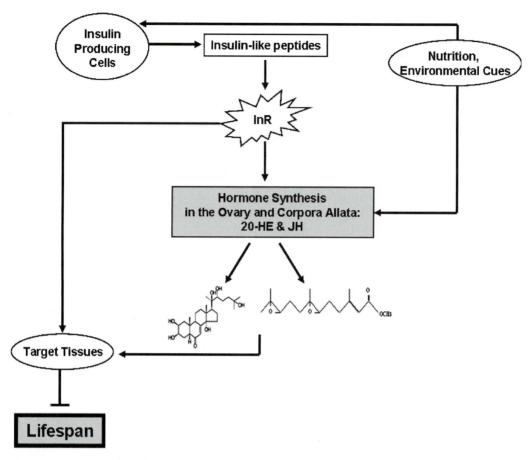

Figure 15.1 Integrated model for the endocrine regulation of aging, based on studies in *D. melanogaster* (see Hwangbo *et al.*, 2004; Tatar, 2004; Tatar *et al.*, 2003) External cues like nutrition stimulate insulin-producing cells (IPCs) to secrete insulin-like peptides (DILPs), which bind and activate the insulin-like receptor at the target tissues (InR in *D. melanogaster*, DAF-2 in *C. elegans*). Ligand binding at InR in turn induces the insulin/IGF-1 signaling cascade in cells of the CNS and other tissues, such as the fat body (primary insulin signaling). Induction of insulin/IGF-1 signaling suppresses a forkhead transcription factor downstream of insulin signaling (dFOXO in *D. melanogaster*, DAF-16 in *C. elegans*) required for life-span extension by slowed insulin signaling. Activation of this transcription factor (or inactivation of InR or ablation of IPCs) extends life span (Broughton *et al.*, 2005; Hwangbo *et al.*, 2004; Kenyon *et al.*, 1993; Tatar *et al.*, 2001b; Wessells *et al.*, 2004). Insulin signaling also has secondary effects: (1) insulin signaling affects insulin production by participating in endocrine and paracrine regulatory feedback circuits to regulate DILP transcription (Hwangbo *et al.*, 2004) and (2) insulin signaling affects the production of secondary aging regulatory signals such as JH from the CA or 20E from the gonads (Simon *et al.*, 2003; Tatar, 2004; Tatar *et al.*, 2001b, 2003; Tu *et al.*, 2002b;). In *Drosophila* and other insects, these secondary endocrine signals (unknown hormones in *C. elegans*, but see Gill *et al.*, 2004) suppress life-span extension (as well as stress resistance, immunity, and somatic maintenance) and upregulate gonad activity and reproduction (Tatar, 2004; Tatar *et al.*, 2003). Note that external cues may also directly affect the production of JH and 20E. Thus, insulin signaling may either directly affect aging (through dFOXO) or indirectly (through secondary pro-aging hormones). See text for further details.

mutation) have multiple hormonal defects, but whether these deficiencies are causally responsible for the slow aging phenotype has remained unclear (Tatar *et al.*, 2003).

Vergara and colleagues (2004) show that treatment with the T4 restores the reduced senescence phenotype in the long-lived Snell mice. Although it cannot be ruled out that the T4 treatment results in a toxic effect reducing life span (Vergara *et al.*, 2004), the restoration of the anti-aging effects by T4 is highly reminiscent of the life-span reduction seen in long-lived JH-deficient flies when treated with methoprene.

B. Genes Involved in JH Signaling

The genetics of JH signaling are currently not well understood (Dubrovsky, 2005). Moreover, the life-span effects of most *Drosophila* genes involved in JH signaling are unknown. Yet, despite our limited understanding, there exist several interesting candidate genes implicated in JH signaling that may affect the aging phenotype.

A major reason limiting our understanding of JH signaling is the unknown nature of the JH receptor (Dubrovsky, 2005; Gilbert *et al.*, 2000; Henrich & Brown, 1995; Jones & Sharp, 1997; Truman & Riddiford, 2002). Recent evidence suggests that *ultraspiracle (usp)*, encoding a retinoid X receptor, may be a JH receptor because JH is closely related to retinoic acid (RA) and USP protein can bind JH (Gilbert *et al.*, 2000; Jones & Sharp, 1997; Truman & Riddford, 2002). Although USP does not show high-affinity binding to JH (Jones & Sharp, 1997), it forms a heterodimer with the ecdysone receptor (EcR) (Gilbert *et al.*, 2002; Truman & Riddiford, 2002), which is itself known to have effects on *Drosophila* life span (Simon *et al.*, 2003). Thus, given the common interactions between JH and 20E and given that mutations in *EcR* or JH deficiency extend life span, *ultraspiracle* appears to be a promising candidate gene affecting aging. Yet, while *usp* probably plays a functional role in JH signaling, the low binding affinity for JH is not consistent with *usp* encoding a JH receptor (Dubrovsky, 2005).

Another candidate gene for the JH receptor is the X-linked gene *Methoprene-tolerant (Met)*, encoding a 85 kD high-affinity JH binding protein essential for transducing JH signals (Ashok *et al.*, 1998; Pursley *et al.*, 2000; Restifo & Wilson, 1998; Shemshedini & Wilson, 1990; Wilson *et al.*, 2003). *Met* mutant flies produce JH in normal amounts but are up to 100 times less sensitive to JH III and methoprene than *Met*⁺ flies (Pursley *et al.*, 2000; Shemshedini & Wilson, 1990; Shemshedini *et al.*, 1990). In adults, the *Met* gene has important effects on life-history traits, such as developmental time, onset of reproduction, and age-specific fecundity (Flatt & Kawecki, 2004; Minkoff & Wilson, 1992; Wilson & Ashok, 1998; Wilson *et al.*, 2003). Given these pleiotropic life-history effects of *Met*, presumably mediated by JH signaling, one may expect that this locus also affects life span. However, inconsistent with the notion of a JH receptor, *Met* null mutants are completely viable. Thus, the exact role of *Met* in JH signaling remains unclear (Dubrovsky, 2005).

Mutations of the *apterous (ap)* gene result in sterile females due to the development of non-vitellogenic ovaries (Ringo *et al.*, 1991). Mutant males are behaviorally sterile, spend less time courting, and are less likely to perform some elements of courtship behavior than age-matched wildtype males, yet they have fertile gametes. Adult mutant flies are JH deficient (Altaratz *et al.* 1991), and application of JH or methoprene to newly eclosed mutant females results in vitellogenic oocytes (Postlethwait & Weiser 1973), suggesting that the development of oocytes is profoundly affected by JH. A recent study clearly supports the notion that *apterous* is involved in JH signaling; in *apterous* mutants, the levels of two JH-inducible genes (Dubrovsky *et al.* 2002), *JhI-21* and *minidiscs (mdn)*, are strongly reduced, and methoprene treatment can rescue this defect. Thus, since *apterous* mutants are JH-deficient, like long-lived mutants of *InR* and *chico*, *apterous* may be an interesting candidate gene affecting aging.

Flies with a mutation in the *cricklet* (*clt*) gene have reduced yolk protein synthesis, larval fat bodies persisting into the adult stage, and an arrested oocyte development in the pre-vitellogenic stage (Shirras & Bownes, 1989). Methoprene has no effect on the fat body synthesis of yolk and vitellogenesis in the mutants; ovarian transplant experiments suggest that females have sufficient JH concentrations to promote oogenesis (Shirras & Bownes, 1989). This indicates that the gene may encode a protein downstream of JH synthesis, such as a receptor or transcription factor, which is nonfunctional in the mutants (Shirras & Bownes, 1989). However, as for many other genes affecting JH signaling, the potential effects of *clt* on aging await further study.

In female *Drosophila*, the post-mating response consists of increased egg deposition and reduced receptivity to males and is regulated by sex peptide (SP), contained in the male seminal fluid and transferred to the female upon mating. SP is known to stimulate JH synthesis in the mature CA (Moshitzky *et al.*, 1996). Consequently, JH appears to be a downstream component in the SP response cascade, causing the progression of vitellogenic oocytes after mating or SP application (Moshitzky *et al.*, 1996; Soller *et al.*, 1999). Remarkably, work by Geiger-Thornsberry & Mackay (2004) shows that the *sex peptide* locus (*Acp70, accessory protein 70*) harbors genetic variation for life span. Thus, the *sex peptide* gene is another promising candidate gene for aging studies, in particular since it may affect life span through its effects on female JH signaling (Flatt, 2004).

Biogenic amines, such as dopamine, octopamine, and serotonin, are known to affect JH synthesis in insects (Lafon-Cazal & Baehr, 1988; Rachinsky, 1994; Roeder, 1999). For example, octopamine

stimulates JH production in locusts (Lafon-Cazal & Baehr, 1988), and both octopamine and serotonin promote JH synthesis in honeybees (Rachinsky, 1994). In *D. melanogaster* and *D. virilis*, dopamine seems to stimulate synthesis of JH in immature females but inhibits its synthesis in mature, intensely reproducing females; similarly, octopamine appears to block JH production (Chentsova *et al.* 2002; Grutenko *et al.*, 2001; Rauschenbach *et al.*, 2002). Two recent experiments suggest that biogenic amines are important determinants of life span. Sze and colleagues (2000) found that a serotonin-synthesis mutant in *C. elegans* exhibits extended reproductive life span, and De Luca and colleagues (2003) report that the gene coding for the enzyme dopa decarboxylase (DDC), required for the final catalytic step in the synthesis of dopamine and serotonin, harbors significant amounts of variation for *Drosophila* longevity. Thus, although *C. elegans* is not known to produce JH, these results suggest that biogenic amine metabolism may affect the levels of secondary endocrine hormone with effects on aging. However, it remains to be determined whether *ddc* mutants in *Drosophila* exhibit variation in JH signaling that may, at least partially, account for the variation in life span attributed to this locus.

Table 15.1 summarizes information on some *Drosophila* genes involved in JH signaling; these genes may be promising candidate genes affecting aging.

C. Genes Involved in 20E Signaling

In contrast to JH, we have a fairly good understanding of the molecular mechanisms of both ecdysteroid synthesis and 20E action, particularly at the onset of metamorphosis (Dubrovsky, 2005). For example, 20E binds to the ecdysone receptor (EcR), which forms a heterodimer receptor complex with USP (Gilbert *et al.*, 2002; Truman & Riddiford, 2002), and recent work

Table 15.1

Examples of *Drosophila* Genes Involved in JH Signaling. Because JH is known to have major effects on insect life span, these genes represent candidate genes for aging. Further information on each of these and further candidate genes, including references, can be found on the flybase Website at: http://flybase.bio.indiana.edu; this database is searchable using gene names, flybase accession numbers, or keywords.

Gene	Function	Mutant Phenotype and Biological Processes	Flybase Accession
Acp70 (sex peptide; accessory gland peptide 70A)	Male product contained in seminal fluid; has hormone activity; negatively regulates female receptivity and post-mating response	Female mating defective; injection of *Acp70A* stimulates JH synthesis in the female, increases egg production and mimics the effects of mating; genetic variation for life span detected as a function of this gene	FBgn0003034
adp (adipose)	Involved in carbohydrate and lipid metabolism	Mutations result in hypertrophied adult fat body with enlarged lipid vesicles and hypertrophied female corpora allata; mutants are viable, starvation resistant, male and female fertile, yet egg hatchability is reduced and eclosion delayed	FBgn0000057
ap (apterous)	Product exhibits zinc ion binding and is involved in neurogenesis	Mutations affect halteres, muscle development, neuroanatomy, ovarian development, oogenesis, and female receptivity; some mutants are JH-deficient; JH application can restore vitellogenesis and positively affects ovarian maturation	FBgn0000099
clt (cricklet)	Carboxylesterase activity	Defective in yolk protein synthesis, histolysis of the larval fat body, vitellogenesis, and synthesis of larval serum protein 2; gene may encode a protein essential for mediating JH signaling in target tissues	FBgn0000326
e (ebony)	Product exhibits beta-alanyl-dopamine synthase activity, involved in cuticle pigmentation	Mutations affect wing and adult cuticle; mutants are locomotor rhythm and body color defective; 1-day-old mutant females show a significantly lower JH-hydrolyzing activity as compared to wildtype	FBgn0000527

(continues)

Table 15.1 (*Cont'd*)

Gene	Function	Mutant Phenotype and Biological Processes	Flybase Accession
Fas2 (fasciclin 2)	Involved in neuronal cell recognition and organ looping and symmetry	Mutations affect the embryonic neurons and 13 other tissues; mutants are larval recessive lethal and have embryonic neuroanatomical defects; the *spin* mutant allele affects neurosecretory cells innervating the corpus allatum, male genitalia rotation, and interacts with the *Met* locus	FBgn0000635
fs(2)B (female sterile (2) Bridges)	Female reproduction; also affects endocrine function	Recessive female sterile; cells of the corpus-allatum-corpus-cardiacum (CA/CC) complex of homozygous mutant females can probably not release hormone product and undergo degenerative changes; enlarged abdominal fat cells	FBgn0000949
ibx (icebox)	Encodes a product involved in female courtship behavior	Various mutant phenotypes, including female mating defective, female courtship defective, yet fertile and viable; treatment with JH analog methoprene results in more mating in homozygous females	FBgn0041750
InR (insulin-like receptor)	Insulin-like receptor; binds *Drosophila* insulin-like peptides	Heterozygous mutants are dwarf, female sterile, and long-lived; some mutants have lowered JH and 20E production	FBgn0013984
jhamt (JH acid methyltransferase)	JH acid methyltransferase activity involved in JH biosynthesis	Unknown	FBgn0028841
Jhbp-30, 63, and 80 (JH binding proteins – 30kD, 63kD, and 80kD)	JH binding activity in larval fat body cell nuclei	Unknown	FBgn0013282; FBgn0013283; FBgn0013284
Jhe (JH esterase)	JH esterase activity involved in JH catabolism	Unknown	FBgn0010052
Jheh1, Jheh2, and Jheh3 (JH epoxide hydrolases 1, 2, 3)	JH epoxide hydrolase activity involved in JH catabolism; maybe involved in defense response	Unknown	FBgn0010053; FBgn0034405; FBgn0034406

(*continues*)

Table 15.1   (*Cont'd*)

Gene	Function	Mutant Phenotype and Biological Processes	Flybase Accession
JhI-1and JhI-26 (JH-inducible proteins 1 and 26)	Unknown; gene expression induced by JH	Unknown	FBgn0028426; FBgn0028424
JhI-21 (JH-inducible protein 21)	L-amino acid transporter activity; amino acid metabolism?	Unknown	FBgn0028425
l(2)gl (lethal (2) giant larvae)	Product with myosin binding, involved in neurotransmitter secretion	Mutations affect the dorsal mesothoracic disc, the larval brain, and 21 other tissues; recessive lethal and tumorigenic; wildtype allele important for onset of vitellogenesis and oocyte growth, follicle cell migration and organization, and germline cell viability; some mutants have reduced size of the larval ring gland (consisting of the corpora cardiaca, the corpora allata, and the prothoracic gland), presumably resulting in endocrine deficiency	FBgn0002121
Methoprene-tolerant (Met 5 Rst(1)JH, Resistance to JH)	Encodes a product with JH binding, a putative JH receptor; involved in regulation of transcription	Loss-of-function alleles have reduced numbers of stage S8 to 9 and stage S10 to 14 oocytes, are methoprene and JH III resistant, viable, but have reduced female fertility; *Met* interacts with *Br* and *Fas2*	FBgn0002723
mama (maternal metaphase arrest)	Unknown	Mutants show lipid accumulation, hypertrophied corpora allata, are viable, recessive female sterile, maternal effect recessive lethal, and reduced male fertile	FBgn0000988
Mdh1 (malate dehydrogenase 1)	L-malate dehydrogenase activity	Unknown; response of Mdh1 to JH depends on ecdysteroids; during interecdysial period of the last instar *Mdh1* rapidly responds to JH by increasing activity	FBgn0002699

(*continues*)

Table 15.1 *(Cont'd)*

Gene	Function	Mutant Phenotype and Biological Processes	Flybase Accession
Rbp9 (RNA binding protein 9)	RNA binding, involved in egg chamber formation	Loss-of-function mutations affect the ovariole, the cystocyte, and the egg chamber and are female sterile; cells of the corpus-allatum corpus-cardiacum complex of homozygous mutant females can probably not release their hormone products and undergo degenerative changes	FBgn0010263
Tbh (tyramine β hydroxylase)	Tyramine-β hydroxylase activity involved in behavioral response to ethanol	Loss-of-function mutations are viable, male fertile and female sterile; under normal conditions, young mutant females have a higher JH-hydrolyzing activity than wildtype	FBgn0010329
usp (ultrapiracle)	Product with ligand-dependent nuclear receptor activity; forms heterodimer with ecdysone receptor; binds JH with low affinity; has cell-autonomous role in controlling neuronal remodeling	Mutations affect the embryonic/larval anterior spiracle, the imaginal discs, the embryonic larval midgut, and are recessive lethal, hypoactive and touch sensitivity defective; mutations show a range of imaginal disc phenotypes	FBgn0003964
Vha44 (vacuolar H[+] ATPase)	Hydrogen-exporting ATPase activity, phosphorylative mechanism, involved in JH biosynthesis	Unknown	FBgn0020611
Yp 1, 2, and 3 (yolk proteins 1, 2, and 3)	Structural molecule activity involved in vitellogenesis	Mutations conditionally affect egg production and the adult fat body and are dominant female sterile; the JH analog methoprene upregulates yolk proteins	FBgn0004045; FBgn0005391; FBgn0004047

confirms the importance of this heterodimer complex for *Drosophila* development (Hall & Thummel, 1998; Hodin & Riddiford, 1998; Dubrovsky, 2005). When bound to the receptor, 20E induces a number of early response genes such as *Broad* (*Br*), a gene essential for transducing 20E signals during metamorphic development of larval and imaginal tissues (Restifo & Wilson, 1998; Zhou & Riddiford, 2002), as well as *E74* and *E75*, which seem to be required for oogenesis (Dubrovsky, 2005; Kozlova & Thummel, 2000). In contrast to the genetic control of JH synthesis, the field has recently witnessed major progress in identifying critical genes required for 20E synthesis, involving key enzymes encoded by genes such as *defective in the avoidance of repellents* (*dare*), *disembodied* (*dib*), *ghost* (*gho*), *phantom* (*phm*), *shade* (*shd*), *shadow* (*sad*), *spook* (*spo*), and *Start1* (Buszczak *et al.*, 1999; Chavez *et al.*, 2000; Gilbert *et al.*, 2002; Petryk *et al.*, 2003; Roth *et al.*, 2004; Warren *et al.*, 2002). Because these genes affect 20E synthesis and because 20E deficiency is known to slow aging, some of these genes may be interesting candidate genes affecting aging.

Table 15.2 summarizes information on some fly genes known to be involved in 20E signaling; our future understanding of the endocrine regulation of aging may be improved by studying the effects of these genes on the aging phenotype.

Table 15.2

Examples of *Drosophila* Genes Involved in 20E Signaling. Because 20E affects insect aging, these genes may represent candidate genes for aging. Further information on each of these and other candidate genes can be found at: http://flybase.bio.indiana.edu ; this data base is searchable using gene names, flybase accession numbers, or keywords.

Gene	Function	Mutant Phenotype and Biological Processes	Flybase Accession
EcR (ecdysone receptor)	20E receptor	Constitutive heterozygous mutants extend life span; follicle cell expression of dominant negative for EcR results in female sterility; germline clones have arrested mid-oogenesis	FBgn0000546
E74 and E75 (ecdysone-induced proteins 74 and 75)	Orphan receptors; transcription factors required for mediating 20E response	Germline clones have arrested mid-oogenesis, degenerate egg chambers; some mutants have low 20E titers	FBgn0000567; FBgn0000568
Br (broad)	Transcription factor; a major 20E inducible gene; also interacts with the *Met* locus	Various mutant phenotypes, including developmental arrest, metathoracic tarsal segment formation, optic lobe formation, effects on adult brain, and reduced transcription rate or stability of the small heat shock protein mRNAs	FBgn0000210

(continues)

Table 15.2   (*Cont'd*)

Gene	Function	Mutant Phenotype and Biological Processes	Flybase Accession
dare (defective in the avoidance of repellents)	Adrenodoxin reductase required for ecdysteroid synthesis	Various mutant phenotypes; blocked ecdysteroid synthesis; abnormal response to olfactory stimuli, degenerate nervous system; germ-line clones arrest oogenesis at stage 8/9	FBgn0015582
dib (disembodied)	Mitochondrial cytochrome P450 required for hydroxylation in ecdysteroid biosynthesis	Low ecdysteroid synthesis and various other mutant phenotypes, including no differentiation of the cuticle or the head skeleton	FBgn0000449
gho (ghost)	Unknown involved in ecdysteroid biosynthesis pathway	Mutants have undifferentiated cuticle due to defect in 20E signaling but normal embryonic ecdysteroid titers	FBgn0001106
InR (insulin-like receptor)	Insulin-like receptor, binding *Drosophila* insulin-like peptides	Heterozygous mutants are dwarf, female sterile, and long-lived; some mutants have lowered JH and 20E production	FBgn0013984
phm (phantom)	Ecdysteroid 25-hydroxylase required for ecdysteroid biosynthesis	Mutations affect the embryonic cuticle, the embryonic head, and oogenesis; embryonic recessive lethal; mutants display a posterior contraction and poorly differentiated cuticle	FBgn0004959
sad (shadow)	Mitochondrial cytochrome P450 required for hydroxylation in ecdysteroid synthesis	Mutants have low larval ecdysteroid titers; no differentiation of the cuticle or the head skeleton	FBgn0003312
shd (shade)	P450 enzyme, converting ecdysone to 20E	Mutants have no differentiation of cuticle or head skeleton; ovarian enzyme activity required for female fertility; low embryonic 20E production	FBgn0003388
spo (spook)	Cytochrome P450 required for electron transport in ecdysteroid synthesis pathway	Mutants with low embryonic ecdysteroid titers; no differentiation of the cuticle or the head skeleton	FBgn0003486

D. Interactions between JH and 20E Signaling

As discussed above (section IV.B), the interactive effects of JH and 20E are supported by the finding that the ecdysone receptor (EcR), affecting fly life span, dimerizes with the USP, which is a candidate receptor for JH (Dubrovsky, 2005; Truman & Riddiford, 2002). The potential importance of this receptor complex for aging is underscored by the suggestion that the molecular chaperones Hsp70 and Hsp90 and the histone deacetylases Sin3A/Rpd3 interact with EcR/USP (Arbeitmann & Hogness, 2000; Tsai *et al.*, 1999). These genes are known to affect life span: overexpression of chaperones extends longevity in *D. melanogaster* and *C. elegans* (Tatar *et al.*, 1997; Yokoyama *et al.*, 2002), and mutation of the gene encoding Rpd3 increases the life span of yeast and *D. melanogaster* (Kim *et al.*, 1999; Rogina *et al.*, 2003). It is thus interesting to speculate that the aging effects of EcR, and potentially those of the EcR/USP complex, may be mediated by these genes.

Interestingly, two 20E-induced transcription factors, *Br* and *E75*, seem to be intimately involved in the cross-talk between JH and 20E signaling (Dubrovsky, 2005). JH and 20E are known to regulate the expression of *Br* (Dubrovsky, 2005, and references therein), and preliminary data suggest that *Br* interacts epistatically with the putative JH receptor gene *Met* (Restifo & Wilson, 1998). In view of this interaction, it would be interesting to study the effects of *Br* on aging. The *E75* gene can be activated by both JH and 20E, and the isoform *E75A* is the first transcription factor whose expression is known to be directly induced by JH (Dubrovsky, 2005, and references therein). Thus, E75 may be an important mediator of the interaction between JH and 20E (Dubrovsky, 2005), and it would be important to examine whether this locus affects aging.

V. Hormones, Nutrition, and Life Span

A. Nutrition Regulates JH and 20E Synthesis

In insects, nutritional status is well known to affect both development and reproduction. Proper nutrition provides an organism with the energy required for development, growth, reproduction, and somatic maintenance. In some insects, insufficient nutrition suppresses egg development by inhibiting CA or ovarian function, as seen in mosquitoes and some higher dipterans (Wheeler, 1996). For example, vitellogenesis in the mosquito *Aedes aegypti* depends on interactions among JH, 20E, and other endocrine factors. These hormones, however, are released only after a blood meal (Dhadialla & Raikhel, 1994). A protein-rich diet is also necessary to initiate JH and 20E synthesis in other higher flies, such as the house fly *M. domestica* (Adams & Gerst, 1991, 1992) and the black blow fly *Phormia regina* (Liu *et al.*, 1988; Yin & Stoffolano, 1990; Yin *et al.*, 1990; Zou *et al.*, 1989).

In *D. melanogaster*, yeast appears to be a major stimulus in activating the endocrine system. For example, DILP production by the IPCs is activated upon yeast feeding in adult flies that were yeast-deprived as third instar larvae (Tu & Tatar, 2003). DILPs may be required for JH and 20E synthesis because reduced insulin signaling, as observed in *InR* and *chico* mutants, is known to result in JH and 20E deficiency. This hypothesis may be supported by the observation that JH synthesis is elevated upon adult yeast feeding in flies that were yeast-deprived as third instar larvae as compared to control flies yeast-starved both during third larval instar and adulthood (Tu & Tatar, 2003). Thus, these results suggest that JH production is directly regulated by adult feeding, not larval feeding. 20E also responds to nutrition in the fruit fly. For instance, flies fed on a diet consisting only of sugar and water produce much less ecdysteroids at both 24 hours and 48 hours of adulthood than yeast-fed control flies, whereas re-feeding female yeast after a 24-hour yeast starvation period induces a high ovarian ecdysteroid production (Schwartz et al., 1985). The above results therefore suggest that the effects of dietary manipulation on life span may be mediated by nutrition-induced changes of pro-aging hormones such as JH and 20E.

B. Nutrient Sensing Pathways Affect Aging Through Hormones

An adequate physiological response to nutrient levels is a key determinant of survival and somatic maintenance. In *Drosophila*, responses to nutrition are mediated by highly conserved nutrient sensing pathways, such as the insulin/IGF signaling pathway and the target of rapamycin (TOR) pathway, both of which are major growth regulators (Chen et al., 1996; Ikeya et al., 2002; Oldham et al., 2000).

For the case of insulin signaling, the gene expression of *dilp3* and *dilp5*, but not *dilp2*, is regulated by nutrient availability, and overexpressing *dilp1–7* promotes growth (Ikeya et al., 2002). Interestingly, recent work shows intimate connections between DILP expression, insulin signaling, and the fat body, which presumably represents a major nutrient sensing tissue in the fly. The fat body is an important target for both JH and 20E, a major organ for the synthesis of vitellogenins and antibacterial peptides, and also has essential nutrient storage functions.

In *C. elegans*, activation of the gene *daf-16*, a forkhead transcription factor downstream of insulin signaling, is required for the life-span extension induced by reduced insulin signaling (Kenyon et al., 1993). Interestingly, in adult *Drosophila*, limited activation of *dFOXO*, the homolog of *C. elegans daf-16*, in the head (pericere-

bral) fat body uniquely reduces expression of neuronally synthesized DILP2 (but not that of DILP3 and DILP5), represses endogenous insulin-dependent signaling in the abdominal fat body, and extends life span (Hwangbo et al., 2004). These nonautonomous and systemic effects suggest that the adult head fat body is a major endocrine site (Hwangbo et al., 2004). Furthermore, these studies indicate that DILPs 2, 3, and 5 may have different physiological functions (Hwangbo et al., 2004; Ikeya et al., 2002). DILP2 responds to long-term downregulation of insulin signaling, whereas DILP3 and DILP5 do not. In contrast, DILP3 and DILP5 respond to acute starvation, whereas DILP2 does not. Thus, DILP3 and DILP5 may mediate the short-term response to changes in nutrient levels, whereas DILP2 may adjust a fly's life history in response to sustained periods of reduced insulin signaling. Clearly, it would be very informative to examine the effects of individual DILPs on aging and on the production of JH and 20E in different developmental stages and under different nutritional conditions (also see Figure 15.1).

In addition to insulin signaling, the *TOR* and the *slimfast* pathways are major nutrition sensing pathways regulating growth through the fat body (Colombani et al., 2003). The involvement of the fat body in insulin, *slimfast*, and *TOR* signaling and its response to nutrition challenge suggest that this tissue is important for both development and the regulation of aging. It is thus conceivable that downregulating the *slimfast* and *TOR* pathways in the fat body may increase longevity. Indeed, recent work demonstrates that constitutive suppression of the *dTOR* pathway, either ubiquitously or in the fat body only, can extend life span (Kapahi et al., 2004). This life-span extension depends on nutritional conditions, suggesting a possible link between the *TOR* pathway and dietary restriction (Kapahi et al., 2004). For example, in yeast

(*Saccharomyces cerevisiae*), the *TOR* pathway mediates cell growth in response to nutrient availability, in part by inducing ribosomal protein gene expression through histone acetylation (Rohde & Cardenas, 2003). Thus, although the longevity extension by downregulation of *TOR* may relate to caloric restriction, the underlying mechanisms remain unclear. Interestingly, the *dTOR* and *slimfast* pathways are known to interact with the insulin signaling pathway (Colombani *et al.*, 2003; Hafen, 2004; Oldham & Hafen, 2003), but whether and how *dTOR* and *slimfast* affect hormones such as JH and 20E remains unknown.

C. Connection Between Caloric Restriction, Hormones, and Life Span

To date, caloric restriction has been one of the most effective interventions extending life span in model organisms, including yeast, nematodes, flies, and rodents (Kenyon, 2001; Masoro, 2000; but see Carey *et al.*, 2002). Similarly, as discussed above, nutrition has major effects on the production of hormones (DILPs, JH, and 20E) that are intimately involved in the regulation of aging. It is thus interesting to speculate that the longevity effects of caloric restriction may be mediated by hormones.

In *Drosophila*, dietary restriction affects both reproduction and age-specific mortality (Good & Tatar, 2001). For instance, low adult nutrition induces an arrest in early stem-cell proliferation and alters the frequency of cell death at two pre-vitellogenic checkpoints; this response requires intact insulin signaling (Drummond-Barbosa & Spradling, 2001). Similarly, caloric (or dietary) restriction can dramatically extend fly life span (Chapman & Partridge, 1996; Chippindale *et al.*, 1993). In contrast, complete yeast starvation of adult flies shortens life span (Chippindale *et al.*, 1993; Good & Tatar, 2001; Tu & Tatar, 2003), suggesting that yeast is a crucial dietary component for survival and somatic maintenance.

Yeast restriction during late development may silence insulin signaling throughout metamorphosis into adulthood, and thereby extend life span. To test this hypothesis, Tu and Tatar (2003) studied aging in adult flies that were yeast-deprived as third instar larvae. As expected, adult flies from yeast-deprived larvae phenocopied insulin signaling mutants by exhibiting prolonged developmental time, small body size, reduced ovariole number, and reduced fecundity (Tu & Tatar, 2003). Furthermore, yeast deprivation reduced insulin signaling: adult flies from yeast deprived larvae had reduced numbers of insulin-positive vesicles. However, unlike constitutive insulin signaling mutants of *InR* or *chico*, adults from yeast-deprived larvae did not exhibit decreased age-specific mortality. Interestingly, yeast feeding increased both insulin-like peptide and JH levels in adult flies from yeast-deprived larvae as compared to flies that were yeast-deprived throughout both their larval and adult life (Tu & Tatar, 2003). This suggests that adult insulin and JH are regulated by adult nutritional state and that slowed aging specifically requires reduced insulin signaling or JH deficiency in the adult.

A better understanding of the interplay between nutrition and hormones in affecting aging is likely to come from genetic analysis. For example, recent findings show that mutations in the gene encoding the Rpd3 histone deacetylase, likely to be involved in caloric restriction, promote life span (Rogina *et al.*, 2003). Interestingly, the histone deacetylases Sin3A/Rpd3 interact with the EcR/USP complex (Tsai *et al.*, 1999), suggesting that they may respond to JH and 20E signaling. Furthermore, in yeast, caloric restriction extends life span by activating Sir2, a member of the sirtuin family of NAD^+-dependent protein deacetylases.

In *C. elegans*, a homolog of Sir2 appears to act in the insulin signaling pathway upstream of DAF-16; overexpression of the *Sir2* gene extends worm life span in a *daf-16* dependent manner (Tissenbaum & Guarente, 2001). Sir2 can also be activated by several sirtuin-activating compounds (STACs) found in plants. For example, the natural compound resveratrol, found in red wine, activates sirtuins in both *C. elegans* and *Drosophila* and extends both worm and fly life span (Wood *et al.*, 2004). The life-span extension induced by resveratrol seems to be independent of caloric restriction: resveratrol does not increase life span in calorically restricted long-lived worms and flies, suggesting that resveratrol affects life span through a mechanism related to caloric restriction (Wood *et al.*, 2004). It is noteworthy that the structure of resveratrol is somewhat similar to that of JH or 20E, with multiple six-carbon rings and long carbon chain branches, and it will be interesting to determine whether and how JH and 20E signal through a sirtuin pathway to regulate aging under starvation conditions. However, in summary, our current understanding of how nutrition and hormonal signaling interact in affecting life span remains very limited.

VI. Hormonal Effects on Stress Resistance and Immunity

A. Hormones and Stress Resistance

Upregulation of stress resistance is thought to be one of the major ways for organisms to regulate senescence (Jazwinski, 1996; Johnson *et al.*, 1996; Lithgow, 1996). During the aging process, molecular chaperones such as heat-shock proteins are thought to combat stress-related senescent dysfunction. For example, transgenic *Drosophila* with extra copies of the heat shock protein gene *hsp70* show increased life span upon heat shock induction (Tatar *et al.*, 1997). Similarly, long-lived *InR*

mutants or transgenic flies overexpressing *dFOXO* have elevated resistance to paraquat, a commonly used free-radical reagent (Hwangbo *et al.*, 2004; Tatar *et al.*, 2001b). Since *InR* mutants have low JH and 20E synthesis, it is possible that JH and 20E negatively regulate stress response in flies. For example, high JH and 20E levels may increase reproduction at the cost of decreased stress resistance and shortened life span. This model is indeed supported by recent experiments. For example, Salmon and colleagues (2001) found that methoprene application increased reproduction in female fruit flies yet decreased stress resistance, measured as the susceptibility to starvation and oxidative stress. Another good example comes from burying beetles (*Nicrophorus spp.*), in which starvation stress decreases both the JH titer and fecundity, whereas treatment with JH or a JH analog reduces starvation resistance (Trumbo & Robinson, 2004).

B. Hormonal Effects on Immunity

The optimal function of the immune system is of crucial importance for survival and somatic maintenance (Arlt & Hewison, 2004). For example, there are many well-known links between longevity and immune-response genes in mammals (Flurkey *et al.*, 2001), such as genes of the major histocompatibility complex (MHC, see review by Ginaldi & Sternberg, 2003). In contrast to mammals, insects such as *Drosophila* do not possess adaptive immunity but exhibit innate immunity to combat microbial infections (Hoffmann, 2003; Tzou *et al.*, 2002).

How hormones in general modulate immune function in insects is not well understood, but recent studies suggest that JH regulates immunity (Rantala *et al.* 2003; Rolff & Siva-Jothy, 2002). In the mealworm beetle (*Tenebrio molitor*) immunity (phenoloxidase levels) is reduced by mating activity, and this trade-off seems to be regulated by JH (Rolff &

Siva-Jothy, 2002). Application of the JH inhibitor fluvastatin increases immune activity; thus, JH specifically downregulates immune function (Rolff & Siva-Jothy, 2002). Similarly, Rantala and colleagues (2003), using the same species, have shown that the tradeoff between immune function and sexual advertisement (i.e., pheromone production) is mediated by JH. Thus, JH, a major gonadotropic hormone, has negative effects on immune function. This observation is interesting in view of the fact that reproductive hormones in vertebrates can often have negative effects on the immune system, as is the case for testosterone (e.g., Casto *et al.*, 2001).

To initiate an improved understanding of hormonal effects on immunity, our laboratory has recently begun to explore the effects of JH on primary immune response genes in *Drosophila* (M. Tatar, unpublished). In this preliminary experiment, flies were yeast-starved for 5 days to lower their endogenous JH titer and to synchronize their physiology. Subsequently, the JH analog methoprene was topically applied to individual flies, using ethanol-treated flies as control. RNA transcript levels from these two groups were then analyzed using Affymetrix gene chips (two replicate chips per group). From these data, with the FatiGO software (Al-Shahrour *et al.*, 2004), we find that genes with functions for response to biotic stimuli are relatively enriched by JH treatment. This gene ontology category includes genes involved in response to microbial infection, starvation, and oxidative stress. Our set of JH responsive genes (criterion: at least two-fold change in gene expression as compared to the untreated control) consisted of 270 probe sets (160 downregulated and 110 upregulated, of a total 14,009 sets with 6,142 annotated). Noticeably, for this set, 12.9 percent of the genes showing changes in gene expression belong to the category "response to biotic stimuli."

To test whether different categorical responses represent the biological effect of JH as distinct from a chance observation, we compared the observed representation within gene ontology categories to the expected representation assuming a process of random sampling. Genes involved in "monosaccharide metabolism" were significantly over-represented (3.91 percent observed relative to 1.21 percent expected from the annotated genome; Fisher's Exact Test, $P = 0.0032$). As well, the categories "response to pest/pathogen/parasite" and "response to biotic stimuli" were enriched relative to chance expectation (respectively: 3.91 percent versus 1.25 percent, $P = 0.0040$; 13.04 percent versus 7.55 percent, $P = 0.0051$). Genes involved in response to biotic stimuli (including parasites and pathogens) are thus significantly over-represented, suggesting that JH influences the state of adult defense response, including immune function.

Among the genes that show a response to biotic stimuli, is there any bias toward upregulation versus downregulation? For instance, among "cell organization and biogenesis" genes, 16.84 percent were upregulated relative to 4.41 percent downregulated (Fisher's Exact Test, $P = 0.0024$). In contrast, among genes in the "biotic response" category, 17.65 percent were downregulated compared to only 6.32 percent in the upregulated set (Fisher's Exact Test, $P = 0.0159$). Thus, although JH stimulates the expression of some of these genes, these data overall suggest that JH functions to suppress many aspects of cellular and systemic stress response (see Table 15.3).

VII. Conclusions

Here we have reviewed the effects of hormones on fly aging. The hormonal mechanisms affecting aging are manifest both as genetic polymorphisms (as seen in endocrine deficient mutants) and as phenotypic/physiological plasticity (as seen

Table 15.3

JH-Induced *Drosophila* Genes Involved in Defense or Immune Response. The table provides information on genes involved in defense, stress, or immune response whose expression is either upregulated or downregulated by application of the JH analog methoprene (M. Tatar, unpublished data). Further information on each of these genes can be found at: http://flybase.bio.indiana.edu.

Gene Name	Function in Reaction to Biological Stimulus	Downregulated or Upregulated	Flybase Accession
Dorsal-related immunity factor	Defense and immune response, response to fungi	Up	FBgn0011274
Turandot M	Humoral defense mechanism	Up	FBgn0031701
Tetraspanin 96F	B-cell mediated immunity	Up	FBgn0027865
Traf3	Defense response	Up	FBgn0030748
CG6662	Defense response	Up	FBgn0035907
Tetraspanin 74F	Defense response	Up	FBgn0036769
CG6435	Defense response, defense response to bacteria	Down	FBgn0034165
CG7627	Defense response, response to toxin	Down	FBgn0032026
JH expoxide hydrolase 2	Defense response, response to toxin	Down	FBgn0034405
Drosocin	Defense response to gram-positive and -negative bacteria	Down	FBgn0010388
Immune induced molecule 23	Defense response	Down	FBgn0034328
PHGPx	Defense response, response to toxin	Down	FBgn0035438
Ejaculatory bulb protein III	Response to virus	Down	FBgn0011695
CG12780	Gram-negative bacterial binding, defense response	Down	FBgn0033301
Metchnikowin	Antibacterial and antifungal humoral response	Down	FBgn0014865
CG1702	Defense response, response to toxin	Down	FBgn0031117
CG6426	Defense response to bacteria	Down	FBgn0034162
CG5397	Defense response	Down	FBgn0031327
CG13422	Defense response to gram-negative bacteria	Down	FBgn0034511
CG10307	Defense response	Down	FBgn0034655
Transferrin 1	Defense response	Down	FBgn0022355
18 wheeler	Antibacterial humoral response, immune response	Down	FBgn0004364
Diptericin B	Antibacterial humoral response	Down	FBgn0034407
Hemolectin	Defense response	Down	FBgn0029167
Diptericin	Defense response to gram-negative bacteria	Down	FBgn0004240

(continues)

Table 15.3   *(Cont'd)*

Gene Name	Function in Reaction to Biological Stimulus	Downregulated or Upregulated	Flybase Accession
CG1681	Defense response	Down	FBgn0030484
CG2736	Defense response	Down	FBgn0035090
CG8336	Defense response	Down	FBgn0036020
takeout	Behavioral response to starvation	Down	FBgn0039298
CG18522	Defense response; reactive oxygen species metabolism	Down	FBgn0038347

in reproductive diapause and senescence plasticity). These sources of variation are likely to involve common endocrine regulatory mechanisms.

As in worms and rodents, reduced insulin signaling can slow aging in the fly (see Figure 15.1). Downstream of insulin signaling, fly aging seems to be regulated by secondary hormones, such as the sesquiterpenoid JH and the steroid 20E. Several lines of evidence indicate that both JH and 20E deficiency can dramatically slow aging while increasing stress resistance or immune function. Insects such as *Drosophila* may use JH and 20E to adaptively coordinate (and, if necessary, trade off) the expression of the "reproductive function" versus the "survival function" in response to environmental cues such as temperature or nutrition. Yet, although in some cases JH and 20E co-affect life span and reproduction, endocrine interventions typically slow aging without causing costs in reproduction. The conditional uncoupling of reproduction and survival will thus require us to rethink classical models for the evolution of senescence, including Williams' (1957) antagonistic pleiotropy hypothesis and the concept of senescence tradeoffs caused by costs of reproduction. Recent work on the *Drosophila* fat body has also advanced our understanding of the tissue specificity of endocrine effects on life span. The fat body appears to regulate aging both autonomously and non-autonomously by affecting insulin sig-

naling and probably secondary hormones such as JH and 20E.

Despite these insights into the endocrine control of aging in *Drosophila* and other insects, there remain many unresolved and difficult questions. For instance, we need to know how general the effects of JH and 20E upon aging are: Does JH or 20E deficiency invariably extend life span, or is this a conditional effect, for instance depending on species, nutrition, temperature, and sex? Do both JH and 20E have identical effects on life span, or do they differ and how? Answering these questions will depend on suitable tools for manipulating JH and 20E signaling. For example, do synthetic JH and 20E inhibitors or inhibitory neuropeptides such as allatostatins extend life span? Does overexpression of JH- or 20E-degrading enzymes in transgenically engineered insects slow aging? Similarly, the molecular details of JH and, to a lesser extent, 20E signaling remain relatively poorly understood. This raises many difficult questions: What is the molecular nature of the JH receptor, and how does it modulate aging? Do most, if not all, JH and 20E signaling genes affect aging? Through which downstream genes do the JH and 20E signaling pathways regulate aging? How exactly does insulin signaling affect JH and 20E signaling? What is the nature of the secondary hormones mediating the effects of fat body insulin signaling on whole-animal life span? How do caloric restriction and hormones interact at the molecular level to affect longevity? We can make further observations and ask related questions. For example, JH and 20E seem to modulate evolutionarily relevant tradeoff relationships between fitness components. How, mechanistically, do JH and 20E modulate these tradeoffs between reproduction and survival, stress resistance, and somatic maintenance? Are the endocrine loci affecting these tradeoffs genetically variable and subject to natural selection in wild populations? Finally, we may ask: Do other insect hormones than JH and 20E have major effects on the aging phenotype? What are the functional equivalents of JH and 20E in other organisms and how do they affect aging?

These are but a few of the most pressing questions to be addressed in the near future. To address them, we will need to combine molecular and evolutionary genetics, endocrinology, nutritional physiology, and biodemography. We have many hypotheses, patterns, and models, but little solid data. Understanding the genetic and endocrine regulation of aging remains a fundamental, yet promising, challenge for modern molecular biogerontology.

Acknowledgements

We thank Kyung-Jin Min for helpful discussions, James Cypser for help with the JH gene chip study, and Faye Lemieux and the other members of the Tatar Lab for producing many of the data we have summarized. This work was supported by the American Federation for Aging Research (MPT); the Swiss National Science Foundation, the Roche Research Foundation, and the Swiss Study Foundation (TF); the National Institute of Health; and the Ellison Medical Foundation (MT).

References

Adams, T. S., & Gerst, J. W. (1991). The effect of pulse-feeding a protein diet on ovarian maturation, vitellogenin levels, and ecdysteroid titre in houseflies, *Musca domestica*, maintained on sucrose. *International Journal of Invertebrate Reproduction and Development*, 20, 49–57.

Adams, T. S., & Gerst, J. W. (1992). Interaction between diet and hormones on vitellogenin levels in the housefly, *Musca domestica*. *International Journal of Invertebrate Reproduction and Development*, 21, 91–98.

Al-Shahrour, F., Diaz-Uriarte, R., & Dopazo, J. (2004). FatiGO: a web tool for finding significant associations of gene ontology terms with groups of genes. *Bioinformatics*, 20, 578–580.

Altaratz, M., Applebaum, S. W., Richard, D. S., Gilbert, L. I., & Segal, D. (1991). Regulation of juvenile hormone synthesis in wild-type and apterous mutant *Drosophila*. *Molecular and Cellular Endocrinology*, 81, 205–216.

Arbeitman, M. N., & Hogness, D. S. (2000). Molecular chaperones activate the *Drosophila* ecdysone receptor, an RXR heterodimer. *Cell*, 101, 67–77.

Arlt, W., & Hewison, M. (2004) Hormones and immune function: implications of aging. Aging Cell, 3, 209–216.

Ashok, M., Turner, C., & Wilson, T. G. (1998). Insect juvenile hormone resistance gene homology with the bHLH-PAS familiy of transcriptional regulators. *Proceedings of the National Academy of Sciences of the USA*, 95, 2761–2766.

Barnes, A. I., & Partridge, L. (2003). Costing reproduction. *Animal Behaviour*, 66,199–204.

Bartke, A., & Lane, M. (2001). Endocrine and neuroendocrine regulatory function. In E. Masoro, & S. Austad (Eds.), *Handbook of the biology of aging* (pp. 297–323). San Diego: Academic Press.

Belgacem, Y. H., & Martin, J.-R. (2002). Neuroendocrine control of a sexually dimorphic behavior by a few neurons of the *pars intercerebralis* in *Drosophila*. *Proceedings of the National Academy of Sciences of the USA*, 99, 15154–15158.

Bodenstein, D. (1950). The postembryonic development of *Drosophila*. In M. Demerec (Ed.), *Biology of Drosophila* (pp. 275–367). New York: Hafner Publishing.

Bownes, M. (1982). Hormonal and genetic regulation of vitellogenesis in *Drosophila*. *Quarterly Review of Biology*, 57, 247–274.

Bownes, M. (1989). The roles of juvenile hormone, ecdysone and the ovary in the control of *Drosophila* oogenesis. *Journal of Insect Physiology*, 35, 409–413.

Brogiolo, W., Stocker, H., Ikeya, T., Rintelen, F., Fernandez, R., & Hafen, E. (2001). An evolutionarily conserved function of the *Drosophila* insulin receptor and insulin-like peptides in growth control. *Current Biology*, 11, 213–221.

Broughton, S. J., Piper, M. D. W., Ikeya, T., Bass, T. M., Jacobson, J., Driege, Y., Martinez, P., Hafen, E., Withers, D. J., Leevers, S. J., & Partridge, L. (2005). Longer lifespan, altered metabolism, and stress resistance in *Drosophila* from ablation of cells making insulin-like ligands. *Proceedings of the National Academy of Sciences of the USA*, 102, 3105–3110.

Buszczak, M., Freeman, M. R., Carlson, J. R., Bender, M., Cooley, L., & Segraves, W. A. (1999). Ecdysone response genes govern egg chamber development during mid-oogenesis in *Drosophila*. *Development*, 126, 4581–4589.

Carey, J. R., Liedo, P., Harshman, L., Zhang, Y., Muller, H. G., Partridge, L., & Wang, J. L. (2002). Life history response of Mediterranean fruit flies to dietary restriction. *Aging cell*, 1, 140–148.

Casto, J. M., Nolan, V. Jr., & Kelterson, E. D. (2001). Steroid hormones and immune function: Experimental studies in wild and captive dark eyed juncas (*Junco hyemalis*). *The American Naturalist*, 157, 408–420.

Chapman, T., & Partridge, L. (1996). Female fitness in *Drosophila melanogaster*: an interaction between the effect of nutrition and of encounter rate with males. *Proceedings of the Royal Society of London B*, 263, 755–759.

Chavez, V. M., Marques, G., Delbecque, J. P., Kobayashi, K., Hollingsworth, M., Burr, J., Natzle, J., & O'Connor, M. B. (2000). The *Drosophila* disembodied gene controls late embryonic morphogenesis and codes for a cytochrome P450 enzyme that regulates embryonic ecdysone levels. *Development*, 127, 4115–4126.

Chen, C., Jack, J., & Garofalo, R. S. (1996). The *Drosophila* insulin receptor is required for normal growth. *Endocrinology*, 137, 846–856.

Chentsova, N. A., Grutenko, N. E., Bogomolova, E. V., Adonyeva, N. V.,

Karpova, E. K., & Rauschenbach, I. Y. (2002). Stress response in *Drosophila melanogaster* strain *inactive* with decreased tyramine and octopamine contents. *Journal of Comparative Physiology B*, 172, 643–650.

Chippindale, A. K., Leroi, A. M., Kim, S. B., & Rose, M. R. (1993). Phenotypic plasticity and selection in *Drosophila* life-history evolution. I. Nutrition and the cost of reproduction. *Journal of Evolutionary Biology*, 6, 171–193.

Clancy, D. Gems, J. D., Harshman, L. G., Oldham, S., Stocker, H., Hafen, E., Leevers, S. J., & Partridge, L. (2001). Extension of life-span by loss of CHICO, a *Drosophila* insulin receptor substrate protein. *Science*, 292, 104–106.

Colombani, J., Raisin, S., Pantalacci, S., Radimerski, T., Montagne, J., & Leopold, P. (2003). A nutrient sensor mechanism controls *Drosophila* growth. *Cell*, 114, 739–749.

Cook, R. M. (1973). Physiological factors in the courtship processing of *Drosophila melanogaster*. *Journal of Insect Physiology*, 19, 397–406.

Darrouzet, E., Mauchamp, B., Prestwich, G. D., Kerhoas, L., Ujvary, I., and Couillaud, F. (1997). Hydroxy juvenile hormones: new putative juvenile hormones biosynthesized by locust corpora allata *in vitro*. *Biochemical and Biophysical Research Communication*, 240, 752–758.

Davey, K. G. (2000). Do thyroid hormones function in insects? *Insect Biochemistry and Molecular Biology*, 30, 877–884.

Debernard, S., Rossignol, F., & Couillaud, F. (1994). The HMG-CoA reductase inhibitor fluvastatin inhibits insect juvenile hormone biosynthesis. *General and Comparative Endocrinology*, 95, 92–98.

De Luca, M., Roshina, N. V., Geiger-Thornsberry, G. L., Lyman, R. F., Pasyukova, E. G., & Mackay, T. F. C. (2003). *Dopa decarboxylase* (*Ddc*) affects variation in *Drosophila* longevity. *Nature Genetics*, 34, 429–433.

DeSalle, R., & Templeton, A. R. (1986). The molecular through ecological genetics of *abnormal abdomen*. III. Tissue-specific differential replication of ribosomal genes modulates the abnormal abdomen phenotype in *Drosophila mercatorum*. *Genetics*, 112, 877–886.

Dhadialla, T. S., & Raikhel, A. S. (1994). Endocrinology of mosquito vitellogenesis. In K. G. Davey, R. E. Pratt, & S. S. Tobe (Eds.), *Perspectives in comparative endocrinology* (pp. 275–281). Ottawa: National Research Council of Canada.

Dingle, H., & Winchell, R. (1997). Juvenile hormones as a mediator of plasticity in insect life histories. *Archives of Insect Biochemistry and Physiology*, 35, 359–373.

Dorman, J. B., Albinder, B., Shroyer, T., & Kenyon, C. (1995). The *age-1* and *daf-2* genes function in a common pathway to control the lifespan of *Caenorhabditis elegans*. *Genetics*, 141, 1399–1406.

Drummond-Barbosa, D., & Spradling, A. C. (2001). Stem cells and their progeny respond to nutritional changes during *Drosophila* oogenesis. *Developmental Biology*, 231, 265–278.

Dubrovsky, E. B. (2005). Hormonal cross talk in insect development. *Trends in Endocrinology and Metabolism*, 16, 6–11.

Dubrovsky, E. B., Dubrovskaya, V. A., & Berger, E. M. (2002). Juvenile hormone signaling during oogenesis in *Drosophila melanogaster*. *Insect Biochemistry and Molecular Biology*, 32, 1555–1565.

Engelmann, F. (2002). Ecdysteroids, juvenile hormone and vitellogenesis in the cockroach *Leucophaea maderae*. *Journal of Insect Science*, 2(20), 1–8.

Finch, C. E., & Rose, M. R. (1995). Hormones and the physiological architecture of life history evolution. *Quarterly Review of Biology*, 70, 1–52.

Flatt, T. (2004). Assessing natural variation in genes affecting *Drosophila* lifespan. *Mechanisms of Ageing and Development*, 125, 155–159.

Flatt, T., & Kawecki, T.J. (2004). Pleiotropic effects of *Methoprene-tolerant* (*Met*), a gene involved in juvenile hormone metabolism, on life history traits in *Drosophila melanogaster*. *Genetica*, 122, 141–160.

Flurkey, K., Papaconstantinou, J., Miller, R. A., & Harrison, D. E. (2001). Life span extension and delayed immune and collagen aging in mutant mice with defects in growth hormone. *Proceedings of the National Academy of Sciences of the USA*, 98, 6736–6741.

Gäde, G., Hoffmann, K.-H., & Spring, J. H. (1997). Hormonal regulation in insects: facts, gaps, and future directions. *Physiological Reviews*, 77, 963–1032.

Gavin, J. A., & Williamson, J. H. (1976). Juvenile hormone-induced vitellogenesis in *apterous*[4], a non-vitellogenic mutant in *Drosophila melanogaster*. *Journal of Insect Physiology*, 22, 1737–1742.

Geiger-Thornsberry, G. L., & Mackay, T. F. C. (2004). Quantitative trait loci affecting natural variation in *Drosophila* longevity. *Mechanisms of Ageing and Development*, 125, 179–189.

Gilbert, L. I., Granger, N. A., & Roe, R. M. (2000). The juvenile hormones: historical facts and speculations on future research directions. *Insect Biochemistry and Molecular Biology*, 30, 617–644.

Gilbert, L. I., Rybczynski, R., & Warren, J. T. (2002). Control and biochemical nature of the ecdysteroidogenic pathway. *Annual Review of Entomology*, 47, 883–916.

Gill, M. S., Held, J. M., Fisher, A. L., Gibson, B. W., & Lithgow, G. J. (2004). Lipophilic regulator of a developmental switch in *Caenorhabditis elegans*. *Aging Cell*, 3, 413–421.

Ginaldi, L., & Sternberg, H. (2003). The immune system. In P. Timiras (Ed.), *Physiological basis of aging and geriatrics* (pp. 265–283). New York: CRC Press.

Good, T. P., & Tatar, M. (2001). Age-specific mortality and reproduction to adult dietary restriction in *Drosophila melanogaster*. *Journal of Insect Physiology*, 47, 1467–1473.

Graf, R., Neuenschwander, S., Brown, M. R., & Ackermann, U. (1997). Insulin-mediated secretion of ecdysteroids from mosquito ovaries and molecular cloning of the insulin receptor homologue from ovaries of bloodfed *Aedes aegypti*. *Insect Molecular Biology*, 6,151–163.

Grutenko, N. E., Monastirioti, M., & Rauschenbach, I. Y. (2001). Juvenile hormone metabolism in *Drosophila melanogaster* imago is controlled by biogenic amines. *Doklady Biological Sciences*, 376, 72–74.

Gu, S.-H., & Chow, Y.-S. (2003). Stimulation of juvenile hormone biosynthesis by different ecdysteroids in *Bombyx mori*. *Zoological Studies*, 42, 450–454.

Hafen, E. (2004). Cancer, type 2 diabetes, and ageing: news from flies and worms. *Swiss Medical Weekly*, 134, 711–719.

Hagedorn, H. H. (1985). The role of ecdysteroids in reproduction. In G. A. Kerkut & L. I. Gilbert (Eds.), *Comparative insect physiology, biochemistry, and pharmacology* (Vol. 8, pp. 205–262). New York: Pergamon Press.

Hall, B. L., & Thummel, C. S. (1998). The RXR homolog ultraspiracle is an essential component of the *Drosophila* ecdysone receptor. *Development*, 125, 4709–4717.

Hammock, B. D., Bonning, B. C., Possee, R. D., Hanzlik, T. N., and Maeda, S. (1990). Expression and effects of the juvenile hormone esterase in a baculovirus vector. *Nature*, 334, 458–460.

Harshman, L. G. (1999). Investigation of the endocrine system in extended longevity lines of *Drosophila melanogaster*. *Experimental Gerontology*, 34, 997–1006.

Hartfelder, K. (2000). Insect juvenile hormone: from "status quo" to high society. *Brazilian Journal of Medical and Biological Research*, 33, 157–177.

Hayflick, L. (1994). *How and why we age.* New York: Ballantine Books.

Henrich, V. C., & Brown, N. E. (1995). Insect nuclear receptors: a developmental and comparative perspective. *Insect Biochemistry and Molecular Biology*, 25, 881–897.

Herman, W. S., & Tatar, M. (2001). Juvenile hormone regulation of aging in the migratory monarch butterfly. *Proceedings of the Royal Society of London B*, 268, 2509–2514.

Hiruma, K., Shimada, H., & Yagi, S. (1978). Activation of the prothoracic gland by juvenile hormone and prothoracicotropic hormone in *Mamestra brassicae*. *Journal of Insect Physiology*, 24, 215–220.

Hodin, J., & Riddiford, L. M. (1998). The ecdysone receptor and ultraspiracle regulate the timing and progression of ovarian morphogenesis during *Drosophila* metamorphosis. *Development Genes Evolution*, 208, 304–317.

Hoffmann, J. A. (2003). The immune response of *Drosophila*. *Nature*, 426, 33–38.

Hollocher, H., & Templeton, A. R. (1994). The molecular through ecological genetics of *abnormal abdomen* in *Drosophila*

mercatorum. VI. The non-neutrality of the Y chromosome rDNA polymorphism. *Genetics*, 136, 1373–1384.

Hwangbo, D. S., Gershman, B., Tu, M.-P., Palmer, M., & Tatar, M. (2004). Regulation of aging and neuronal insulin by dFOXO in fat body of adult *Drosophila*. *Nature*, 429, 562–566.

Ikeya, T., Galic, M., Belawat, P., Nairz, K., & Hafen, E. (2002). Nutrient-dependent expression of insulin-like peptides from neuroendocrine cells in the CNS contributes to growth regulation in *Drosophila*. *Current Biology*, 12, 1293–1300.

Jazwinski, S. M. (1996). Longevity, genes, and aging. *Science*, 273, 54–59.

Johnson, T., Lithgow, G., & Murakami, S. (1996). Hypothesis: interventions that increase the response to stress offer the potential for effective life prolongation and increased health. *Journal of Gerontology A: Biological Sciences and Medical Sciences*, 51B, 392–395.

Jones, G., & Sharp, P. A. (1997). Ultraspiracle: an invertebrate nuclear receptor for juvenile hormones. *Proceedings of the National Academy of Sciences of the USA*, 94, 13499–13503.

Kambysellis, M. P., & Heed, W. B. (1974). Juvenile hormone induces ovarian development in diapausing cave-dwelling *Drosophila* species. *Journal of Insect Physiology*, 20, 1779–1786.

Kapahi, P., Zid, M. B., Harper, T., Koslover, D., Sapin, V., & Benzer, S. (2004). Regulation of lifespan in *Drosophila* by modulation of genes in the TOR signaling pathway. *Current Biology*, 14, 885–890.

Kenyon, C.A. (2001). A conserved regulatory mechanism for aging. *Cell*, 105, 165–168.

Kenyon, C., Chang, J., Gensch, E., Rudner, A., & Tabtiang, R. (1993). A *C. elegans* mutant that lives twice as long as wild type. *Nature* 366:461–464.

Ketterson, E. D., & Nolan, V. (1992). Hormones and life histories: an integrative approach. *American Naturalist*, 140 (Supp), S33–S62.

Kim, S., Benguria, A., Lai, C.-Y., & Jazwinski, S. M. (1999). Modulation of life-span by histone deacetylase genes in *Saccharomyces cerevisiae*. *Molecular Biology of the Cell* 10, 3125–3136.

Kozlova, T., & Thummel, C. S. (2000). Steroid regulation of postembryonic development and reproduction in *Drosophila. Trends in Endocrinology and Metabolism*, 11, 276–280.

Lafon-Cazal, M., & Baehr, J. C. (1988). Octopaminergic control of corpora allata activity in an insect. *Experientia* 44, 895–896.

Leroi, A. M. (2001). Molecular signals versus the Loi de Balancement. *Trends in Ecology and Evolution*, 16, 24–29.

Liu, M.-A., Jones, G. L., Stoffolano, J. G., Jr., & Yin, C.-M. (1988). Conditions for estimation of corpus allatum activity in the blowfly, *Phormia regina*, in vitro. *Physiological Entomology*, 13, 69–79.

Lithgow, G. J. (1996). Invertebrate gerontology: the age mutations of *Caenorhabditis elegans. BioEssays*, 18, 809–815.

Manning, A. (1966). Corpus allatum and sexual receptivity in female *Drosophila melanogaster. Nature*, 211, 1321–1322.

Manning, A. (1967). The control of sexual receptivity in female *Drosophila. Animal Behaviour* 15: 239–250.

Marden, J. H., Rogina, B., Montooth, K. L., & Helfand, S. L. (2003). Conditional tradeoffs between aging and organismal performance of *Indy* long-lived mutant flies. *Proceedings of the National Academy of Sciences of the USA*, 100, 3369–3373.

Masoro, E.J. (2000). Caloric restriction and aging: an update. *Experimental Gerontology*, 35, 299–305.

Minkoff, C., & Wilson, T. G. (1992). The competitive ability and fitness components of the methoprene-tolerant (Met) *Drosophila* mutant resistant to juvenile hormone analog insecticides. *Genetics*, 131, 91–97.

Moshitzky, P., Fleischmann, I., Chaimov, N., Saudan, P., Klauser, S., Kubli, E., & Applebaum, S. W. (1996). Sex-peptide activates juvenile hormone biosynthesis in the *Drosophila melanogaster* corpus allatum. *Archives of Insect Biochemistry and Physiology*, 32, 363–374.

Nagasawa, H. (1992). Neuropeptides of the silkworm, *Bombyx mori. Experientia*, 48, 425–430.

Nijhout, H. F. (1994). *Insect Hormones.* Princeton, NJ: Princeton University Press.

Nijhout, H. F. (2003). The control of growth. *Development*, 130, 5863–5867.

Oldham, S., & Hafen, E. (2003). Insulin/IGF and target of rapamycin signaling: a TOR de force in growth control. *Trends in Cell Biology*, 13, 79–85.

Oldham, S., Montagne, J., Radimerski, T., Thomas, G., & Hafen, E. (2000). Genetic and biochemical characterization of *dTOR*, the *Drosophila* homolog of the target of rapamycin. *Genes and Development*, 14, 2689–2694.

Partridge, L., & Gems, D. (2002). Mechanisms of ageing: public or private? *Nature Reviews Genetics*, 3, 165–175.

Pener, M. P. (1972). The corpus allatum in adult acridids: the inter-relation of its functions and possible correlations with the life cycle. In C. F. Hemming & T. H. C. Taylor (Eds.), *Proceedings of the International Study Conference on the Current and Future Problems of Acridology* (pp. 135–147). London: Centre for Overseas Pest Research.

Petryk, A., Warren, J. T., Marques, G., Jarcho, M. P., Gilbert, L. I., Kahler, J., Parvy, J.-P., Li, Y., Dauphin-Villemant, C., & O'Connor, M. B. (2003). Shade is the *Drosophila* P450 enzyme that mediates the hydroxylation of ecdysone to the steroid insect molting hormone 20-hydroxyecdysone. *Proceedings of the National Academy of Sciences of the USA*, 100, 13773–13778.

Postlethwait, J.H., & Weiser, K. (1973). Vitellogenesis induced by juvenile hormone in the female sterile mutant *apterous*[4] in *Drosophila melanogaster. Nature*, 244, 284–285.

Pursley, S., Ashok, M., & Wilson, T. G. (2000). Intracellular localization and tissue specificity of the Methoprene-tolerant (Met) gene product in *Drosophila melanogaster. Insect Biochemistry and Molecular Biology*, 30, 893–845.

Rachinsky, A. (1994). Octopamine and serotonin influence on corpora allata activity in honey bee (*Apis mellifera*) larvae. *Journal of Insect Physiology*, 40, 549–554.

Rantala, M. J., Vainikka, A., & Kortet, R. (2003). The role of juvenile hormone in immune function and pheromone production trade-offs: a test of the immunocompetence handicap principle. *Proceedings of the Royal Society London B,* 270, 2257–2261.

Rauschenbach, I. Y., Adon'eva, N. V., Grutenko, N. E., Karpova, E. K., Chentsova, N. A., & Faddeeva, N. V. (2002). The synthesis and degradation of juvenile hormone in *Drosophila* are under common control. *Doklady Biological Sciences,* 386, 448–450.

Restifo, L. L., & Wilson, T. G. (1998). A juvenile hormone agonist reveals distinct developmental pathways mediated by ecdysone-inducible broad complex transcription factors. *Developmental Genetics,* 22, 141–159.

Richard, D. S., Applebaum, S. W., Sliter, T. J., Baker, F. C., Schooley, D. A., Reuter, C. C., Henrich, V. C., & Gilbert, L. I. (1989). Juvenile hormone bisepoxide biosynthesis in vitro by the ring gland of *Drosophila melanogaster*: a putative juvenile hormone in the higher Diptera. *Proceedings of the National Academy of Sciences of the USA,* 86, 1421–1425.

Richard, D. S., Jones, J. M., Barbarito, M. R., Cerula, S., Detweiler, J. P., Fisher, S. J., Brannigan, D. M., & Scheswohl, D. M. (2001). Vitellogenesis in diapausing and mutant *Drosophila melanogaster*: further evidence for the relative roles of ecdysteroids and juvenile hormones. *Journal of Insect Physiology,* 47, 905–913.

Richard, D. S., Watkins, N. L., Serafin, R. B., & Gilbert, L. I. (1998). Ecdysteroids regulate yolk protein uptake by *Drosophila melanogaster* oocytes. *Journal of Insect Physiology,* 44, 637–644.

Riddiford, L. M. (1985). Hormone action at the cellular level. In G. Kerkut & L. I. Gilbert (Eds.), *Comprehensive insect biochemistry, physiology, and pharmacology* (Vol. 8, pp. 37–84). New York: Pergamon Press.

Riddiford, L. M. (1993). Hormones and *Drosophila* development. In M. Bate & A. Martinez Arias (Eds.), *The development of Drosophila melanogaster* (pp. 899–939). Cold Spring Harbor, NY: Cold Spring Harbor Laboratory Press.

Riddiford, L. M. (1994). Cellular and molecular actions of juvenile hormone. I. General considerations and premetamorphic actions. In P. D. Evans (Ed.), *Advances in insect physiology* (pp. 213–274). San Diego: Academic Press.

Riddiford, L. M. (1996). Juvenile hormone: the status of its "status quo" action. *Archives of Insect Biochemistry and Physiology,* 32, 271–286.

Riddiford, L. M., & Ashburner, M. (1991). Effects of juvenile mimics on larval development and metamorphosis of *Drosophila melanogaster. General and Comparative Endocrinology,* 82, 172–183.

Riehle, M. A., & Brown, M. R. (1999). Insulin stimulates ecdysteroid production through a conserved signaling cascade in the mosquito *Aedes aegypti. Insect Biochemistry and Molecular Biology,* 29, 855–860.

Ringo, J., Werczberger, R., Altaratz, M., & Segal, D. (1991). Female sexual receptivity is defective in juvenile-hormone deficient mutants of the *apterous* gene of *Drosophila melanogaster. Behavioral Genetics,* 21, 453–469.

Roeder, T. (1999). Octopamine in invertebrates. *Progress in Neurobiology,* 59, 533–561.

Rogina, B., Helfand, S. L., & Frankel, S. (2003). Longevity regulation by *Drosophila* rpd3 deacetylase and caloric restriction. *Science,* 298, 1745.

Rohde, J. R., & Cardenas, M. E. (2003). The *Tor* pathway regulates gene expression by linking nutrient sensing to histone acetylation. *Molecular and Cellular Biology,* 23, 629–635

Rolff, J., & Siva-Jothy, M. T. (2002). Copulation corrupts immunity: a mechanism for a cost of mating in insects. *Proceedings of the National Academy of Sciences USA,* 99, 9916–9918.

Roth, G. E., Gierl, M. S., Vollborn, L., Meise, M., Lintermann, R., & Korge, G. (2004). The *Drosophila* gene Start1: a putative cholesterol transporter and key regulator of ecdysteroid synthesis. *Proceedings of the National Academy of Sciences of the USA,* 101, 1601–1606.

Rulifson, E. J., Kim, S. K., & Nusse, R. (2002). Ablation of insulin-producing neurons in flies: growth and diabetic phenotypes. *Science,* 296, 1118–1120.

Salmon, A. B., Marx, D. B., & Harshman, L. G. (2001). A cost of reproduction in *Drosophila melanogaster*: stress susceptibility. *Evolution,* 55, 1600–1608.

Saunders, D. S., Henrich, V. C., & Gilbert, L. I. (1989). Induction of diapause in *Drosophila melanogaster*: photoperiodic regulation and the impact of arrhythmic clock mutations on time measurement. *Proceedings of the National Academy of Sciences of the USA*, 86, 3748–3752.

Schwartz, M. B., Kelly, T. J., Imberski, R. B., & Rubenstein, E. C. (1985). The effects of nutrition and methoprene treatment on ovarian ecdysteroid synthesis in *Drosophila melanogaster*. *Journal of Insect Physiology*, 31, 947–957.

Schwartz, M. B., Kelly, T. J., Woods, C. W., & Imberski, R. B. (1989). Ecdysteroid fluctuations in adult *Drosophila melanogaster* caused by elimination of pupal reserves and synthesis by early vitellogenic ovarian follicles. *Insect Biochemistry*, 19, 243–249.

Shemshedini, L., & Wilson, T. G. (1990). Resistance to juvenile hormone and an insect growth regulator in *Drosophila* is associated with an altered cytosolic juvenile hormone binding protein. *Proceedings of the National Academy of Sciences of the USA*, 87, 2072–2076.

Shemshedini, L., & Wilson, T. G. (1993). Juvenile hormone binding proteins in larval fat body nuclei of *Drosophila melanogaster*. *Journal of Insect Physiology*, 39, 563–569.

Shemshedini, L., Lanoue, M., & Wilson, T.G. (1990). Evidence for a juvenile hormone receptor involved in protein synthesis in *Drosophila melanogaster*. *Journal of Biological Chemistry*, 265, 1913–1918.

Shirras, A. D., & Bownes, M. (1989). *cricklet*: a locus regulating a number of adult functions of *Drosophila melanogaster*. *Proceedings of the National Academy of Sciences of the USA*, 86, 4559–4563.

Siegmund, T., & Korge, G. (2001). Innervation of the ring gland of *Drosophila melanogaster*. *Journal of Comparative Neurology*, 431, 481–491.

Simon, A. F., Shih, A., Mack, A., & Benzer, S. (2003). Steroid control of longevity in *Drosophila melanogaster*. *Science*, 299, 1407–1410.

Soller, M., Bownes, M., & Kubli, E. (1999). Control of oocyte maturation in sexually mature *Drosophila* females. *Developmental Biology*, 208, 337–351.

Stay, B., Friedel, T., Tobe, S. S., & Mundall, E. C. (1980). Feedback control of juvenile hormone synthesis in cockroaches: possible role for ecdysterone. *Science*, 207, 898–900.

Stearns, S. C., & Partridge, L. (2001). The genetics of aging in *Drosophila*. In E. Masoro & S. Austad (Eds.), *Handbook of the biology of aging* (pp. 353–368). San Diego: Academic Press.

Sze, J. Y., Victor, M., Loer, C., Shi, Y., & Ruvkun, G. (2000). Food and metabolic signaling defects in a *Caenorhabditis elegans* serotonin-synthesis mutant. *Nature*, 403, 560–564.

Tatar, M. (2004). The neuroendocrine regulation of *Drosophila* aging. *Experimental Gerontology*, 39, 1745–1750.

Tatar, M., & Yin, C.-M. (2001). Slow aging during insect reproductive diapause: why butterflies, grasshoppers and flies are like worms. *Experimental Gerontology*, 36, 723–738.

Tatar, M., Bartke, A., & Antebi, A. (2003). The endocrine regulation of aging by insulin-like signals. *Science*, 299, 1346–1351.

Tatar, M., Chien, S. A., & Priest, N. K. (2001a). Negligible senescence during reproductive diapause in *Drosophila melanogaster*. *American Naturalist*, 158, 248–258.

Tatar, M., Khazaeli, A. A., Curtsinger, J. W. (1997). Chaperoning extended life. Nature, 390, 30.

Tatar, M., Kopelman, A., Epstein, D., Tu,M.-P., Yin, C.-M., & Garofalo, R. S. (2001b). A mutant *Drosophila* insulin receptor homolog that extends life-span and impairs neuroendocrine function. *Science*, 292, 107–110.

Teal, P. E. A., & Gomez-Simuta, Y. (2002). Juvenile hormone: action in regulation of sexual maturity in Caribbean fruit flies and potential use in improving efficacy of sterile insect control technique for tephritid fruit flies. *IOBC wprs Bulletin*, 25, 1–15.

Teal, P. E. A., Gomze-Simuta, Y., & Proveaux, A. T. (2000). Mating experience and juvenile hormone enhance sexual signaling and mating in male Caribbean fruit flies. *Proceedings of the National Academy of Sciences of the USA*, 97, 3708–3712.

Templeton, A. R. (1982). The prophecies of parthenogenesis. In H. Dingle & J. P. Hegmann (Eds.), *Evolution and genetics of life histories* (pp. 75–101). Berlin: Springer.

Templeton, A. R. (1983). Natural and experimental parthenogenesis. In M. Ashburner, H. L. Carson, & J. R. Thompson (Eds.), *The genetics and biology of Drosophila* (pp. 343–398). London: Academic Press.

Templeton, A. R., & Rankin, M. A. (1978). Genetic revolutions and the control of insect populations. In R. H. Richardson (Ed.), *The screw-worm problem* (pp. 83–112). Austin: University of Texas Press.

Templeton, A. R., Hollocher, H., & Johnston, J. S. (1993). The molecular through ecological genetics of *abnormal abdomen* in *Drosophila mercatorum*. V. Female phenotypic expression on natural genetic backgrounds and in natural environments. *Genetics*, 134, 475–485.

Thomas, R. B. (1991). *Ecological aspects of longevity, fertility and desiccation and the role of juvenile hormone in the abnormal abdomen syndrome in Drosophila mercatorum (Diptera: Drosophilidae).* Unpublished doctoral dissertation, Texas A& M University, Texas.

Tissenbaum, H. A., & Guarente, L. (2001). Increased dosage of a sir-2 gene extends lifespan in *Caenorhabditis elegans*. *Nature*, 410, 227–230.

Tobe, S. S., & Bendena, W. G. (1999). The regulation of juvenile hormone production in arthropods: functional and evolutionary perspectives. *Annals of the New York Academy of Sciences*, 897, 300–310.

Tobe, S. S., & Stay, B. (1985). Structure and regulation of the corpus allatum. *Advances in Insect Physiology*, 18, 305–432.

Truman, J. W., & Riddiford, L. M. (2002). Endocrine insights into the evolution of metamorphosis in insects. *Annual Review of Entomology*, 47, 467–500.

Trumbo, S. T., & Robinson, G. E. (2004). Nutrition, hormones and life history in burying beetles. *Journal of Insect Physiology*, 50, 383–391.

Tsai, C.-C., Kao, H.-Y., Yao, T.-P., McKeown, M., & Evans, R.M. (1999). SMRTER, a *Drosophila* nuclear receptor coregulator, reveals that EcR-mediated repression is critical for development. *Molecular Cell*, 4,175–186.

Tu, M.-P., & Tatar, M. (2003). Juvenile diet restriction and the aging and reproduction of adult *Drosophila melanogaster*. *Aging Cell*, 2, 327–333.

Tu, M.-P., Epstein, D., & Tatar, M. (2002a). The demography of slow aging in male and female *Drosophila* mutant for the insulin-receptor substrate homologue *chico*. *Aging Cell*, 1, 75–80.

Tu, M.-P., Yin, C.-M., & Tatar, M. (2002b). Impaired ovarian ecdysone synthesis of *Drosophila melanogaster* insulin receptor mutants. *Aging Cell*, 1, 158–160.

Tu, M.-P., Yin, C.-M., & Tatar, M (2005). Mutations in insulin signaling pathway alter juvenile hormone synthesis in *Drosophila melanogaster*. *General and Comparative Endocrinology*, 142, 347–356.

Tzou, P., De Gregorio, E., & Lemaitre, B. (2002). How *Drosophila* combats microbial infection: a model to study innate immunity and host-pathogen interactions. *Current Opinion in Microbiology*, 5, 102–110.

Vergara, M., Smith-Wheelock, M., Harper, J. M., Sigler, R., & Miller, R. A. (2004). Hormone-treated Snell dwarf mice regain fertility but remain long lived and disease resistant. *Journal of Gerontological Sciences: Biological Sciences*, 59A, 1244–1250.

Warren, J. T., Petryk, A., Marques, G., Jarcho, M., Parvy, J.-P., Dauphin-Villemant, C., O'Connor, M. B., & Gilbert, L. I. (2002). Molecular and biochemical characterization of two P450 enzymes in the ecdysteroidogenic pathway of *Drosophila melanogaster*. *Proceedings of the National Academy of Sciences of the USA*, 99, 11043–11048.

Wessells, R. J., Fitzgerald, E., Cypser, J.R., Tatar, M., & Bodmer, R. (2004). Insulin regulation of heart function in aging fruit flies. *Nature Genetics*, 36, 1275–1281.

Wheeler, D. (1996). The role of nourishment in oogenesis. *Annual Review of Entomology*, 41, 407–431.

Wheeler, D. E., & Nijhout, H. F. (2003). A perspective for understanding the modes of juvenile hormone action as a lipid signaling system. *BioEssays*, 25, 994–1001.

Williams, G. C. (1957). Pleiotropy, natural selection, and the evolution of senescence. *Evolution*, 11, 398–411.

Wilson, T. G. (2004). The molecular site of action of juvenile hormone and juvenile hormone insecticides during metamorphosis: how these compounds kill insects. *Journal of Insect Physiology*, 50, 111–121.

Wilson, T. G., & Ashok, M. (1998). Insecticide resistance resulting from an absence of target-site gene product. *Proceedings of the National Academy of Sciences of the USA*, 95, 14040–14044.

Wilson, T. G., DeMoor, S., & Lei, J. (2003). Juvenile hormone involvement in *Drosophila melanogaster* male reproduction as suggested by the *Methoprene-tolerant 27* phenotype. *Insect Biochemistry and Molecular Biology*, 33, 1167–1175.

Wilson, T. G., Landers, M. H., & Happ, G. M. (1983). Precocene I and II inhibition of vitellogenic oocyte development in *Drosophila melanogaster*. *Journal of Insect Physiology*, 29, 249–254.

Wood, J. G., Rogina, B., Lavu, S., Howitz, K., Helfand, S. L., Tatar, M., & Sinclair, D. (2004). Sirtuin activators mimic caloric restriction and delay ageing in metazoans. *Nature*, 430, 686–689.

Wyatt, G. R., & Davey, K. G. (1996). Cellular and molecular actions of juvenile hormone. II. Roles of juvenile hormone in adult insects. In P. D. Evans (Ed.), *Advances in insect physiology* (pp. 1–155). San Diego: Academic Press.

Yin, C.-M., & Stoffolano, J. G. Jr. (1990). The interactions among nutrition, endocrines and physiology on the reproductive development of the black blowfly, *Phormia regina* Meigen. In Y. S. Chow (Ed.), *Molecular entomology symposium* (pp. 87–108). Taipei, Taiwan: Institute of Zoology, Academia Sinica.

Yin, C.-M., Zou, B.-X., Jiang, M., Li, M.-F., Qin, W., Potter, T. L., & Stoffolano, J. G. Jr. (1995). Identification of juvenile hormone III bisepoxide (JHB3), juvenile hormone III and methyl farnesoate secreted by the corpus allatum of *Phormia regina* (Meigen), in vitro and function of JHB3 either applied alone or as a part of a juvenoid blend. *Journal of Insect Physiology*, 41, 473–479.

Yin, C.-M., Zou, B.-X., Yi, S.-X., & Stoffolano, J. G. Jr. (1990). Ecdysteroid activity during oogenesis in the black blow fly, *Phormia regina* (Meigen). *Journal of Insect Physiology*, 36, 375–382.

Yokoyama, K., Fukumoto, K., Murakami, T., Harada, S.-I., Hosono, R., Wadhwa, R., Mitsui, Y., & Ohkuma, S. (2002). Extended longevity of *Caenorhabditis elegans* by knocking in extra copies of hsp70F, a homolog of mot-2 (mortalin)/mthsp70/Grp75. *FEBS Letters*, 516, 53–57.

Zera, A. J. (2004). The endocrine regulation of wing polymorphism in insects: state of the art, recent surprises, and future directions. *Integrative and Comparative Biology*, 43, 607–616.

Zera, A. J., & Harshman, L. G. (2001). The physiology of life history trade-offs in animals. *Annual Review of Ecology and Systematics*, 32, 95–126.

Zhou, X., & Riddiford, L. M. (2002). *Broad* specifies pupal development and mediates the 'status quo' action of juvenile hormone on the pupal-adult transformation in *Drosophila* and *Manduca*. *Development*, 129, 2259–2269.

Zou, B.-X., Yin, C.-M., Stoffolano J. G. Jr., & Tobe, S. S. (1989). Juvenile hormone biosynthesis and release during oocyte development in *Phormia regina* Meigen. *Physiological Entomology*, 14, 233–239.

Chapter 16

A Critical Evaluation of Nonmammalian Models for Aging Research

Steven N. Austad and Andrej Podlutsky

I. Introduction

The widespread implementation of model invertebrate species for aging research has greatly accelerated progress in identifying genes and biochemical processes that can modify longevity and perhaps aging rate (see Chapters 3, 7, and 13–15, this volume). The great unanswered question, however, is the extent to which underlying mechanisms of aging will overlap among invertebrate models, in which the majority of progress has been made, and the species of ultimate interest to most researchers: humans. Put another way, to what extent will aging mechanisms turn out to be public—that is, shared across the vast sweep of species versus private, or idiosyncratic among species (to use George Martin's felicitous terminology)? To the extent that aging mechanisms, or their regulation, is private, invertebrate or even short-lived mammalian models will not be greatly informative about human aging, so everyone hopes that such mechanisms will be largely public.

The widespread senescence-retarding effect of caloric restriction across animal taxa (Weindruch & Walford, 1988) has been adduced as evidence that at least some aging mechanisms will be general. In addition, at least one biochemical pathway of longevity modulation—the sir2 pathway—appears conserved among yeast, flies, worms, and perhaps mammals (Cohen *et al.*, 2004; Picard *et al.*, 2004; Rogina & Helfand, 2004; Tissenbaum & Guarente, 2001), and another—the insulin-IGF pathway—seems to be conserved among nematodes, flies, and mice (Tatar *et al.*, 2003), although its impact is substantially smaller in mice than in invertebrates. Whether that pathway is also involved in human longevity is still unclear (see Chapter 19, this volume). On the other hand, the ubiquity of the caloric restriction effect may have been overstated. Careful studies in medflies (Carey *et al.*, 2002), some species of rotifers (Kirk, 2001), and some populations of fish (Reznick *et al.*, 2004), as well as some mouse genotypes (Forster *et al.*, 2003)

Handbook of the Biology of Aging, Sixth Edition

fail to find life extension with caloric restriction.

Given that the generality of aging mechanisms is still largely unknown, many biomedical researchers who use mice, rats, humans, or other primates in their research express private doubt that studies of insects or nematodes—with their distant evolutionary relationship to humans and their peculiarities of growth, development, and physiology *vis à vis* mammals—will contribute significantly to understanding aging and/or the development of late-life diseases in humans. Regardless of whether these doubts turn out to be justified, the arguments underlying them deserve to be brought out into the open and discussed rather than whispered about. The purpose of this chapter is to do just that. It is not the purpose of this chapter to question whether research efforts on the current invertebrate models are worthwhile. They unquestionably are worthwhile and will continue to contribute to our understanding of many biological processes in the future as they have in the past. A fair question though is, what, if any, are the limitations on what we may be able to learn from them (Gershon & Gershon, 2002)?

The primary nonmammalian organisms used as models for aging research are a single-cell fungus, the budding yeast (*Saccharomyces cerevisiae*), a free-living soil nematode (*Caenorhabditis elegans*, hereafter called "the worm"), and a dipteran insect (*Drosophila melanogaster*, hereafter called "the fly"). Sporadic aging research has been performed with other nonvertebrates, but no others have multiple major laboratories devoted to their study with respect to aging and longevity. It is worth noting that even within their own taxa, the model species above are exceptionally short-lived. Some nematodes, for instance, can live more than a decade compared to the several weeks of *C. elegans* (Gems, 2000). Some insects can also live more than a decade, and of course numerous mammal species live numerous decades compared with the 2 to 3 years of the laboratory mouse (Finch, 1990). If there are fundamental differences in the modulation of aging among short- and long-lived species, we will be likely to overlook them given the range of animal species most typically studied.

Aging is not straightforward to define or identify in budding yeast, a single-cell eukaryotic organism with little in the way of observable behavior. As a consequence, two utterly different approaches have been taken. Most thoroughly investigated is yeast replicative life span. Because cell division is asymmetrical, each mitotic episode yields an easily identifiable mother and smaller daughter cell that eventually grows to the size of the mother. Mother cells produce a finite number of daughters before permanently ceasing to divide. The number of daughters produced in a mother's life, rather than the length of time a mother cell survives, defines replicative longevity. Replicative longevity, in other words, equals lifetime reproductive success or Darwinian fitness. As more and more daughter cells are produced, mother cells undergo a series of phenotypic changes, such as alterations in cell size and shape, the appearance of surface wrinkles, and a decrease in protein-synthesis rate, which might be interpreted as symptoms of senescence (Jazwinski, 1995). Replicative longevity is dependent on genotype, nutrient conditions, and perhaps temperature.

An alternative paradigm has been called "chronological aging" of yeast. In this case, cells are maintained in a nondividing state by placing them in exhausted or minimal glucose medium or distilled water. Aging is measured by periodically moving cell samples from the static population to growth medium and assessing their declining ability over time to renew cell division (Fabrizio & Longo, 2003).

The extent to which either of these experimental paradigms are relevant to one another or to the organismic longevity of multicellular animals is not clear. Some genetic mutations, such as those that reduce activity in the Ras/PKA (cAMP-dependent protein kinase) pathway, extend both types of life span. Also, ablation of SOD1 activity shortens both types of life spans. On the other hand, SIR2 activity, although directly related to replicative life span, has not been reported to affect chronological aging, and deletion of RAS2, which activates a stress-resistance pathway, shortens replicative, but lengthens chronological, life span (Fabrizio & Longo, 2003). The strongest evidence that replicative longevity in yeast is relevant to longevity in multicellular animals is that overexpression of *sir2*, which lengthens replicative life span in yeast, also increases chronological life span in worms (Tissenbaum & Guarente, 2001) and flies (Rogina & Helfand, 2004).

Because the relationship between aging in either yeast experimental paradigm and organismal aging is still unclear, and because the issue of this relationship is part of a larger, continuing debate concerning what can be learned about organismal aging from the study of senescence of individual cells (Hornsby, 2001), we will concentrate in this chapter on the less controversial relation between longevity and its modulation in multicellular invertebrates compared with that in endothermic vertebrates such as mice, rats, and humans. There is less controversy because the major phenotype of interest, how long individuals in a population survive, is identical between vertebrates and invertebrates.

II. Key Evolutionary Relationships

The spread of newly developed analytical techniques for reconstructing evolutionary divergence patterns from molecular sequence data, combined with the virtual avalanche of new DNA sequences from a multitude of organisms, has altered traditional views of large-scale phylogenetic relationships within multicellular animals (e.g., Aguinaldo *et al.*, 1997; Mallatt & Winchell, 2002; Murphy *et al.*, 2001). Traditional studies by necessity characterized evolutionary relationships among major multicellular animal (=metazoan) groups primarily by morphological traits, such as patterns of body symmetry and embryonic development, morphology of body cavities, and the presence or absence of segmented body regions (see Figure 16.1A) (Hickman *et al.*, 2000). However, recent molecular analyses employing extensive sequence data support a different configuration of relationships among the major animal groups. This new phylogeny is broadly (Copley *et al.*, 2004; Philippe *et al.*, 2005), but not universally (Philip *et al.*, 2005), accepted by evolutionary systematists. Of particular relevance for the topic of how molecular genetic discoveries from invertebrate model organisms might extend to mammals is that the new phylogeny identified an evolutionary branch (=clade), the Ecdysozoa or molting animals (see Figure 16,1B), which includes both insects such as flies and nematodes such as worms (Aguinaldo *et al.*, 1997; Anderson *et al.*, 2004; Mallatt & Winchell, 2002).

The significance of this altered phylogeny is that according to the traditional view, the experimentally tractable worm and fly species shared their last common ancestor with mammals. Therefore, a trait that evolved ancestral to the split between nematodes and insects (bar 1 in Figure 16.1A), for instance the impact of a particular gene on longevity modulation, necessarily existed in the ancestry of humans as well. Consequently, unless the trait has been lost secondarily (always a possibility in groups that

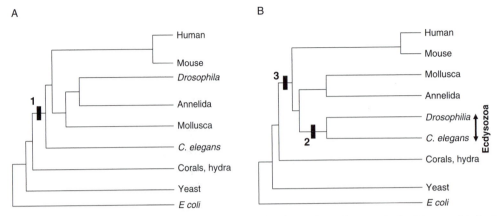

Figure 16.1 Recent changes in our view of evolutionary relationships changes the legitimacy of inferring conservation of traits from *C. elegans* and *Drosophila* to humans. (A) Traditional taxonomy largely based on morphology and embryonic development patterns (after Hickman *et al.*, 2000). (B) Revised taxonomy based on molecular data (after Aguinaldo *et al.*, 1997). 1 = Trait evolving here will be shared among humans, insects, and nematodes unless secondarily lost. 2 = Last common ancestor among insects and nematodes. 3 = Last common ancestor among humans, insects, and nematodes. Branch lengths not drawn to scale.

differ so dramatically in biological organization), the same genetic effect might be expected to exist in mammals today. Implicitly then, molecular mechanisms of aging conserved between worms and flies were likely to be conserved in humans as well.

The new phylogeny, if valid, changes all that. Because nematodes and insects are now considered members of the same phylogenetic branch or clade (see Figure 16.1B), the Ecdysozoa, a trait shared by both could plausibly have arisen after their divergence from the mammal lineage (bar 2, Figure 16.1B). Thus, finding that a similar gene or process modulates longevity in both worms and flies gives little indication of its degree of conservation outside the Ecdysozoa (Fitch & Thomas, 1997). By contrast, a trait, such as life extension by overexpression of *sir2*, shared by yeast (Sinclair *et al.*, 1998), nematodes (Tissenbaum & Guarente, 2001), and insects (Wood *et al.*, 2004) does indeed suggest an ancient ancestry, in which the common ancestor of all multicellular animals likely possessed the same trait.

Unless it was secondarily lost during later evolution, it would also be shared with mammals such as ourselves.

The general message, however, is that to the extent that the new phylogeny stands up to further investigation, demonstrating conservation of traits among nematodes and insects adds little information about conservation of the same traits among the rest of the metazoans.

III. Genomic Properties

Current estimates of the number of genes in the human genome (International Human Genome Sequencing Consortium, 2004) suggest that humans, despite having about 30-fold more nucleotides in their genome than worms, possess only marginally more actively transcribed genes (see Table 16.1). A naïve interpretation of these numbers might indicate that virtually all genes and gene function are likely to be highly conserved across metazoans. However, this is not true. The best guesses are that somewhere between about 36 percent

Table 16.1
Genomic Comparison Among Major Invertebrate Models of Aging

Organism	Estimated Genome Size ($\times 10^6$ bp)	Estimated Gene Number	Average Gene Length (Bases per Gene)	Diploid Chromosome Number
Human	2900	20–25,000	100,000	46
Drosophila melanogaster	180	13,600	9,000	8
C. elegans	97	19,100	5,000	12
Saccharomyces cerevisiae	12	6,300	2,000	16

Source: International Human Genome Sequencing Consortium, 2004; Functional and Comparative Genomics Fact Sheet [Human Genome Projection Information, 2004]

(Rubin *et al.*, 2000) and 60 percent (Harris *et al.*, 2004) of worm genes have identifiable similarities to human genes—depending on how stringently one defines "identifiable similarities." Using a single comparative criterion, Rubin and colleagues (2000) identified about 50 percent of fly genes and 36 percent of worm genes with human orthologs. This contrasts with approximately 99 percent human orthologs in mice (Mouse Genome Sequencing Consortium, 2002). Given the new phylogeny in which worms and flies are equally distant from humans, and the fact that flies have 30 percent fewer genes in their genome than *C. elegans* (see Table 16.1), it is somewhat surprising that they apparently have more human orthologs than worms. Even confining the discussion only to known human disease-related genes, flies still have more orthologs. Specifically, a recently compiled database of human disease gene orthologs finds 724 matches in flies and 533 in worms compared with 1,354 in mice (O'Brien *et al.*, 2004). Possible reasons for this difference will emerge in the remainder of this chapter.

If flies and worms share approximately one-half and one-third of their genes with humans, respectively, then other, nonshared genes will be a combination of newly arisen genes and lineage-specific

loss of ancestral genes. The exceptionally rapid rate of molecular evolution in worms and flies, some thousand-fold higher than in mammals (Denver *et al.*, 2004; Kumar & Subramanian, 2002) has seemingly led to exceptional gene loss as well as gene gain in the Ecdysozoan lineage (Raible & Arendt, 2004). Exacerbating this degree of evolutionary divergence from mammals, genetic innovation in vertebrates seems to have been substantial. For instance, our chordate relative, the tunicate *Ciona intestinalis*, has been reported to share as many as one-sixth of its genes only with other chordates, suggesting that a significant fraction of mammalian genes are likely to lack orthologs in any invertebrate species (Dehal *et al.*, 2002).

The situation is probably more complicated than this, though. It is becoming apparent that phyla such as the Cnidaria (hydra, corals, jellyfish, anemones) that are more distantly related to us than either flies or worms under either phylogenetic scenario (see Figure 16.1) contain a number of presumptive chordate-specific genes! Kortschak and colleagues (2003), for instance, examined 500 expressed sequence tag (EST) clusters from a coral species, *Acropora millepora*. Focusing only on genes that gave at least one strong match from any of the fully sequenced genomes of humans, flies, or worms, they found about 11 percent of the coral ESTs appeared to be shared only with humans, compared with about 1 percent that were shared exclusively with either worms or flies. The absence of clear fly or worm homologs of many genes represented in both human and coral genomes reflects more than a 10-fold higher rate of secondary gene loss in these model organisms relative to the vertebrate lineage. The insulin pathway, clearly involved in longevity modulation, appears particularly well conserved among animal lineages compared with other pathways. On the other hand, among the important human genes not represented in flies or worms are the estrogen receptor and its close relatives androgen, progestin, glucocorticoid, and mineralocorticoid receptors (Thornton et al, 2003), growth hormone and thyroid hormone pathway genes, and body mass regulators such as leptin (Rubin et al., 2000). Some of the genes known to alter longevity in worms do not have apparent mammalian homologs (Rikke et al., 2000), although the lack of precise orthologs need not necessarily mean that a function has been lost.

Furthermore, even among coral genes that appear to be represented in humans as well as flies or worms, about five times as many genes exhibited greater similarity to humans (at least a thousand-fold higher E-value by BLAST (Basic Local Alignment Search Tool) criteria) than to flies and worms compared with the reverse. The genes that were more similar between corals and humans than corals versus worms/flies were not confined to a few categories. They include a number of transcription factors, components of cellular signaling pathways such as DPP (Decapentaplegic) and Smads, and house-keeping proteins such as methyl CpG binding protein and WASp (Kortschak et al., 2003). In sum, these data suggest that divergence from the ancestral genome has been much more rapid in

worms and flies than in vertebrates. The data also suggest that model organisms from more ancient human ancestors than flies and worms are likely to be more informative than either for some as yet unidentified biological functions.

This seems to be a classic glass-half-empty, glass-half-full scenario. Many genes and gene pathways are clearly conserved among humans and model invertebrates, yet just as clearly, many are not. The key question is the functional consequences of these differences with respect to aging and longevity. Genes that exhibit a propensity to be lost during evolution are not a random sample of genes. Typically, genes that are lost at a high rate during evolution perform less critical functions in an organism. Also, those genes tend to evolve at a high rate. Genes with a low propensity for evolutionary loss interact with more proteins than genes with a high loss rate (Krylov et al., 2003). From the perspective of gene networks, how might deleting a number of network members affect regulation of the network as a whole, particularly since proteins associated with senescence seem to have greater connectivity with other proteins than one would expect by chance (Promislow, 2004)?

One way to begin conceptually organizing the significance of these differences might be to categorize them as follows: (1) differences in generalized genome organization, (2) absence or presence of specific genes, (3) importance of presence or absence of specific genes for species pathways or networks, and (4) homologous genes that have different roles in different species.

Differences in genome organization between vertebrates and worms/flies are substantial. That is, there are more differences among genomes than can be captured by differences in coding gene sequences. In terms of evolution, mutations fixed by evolution tend to be insertions in C. elegans compared with base pair substitutions in mammals. Also, due to much more noncoding sequence in mammals, gene length is approximately 20-fold lower in the *C. elegans* genome and 10-fold lower in *Drosophila* than in the human genome (see Table 16.1). As much as 97-plus percent of the transcriptional output of the human genome is noncoding RNA. Yet transcription is expensive and time-consuming. Approximately 20 nucleotides can be transcribed per second at a cost of at least two ATPs per nucleotide (Castillo-Davis *et al.*, 2002). The evolutionary implications of such an energetic burden, combined with the emerging realization that nontranslated RNA directs a variety of genetic and epigenetic phenomena in higher eukaryotes, suggests that differences in the amount of noncoding RNA in mammals and invertebrates may represent very different modes and methods of gene regulation (Mattick, 2003). Introns of highly expressed genes in the human genome, for instance, are only one-fourteenth as long as those of genes with low expression. Highly expressed genes in *C. elegans* also have shorter introns than genes with low expression, but the difference is smaller—only twofold difference (Castillo-Davis *et al.*, 2002). The functional significance of these differences, if any, has yet to be adequately understood, however.

We have already mentioned some human genes do not seem to appear in worms and flies and vice versa. A related issue is that some gene families are considerably more complex in humans than worms or flies (and vice versa). Consider the Forkhead (Fox) gene family. These genes encode transcription factors containing an approximately 100 amino acid DNA-binding domain known as the *forkhead domain* (Mazet *et al.*, 2003). There are 16 Fox genes in *Drosophila*, at least 14 in *C. elegans*, compared with 42 in humans. Recently, vertebrate Fox genes have been classified into 17 groups

named FoxA to FoxQ (Klaus *et al.*, 2000). And while some *C. elegans* and human forkhead genes show a certain degree of homology, for example DAF-16 (Cel 18378) and FOXO1A (Hs 170133) have about 40 percent similarity at the amino-acid level, the majority of forkhead genes do not have apparent orthologs in worm or fly genomes. Possibly the novel vertebrate genes have overlapping roles with the smaller number of invertebrate roles, in which case one could argue that the system can be more easily dissected in worms and flies. On the other hand, it is also possible that they represent critical new pathways, some of which may be involved in senescence.

Another key gene that appears to have an ortholog in flies/worms and mammals is p53, but it isn't clear to what extent it is a functional ortholog or not. p53 is of considerable interest to the study of senescence because of its role as a tumor suppressor and as a possible modulator of senescence (see Chapter 6, this volume). Human p53 is a transcription factor consisting of an N-terminal transactivation domain, a central sequence-specific DNA binding domain, and a C-terminal oligomerization domain. The *Drosophila* ortholog (dmp53) has very low sequence similarity with the human gene, mainly in the DNA binding domain (25 percent identity, 43 percent similarity), and its orthologous status is due to similarity in domain function (Sutcliffe, & Brehm, 2004). In mammalian cells, the level of p53 is tightly regulated by interaction with MDM2 protein, which in turn binds to p19ARF (cyclin-dependent kinase inhibitor). Both MDM2 and p19ARF apparently lack *Drosophila* orthologs. Moreover unlike in mammalian cells, overexpression of dmp53 does not induce G1 arrest in *Drosophila* cells, likely because in fails to activate *dacapo*, the *Drosophila* homolog of the CIP/KIP-type inhibitors responsible for p53-mediated G1 arrest in mammals. Although overexpression does not provoke cell cycle arrest, it does induce apoptosis in certain cell types and in response to some cellular insults (Sutcliffe & Brehm, 2004). Thus, some p53 functions appear conserved, some do not. The closest p53 ortholog in worms appears more similar in function to flies than to humans.

The key question in regard to these differences in gene function (and others not mentioned) among various model systems will be how well conserved are specific genes' roles in the aging process.

IV. Physiological and Pathophysiological Properties

Aging is the progressive deterioration of virtually every physiological function in the body. If there are such things as fundamental aging processes independent of diseases of aging (see Chapter 2 this volume for a discussion of this issue), then we might expect that at least many of these processes will be independent of the precise pathologies that aging entails. This is a reasonable hypothesis to be sure. However, if general processes of aging are not independent of disease processes, then specific types of pathologies shared among aging models become important. For instance, atherosclerotic vascular wall changes may be close to a universal feature of aging in humans (Chapter 2, Lakatta, 2003). Vascular lesions appear as early as childhood, although functional consequences may not be evident for many decades. *C. elegans* of course has no circulatory organ system. Lacking a heart or vascular system, cardiovascular pathology, the number one cause of death and debility in humans, is irrelevant to aging in *C. elegans*. In fairness, each mammal species has its special pathologies as well. In rats, for instance, atherosclerosis is very rare and can only be induced with Herculean efforts.

There is a multitude of such differences, of course, between organisms as distantly related as worms/flies and humans. In this section, we review a few of these fundamental differences in life history, organs, and organ systems that may indicate differences in the aging process between humans versus worm and fly model systems. We emphasize differences here because the many commonalities have been discussed extensively in many other places (Riddle et al., 1997).

One striking difference between humans and worms/flies is that both worms and flies can experience a period of facultative non-aging diapause as part of their normal lives (Riddle, 1988; Tatar et al., 2001). In the case of worms, an entire phase of the life history, the dauer larva—an alternative third larval stage—is specialized for diapause, which occurs in response to crowding or food shortage. In flies, diapause occurs in adulthood in response to low temperature. Although humans do not, some mammal species, specifically those that enter hibernation or torpor, may experience an analogous state. Interestingly, some evidence suggests that hibernation retards aging (Lyman et al., 1981; Wilkinson & South, 2002) and certain aspects of the physiological state of caloric restriction resembles hibernation (Walford & Spindler, 1997).

A clear pattern in comparing life-extending genetic alterations in worms, flies, and mice is that mutations in worms and flies typically have a greater effect on longevity. For instance, mutations in the insulin/IGF receptor can extend life as much as two-fold and six-fold in hermaphrodite and male *C. elegans*, respectively (Partridge & Gems, 2002) compared with increases of no more than 85 percent in *Drosophila melanogaster* (Tatar et al., 2001) and 26 percent in mice (Coschigano et al., 2003). Greater mammalian longevity extension than this has been observed, but only for multiple hormone deficiencies (Brown-Borg *et al.*, 1996). It is at least possible that much of the more dramatic effect in worms/flies is due to induction of a diapause pathway that operates somewhat differently in mammals generally and humans specifically. Indeed, in *C. elegans* there appears to be a shared transcriptional signature between dauer larvae and long-lived *daf-2* mutants (McElwee *et al.*, 2004).

Another feature of fly and worm biology that is common in molting animals is that adult somatic cells are virtually all post-mitotic. As a result, these models do not face one of the major problems of aging mammals: loss of proliferative homeostasis. Proliferative homeostasis is the maintenance of tissue or organ functional integrity by a precise balance between cell loss and cell replacement. Loss of this homeostasis can lead to critical tissue atrophy or, more commonly, the development of tumors. Not surprisingly, neither worms nor flies develop malignant tumors or tumors of any sort that arise with aging. Underlying this major difference in cell biology presumably lie significant differences in the control of proliferation and apoptosis. The apoptosis pathway in worms and humans, like the action of p53, appears partially conserved, partially unique, and not surprisingly less complex in worms than in mammals. One of the best-understood pathways is the worm apoptotic pathway, in which two BCL-2 related proteins (pro-apoptotic EGL-1 and anti-apoptotic CED-9) are essential for controlling developmentally programmed somatic cell death. Mammals bear at least at least nine homologs of EGL-1 and at least five homologs of CED-9 (Willis *et al.*, 2003). There are some known significant differences in the details of the killing machinery in worms and humans. For instance, in worms, the death machinery is activated when EGL-1 binds CED-9 at the mitochondria and displaces an adaptor molecule, CED-4, which translocates to the perinuclear region, where its proximity helps activate the effector CED-3. The mammalian homolog of CED-4, APAF-1, forms a complex with cytochrome c (after its release from the mitochondria) and an initiator, caspase-9, which in turn activate the effector, caspase-3. Unlike worm CED-4, APAF-1 is not localized to the mitochondria and does not bind BCL-2. That is, there are alternative modes of activating effector caspases in mammalian cells (Danial & Korsmeyer, 2004).

Worms also display the very unusual property of eutely, or determinate somatic cell (more precisely, nucleus) number in any life stage. This phenomenon is unusual even within nematodes (Cunha *et al.*, 1999). It is also seen in some rotifers but very other few animal groups (Hickman *et al.*, 2000). Thus, all adult worm hermaphrodites have 959 somatic nuclei, of which 302 are neurons and 95 are striated muscle cells. During development, 131 cells die. The lineage of each cell in the adult body is nearly invariant (Riddle *et al.*, 1997). These properties—eutely and determinate cell lineages—might be expected to be accompanied by idiosyncrasies of cell cycle regulation. The extent to which this is true is not yet known; however, there are clear differences between worms as compared with flies and humans in a variety of cellular processes. For instance, orthologs of cell cycle and transcription-related cyclins have been found in humans and flies. Apparent orthologs of these have also been inferred in worms, but the similarity is substantially less. Indeed, BLAST comparisons suggest that vertebrate and fly CycA and CycB are more similar to yeast orthologs than to the proposed worm orthologs (Rubin *et al.*, 2000). The retinoblastoma gene product pRb is a cell cycle regulator in mammals, and many components of the Rb pathway have been found in *Drosophila*. The *C. elegans* Rb-related gene has not yet been shown to play a direct role in cell cycle regulation, however. A variety of other differences in fundamental cellular processes in worms as compared with flies and humans have also been observed (Rubin *et al.*, 2000).

Why might flies frequently show more genetic similarity to humans than worms if their evolutionary lineages diverged at the same time? Part of the answer may lie in the greater similarity of flies (compared with worms) to humans in fundamental organ types. For instance, neither flies nor worms have bones, but flies like humans have organs devoted to vision and hearing, although these differ dramatically in organization, whereas worms don't. Flies and humans have a heart and vascular system, but worms don't. Flies and humans have cells highly specialized for phagocytosis, worms don't. The excretory system of a worm consists of three cells, whereas that of flies and humans consists of multiple integrated cell types. If the common ancestor of worms, flies, and humans (the protostome-deuterostome ancestor, or PDA) possessed eyes, a hearing apparatus, a circulatory system, and specialized phagocytic cells, then flies and humans are likely to have retained genetic pathways devoted to the development of these organs, whereas worms may have lost them. This would explain the seeming evolutionary paradox of equivalent ancestry but greater similarity to humans of flies compared with worms (Carroll *et al.*, 2001).

According to the new phylogeny, the last PDA was also the last common bilaterian ancestor (see Figure 16.1b). A key question for understanding the implications of these shared organ systems then becomes, what was the nature of this ancestor? Are genes and pathways associated with vision or hearing or heart function really conserved, or have such functions arisen independently in flies and humans and been secondarily lost or modified for other purposes in worms (Erwin & Davidson, 2002)?

Many discussions of the issue accept the view that the last common PDA was indeed a highly complex organism equipped with head, eyes, heart, appendages, and many other advanced characteristics (Carroll *et al.*, 2001; Coates & Cohn, 1998; Holland, 2002). Supporting this view is the astonishing conservation of genetic apparatus among the Bilateria, especially genes encoding transcription factors and signaling molecules. A canonical case is *pax6*, a transcriptional regulator utilized in the morphogenesis of both insect and vertebrate eyes. In eyeless nematodes, its function has been co-opted for a role in development of the sensory organ of the male tail (Lints *et al.*, 2004). The common view is that the morphogenetic function of *pax6* has been inherited from the common fly-vertebrate ancestor and its function conserved in the strictest sense.

There are two potential difficulties with the interpretation above. If indeed such a complex PDA existed, no fossil evidence of it has been uncovered in the well-studied Neoproterozoic strata. Second, for many developmental regulatory systems there is little in the way of convincing evidence that it is specific *morphogenetic* pathways per se that is conserved rather than cell-type specification and differentiation processes (Erwin & Davidson, 2002). That is, differentiation programs into specific cell types is conserved, but the design of gene networks controlling the formation of what, in this interpretation, are the analogous (not homologous) body parts will be specific to different animal evolutionary lineages. Under this interpretation, the common bilaterian ancestor could have been much simpler in design, requiring, for instance, only the existence of photosensitive molecules rather than fully developed photoreceptors or eyes. In the case of *pax6*, what is conserved then would be its function in the control of genes encoding visual pigments. By implication, the gene was then later co-opted for use in the various morphogenetic programs that produce the wide variety of eyes in nature (Erwin & Davidson, 2002). This evolutionary scenario suggests that there may be much greater conservation of cell types than organ function among multicellular animals. If true, the logical conclusion is that just because contractile heart cell types are shared between insects and vertebrates (Bodmer & Venketesh, 1998) does not mean that the genetics underlying integrated heart function or, more importantly for aging, failure are shared as well.

Several problems in assessing similarities and differences among model invertebrates and mammals stem from their small body size, the large laboratory populations typically studied, and the consequent difficulty in following the fates and behaviors of individuals (Johnson, 2003). There are obvious difficulties in judging the health and functional status of individuals, but more subtle interpretational problems also exist. To pick one example of why this can potentially matter, consider that food consumption rate is difficult to determine in worms and flies (although see Carey *et al.*, 2002). Because reducing food availability lengthens life in worms (Lakowski & Hekimi, 1998) and flies (Mair *et al.*, 2003; Nusbaum *et al.*, 1996), it would be informative to know whether or not the action of putative longevity genes might have their effect through appetite suppression rather than the more direct effect on aging that most researchers assume. Precedents exist for this effect in the mammal caloric restric-

tion literature. For instance, two early studies found that supplementing mouse food with the antioxidant ethoxyquin lengthened life (Comfort *et al.*, 1971; Harman, 1968). However, food consumption was not measured in these experiments. Later, when food intake was measured and manipulated, it turned out that there was no longevity effect of this substance without caloric restriction (Harris *et al.*, 1990). At least one of the longevity mutations in fruit flies may be due to the same effect, as suggested by the observation that longevity follows the same trajectory and same elevation as a function of food availability in *chico* mutants and controls (Clancy *et al.*, 2002). The curve of the *chico* mutant is simply shifted right (see Figure 16.2).

A final issue particularly with *C. elegans* regards the relevance of standard laboratory husbandry and how it might affect the outcome of experiments. This issue stems from our ignorance about the field ecology of this soil-dwelling nematode. For instance, its standard laboratory diet is *E. coli*, a bacterium

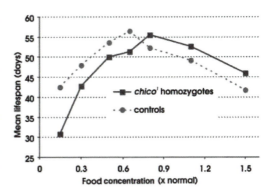

Figure 16.2 Effect of food concentration on mean longevity in control versus long-lived *chico* mutant of *Drosophila melanogaster*. Reprinted with permission of the authors and publisher from *Science*, *296*, p. 319, Copyright 2002. Note that maximum longevity for any food level is not different between mutant and controls. The mutant curve resembles the control curve except it is shifted to the right as might be expected if mutant flies ate less.

that is potentially pathogenic to *C. elegans* and that is not found in its natural soil habitat. Worms live somewhat longer when grown on *Bacillus subtilis*, which is a potential food source in nature (Garsin *et al.*, 2003). It is reassuring to find that *daf-2* longevity mutants also live longer than controls on *B. subtilis*. However, the situation is more worrisome when considering the standard laboratory substrate on which *C. elegans* is maintained. Van Voorhies and colleagues (2005) find that worms are as much as 10-fold shorter-lived when reared in soil (containing either native soil bacterial fauna or heat-pasteurized and supplemented with *E. coli*) as opposed to agar; moreover, wildtype worms live *longer* in soil than a standard *daf-2* longevity mutant when both are raised on soil. The significance of this experiment is not that worms are typically reared in "unnatural" conditions. Rodents in a pathogen-, temperature-, and humidity-controlled laboratory are also in an "unnatural" environment. The worry is that we don't know *why* even sterilized soil is toxic to the worms and why it might reverse the longevity relations between two genotypes. That is, we have no clue how relevant or irrelevant our findings are without understanding these issues.

V. Empirically Investigating the Similarities and Differences Among Model Organisms

One cannot help but be impressed by the degree of conservation of fundamental processes across eukaryotes generally and metazoans in particular. Many reviews emphasizing such conservation have quite appropriately been produced in recent years. However, for this chapter, I have deliberately emphasized potentially significant nonconserved traits and functions with respect to the study

of senescence in order to bring into the open a critically important and as yet unresolved issue: How conserved are mechanisms and modulators of senescence across animals? And therefore, what limitations if any are there on what we can understand about human aging from the study of worms and flies? Put crudely, to what extent are worms and flies like humans with a cuticle or wings? More importantly, how can we move beyond idly speculating about critical similarities and differences among organisms to identifying and understanding them? I have three suggestions. First is to note that simply continuing existing research trajectories will begin to clarify these issues in time. As the genetic modulators of aging in worms and flies are moved into mice, the answers will gradually begin to emerge. However, because the pace of aging research in mice is necessarily so slow compared with model invertebrates, answers will be comparatively slow in coming unless aging biomarkers detectable in early adulthood are developed. Also, although I haven't emphasized it for this essay, mice are not humans either. One could easily produce a similar chapter emphasizing differences among rodents and humans. However, as more and more similarities among worms, flies, and mice appear, confidence should rightly increase that whatever similarities remain will extend to humans.

Second, it would be useful to develop an animal model for aging research that diverged from the human lineage prior to worms and flies. As I've noted, organisms such as cnidarians possess a number of genes that exist in humans but not in worms or flies, and even when genes are shared with worms or flies, they still have more sequence similarity to humans. Yeast to a certain extent already fill that role but do not possess a host of genes involved in, for instance, cell-cell interactions. In addition we might like to employ another multicellular organism in which death can be cleanly separated from reproduction.

Third, progress would be greatly accelerated, and the minds of skeptics greatly relieved, if we knew more about the phenotypic details of deterioration and death in our model organisms (Johnson, 2003). Why are the details of deterioration and death important to know? In laboratory rodents for which there is extensive documentation of pathological changes with age and causes of death, certain genotypes are purposefully avoided for aging research, usually because inbreeding has fixed specific alleles with the effect that their pathology profile is dominated by one type of lesion. For instance, AKR/J mice invariably die from thymic lymphoma, as many as 90 percent of SJL/J mice develop reticulum cell sarcoma by 13 months of age, middle-age in most mice (Miller & Nadon, 2000). Studying the genetics of longevity and its alteration in these genotypes would in reality be studying the genetics of lymphoma and sarcoma respectively—informative admittedly, but not for the study of aging *per se* either. Until we know more about the details of deterioration and death in our model organisms, we have no way of knowing whether we are studying a worm or fly equivalent of an AKR/J mouse. Indeed, there may be reason to worry about this. A landmark paper from the Driscoll lab found by a series of elegant microscopic investigations that along with the increasing dispersion of yolk protein throughout the body, virtually every worm exhibited extensive muscle deterioration with age (Herndon et al., 2002). Surprisingly, there was no ultrastructural evidence of an age-related decline in neuron number or function, and the *age-1* longevity mutant only appeared to affect the timing of muscle deterioration, not yolk dispersion. Thus

it is possible that standard studies of the genetics of *C. elegans* longevity, including a number of long-lived mutants, are mostly about muscle deterioration.

The fact that true wildtype flies live substantially longer than their laboratory-adapted relatives also suggests that deleterious alleles potentially associated with specific pathologies may lurk in laboratory populations (Sgrò & Partridge, 1999; Linnen et al., 2001). The situation is less clear with worms, as a number of the substrains of the original wildtype N2 strain have evolved shorter lives over time due to drift or selection (Gems & Riddle, 2000). The original strain still exists, however, and can be used for authentic wildtype comparisons (Johnson & Hutchinson, 1993).

Proven longevity mutations may not have the same effect in these wildtype animals. For instance, flies overexpressing human SOD1 in motor neurons lived 25 to 40 percent longer than controls in a laboratory-adapted genetic background (Parkes et al., 1998; Spencer et al., 2003). Putting the same construct in 50 to 100 percent longer-lived wild-caught backgrounds reduced or obliterated the longevity effect. Specifically, in 10 wild-caught backgrounds with 450 flies per longevity group, female SOD overexpressors were statistically longer-lived in six backgrounds, nonsignificantly longer-lived in three backgrounds, and nonsignificantly shorter-lived in one. The biggest longevity difference between overexpressors and controls in any background was about 15 percent compared with about a 40 percent difference in the laboratory background. Male overexpressors were significantly longer-lived only in one of 10 wild-caught backgrounds. They were nonsignificantly longer-lived in five backgrounds, nonsignificantly shorter-lived in four backgrounds (Spencer et al., 2003). The largest longevity extension in a wild-caught background was 10 to 15 percent compared with about a

25 percent difference in the laboratory background. In sum, the *large* impact of human SOD1 overexpression on fly longevity seems largely confined to laboratory populations.

The easiest way to address many of these issues, to see if they are relatively significant or trivial, is to further refine our knowledge of the phenotypic degenerative changes with aging in all our model organisms. We should work to develop more measures of aging than length of life. After all, what we seek in humans is to increase health span rather than simply life span.

VI. Conclusions

Worms, flies, and human bodies consist to a first approximation of 10^3, 10^6, and 10^{14} cells, respectively. Put another way, the human body contains 100 million times as many cells as a *Drosophila* body and 100 *billion* times as many cells as a worm body. The worm and fly evolutionary lineage diverged from the human lineage somewhere between 600 million and 1 billion years ago (Hickman *et al.*, 2000). Although all species eat and reproduce, worms are highly specialized for slipping among soil particles and foraging on clumps of bacteria; flies for aerially foraging on patches of fruit; and humans for plodding along the ground in pursuit of who-knows-what? Given these fundamental differences, it is remarkable that any of their fundamental biological processes are conserved, and yet many, even most, are.

Because of their short lives, greater simplicity, and ease of experimental and genetic manipulation, worm and flies have become the invertebrate models of choice for dissecting many properties of multicellular animals. They have been wildly successful in this role. And yet at some point, the biological differences begin to matter. How much they matter

for understanding senescence and its modulation in humans is as yet unclear. Worms and flies do not get some of the hallmarks of human aging. They do not get cancer. They do not get Alzheimer's disease, osteoporosis, or chronic obstructive pulmonary disease. This does not mean that they may not be useful in understanding some of the cellular processes underlying, for instance, Alzheimer's disease (Link, 1995) or carcinogenesis. Cancer cells are characterized among other things by evasion of apoptosis and tissue invasiveness. Both of these processes have been modeled in *C. elegans* (Poulin *et al.*, 2004).

However, aging is somewhat different than a particular process of a specific human disease. It is the synchronized loss of function in virtually every physiological process as well as the development of multiple diseases. In order to determine the extent to which aging as observed and altered in worms and flies is likely to resemble aging in humans, we will need to know considerably more about the details of physiological deterioration in both invertebrate species. Likely, there will be certain critical processes that will not be replicated in worms and flies. Inflammation comes to mind as a candidate. Data from diverse sources now suggests that aging in mammals resembles a pro-inflammatory state (Chung *et al.*, 2001; Finch & Crimmins, 2004; Kletsas *et al.*, 2004; Tracy, 2003,). What will we look for as an analogy to this in worms and flies, neither of which has an inflammatory response? Perhaps the increased expression of other immunity-related processes with age (Murphy *et al.*, 2003) is a functional equivalent, perhaps not. These are more than abstract questions. We would like to know, for instance, as we begin to evaluate senescence-retarding therapies, will worms and flies be useful as preliminary models? The answers, however they turn out, will be of interest in terms of understanding fundamental biological processes as well as clinical therapeutics.

Acknowledgments

We thank Pamela Larsen, Tom Johnson, Caleb Finch, Ed Masoro, and an anonymous reviewer for helpful comments on the manuscript. The opinions expressed in this chapter, however, reflect only the views of the authors. Preparation of this manuscript was supported by NIH Grant AG022873 and by the Glenn/AFAR Research Grant Program.

References

Aguinaldo, A. M., Turbeville, J. M., Linford, L. S., Rivera, M. C., Garey, J. R., Raff, R. A., & Lake, J. A. (1997). Evidence for a clade of nemtodes, arthropods, and other moulting animals. *Nature*, 387, 489–493.

Anderson, F. E., Cordoba, A. J., & Thollesson, M. (2004). Bilaterian phylogeny based on analyses of a region of the sodium–potassium ATPase a-subunit gene. *Journal Molecular Evolution*, 58, 252–268.

Anonymous (2004). Functional and Comparative Genomics Fact Sheet. Human Genome Project Information. http://www.ornl.gov/sci/techresources/Human_Genome/faq/compgen.shtml.

Bodmer, R., & Venkatesh, T. V. (1998). Heart development in *Drosophila* and vertebrates: conservation of molecular mechanisms. *Developmental Genetics*, 22, 181–186.

Brown-Borg, H., Borg, K. E., Meliska, C. J., & Bartke, A. (1996). Dwarf mice and the ageing process. *Nature*, 384, 33.

Carey, J. R., Liedo, P., Harshman, L., Zhang, Y., Muller, H. G., Partridge, L., & Wang, J. L. (2002). Life history response of Mediterranean fruit flies to dietary restriction. *Aging Cell*, 1, 140–148.

Carroll, S. B., Grenier, J. K., & Weatherbee, S. D. (2001). *From DNA to diversity*. Malden, MA: Blackwell Science.

Castillo-Davis, C. I., Mekhedov, S. L., Hartl, D. L., Koonin, E. V., & Kondrashov, F. A. (2002). Selection for short introns in highly expressed genes. *Nature Genetics*, 31, 415–418.

Chung, H. Y., Kim, H. J., Kim, J. W., & Yu, B. P. (2001). The inflammation hypothesis of aging: molecular modulation by calorie restriction. *Annals of the New York Academy of Sciences*, 928, 327–335.

Clancy, D. J., Gems, D., Hafen, E., Leevers, S. J., & Partridge, L. (2002). Dietary restriction in long-lived dwarf flies. *Science*, 296, 319.

Coates, M. I., & Cohn, M. J. (1998). Fins, limbs and tails: outgrowths and axial patterning in vertebrate evolution. *BioEssays*, 20, 371–381.

Cohen, H. Y., Miller, C., Bitterman, K. J., Wall, M. R., Hekking, B., Kessler, B., Howitz, K. T., Gorospe, M., de Cabo, R., & Sinclair, D. A. (2004). Calorie restriction promotes mammalian cell survival by inducing the SIRT1 deacetylase. *Science*, 305, 390–392.

Comfort, A., Youhotsky-Gore, I., & Pathmanathan, K. (1971). Effect of ethoxyquin on the longevity of C3H mice. *Nature*, 229, 254–255.

Copley, R. R., Aloy, P., Russell, R. B., & Telford, M. J. (2004). Systematic searches from molecular synapomorphies in model metazoan genomes give some support for Ecdysozoa after accounting for the idiosyncrasies of *Caenorhabditis elegans*. *Evolution and Development*, 6, 164–169.

Coschigano, K. T., Holland, A. N., Riders, M. E., List, E. O., Flyvbjerg, A., & Kopchick, J. J. (2003) Deletion, but not antagonism, of the mouse growth hormone receptor results in severely decreased body weights, insulin, and insulin-like growth factor I levels and increased life span. *Endocrinology*, 144, 3799–3810.

Cunha, A., Azevedo, R. B., Emmons, S. W., & Leroi, A. M. (1999). Variable cell number in nematodes. *Nature*, 402, 253.

Danial, N. N., & Korsmeyer, S. J. (2004). Cell death: critical control points. *Cell*, 116, 205–219.

Dehal, P., Satou, Y., Campbell, R. K., *et al.* (2002). The draft genome of *Ciona intestinalis*: insights into chordate and vertebrate origins. *Science*, 298, 2157–2167.

Denver, D. R., Morris, K., Lynch, M., & Kelley, T. W. (2004). High mutation rate and predominance of insertions in the *Caenorhabditis elegans* nuclear genome. *Nature*, 430, 679–682.

Erwin, D. H., & Davidson, E. H. (2002). The last common bilaterian ancestor. *Development*, 129, 3021–3032.

Fabrizio, P., & Longo, V. D. (2003). Chronological aging in *Saccharomyces cerevisiae*. *Aging Cell*, 2, 73–81.

Finch, C. E. (1990). *Longevity, senescence, and the genome*. Chicago: University of Chicago Press.

Finch, C. E., & Crimmins, E. M. (2004). Inflammatory exposure and historical changes in human life-span. *Science*, 305, 1736–1739.

Fitch, D. H. A., & Thomas, W. K. (1997). Evolution. In D. L. Riddle, T. Blumenthal, B. J. Meyer, & J. R. Priess (Eds.), *C. elegans II: monograph 33* (pp. 815–850). Plainview, NY: Cold Spring Harbor Laboratory Press.

Forster, M. J., Morris, P., & Sohal, R. S. (2003). Genotype and age influence the effect of caloric intake on mortality in mice. *FASEB Journal*, 17, 690–692.

Garsin, D. A., Villanueva, J. M., Begun, J., *et al.* (2003). Long-lived *C. elegans daf-2* mutants are resistant to bacterial pathogens. *Science*, 300, 1921.

Gems, D. (2000). Longevity and ageing in parasitic and free-living nematodes. *Biogerontology*, 1, 289–307.

Gems, D., & Riddle, D. L. (2000). Defining wild-type life span in *Caenorhabditis elegans*. *Journals of Gerontology: Biological Sciences & Medical Sciences*, 55, B215–B219.

Gershon, H., & Gershon, D. (2002). *Caenorhabditis elegans*—a paradigm for aging research: advantages and limitations. *Mechanisms of Ageing and Development*, 123, 261–274.

Harman, D. (1968). Free radical theory of aging: effect of free radical inhibitors on the life span of male LAF1 mice—second experiment (abstract). *Gerontologist*, 8, 13.

Harris, S. B., Weindruch, R., Smith, G. S., Mickey, M. R., & Walford, R. L. (1990). Dietary restriction alone and in combination with oral ethoxyquin/ 2-mercaptoethylamine in mice. *Journal of Gerontology: Biological Sciences*, 45, B141–B147.

Harris, T. W., Chen, N., Cunningham, F., *et al.* (2004). WormBase: a multi-species resource for nematode biology and genomics. *Nucleic Acids Research*, 32, D411–D417.

Herndon, L. A., Schmeissner, P. J., Dudaronik, J. M., *et al.* (2002). Sotchastic and genetic factors influence tissue-specific decline in ageing *C. elegans*. *Nature*, 419, 808–814.

Hickman, C. P. Jr, Roberts, L. S., & Larson, A. (2000). *Integrated principles of zoology*, 11th ed. New York: McGraw-Hill.

Holland, L. Z. (2002). Heads or tails? Amphioxus and the evolution of anterior-poterior patterning in deuterostomes. *Developmental Biology*, 241, 209–228.

Hornsby, P. J. (2001). Cell proliferation in mammalian aging. In E. J. Masoro & S. N. Austad (Eds.), *Handbook of the biology of aging* (5th ed., pp. 207–245). San Diego, CA: Academic Press.

International Human Genome Sequencing Consortium. (2004). Finishing the euchromatic sequence of the human genome. *Nature*, 431, 931–945.

Jazwinski, S. M. (1995). Longevity-assurance genes and mitochondrial DNA alterations: yeast and filamentous fungi. In E. L. Schneider & J. W. Rowe (Eds.), *Handbook of the biology of aging* (4th ed., pp. 39–54). San Diego, CA: Academic Press.

Johnson, T. E. (2003). Advantages and disadvantages of *Caenorhabditis elegans* for aging research. *Experimental Gerontology*, 38, 1329–1332.

Johnson, T. E., & Hutchinson, E. W. (1993). Absence of strong heterosis for life span and other life history traits in *Caenorhabditis elegans*. *Genetics*, 134, 465–474.

Kirk, K. L. (2001). Dietary restriction and aging: comparative tests of evolutionary hypotheses. *Journals of Gerontology: Biological Sciences and Medical Sciences*, 56, B123–B129.

Klaus, H., Kaestner, W. K., & Martinez, D. E. (2000). Unified nomenclature for the winged helix/forkhead transcription factors. *Genes and Development*, 14, 142–146.

Kletsas, D., Pratsinis, H., Mariatos, G., Zacharatos, P., & Gorgoulis, V. G. (2004). The proinflammatory phenotype of senescent cells: the p53-mediated ICAM-1 expression. *Annals of the New York Academy of Sciences*, 1019, 330–332.

Kortschak, R. D., Samuel, G., Saint, R., & Miller, D. J. (2003). EST analysis of the cnidarian *Acropora millepora* reveals extensive gene loss and rapid sequence divergence in the model invertebrates. *Current Biology*, 13, 2190–2196.

Krylov, D. M., Wolf, Y. I., Rogozin, I. B., & Koonin, E. V. (2003). Gene loss, protein sequence divergence, gene dispensability, expression level, and interactivity are correlated in eukaryotic evolution. *Genome Research*, 13, 2229–2235.

Kumar, S., & Subramanian, S. (2002). Mutation rates in mammalian genomes. *Proceedings of the National Academy of Sciences of the USA*, 99, 803–808.

Lakatta, E. G. (2003). Arterial and cardiac aging: major shareholders in cardiovascular disease enterprise: Part III: cellular and molecular clues to heart and arterial aging. *Circulation*, 107, 490–497.

Lakowski, B., & Hekimi, S. (1998). The genetics of caloric restriction in *Caenorhabditis elegans*. *Proceedings of the National Academy of Sciences of the USA*, 95, 13091–13096.

Link, C. D. (1995). Expression of human beta-amyloid peptide in transgenic *Caenorhabditis elegans*. *Proceedings of the National Academy of Sciences of the USA*, 92, 9368–9372.

Linnen, C., Tatar, M., & Promislow, D. E. L. (2001). Cultural artifacts: a comparison of senescence in natural, lab-adapted and artificially selected lines of *Drosophila melanogaster*. *Evolutionary Ecology Research*, 3, 877–888.

Lints, R., Jia, J., Kim, K., Li, C., & Emmons, S. W. (2004). Axial patterning of *C. elegans* male sensilla identities by selector genes. *Developmental Biology*, 269, 137–151.

Lyman, C. P., O'Brien, R. C., Greene, G. C., & Paparangos, E. D. (1981). Hibernation and longevity in the Turkish hamster *Mesocricetus brandti*. *Science*, 212, 668–670.

McElwee, J. J., Schuster, E., Blanc, E., Thomas, J. H., & Gems, D. (2004). Shared transcriptional signature in *Caenorhabditis elegans* dauer larvae and long-lived daf-2 mutants implicates detoxification system in longevity assurance. *Journal of Biological Chemistry*, 279, 44533–44543.

Mair, W., Goymer, P., Pletcher, S. D., & Partridge, L. (2003). Demography of dietary restriction and death in *Drosophila*. *Science*, 301, 1731–1733.

Mallatt, J., & Winchell, C. J. (2002). Testing the new animal phylogeny: first use of combined large-subunit and small-subunit rRNA gene sequences to classify the protostomes. *Molecular Biology and Evolution*, 19, 289–301.

Mattick, J. S. (2003). Challenging the dogma: the hidden layer of non-protein-coding RNAs in complex organisms. *BioEssays*, 25, 930–939.

Mazet, F., Yu, J. K., Liberles, D. A., Holland, L. Z., & Shimeld, S. M. (2003). Phylogenetic relationships of the Fox (Forkhead) gene family in the bilateria. *Gene*, 316, 79–89.

Miller, R. A., & Nadon, N. L. (2000). Principles of animal use for gerontological research. *Journal of Gerontology: Biological Sciences*, 55A, B117–B123.

Mouse Genome Sequencing Consortium. (2002). Initial sequencing and comparative analysis of the mouse genome. *Nature*, 420, 520–562.

Murphy, C. T., McCarroll, S. A., Bargmann, C. I., Fraser, A., Kamath, R. S., Ahringer, J., Li, H., & Kenyon, C. (2003). Genes that act downstream of DAF-16 to influence the lifespan of *Caenorhabditis elegans*. *Nature*, 424, 277–283.

Murphy, W. J., Eizirik, E., Johnson, W. E., Zhange, U. P., Ryder, O. A., & O'Brien, S. J. (2001). Molecular phylogenetics and the origins of placental mammals. *Nature*, 409, 614–618.

Nusbaum, T. J., Mueller, L. D., & Rose, M. R. (1996). Evolutionary patterns among measures of aging. *Experimental Gerontology*, 31, 507–516.

O'Brien, K. P., Westerlund, I., & Sonnhammer, E. L. L. (2004). OrthoDisease: a database of human disease orthologs. *Human Mutation*, 24, 112–119.

Parkes, T. L., Elia, A. J., Dickinson, D., Hilliker, A. J., Phillips, J. P., &

Boulianne, G. L. (1998). Extension of *Drosophila* lifespan by overexpression of human SOD1 in motorneurons. *Nature Genetics*, 19, 171–174.

Partridge, L., & Gems, D. (2002). Mechanisms of ageing: public or private? *Nature Reviews Genetics*, 3, 165–175.

Philip, G. K., Creevey, C. J., & McInerney, J. O. (2005). The opisthokonta and the ecdysozoa may not be clades: strong support for the grouping of plant and animal than for animal and fungi and stronger support for the Coelomata than Ecdysozoa. *Molecular Biology and Evolution*, 22, 1175–1184.

Philippe, H., Lartillot, N., & Brinkmann, H. (2005). Multigene analyses of bilaterian animals corroborate the monophyly of Ecdysozoa, Lophotrochozoa and Protostomia. *Molecular Biology and Evolution*, 22, 1246–1253.

Picard, F., Kurtev, M., Chung, N., Topark-Ngarm A., Senawong, T., Machado De Oliveira, R., Leid, M., McBurney, M. W., & Guarente, L. (2004). Sirt1 promotes fat mobilization in white adipocytes by repressing PPAR-gamma. *Nature*, 429, 771–776.

Poulin, G., Nandakumar, R., & Ahringer, J. (2004). Genome-wide RNAi screens in *Caenorhabditis elegans*: impact on cancer research. *Oncogene*, 23, 8340–8345.

Promislow, D. E. (2004). Protein networks, pleiotropy and the evolution of senescence. *Proceedings of the Royal Society of London B-Biological Science*, 271, 1225–1234.

Raible, F., & Arendt, D. (2004). Metazoan evolution: some animals are more equal than others. *Current Biology*, 14, R106–R108.

Reznick, D. N., Bryant, M. J., Roff, D., Ghalambor, C. K., & Ghalambor, D. E. (2004). Effect of extrinsic mortality on the evolution of senescence in guppies. *Nature*, 431, 1095–1099.

Riddle, D. L. (1988). The dauer larva. In W. B. Wood (Ed.), *The nematode Caenorhabditis elegans: monograph 17* (pp. 393–414). Plainview, NY: Cold Spring Harbor Laboratory Press.

Riddle, D. L., Blumenthal, T., Meyer, B. J., & Priess, J. R. (Eds.). (1997). *C. elegans II:*

monograph 33. Plainview, NY: Cold Spring Harbor Laboratory Press.

Rikke, B. A., Murakami, S., & Johnson, T. E. (2000). Parology and orthology of tyrosine kinases that can extend the life span of *Caenorhabditis elegans. Molecular Biology and Evolution*, 17, 671–683.

Rogina, B., & Helfand, S. L (2004). Sir2 mediates longevity in the fly through a pathway related to calorie restriction. *Proceedings of the National Academy of Sciences of the USA*, 101, 15998–16003.

Rubin, G. M., Yandell, M. D., Wortman, J. R., et al. (2000). Comparative genomics of the eukaryotes. *Science*, 287, 2204–2215.

Sgrò, C., & Partridge, L. (2002). Laboratory adaptation of life history in *Drosophila. American Naturalist*, 158, 657–658

Sinclair, D. A., Mills, K., & Guarente, L. (1998). Molecular mechanisms of yeast aging. *Trends in Biochemical Sciences*, 23, 131–134.

Spencer, C. C., Howell, C. E., Wright, A. R., & Promislow, D. E. (2003). Testing an "aging gene" in long-lived *Drosophila* strains: increase in longevity depends on sex and genetic background. *Aging Cell*, 2, 123–130.

Sutcliffe, J. E., & Brehm, A. (2004). Of flies and men: p53, a tumour suppressor. *FEBS Letters*, 567, 86–91.

Tatar, M., Bartke, A., & Antebi, A. (2003). The endocrine regulation of aging by insulin-like signals. *Science*, 299, 1346–1351.

Tatar, M., Chien, S. A., & Priest, N. F. (2001). Negligible senescence during reproductive dormancy in *Drosophila melanogaster. American Naturalist*, 158, 248–258.

Thornton, J. W., Need, E., & Drews, D. (2003). Resurrecting the ancestral steroid receptor: ancient origin of estrogen signaling. *Science*, 301, 1714–1717.

Tissenbaum, H. A., & Guarente, L. (2001). Increased dosage of sir-2 gene extends lifespan in *Caenorhabditis elegans. Nature*, 410, 154–155.

Tracy, R. P. (2003). Emerging relationships of inflammation, cardiovascular disease, and chronic diseases of aging. *International Journal of Obesity and Related Metabolic Disorders*, 27 (Suppl 3), S29–S34.

Van Voorhies, W. A., Fuchs, J., & Thomas, S. The longevity of *Caenorhabditis elegans* in soil. *Biology Letters*, 1, 247–249.

Walford, R. L., & Spindler, S. R. (1997). The response to caloric restriction in mammals shows features also common to hibernation: a cross-adaptation hypothesis. *Journals of Gerontology A: Biological Sciences and Medical Sciences, 52,* B179–B183.

Weindruch, R., & Walford, R. L. (1988). *The retardation of aging and disease by dietary restriction.* Springfield, IL: Charles C. Thomas.

Wilksinson, G. S., & South, J. M. (2002). Life history, ecology, and longevity in bats. *Aging Cell, 1,* 124–131.

Willis, S., Day, C. L., Hinds, M. G., & Huang, D. C. S. (2003). The Bcl-2-regulated apoptotic pathway. *Journal of Cell Science,* 116, 4053–4056.

Wood, J. G., Rogina, B., Lavu, S., *et al.* (2004). Sirtuin activators mimic caloric restriction and delay ageing in metazoans. *Nature,* 430, 686–689.

Section III:

Mammalian Models

Chapter 17

Differential Aging Among Skeletal Muscles

Roger J. M. McCarter

I. Introduction

Sarcopenia, defined as the age-related loss of mass and function of skeletal muscle, has been well documented in men, women, and in various animal models (Frontera et al., 2000a; Holloszy et al., 1991; Rogers & Evans, 1993). Consequences of these losses are severe, including decreased mobility, increased risk of falls, and increased susceptibility to the development of frailty in the elderly. This condition is therefore of practical importance, and understanding its etiology has some urgency (Dutta et al., 1997; Roubenoff, 2003).

The large volume of scientific literature in the area reveals many inconsistencies, however, rendering a consistent view of predictable changes with age in muscle difficult. The difficulty arises naturally from the remarkable plasticity of skeletal muscle fibers: these postmitotic, multi-nucleated cells respond, even at advanced age of the host, to changes in their environment and to changes in the demands placed upon

them (Dedkov et al., 2003; Pette, 1980). For example, surgically induced sustained change of length (increase or decrease) of the muscle in vivo results in the addition or subtraction of contractile units (sarcomeres) to constituent fibers, allowing optimal performance in the new setting. Similarly, sustained activity (aerobic or strength training) results in the well-known adaptations of increased oxidative capacity and/or increased numbers of sarcomeres in parallel (Rogers & Evans, 1993). Given all of the changes in hormonal profiles, central nervous system activity, physical activity, and in body composition that accompany advancing age, it is not surprising that muscle fibers alter their size and function in response. However, altered environment and functional demand depend on local factors. For example, a muscle involved mainly in maintenance of posture will respond primarily to changes in body weight and will be less affected by changes in levels of physical activity with age. Conversely, altered levels or patterns of activity will have a greater impact on fibers participating in these activities. The health status of the host also may play a role in loss of muscle function. So, for example, Florini (1989) suggested that differences reported in the literature regarding loss of function with age in muscles of laboratory rodents are associated with whether animals were maintained under specific pathogen-free (SPF) conditions. Whole muscles of adult animals or people are comprised of several different types of fiber, broadly classified as fast (Type II) and slow (Type I) fibers. The Type II fibers may be further subdivided into those that are fatigue-resistant (Type IIA) and those that fatigue rapidly (Type IIB or IIX). The importance of this classification for understanding sarcopenia is that motor units (a motor neuron and all the muscle fibers it innervates) are comprised of a single type of fiber. During movement, motor units are activated by the central nervous system according to the size principle, from small (usually Type I fibers) to large (usually Type IIB or IIX fibers). Thus, routine activities involve mainly Type I (slow) fibers, whereas forceful activities involve Type II (fast) fibers. Decreased intense physical activity with age will therefore preferentially affect Type II rather than Type I fibers. The type of activity is also of importance: concentric (shortening) muscle contractions involve high-energy expenditure (ATP consumption), whereas eccentric activity (stretch of an active muscle) uses very little energy above the resting level (low ATP consumption). Bodily movement usually involves muscles operating in paired groups (agonist, antagonist), and those muscles undergoing mainly eccentric activity may age differently from those undergoing mainly concentric activity.

In determining mechanisms of sarcopenia using different animal models, it is important to use animals at comparable stages of their life span and muscles

or muscle fibers under appropriate physiological conditions. For example, comparison of the muscles of 24-month-old rats with those of 24-month-old humans is not useful. Even different strains of rodents have very different longevities: The work of Turturo and colleagues (1999) shows that *ad libitum*-fed male F344 rats have median life span (50 percent survival) of about 25 months and maximum life span (10 percent survival) of about 30 months. In contrast, male F344XBNF1 rats raised under identical conditions have median and maximum life spans of 33 and 38 months, respectively. Life spans of female rats were also found to be different (usually less) than those of male rats of comparable genotype. The authors reported similar effects in different mouse strains. Differences in life expectancy of men and women (women greater than men) are also commonly reported. It is important therefore that differences in longevity should be taken into account when comparing age-related decline in muscle function in various genders, strains, and species. In particular, decline of function should be measured over comparable stages of the life span. So, for example, muscle function in male F344 rats aged 25 months should be compared with muscle function of male F344XBNF1 rats aged 33 months because these ages represent the respective median life span of each strain. Also, comparison of muscle function in 30-month-old male F344 and F344XBNF1 rats would be inappropriate because this age represents the maximum life span of the F344 rats but not even median life span of the F344XBNF1 rats. Similarly, measurement of muscle function under conditions that are known to be damaging (such as in hyper- or hypoxic environments) is not instructive for understanding usual aging. Much of the scientific literature in this area involves studies of muscles of the legs. This is of great practical importance since gait, movement and independent living depend on muscles of the legs. However, it should be noted that for the several reasons outlined later, results obtained for muscles from these anatomical locations may not be generalizable to aging of muscles from other locations. The work of Fujisawa (1974) demonstrates very different rates of atrophy in lower leg versus thigh muscles of rats with age, as shown in Figure 17.1, consistent with this view. The goal of this chapter is to review results obtained for muscles and fibers from different species and different anatomical locations, and to assess their similarities and differences.

The approach adopted in this chapter is to begin by comparing changes in lean body mass (LBM) of humans and rodents. This is because skeletal muscle is the major component of LBM, and rodents have been the major animal model utilized in characterizing mechanisms of muscle aging. Then, the various components of the neuromuscular system and their variability with age are examined.

The importance of this systematic approach is that these elements operate in series. Hence, compromised function of one element further compromises the function of all other components of the chain. Decreased function of each of several elements in series therefore compounds, resulting in magnified changes in performance of the system as a whole. For example, decreased magnitude of action potentials in skeletal muscle membranes, or decreased numbers of Ca^{++} ion channels of the sarcoplasmic reticulum, would result in the formation of smaller numbers of force-producing links (crossbridges) between actin- and myosin-containing filaments of sarcomeres during contraction. If some of these activated crossbridges have been further compromised by age-related alterations in protein structure (by, for example, oxidative damage or non-enzymatic glycosylation), then

force production is further compromised in these fibers. Available literature documents decreased performance with age in almost every single component of the chain of events necessary for muscle contraction. If all of these events occurred during aging, the result would be a rapid onset of failure of fibers and mortality due to failure of the diaphragm muscle or of the heart. Since most skeletal muscles appear to lose function gradually rather than precipitously, it appears that age-related changes occur with different time courses and in different fibers. It should be noted that the rate of progression of sarcopenia is not linear; that is, the results of Lexell and colleagues (1988) and others demonstrate relatively stable muscle mass during adulthood followed by ever-increasing levels of sarcopenia beyond about 60 years of age in men and women. Factors responsible for the onset of decline have not been identified, but there are many possibilities, as discussed in subsequent sections. Loss, rather than atrophy, of fibers has more serious consequences for the individual. In this case, therapeutic interventions such as various regimens of exercise will be less effective in alleviating the problem. Determination of the mechanism of the loss in mass of muscle with age is therefore important because this can occur as a result of fiber atrophy and/or fiber loss.

II. Changes in Muscle Mass and Composition

A. Lean Body Mass

In men and women, there is a linear loss of lean body mass with age from about 30 years onwards (Holloszy & Khort, 1995). Also, there is evidence that the decrease in muscle mass accompanying the loss of lean mass is greater in men than in women and greater in the lower than in the upper body (Janssen et al., 2000). However, the loss of the cellular

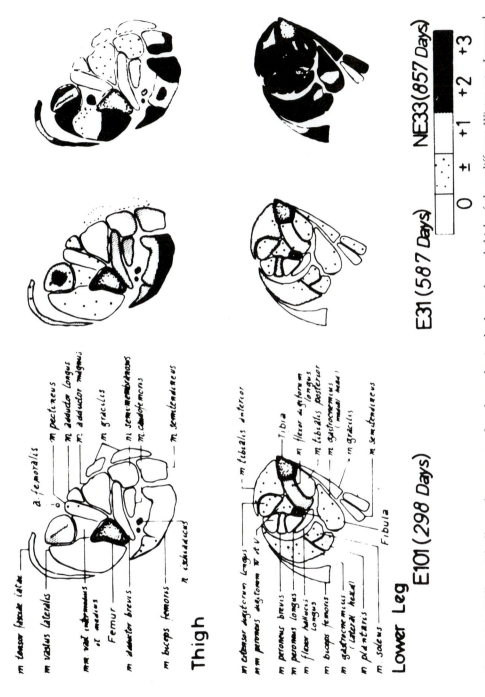

Figure 17.1 Differential effects of age on atrophy of muscles in the lower leg and thigh of three different Wistar rats. Increased severity of atrophy is indicated by increased shading. Note the different rates of progression of atrophy in the different rats and in the different muscles of the same rat. Reproduced from McCarter, 1990, as modified from Fujisawa, 1974. Reproduced by permission.

component of lean mass is greater than that of extracellular components, such as collagen. Thus, there is a change in composition of LBM toward decreased contractile material and an increased fraction of noncontractile material in muscles with age. Frontera and colleagues (2000a) estimate that more than 90 percent of the age-related variability of tension development in muscles of 130 healthy men and women aged 60 and older can be explained on the basis of altered quantity of muscle rather than quality.

Literature dealing with rodents suggests a different life course of LBM, with increasing lean mass over most of the life span, followed by a terminal decline at about 80 percent of the life span (Yu et al., 1982). The frequently reported decrease with age in the mass of leg muscles of rodents is thus probably not representative of muscles in the remainder of the body of these animals. These data are particularly compelling because they were obtained in a longitudinal manner from individual rats over their entire life span, with animals housed under barrier conditions and of known pathology. The different life courses of change in LBM between humans and rats thus suggest that most muscles of men and women decline in mass from adulthood onward, whereas in rats, most muscles increase in mass with age and then decrease during the terminal stages of life (the final 20 percent of life span). However, it should be noted that data obtained by Olfert and colleagues (2004) in a cross-sectional study of male F344XBNF1 rats suggests results more similar to those reported in men and women. They found stable lean body mass between 12 and 24 months of age but a significant decrease in lean mass between 24 and 35 months of age. The authors also reported significant loss of mass in tibialis anterior, gastrocnemius, and plantaris muscles over the age range of 12 to 35 months. The

results demonstrate the great heterogeneity in response to age, even in different strains of laboratory rodents. Further, they suggest that sarcopenia in muscles of F344XBNF1 rats more closely approximates characteristics of human sarcopenia than does that reported for F344 rats.

B. Muscle Fiber Number and Area

The age-related loss of mass has been shown to be a function of both decreased numbers of muscle fibers as well as atrophy, or decreased diameter, of remaining fibers. Such changes are difficult to determine precisely in men and women because their muscles contain very large numbers of fibers. However, Lexell and colleagues (1988) have executed such measurements on vastus lateralis (thigh) muscles of men using autopsy material. Their results show progressive decrease in the total number of fibers and in the cross-sectional area of these fibers from age 50 onward (Lexell et al., 1988). This study, together with results from others, suggests loss of Type I and/or Type II fibers with age in men and women. The overall result is a reduction of about 25 percent in fiber number in men and women between the ages of 25 and 70 (Rogers & Evans, 1993). Atrophy, as measured by decreased fiber area, does have fiber specificity in humans. There is little change in the area of Type I fibers with age but a reduction of about 26 percent in area of Type II fibers between young adulthood and 80 years of age (Lexell et al., 1988). These definitive data from whole muscle cross-sections are consistent with those of many other studies in this area. Gender differences also arise: there is evidence of Type I fibers having greater area, and Type II fibers having smaller area with age in women than in men (Doherty et al., 1993; Aniansson et al., 1981).

A more complicated picture arises in rodent muscles, even though most results have been obtained using muscles of the legs. For example, Degens and colleagues (1995) found no change with age over the range 5 to 25 months for plantaris muscles (PL muscles, mainly Type II fibers) of female Wistar rats. These authors also found only small age-related changes in the amount of contractile versus noncontractile material in the muscles, in agreement with previously mentioned human muscle data. In contrast, Payne and colleagues (2003) found large increases of extracellular space (28 percent and 55 percent, respectively) in soleus (mainly Type I fibers) and extensor digitorum longus muscles (EDL muscles, mainly Type II fibers) of male F344 rats over the age range 12 to 28 months. The mass of both muscles declined significantly with age, but only by 13 percent, so there was a larger effect in these muscles of a decrease in contractile material than suggested by altered muscle mass. Using the same strain (F344 male SPF rats), Urbanchek and colleagues (2001) found no age-related change in mass of EDL muscles from rats aged 3 and 29 months. However, the conclusion of Payne and colleagues (2003) is supported by studies in men and women utilizing noninvasive imaging techniques such as nuclear magnetic resonance (NMR) spectroscopy and computed tomography (e.g., Hatakenaka et al., 2001; Overend et al., 1992). These studies also suggest that the effect may be fiber-type-specific because major effects were found only in muscles having high percentages of Type II fibers. In contrast to these suggestions, Brooks and Faulkner (1988) found significant numbers of small, atrophic fibers in both soleus and EDL muscles of male C57BL/6 mice aged 26 to 27 months, indicating atrophy of both Type I and Type II fibers with age in mice. In these mice, mass of soleus (SOL) muscles of young (2- to 3-month-old) and old (26- to 27-month-old) mice was similar, whereas EDL mass was significantly lower in old

versus young mice. Rather different results were reported in an impressive and comprehensive study by Larsson and Edstrom (1986). These authors studied SOL, EDL, and tibialis anterior muscles (TA muscles, mainly Type II fibers) of male Wistar rats over the age range of 6 to 24 months (Larsson & Edstrom, 1986). They found a significant decrease in mass, fiber number, and fiber area of SOL muscles with age. However, in EDL and TA muscles, there was no change in fiber number or fiber area, and the mass of TA muscles actually increased with age. Similarly, Walters and colleagues (1990) found no change in fiber number, area, mass, and composition of FDL muscles (flexor digitorum longus muscles, mainly Type II fibers) of male F344 rats over the age range of 6 to 28 months. Finally, Brown and Hasser (1996) studied SOL, EDL, plantaris (PL), and gastrocnemius (GASTR) muscles of male long-lived F344XBN rats over the age range of 6 to 36 months. Most of the previously cited rodent strains have a median (or mean) survival of about 24 months. The F344XBN strain has a mean survival of about 33 months and 10 percent survival at 38 months, so examining muscles of animals 36 months of age provides data relating to the terminal stage of life for these animals. Mass of EDL muscles nevertheless did not change significantly with age. SOL, PL, and GASTR muscles decreased significantly with age only between 28 and 36 months of age; that is, muscle mass did not change over the age range of 6 to 28 months, or from adulthood until the time of mean survival for this strain of rat. A similar overall trend was found for fiber area, with little change occurring between 6 and 28 months. Exceptions were Type II fibers of GASTR and SOL muscles, which decreased significantly with age. Indeed, in rapidly contracting muscles (EDL, PL, GASTR), Types I and IIA fiber areas were relatively constant with age, but Type IIB fibers decreased in area with age. In slow SOL muscles, Types I and IIA fibers atrophied significantly with age. In these muscles also, muscle fiber area decreased to a greater extent with age than did muscle mass (5 to 16 percent more). This indicates again the increased presence of extracellular, noncontractile material in muscles with advancing age. There is clearly great variability of change with age in muscle fiber area in both human and rodent muscles. For example, Aniansson and colleagues (1992) found increased fiber size with age in longitudinal measurements of muscles of 11 physically active men over the age range of 69 to 80 years. Hepple and colleagues (2004) demonstrated decreased fiber size of the "white" compartment but increased fiber size in the "red" compartment of gastrocnemius muscles of F344XBNF1 rats with age. Such data suggest compensatory hypertrophy of remaining muscle fibers when other fibers atrophy or are lost entirely in a given muscle.

One major factor in this array of discordant results may be that identified by Holloszy and colleagues (1991). These investigators specifically addressed the issue of atrophy in weight-bearing versus non-weight-bearing muscles, using male SPF Long-Evans rats aged 9 to 28 months. They found the mass of weight-bearing muscles of the legs (SOL, PL, GASTR, and quadriceps) all declined significantly with age, whereas non-weight-bearing muscles (epitrochlearis, forearm muscle, and adductor longus, thigh muscle) did not. Fiber typing and area assessment were executed only for PL muscles. In these muscles, there were significant decreases in average areas of Type I and Type IIB fibers but not in Type IIA fibers. However, there was a decrease of almost 50 percent in the number of Type IIA fibers of these muscles in old rats.

In summary, for most but not all muscles, there is a decrease in mass with age, even if this only occurs in the final stages of life. The different trajectories of lean body mass with age in humans and in different strains of rodents suggest diversity in muscle loss with age. The loss of contractile material is greater than the loss of lean body mass with age, due to increased accumulation of extracellular components (and probably also of intracellular, noncontractile components) with age. However, the functional significance of the increased extracellular components remains controversial. Loss of muscle fibers and/or fiber area does occur, and this may be compensated by increased area of remaining fibers and be related to load-bearing status and anatomical location, but there is no obviously consistent pattern that has been identified at this time. Permutations and combinations of change with age in fiber number, fiber area, and extracellular space have been reported in fast and slow muscles. There is evidence for greater loss of Type II fiber area than that of other fibers. Gender differences in these effects have not been systematically investigated. In addition, there is clear need for more information related to aging of muscles in locations other than the leg, in both humans and in rodents.

III. Loss of Motor Units with Age

There is strong evidence for the loss of motor neurons and hence loss of motor units with advancing age in both humans and in animal models. All of the muscle fibers innervated by a given motor neuron are of the same type. Following denervation, these fibers may become re-innervated as a result of terminal sprouting from neighboring axons. The muscle fibers then may assume a different character from their earlier form, following the different neural input. This process was identified by Gutman and Hanzlikova (1972) as "fiber-type grouping" in cross-sections of muscles of older animals. The characteristic appearance of many fibers of similar type in a well-defined area of a whole muscle cross-section is in contrast to the usual mosaic appearance of several different types of fiber, seemingly randomly distributed across muscle cross-sections in muscles of young and adult animals.

The recent study of Dedkov and colleagues (2003) is relevant to this issue. These authors examined the response to denervation of various muscles of male WI/Hickscar rats aged 4 and 24 months. The now-familiar SOL, EDL, and tibialis anterior (TA) muscles were studied following one and two months of denervation. In general, Type II muscle fibers atrophied rapidly, but there were muscle-specific differences in the rate of atrophy. In SOL muscles, rate of atrophy of Type I fibers was similar to that of Type II fibers, whereas in TA muscles, the area of Type I fibers actually increased after two months of denervation. The authors concluded that "the reaction of muscle fibers to denervation relates more closely to the type of muscle than to the type of muscle fiber" and that "caution should be used in extrapolating results from one muscle to the other and from one age group to the next (Page 990)" (Dedkov et al., 2003). Similar conclusions were drawn by Kanda and Hashizume (1989), who studied fast and slow motor units of medial gastrocnemius muscles of 10- to 14-month-old and 23- to 30-month-old male SPF F344 Du Cri rats. They found increased size of slow units, decreased size of fast units, and decreased conduction velocity of all units with age. However, there was no age-related difference in the distribution of fast and slow units and no significant transformation of one type of muscle fiber into another. The authors emphasized the importance of muscle specificity in age-related change because altered motor unit distribution may depend on the location and function of a particular muscle. Urbanchek and

colleagues (2001) measured the numbers of denervated fibers in EDL muscles of male SPF F344 rats aged 3 months and 27 to 29 months. They found the number of denervated fibers in these muscles increased approximately five times over this age range and that the increased presence of denervated fibers could explain about 10 percent of the decreased performance with age of these muscles, although this small effect (10 percent) is not statistically significant. The authors stressed that "muscle fiber denervation and re-innervation is a lifelong, ongoing process that accelerates with aging" and that "though axonal regeneration and re-innervation are maintained throughout life, they are delayed and less effective with increased age." Brown and Hasser (1996) found no influence of denervation on the performance of SOL, EDL, and PL muscles of F344XBN rats aged 6, 12, 28, and 36 months. These authors found no change in muscle performance when muscles were electrically stimulated via the motor nerve or directly, even for muscles from very aged rats. Similarly, Walters and colleagues (1990) found no difference in the performance of FDL (flexor digitorum longus) muscles of male SPF F344 rats aged 6 to 8, 16 to 18, and 26 to 28 months, whether the muscles were stimulated directly or via the motor nerve. The conclusion seems therefore that aging of motor units is as variable and complex as is the change of muscle mass and composition with age discussed earlier. The results suggest that denervation and re-innervation are occurring throughout life but that the effect of denervation on muscle function at a given age is small. The results of Wineinger and colleagues (1995) underscore this conclusion. These authors studied peripheral nerve and muscle function in tibialis anterior (TA) muscles of male SPF F344XBN rats aged 6, 18, and 30 to 32 months. Their results suggest no loss of motor neurons with age but rather the presence of peripheral neuropathy leading to delayed activation of muscle fibers and delayed proprioceptive reflexes. Studies of neuromuscular development are also instructive in this regard: the work of Buffelli and colleagues (2004) demonstrates the importance of activity-dependent synaptic competition at neuromuscular junctions. Synaptic connections remain in dynamic equilibrium throughout development and throughout life. Because there is an earlier onset of asynchronous motor nerve activity in motor neurons innervating developing TA muscles than in neurons innervating developing SOL muscles, synapse elimination and muscle function develop earlier in TA muscles than in SOL muscles. With advanced age it seems possible therefore that variable degeneration of neurons within the central nervous system would produce variable effects on motor units and in turn variable effects on muscle fibers.

The situation appears less complicated in the case of aging men and women. There are, however, fewer studies in this area, and subjects are usually carefully screened for health status, limiting inter-subject variability. Available evidence is strong for the loss of motor neurons with age and for incomplete re-innervation of denervated muscle fibers. Figure 17.2 (Campbell et al., 1973) demonstrates the profound loss of functioning motor units after age 60 years in extensor digitorum brevis (EDB) muscles in individuals aged 3 to 96 years. Most studies report significant losses of fast motor units, but there may be a gender difference in these decreases with age. Results in women suggest increased area occupied by slow fibers, whereas in men there is an increased area of fast fibers (Doherty et al. 1993, Anianson et al., 1981; Essen-Gustavsson et al., 1986; Frontera et al., 2000b).

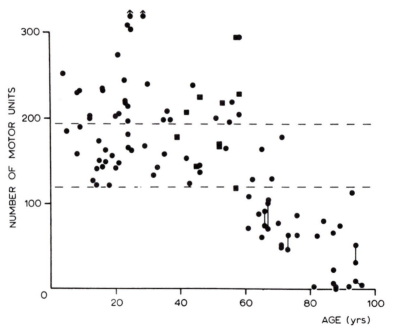

Figure 17.2   Variation with age in the number of intact motor units of extensor digitorum brevis muscles of 94 individuals between the ages of 3 and 96 years. The upper dashed line represents the mean number of intact units in individuals aged 3 to 58 years. The lower dashed line represents the lowest number of functional motor units found in the same age range. From Campbell and colleagues (1973). Reproduced by permission from BMJ Publishing Group.

In particular, the results of Doherty and colleagues (1993) indicate that even 60-year-old healthy men and women have only 50 percent of the alpha motor neurons of young individuals in their 20s. Roubenoff (2003) indeed suggests that loss of motor neurons may be the single most important factor in age-related human sarcopenia. Many earlier studies of neuromuscular performance in the elderly are consistent with this conclusion, such as those of Stålberg and colleagues (1982), Tesch and colleagues (1984) and Tomlinson and Irving (1977).

Thus, in humans, loss of motor units with age may constitute the major mechanism for altered composition, altered function, and loss of muscle mass. In rodents this has been shown to occur in the case of some but not all studies, and the functional consequence of the loss of motor neurons is not clear.

IV. Altered Neuromuscular Junctions with Age

The dynamic nature of neuromuscular interactions was discussed in the preceding section. Studies of synapses between nerve and muscle with advancing age demonstrate an altered balance between denervation and re-innervation and emphasize the individual and local nature of the interactions. This specificity is illustrated by the results of Rosenheimer and Smith (1985) for junctions in SOL, EDL, and diaphragm (DPH) muscles of F344 rats 10 to 30 months of age, with animals maintained under barrier conditions. In DPH muscles, there was increased proliferation of nerve terminal branches with age. However, in EDL and SOL muscles, decreased proliferation occurred with age. Precipitous changes in end-plate morphology occurred in all muscles after 25 months of age. These authors also reported that forced exercise of aging rats increased terminal sprouting in SOL and EDL muscles. Age-related changes in terminal branches at the nerve-muscle junction are shown in Figure 17.3, from this study of Rosenheimer and Smith (1985).

The results of Cardasis and La Fontaine (1987) demonstrate also the abrupt nature of change at neuromuscular junctions. These authors studied junctions in SOL and DPH muscles of male CD-CrL:COBS BR rats. Prior to age 20 months, SOL muscles exhibited gradual loss of synaptic contact. Beyond age 20 months, extensive loss of nerve-muscle junctions was found. DPH muscles exhibited continual remodeling

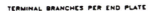

TERMINAL BRANCHES PER END PLATE

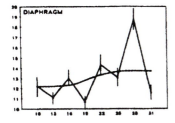
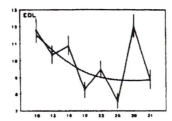
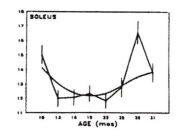

Figure 17.3 Variability with age of nerve terminal branches per end plate in three different muscles of F344 rats. Note the different trajectories of change with age in each muscle and the abrupt increase in terminal branches for all muscles after age 25 months. Modified from Rosenheimer and Smith (1985). Used with permission.

of nerve-muscle junctions throughout the same age range. Jacob and Robbins (1990) found reduced end-plate potentials in mouse skeletal muscles with advancing age. Also, Andonian and Fahim (1987) found significant increase in area, length, and the number of branches of neuromuscular junctions of mice with advancing age. These results together with those of others led Urbanchek and colleagues (2001) to suggest that denervation in old animals is associated with impaired re-innervation, which produces myoneural junctions of marginal function.

The neuromuscular junction is thus a potentially vulnerable link in the linear chain of events required for appropriate motor function. The nerve-muscle junctions of human and animal motor units are constantly remodeling and are the subject of many pharmacologic interventions. However, there is too little information currently available to suggest that this site has any significant responsibility for the differential performance of skeletal muscles with age, in both humans and in animal models. There is evidence, however, of differential changes with age in end-plate morphology of various muscles of the same animal.

V. Excitation-Contraction Coupling

End-plate potentials (EPPs) are generated in post-synaptic muscle membranes as a consequence of activation of nerve-muscle junctions. These EPPs are generated in the region of the junction and are graded depolarizations of the muscle membrane dependent on the number of molecules of acetylcholine released from nerve terminals and on the number subsequently bound to receptors on the muscle membrane. The EPPs in turn lead to propagated action potentials in the surrounding areas of muscle membrane that contain voltage-gated Na^+ and K^+ ion channels. The signals are propagated into the interior of muscle cells via the transevere tubular network, ultimately resulting in the release of intracellular Ca^{++} ion stores from the sarcoplasmic reticulum (SR). The release of Ca^{++} is also a graded phenomenon dependent on the degree of depolarization of the muscle cell membrane and on the coupling between voltage-sensing dihydropyridine receptors (DHPRs) of the muscle membrane and Ca^{++}-release channels of the sarcoplasmic reticulum (the ryanodine receptors, or RyRs). Less membrane depolarization, or decreased coupling of the Ca^{++}-release receptors, leads to decreased activation of the contractile proteins and therefore decreased performance of skeletal muscle fibers. It should be stressed that this mechanism is unique to skeletal muscle fibers because both cardiac muscle cells and smooth muscle cells derive much of the Ca^{++} ions required for activation from extracellular sources rather than the solely intracellular source utilized by skeletal muscle fibers. Thus, compromised or decreased numbers of DHPRs or RyRs would result in decline of skeletal muscle performance in the absence of any significant decline in performance of cardiac and/or smooth muscle tissue. This potential mechanism of sarcopenia has been extensively investigated by the Delbono laboratory (Delbono et al., 1995; Delbono et al., 1997; Wang et al., 2000). In particular, these investigators have established decreased expression of DHPR and RyR as well as decreased peak intracellular Ca^{++} levels in limb muscles of rodents with advancing age (Renganathan et al., 1997, 1998). Recently, the same group reported decreases in peak active tension of single fibers of FDB (flexor digitorum brevis) muscle and of maximum intracellular Ca^{++} levels of old (22- to 24-month-old) versus young (2- to 6-month-old) DBA or FVB SPF mice (Gonzalez et al., 2003). The authors provided additional evidence supporting the notion that it is not the depletion of Ca^{++} ions from the SR of muscle cells of aged mice, but rather the inadequate release of stored Ca^{++} that is responsible for the sarcopenia observed in these muscles. In contrast to this series of consistent experimental results, Ryan and colleagues (2003) recently reported no change with age in DHPR expression in human skeletal muscle. The simplest explanation of this difference in outcome is that it may relate to a species specificity of altered gene expression with age. However, because this field has only recently been developed, it seems equally likely that the difference in outcome may be related to anatomical location, function, and fiber composition of the muscles involved. Such differences in outcome have been previously reported in another step of the process of excitation-contraction coupling: Gafni and Yuh (1989) reported a decline in the capacity to accumulate Ca^{++} ions of SR vesicles prepared from hind-limb muscles of old (28-month-old) versus young (4-month-old) Sprague-Dawley rats. In this case, vesicles of old rats exhibited similar ATPase activities as vesicles of muscles of young rats. However, there was a decrease in the efficiency of Ca^{++} transport; that is, the number of Ca^{++} ions transported per mole of ATP hydrolyzed declined markedly with age. This result, if present in most skeletal muscle fibers, would lead to prolonged contraction and relaxation times as well as to increased energy cost of movement. However, the result is in contrast to the findings of Bertrand and colleagues (1975), who reported an increase with age in the ratio of Ca^{++} ions transported to moles of ATP hydrolyzed in similar SR vesicles. This study was executed using SPF male F344 rats. Because the F344 rats do not exhibit the age-related obesity of Sprague-Dawley rats and were maintained under barrier conditions, it is possible that age-related pathology and health of the elderly rats played a role in the divergent outcomes.

The several processes of excitation-contraction coupling and their potential variability with advancing age clearly deserve more scrutiny. In particular, it is important to establish whether there is decreased expression of DHPR and RyR with advanced age in muscles of different anatomical locations and in muscles of different species. Indeed, it seems advisable to establish *a priori* whether Ca^{++} release and uptake processes and Ca^{++} availability do indeed limit the performance of muscles of the elderly.

VI. Mechanical Properties

The primary function of skeletal muscle is to effect movement. This is accomplished by two particular properties of activated muscle fibers: the ability to develop tension at a level greater than that present in the resting fiber, and the ability to change length while sustaining elevated levels of tension. The changes of length that occur during usual movement are both shortening (of the agonist muscle) and lengthening (of the antagonist muscle). Movements that involve primarily shortening muscles are designated as "concentric," whereas those involving mainly stretch of active muscles are "eccentric." Both are usually described as utilizing muscle "contractions," despite the fact that eccentric contractions involve increased length of the active muscle. The distinction between the two is important because of evidence indicating the effects of age on muscle performance may be different depending on which type of contraction is used to evaluate performance. The energy cost of concentric contraction is much higher than that of eccentric contraction, so altered balance between these two types of contraction may greatly affect the energy cost of movement. The resting elasticity of muscles is also of importance in age-related change because increased resistance to stretch may limit performance of muscles of the elderly. And there is evidence, as described earlier, of the accumulation with age of extracellular components of muscle such as connective tissue, which increase resistance to stretch.

particularly serious consequences with respect to the energy cost of breathing. Decreased efficiency of breathing has indeed been identified in elderly men and women and has been attributed in part to the decreased compliance of respiratory muscles with advanced age (Reddan, 1980).

A. Passive Elasticity

The resistance to stretch of resting muscles comes from elastic elements of both the intracellular (primarily sarcomeric titin molecules) and extracellular (connective tissue and extracellular matrix) compartments (Purslow, 1989; Wang et al., 1991). Altered passive elasticity with age is thought to be a consequence of increased stiffness of the extracellular connective tissue (Alnaqeeb et al., 1984). However, no data are currently available regarding altered stiffness of titin or other intracellular elastic components with age, so this issue remains an open question. Available information indicates altered tensile strength of muscles with age (Yamada, 1970) and altered passive elasticity with age (McCarter and Kelly, 1993). The results of the latter authors demonstrate that these changes in stiffness with age are probably muscle-specific rather than fiber-type-specific. For example, in Figure 17.4, it can be seen that soleus muscles (mainly Type I fibers) exhibit a large increase in passive elasticity with age, in contrast to lateral omohyoideus muscle (LOMO muscle, mainly Type IIB fibers), which remains highly compliant over the age range of 6 to 24 months. However, DPH muscles (mixed fiber-type muscles) exhibit a large increase in stiffness over the same age range. The muscles of hese experiments were obtained from male F344 rats maintained under barrier conditions throughout life. Large increases in passive elasticity with age may have

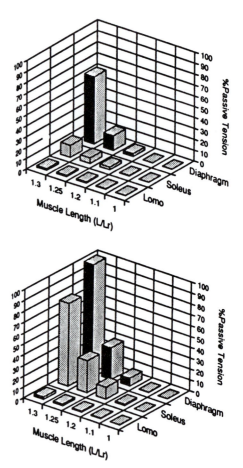

Figure 17.4 Length-passive tension relation of three different muscles at two different ages. Upper figure, muscles from 6-month-old male F344 rats. Lower figure, muscles from 24-month-old male F344 rats. Muscle lengths expressed in terms of length (L_f) at stress of 700 Pascals. Tension is expressed as a percentage of maximum tension recorded in DPH muscles of 24-month rats at a length 30 percent greater than L_f. From McCarter and Kelly (1993). Reproduced by permission.

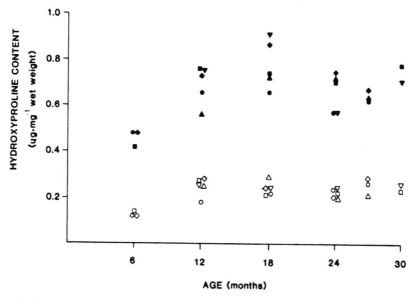

Figure 17.5 Hydroxyproline content of SOL (solid symbols) and lateral omohyoidius (LOMO, open symbols) muscles of male F344 rats with age. Rats were fed *ad libitum* or 40 percent less than *ad libitum* for variable fractions of the life span. Each symbol represents mean +/− standard error of the mean for five muscles sampled with separate symbols assigned to muscles from rats subjected to restriction of food intake ranging from 0 to 36 months. From McCarter and McGee (1987). Copyright 1987, the Gerontological Society of America, reproduced by permission of the publisher.

The muscle-specific character of amount of extracellular collagen is illustrated in Figure 17.5. This shows results obtained by McCarter and McGee (1987) from male SPF Fischer 344 rats that were either fed *ad libitum* or a life-prolonging calorie-restricted diet for various fractions of the life span. Despite different longevity in each of the five groups of rats, muscle collagen content (assessed from measurement of hydroxyproline content) remained muscle-specific, increased from 6 to 12 months of age, and was relatively constant over the remaining life span. Throughout life, SOL muscles having high passive elasticity had significantly higher collagen content than did LOMO muscles, whose passive elasticity remained low (i.e., highly compliant) throughout life.

B. Active Tension Development

Maximum active tension is developed by skeletal muscles when their length is held constant during contraction in so-called isometric contractions. A single stimulus produces a muscle twitch, but this does not permit the sustained cycling of crossbridges between thick and thin filaments of the sarcomeres necessary for maximum performance. Hence, age-related changes in tension development have been measured using repetitive stimulation appropriate to produce a fused and maximum development of force at a given muscle length. The force-generating elements, or sarcomeres, are arranged in series along the length of the muscle fiber in units termed *myofibrils*. The force generated by the entire fiber is then the sum of forces generated by all of the myofibrils, which are arranged in parallel over the cross-section of the fiber. Because of this parallel arrangement of myofibrillar force generators, muscle force is usually expressed per unit of cross-sectional area. Much discussion has appeared in the literature regarding the possible loss of this "area-specific" force with age; that is, the age-related loss of muscle function may be due to not only the loss of entire parallel force generators (muscle fibers and/or myofibrils), but also to the loss of force per unit cross-sectional area. The latter might arise because of the increased presence of noncontractile (i.e., nonsarcomeric) material with age or because of decreased force-generating capacity of the sarcomeres. Such a decrease might be a consequence of altered activation, altered structure, or damaged structure of the contractile proteins comprising the thick and thin filaments of the sarcomeres. Evidence for all of these possibilities has indeed been reported, as has evidence for no change with age in maximum force development, sometimes in the same muscle harvested from similar animals! It should be noted also that muscle strength may be a predictor of mortality in men and women. Rantanen and colleagues (1999) have shown that, regardless of body size, low handgrip strength (measured between the ages of 40 and 50, with a 30-year subsequent follow-up) was associated with high mortality.

In general, muscle weakness is widely regarded as an inevitable consequence of old age, and there is much literature documenting this effect (e.g., Grimby & Saltin, 1983; Roubenoff, 2003). However, there is considerable variability in the decline reported with age, including gender differences. For example, Hughes and colleagues (2001) measured the strength of muscles causing elbow and knee flexion and extension in 130 healthy men and women aged about 60 years. These individuals were then followed over a period of 10 years. For knee muscles, both men and women lost strength at a rate of about 1 percent per year. Women, but not men, maintained elbow muscle strength with age. That is, there was upper and lower extremity sarcopenia in the healthy men but only lower extremity sarcopenia in the women. Somewhat similar results were reported by Lynch and colleagues (1999), who investigated changes in muscle "quality" with age in men and women. Quality was defined as peak torque per unit of muscle mass. This was measured in 703 men and women aged 19 to 93 recruited from the Baltimore Longitudinal Study on Aging. Of these, only 502 subjects had the mass of their arm and leg muscles measured, but all 703 underwent measures of peak torque developed by arm and leg muscles in both concentric and eccentric movements. As reported by others, these authors found greater muscle quality (MQ) for arm than for leg muscles in both men and women. Also, MQ declined similarly with age (by 20 to 40 percent) in both men and women for arm and leg muscles during concentric contraction and for men during all types of movements. However, arm peak torque per unit muscle mass did not change significantly with age in women during eccentric torque development. The latter result is consistent with studies of muscles from animal models, in which stretch of an active muscle eliminates age-associated decline in maximum tension development (Phillips *et al.*, 1991). Several other studies indicate differences at the single fiber level in similar muscles of men and women, including a greater distribution of Type I fibers in women and a greater distribution of Type II fibers in men (Essen-Gustavsson & Borges, 1986; Frontera *et al.*, 2000a). The latter authors found evidence that large muscle fibers from the muscles of men developed more force than large fibers from women's muscles. They also found that Type I and Type II muscle fibers had equal strength in women, whereas Type II fibers were stronger than Type I fibers in men. Clearly, gender differences exist in the active tension developed by muscles of men versus women. Whether such differences are related to behavioral or to genetic factors is unknown at this time.

Longitudinal studies of loss of strength with age are particularly valuable because they document change in the same individual over time. One definitive study in this area is that of Aniansson and colleagues (1986). These authors followed 23 healthy men aged 73 to 83 years over a 7-year period. Isokinetic strength of the vastus lateralis muscles of these individuals decreased by 10 to 22 percent with age, depending on the speed of contraction. Area of Type I muscle fibers was unchanged with age, but Type II fiber area decreased by over 50 percent on a per-decade basis. Because the loss of Type II area was far greater than the loss of muscle strength, presumably denervated Type II fibers were re-innervated by motor neurons associated with slow muscles.

Finally, in a study involving both a cross-sectional and a longitudinal design of 617 men and women, Metter and colleagues (1999) found that "gender accounted for about half of the variance in arm strength and a quarter of the variance in leg strength," whereas "age and gender accounted for about 75 percent of the variance in arm strength and half the variance in leg strength (Page B216)." The authors concluded that age-associated sarcopenia in men and women has different characteristics and may involve different mechanisms. They also point out that, as is the case in many age-related investigations, the results obtained may vary depending on the method of analysis. This point is illustrated by results of these authors, shown in Figure 17.6. Arm strength was expressed as force per unit area or as force per unit total body muscle mass (as assessed from 24-hour urinary

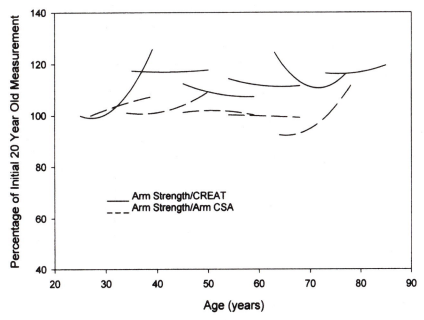

Figure 17.6 Longitudinal change in isometric tension developed by arm muscles of men over periods of at least 10 years. Strength (y-axis) is expressed as a percentage of initial measurement. Age (x-axis) in years with men is grouped in decades based on age at initial measurement. Note that strength is normalized to creatinine clearance (as a measure of total muscle mass) and to measured cross-sectional area. From Metter and colleagues (1999). Copyright 1999, the Gerontological Society of America, reproduced by permission of the publisher.

creatinine excretion). Results of the cross-sectional study showed significant decline in muscle strength if force was normalized to cross-sectional area (CSA). However, longitudinal analysis of individuals over a roughly 15-year period demonstrated no significant decline in normalized muscle strength (see Figure 17.6). Indeed, strength increased on average for the oldest individuals sampled when results were normalized to creatinine and to CSA. These authors concluded that decline of muscle strength with age depends on study design and on normalization procedure.

The general conclusion derived from studies of sarcopenia in men and women is that loss of muscle strength with age is a consequence primarily of loss of muscle mass (e.g., Frontera et al., 2000a). Investigation of the mechanisms associated with this loss and also of mechanisms underlying decreased performance independent of loss of mass, have been pursued using animal models. The laboratory animal of choice has been the rodent, with most studies utilizing rats or mice. The bulk of these studies have been conducted using muscles of the lower leg and, in particular, SOL and EDL as representing slow and fast muscles, respectively. Thus, there exists a wealth of data on these muscles, some of which is conflicting. Earlier studies utilized whole muscles or bundles of muscle fibers; more recent studies have probed cellular and molecular mechanisms utilizing single muscle fibers, either intact or rendered inexcitable by destruction of the excitable membranes by detergent treatment. Although there is controversy surrounding the age-related characteristics of whole muscles or fiber bundles, much of the single-fiber data are consistent in demonstrating significant loss with age of active tension developed per unit cross-sectional area.

The extensive literature in this area will be briefly summarized with a focus on more recent reports, proceeding from multi-fiber to single-fiber preparations and contrasting data obtained from muscles of different locations.

Data on multi-fiber preparations come from whole muscles with intact vascular supply stimulated indirectly via motor nerves (e.g., Brown & Hasser, 1996; Degens et al., 1995; Fitts et al., 1984; Walters et al., 1990) and from whole muscles (Brooks & Faulkner, 1988; Payne et al., 2003) and fiber bundles stimulated directly in vitro (Mardini et al., 1987; McCarter & McGee, 1987; Norton et al., 2001). Muscles studied include SOL, EDL, PL, masseter, omohyoideus, FDL, and TA in rats and mice, and thyroarytenoid muscles in baboons. The studies provide roughly equal numbers of instances in which the active tension developed per unit area declined or did not change with age. The notable study of Brown and Hasser (1996) reported both results, in that total active tension and active tension per unit cross-sectional area remained remarkably constant from 6 to 28 months of age in SOL, EDL, and PL muscles of male, long-lived F344XBN rats. However, by age 36 months, force per unit area decreased significantly in SOL and EDL but not in PL muscles. Payne and colleagues (2003) reported significant decline in specific force (active tension per unit cross-sectional area) in SOL muscles over the age range of 12 to 28 months in F344 rats. In contrast, Larsson and Edstrom (1986) found no difference in specific force of SOL muscles of Wistar rats aged 6 to 24 months. Brooks and Faulkner (1991) found no significant difference with age in specific force of EDL muscles of SPF male C57BL/6 mice over the age range 3 to 27 months. These muscles were stimulated indirectly in situ at 35 °C. However, the same authors reported a significant decrease in specific force of EDL muscles from similar mice (aged 3 to 27 months) when muscles were stimulated directly in vitro at 25 °C

(Brooks & Faulkner, 1988). The specific force of indirectly stimulated EDL muscles of old (27-month-old) mice was the same as that of *directly* stimulated EDL muscles of young (3-month-old) mice, in comparing results of the two different studies. The studies were done at different temperatures (35 °C versus 25 °C) using different cohorts of the same strain of mice. However, the different outcomes illustrate the variability and importance of experimental design in this area. In the same study, the authors reported no significant decrease with age in specific force of SOL muscles.

In two interesting studies using young (3- to 8-month-old) and old (28- to 30-month-old) male C57BL/6 mice, Phillips and colleagues (1991, 1993) reported significant (13 to 20 percent, $p < 0.05$) decreases with age in specific force of SOL muscles at 23 °C to 25 °C. However, they found that stretch of the old active muscles produced the same force as did stretch of muscles from young mice (Phillips *et al*, 1991). This indicates that the weakness of the muscles of old mice may be removed by stretching—a result similar to that discussed previously in the case of eccentric contractions in elderly women. The authors suggested a likely cause of the weakness therefore might reside in less active tension developed per crossbridge, possibly induced by a higher proportion of crossbridges being in the low-force-generating than in the high-force-generating state in muscles of old mice. However, their subsequent work (Phillips *et al.*, 1993) demonstrated that such a transition is not induced by differences in intracellular levels of inorganic phosphate (P_i) and pH because these levels were not affected by age in both SOL and EDL muscles. Remarkably, they also reported no difference with age in levels of intracellular ATP, ADP, and creatine phosphate in these muscles.

Florini (1989) has suggested that animal housing might be a major factor in explaining the different outcomes regarding sarcopenia in these various models and different muscles. His review of the literature indicated that muscles of SPF rodents exhibited less age-related change than muscles of conventionally housed animals. However, many studies have appeared during the past decade in which SPF barrier-protected animals were utilized, and yet the controversy persists. The simplest conclusion seems that aging, especially of plastic skeletal muscle fibers, is highly variable and that all outcomes thus far reported are possible and valid expressions of sarcopenia.

Data obtained from studies of single muscle fibers provide a more coherent picture—this despite the fact that the first publication in this area reported no change with age in specific force of single fibers (Eddinger *et al.*, 1986). These authors studied single fibers of rat SOL muscles whose membranes had been permeabilized by treatment with detergents so that activation of the contractile machinery was effected by altering the Ca^{++} level of the bathing medium. Fibers from old F344 rats were smaller but had similar specific force as fibers from young rats. Hence these authors suggested age-related sarcopenia must arise in processes earlier in the activation process, such as in excitation-contraction coupling or in neuromuscular interaction. Rather different results were reported by Thompson and Brown (1999) who investigated permeabilized SOL single fibers from long-lived F344XBN male rats. They found constant fiber area for rats aged 12 to 36 months. However, there was a significant and progressive decrease (about 50 percent) in specific force from 12, 24, and 37 months of age. The authors concluded that mechanisms underlying this form of sarcopenia must reside within the molecular components of the contractile machinery, perhaps in an altered distribution of the isoforms of myosin.

Yet another possibility has been introduced by work of the Delbono laboratory. These investigators have pioneered the use of intact single muscle fibers for addressing mechanisms of sarcopenia. Their findings have focused attention on the role of excitation-contraction coupling (ECC) as a cause of sarcopenia. The intact single fiber preparation does eliminate possible artifacts due to the detergent treatment present in the previously described work. However, considerable surgical skill is required to not injure fibers during dissection, given the extended length of most muscle fibers and the need to remove as much adhering connective tissue as possible—a particularly difficult task in muscles of old animals where there is increased accumulation of extracellular material. An initial report from this group (Gonzalez *et al.*, 2000) demonstrated significant decrease with age in specific force of muscle fibers from both SOL and EDL muscles of DBA or FVB mice over the age range 2 to 6 (young, Y), 12 to 14 (middle aged, MA), and 20 to 24 (Old, O) months. Of particular interest is the distribution of results obtained at every age, as shown in Figure 17.7 (Gonzalez *et al.*, 2000, Figure 3), in which each point represents a single measurement of maximum tetanic specific force and numbers of fibers sampled ranged from 8 to 25. For mice at any age, there are fibers developing high and low specific force. With advancing age, the distribution includes increasing numbers of fibers of ever lower specific force. However, it is of interest that even the oldest mice had EDL and SOL muscle fibers generating active tensions as great as those found in muscles of the youngest animals. It seems also likely that atrophied fibers might not survive the dissection procedures and that the

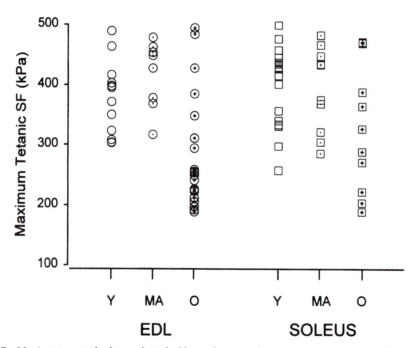

Figure 17.7 Maximum specific force of single fibers of EDL and SOL muscles from young (Y), middle-aged (MA), and old (O) male DBA or FVB mice. Note wide distribution of fiber tensions at every age. From Gonzalez and colleagues (2000), reproduced by permission.

heterogeneity of response is actually greater than indicated in the figure. These results demonstrate the great diversity of sarcopenia at the level of individual muscle fibers.

Overall, studies by this group (Gonzalez et al., 2003; Renganathan, 1997, 1998; Wang et al., 2002) have demonstrated decreased release of intracellular Ca^{++} upon activation of single fibers of FDB muscles of FVB or DBA mice. This occurs in association with decreased expression of DHPR and RyR in muscles of old mice and can be prevented by increased levels of circulating IGF-1 (insulin-like growth factor 1). Thus, in the muscles (FDB, EDL, SOL) of these mice (DBA, FVB), excitation-contraction coupling appears to play a major role in sarcopenia, and declining IGF-1 levels with age appear to be an important factor in this mechanism of sarcopenia. The authors also demonstrated no significant age-related changes in myosin isoforms and in sarcoplasmic stores of Ca^{++} ions, suggesting that mechanisms of sarcopenia do not involve altered crossbridge structure and function.

C. Changes in Muscle Length

1. Shortening

Once skeletal muscles have generated sufficient tension to overcome an external load, movement of load and limb are produced by shortening of the sarcomeres at a particular rate. Muscles are characterized as fast or slow from estimates of their maximum speed of shortening (V_{MAX}), which occurs when the muscles shorten under no load. Less variability has been found in V_{MAX} with age when there is no major change in the fiber composition of the muscle. For example, the preferential loss (as a result of denervation) of Type II fibers with age might lead to muscle speed

slowing with age, resulting from a dominance of Type I fibers in the older muscle. Many studies of intact muscles and fiber bundles have demonstrated no change with age in V_{MAX}, even in cases where significant atrophy and loss of tension-generating capacity have been reported (e.g., Brooks & Faulkner, 1988; Fitts et al., 1984; McCarter & McGee, 1987; Walters et al., 1990). However, a variety of different results have been reported in studies of single muscle fibers with age. Eddinger and colleagues (1986) reported no change with age in V_{MAX} of permeabilized fibers from SOL muscles of rats aged 24 to 30 months. In contrast, in a series of studies, Larsson and colleagues have demonstrated that for several muscles, slowing of single fibers with age is indeed part of the phenotype of sarcopenia. These studies indicate that in leg muscles of rats and humans, slow (Type I) fibers exhibit a decline in V_{MAX} of about 50 percent with advancing age (Larsson et al., 1997; Li & Larsson, 1996; Yu et al., 1998) and that this decline in V_{MAX} is probably a consequence of age-related alterations in the myosin molecules of the sarcomeres (Hook et al., 1999). There is therefore a conflict between these data and those of the studies discussed above in which no change in V_{MAX} was found. If aging inevitably results in the expression of myosin isoforms associated with slower speed of shortening, then this should result in decreased V_{MAX} of fiber bundles and of whole muscles.

Given that the different results were obtained using different strains of rodents and sometimes different muscles, it is possible that there are strain and animal husbandry factors associated with these apparently divergent results. The divergent results are surprising also in view of biochemical studies showing no change with age in myosin ATPase activity (the rate-limiting process in determining V_{MAX}) of EDL and SOL muscles from young and old barrier-raised F344 rats and C67B1/Nnia mice (Florini, 1989; Florini & Ewton, 1989).

2. Lengthening

At least one study shows that stretch of active muscles from old animals eliminates the sarcopenia evident from measurements of maximum isometric tension (Phillips et al., 1991). The age-related performance of men and women during eccentric versus concentric contractions is thus of interest because these animal experiments suggest that eccentric movements might exhibit less decrement in performance with age than those involving concentric activity. Available literature provides marginal support for this possibility. For example, as noted earlier, the study of Lynch and colleagues (1999) found that arm muscle quality (MQ) decreased with age (19 to 93 years) in men but not in women when assessed by measurement of peak torque in eccentric contractions. However, both men and women exhibited age-related decline in arm MQ assessed by peak torque developed in concentric contractions. Also, there was an age-related decline in leg MQ for men and women in eccentric as well as in concentric contractions. Further animal experimentation is needed in this area so as to determine the general applicability of the findings of Phillips and colleagues (1991). If applicable to many muscles of the elderly, eccentric contractions might be used to alleviate some of the debilitating aspects of sarcopenia.

VII. Biochemical Environment

Many studies have demonstrated changes with age in biochemical characteristics of both the extracellular and the intracellular environment of skeletal muscles. One expression of such alteration is the differential ability of skeletal muscle regeneration with age. Gutman and Carlson (1976) demonstrated that skeletal muscles of old rats have significant regenerative capacity. In a series of muscle transplantation experiments, they showed, however, that the environment provided by the old host is the least receptive to muscle regeneration. Increased accumulation of connective tissue in muscles of older individuals and animals has been discussed earlier (e.g., Payne et al., 2003). Age-related changes in hormonal profiles (such as decreased levels of IGF-1, growth hormone, and thyroid hormone) may provide protection from increased neoplasias but may also mitigate against maintenance of homeostasis of muscle fibers. These changes are superimposed on conditions of decreased physical activity and compromised cardiovascular function with age. It is not surprising, therefore, that many age-related changes in the biochemical properties of skeletal muscles have been described (e.g., Florini, 1989). However, these changes differ among muscles, and differentially affect the cellular systems. For example, protein synthesis has been shown to decrease with age in SOL muscles of F344XBN rats but to not change with age in EDL and GASTR muscles of the same animals (Fluckey et al., 1996). Ferrington and colleagues (1998) found RyR and Ca-ATPase turnover decreased with age in muscles of F344 rats but that turnover of calsequestrin (a Ca^{++}-binding protein of the SR) increased with age. Balagopal and colleagues (1997) demonstrated decreased turnover of contractile protein but unchanged turnover of SR protein with age in human muscle. Oxidative enzyme activity has been reported to decrease and to remain unchanged with age depending on the particular muscle being studied (e.g., Cartee & Farrar, 1987; Walters et al., 1990). In general, decreased protein synthesis with age is balanced by decreased protein degradation so that cellular protein content remains constant with age

(Ward, 2000). Similarly, a surprising finding is the evidence that levels of molecules essential for providing energy for muscular contraction are constant with age. For example, Phillips and colleagues (1993) found no difference with age in the levels of ATP, creatine phosphate, pH, and ADP in SOL and EDL muscles of male C57BL/6 mice aged 6 months and 28 months. These experimental data are particularly interesting because they were obtained noninvasively using NMR spectroscopy. In contrast, Drew and colleagues (2003) used conventional sampling methods and reported that ATP content of mitochondria obtained from gastrocnemius muscles of F344 rats decreased by 50 percent with age. More studies are needed of muscles from other locations and from animals of various ages to determine biochemical changes with age under conditions similar to those found *in vivo*.

VIII. Conclusions

The decrease with age in muscle mass and function constituting sarcopenia is clearly a complex phenomenon. The above discussion provides some of many examples of the pitfalls of generalizing these effects. There is evidence for the preferential loss of Type II fibers with age in some muscles and under some conditions. However, there is clearly a loss of Type I fibers or no loss of either fiber type in other muscles under different conditions. The general conclusion to be derived from the huge volume of data in this area is that there is great diversity in the loss of muscle mass and function with age. Very different results have been obtained by careful investigators studying the same muscles in various animal strains. Although there is loss of muscle mass with age, this may occur only in late life in animals whose age is greater than the median survival of a particular

strain. Also, the loss of mass may involve loss of muscle fibers and/or fiber atrophy, and these processes may or may not preferentially affect specific types of fiber, especially the fast Type II fibers. There is evidence for loss of function, both in the ability to develop active tension and in the ability to shorten rapidly. However, although most of the loss of tension-generating ability is a consequence of the loss of muscle mass (contractile units), there is evidence also for loss of tension-generating ability of the remaining contractile units of muscles of the elderly and of old animals. Significant progress is being made in identifying molecular changes with age that underlie the decreased ability of muscle fibers of old animals to generate tension and to shorten rapidly. However, there is diversity in these results also: studies of permeabilized single fibers and of isolated myosin molecules suggest that altered myosin isoforms with age are responsible for decreased fiber performance. In contrast, studies of intact fibers suggest a major role for inadequate release of intracellular Ca^{++} upon stimulation in the etiology of sarcopenia. Other studies of intact muscle preparations suggest a role for decreased nerve-muscle interaction as a mechanism of sarcopenia.

Comparison of results from these many studies is complicated by issues of animal husbandry, muscles studied, experimental protocols, and the fact that tissues of old animals may be more susceptible to injury during any isolation procedure. This is particularly important to consider when evaluating the results obtained in detergent-treated and intact single muscle fibers. Because aging is characterized by increased susceptibility to stress, it seems likely that single fibers isolated from muscles of old individuals and animals will demonstrate diminished performance associated with the isolation procedures, more so than will those isolated from the young. The situation *in vitro* is further compromised by the use of bathing media and conditions that do not resemble conditions *in vivo*. For example, most studies *in vitro* involve muscles at room temperature (23 °C to 25 °C) and utilize solutions containing 95 percent O_2. Both the lower temperature and the hyperoxia would be expected to affect cellular function, more so for cells from old sources than for cells from young hosts. One of the many possible examples of such an effect is the different outcomes reported by Brooks and Faulkner (1988, 1991). The earlier work (1988) demonstrated a significant decrease in specific force of EDL muscles of mice with age when muscles were stimulated directly at room temperature. In contrast, the later work (1991) found higher maximum specific forces and no significant decrease in specific force of EDL muscles of old mice when these were stimulated indirectly *in situ* at body temperature. Other reports (e.g., Payne *et al.*, 2003) deal with muscles in which many fibers would be hypoxic or anoxic, a consequence of using muscles *in vitro* of a thickness far greater than the critical diffusion distance for oxygen. The authors cite the fact that expected levels of muscle active tension were generated, but the effects of the hypoxia may be much more severe on muscles from old than from young animals. Clearly, data are needed in this area obtained using noninvasive techniques *in vivo*. For example, the NMR spectroscopy utilized by Phillips and colleagues (1993) provided the important finding that levels of energy metabolites (ATP, ADP, P_i, and creatine phosphate), although being different in different muscles, did not change with age, at least in the case of the muscles and animals they studied. The greater use of noninvasive spectroscopy for determining muscle function *in vivo* would provide an important means of reconciling the different results in this area.

Animal husbandry is also of concern. Florini (1989) has previously pointed out the need in studies of sarcopenia for all investigators to use animals free of infectious disease. This entails the use of animals maintained under the barrier conditions, and of known pathology and survival. An additional factor of importance (given the plasticity of muscle fibers and their sensitivity to use) is to provide some form of routine exercise for caged laboratory animals. Identification of mechanisms of sarcopenia in rats and mice that are almost completely sedentary throughout their lifetimes may not be relevant to the issue of sarcopenia in free-living men and women. One possibility here would be the routine use of cages with exercise wheels, so as to provide the opportunity of voluntary exercise.

Finally, it appears unlikely on the basis of the evidence available that all of the mechanisms identified in different studies are essential components of sarcopenia (i.e., increased accumulation of noncontractile material, loss or atrophy of fibers, denervation, decreased excitation-contraction coupling, altered isoforms of myosin, etc).

Indeed, the work of Sweeney, Rosenthal, and their collaborators (e.g., Barton-Davis *et al.*, 1998) suggests that sarcopenia may be the result of a generalized failure of muscles of old animals to repair damage arising from repeated contractions. These investigators demonstrated maintenance of mass, composition, and function in TA muscles of 24-month-old C57BL/6 mice overexpressing IGF-1 in the muscles. Later work by Rosenthal and colleagues (e.g., Musaro *et al.*, 2004) indicates that the maintenance of regenerative capacity is associated with the muscle-specific variant of IGF-1. Future studies should determine which of the many possibilities described above are indeed present when sarcopenia is identified—at best in longitudinal rather than cross-sectional studies. In particular, the existence of compromised function should be established under active shortening, isometric, and active lengthening conditions because this will provide insight into possible mechanisms involved. The extent to which such experiments can be executed as noninvasively as possible utilizing the same individuals or physically active laboratory animals will determine the real value of the data obtained.

Acknowledgements

The author gratefully acknowledges the considerable assistance received from Mr. Walter Mejia, Ms. Erica Castillo, Ms. Elana Pyle, and Ms. Toni Auman in the preparation of this manuscript.

References

Alnaqeeb, M. A., Aaid, N. S., & Goldspink, G. (1984). Connective tissue changes and physical properties of developing and ageing skeletal muscle. *Journal of Anatomy*, 139(4), 677–689.

Andonian, M. H., & Fahim, M. A. (1987). Effects of endurance exercise on the morphology of mouse neuromuscular junctions during ageing. *Journal of Neurocytologyy*, 16, 589–599.

Aniansson, A., Grimby, G., Hedberg, H., & Krotkiewski, M. (1981). Muscle morphology, enzyme activity, and muscle strength in elderly men and women. *Clinical Physiology*, 1, 73–86.

Aniansson, A., Hedberg, M., Henning, G-B., & Grimby, G. (1986). Muscle morphology, enzymatic activity, and muscle strength in elderly men: a followup study. *Muscle & Nerve*, 9, 585–591.

Aniansson, A., Grimby, G., & Hedberg, M. (1992). Compensatory muscle hypertrophy in elderly men. *Journal of Applied Physiology*, 73, 812–816.

Balagopal, P., Rooyackers, O. E., Adey, D. B., Ades, P. A., & Nair, K. S. (1997). Effects of aging on in vivo synthesis of skeletal muscle myosin heavy-chain and sarcoplasmic protein in humans. *American Journal of Physiology*, 273, E790–E800.

Barton-Davis, E., Shoturma, D., Musaro, A., Rosenthal, N., & Sweeney, H. L. (1998). Viral mediated expression of insulin-like growth factor 1 blocks the aging-related loss of skeletal muscle function.

Proceedings of the National Academy of Sciences of the USA 95, 15603–15607.

Bertrand, H. A., Yu, B. P., & Masoro, E. J. (1975). The effect of rat age on the composition and functional activities of skeletal muscle sarcoplasmic reticulum preparations. *Mechanisms of Ageing and Development*, 4, 7–17.

Brooks, S. V., & Faulkner, J. A. (1988). Contractile properties of skeletal muscles from young, adult, and aged mice. *Journal of Physiology*, 404, 83–99.

Brooks, S. V., & Faulkner, J. A. (1991). Maximum and sustained power of extensor digitorum longus muscles from young, adult, and old mice. *Journal of Gerontology*, 46, B28–B33.

Brown, M., & Hasser, E. M. (1996). Complexity of age-related change in skeletal muscle. *Journal of Gerontology*, 51A, B117–B123.

Buffelli, M., Busetto, G., Bidoia, C., Favero, M., & Cangiano, A. (2004). Activity-dependent synaptic competition at mammalian neuromuscular junctions. *News in Physiological Sciences*, 19, 85–91.

Campbell, M. J., McComas, A. J., & Petito, F. (1973). Physiological changes in aging muscle. *Journal of Neurology and Neurosurgical Psychiatry*, 36, 174–182.

Cardasis, C. A., & La Fontaine, D. M. (1987). Aging rat neuromuscular junctions: a morphometric study of cholinesterase-stained whole mounts and ultrastructure. *Muscle & Nerve*, 10, 200–213.

Cartee, G. D., & Farrar, R. P. (1987). Composition of muscle respiratory capacity and Vo2max between young and old exercise-trained rats. *Journal of Applied Physiology*, 63, 257–261.

Dedkov, E. I., Borisov, A. B., & Carlson, B. M. (2003). Dynamics of postdenervation atrophy of young and old skeletal muscles: differential responses of fiber types and muscle types. *Journal of Gerontology*, 58, B984–B991.

Degens, H., Hoofd, L., & Binkhorst, R. A. (1995). Specific force of the rat plantaris muscle changes with age, but not with overload. *Mechanisms of Ageing and Development*, 78, 215–219.

Delbono, O., O'Rourke, K., & Ettinger, W. (1995). Excitation-calcium release uncoupling in aged single human skeletal muscle fibers. *Journal of Membrane Biology*, 148, 211–222.

Delbono, O., Renganathan, M., & Messi, M. L. (1997). Excitation-Ca2+ release-contraction coupling in single aged human skeletal muscle fiber. *Muscle & Nerve*, (Suppl) 5, S88–S92.

Doherty, T. J., Vandervoort, A. A., Taylor, A. W., & Brown, W. F. (1993). Effects of motor unit losses on strength in older men and women. *Journal of Applied Physiology*, 74, 868–874.

Drew, B., Phaneuf, S., Dirks, A., Selman, C., Grediklla, R., Lezza, A., Barja, G., & Leeuwenburgh, C. (2003). Effects of aging and caloric restriction on mitochondrial energy production in gastrocnemius muscle and heart. *American Journal of Physiology*, 284, R474–R480.

Dutta, C., Hadley, E. C., & Lexell, J. (1997). Sarcopenia and physical performance in old age: overview. *Muscle & Nerve*, (Suppl.) 5, S5–S9.

Essen-Gustavsson, B., & Borges, O. (1986). Histochemical and metabolic characteristics of human skeletal muscle in relation to age. *Acta Physiologica Scandinavica*, 126, 107–114.

Eddinger, T. J., Cassens, R. G., & Moss, R. L. (1986). Mechanical and histochemical characterization of skeletal muscles from senescent rats. *American Journal of Physiology*, 251, C421–C430.

Ferrington, D. A., Krainev, A. G., & Bigelow, D. J. (1998). Altered turnover of calcium regulatory proteins of the sarcoplasmic reticulum in aged skeletal muscle. *Journal of Biological Chemistry*, 273, 5885–5991.

Fitts, R. H., Troup, J. P., Witzmann, F. A., & Holloszy, J. O. (1984). The effect of ageing and exercise on skeletal muscle function. *Mechanisms of Ageing and Development*, 27, 161–172.

Florini, J. R. (1987). Effect of aging on skeletal muscle composition and function. *Review of Biological Research in Aging*, 3, 337–358.

Florini, J. R. (1989). Minireview: limitations of interpretation of age-related changes in hormone levels: illustration by effects of thyroid hormones on cardiac and skeletal muscle. *Journal of Gerontology*, 44, B107–B109.

Florini, J., & Ewton, D. Z. (1989). Skeletal muscle fiber types and myosin ATPase do not change with age or growth hormone administration. *Journal of Gerontology*, 44, B110–B117.

Fluckey, J. D., Vary, T. C., Jefferson, L. S., Evans, W. J., & Farrell, P. A. (1996). Insulin stimulation of protein synthesis in rat skeletal muscle following resistance exercise is maintained with advancing age. *Journal of Gerontology*, 51A, B323–B330.

Frontera, W. R., Hughes, V. A., Rielding, R. A., Fiatarone, M. A., Evans, W. J., & Roubenoff, R. (2000a). Aging of skeletal muscle: a 12-year longitudinal study. *Journal of Applied Physiology*, 88, 1321–1326.

Frontera, W. R., Suh, D., Kirivickas, L. S., Hughes, V.A., Goldstein, R., & Roubenoff, R. (2000b). Skeletal muscle fiber quality in older men and women. *American Journal of Physiology*, 279, C611–C618.

Fujisawa, K. (1974). Some observations on the skeletal musculature of aged rats. Part 1. Histological aspects. *Journal of Neurological Science*, 22, 353–366.

Gafni, A., & Yuh, K. (1989). A comparative study of the Ca2+-Mg2+ dependent ATPase from skeletal muscles of young, adult and old rats. *Mechanisms of Ageing and Development*, 49, 105–117.

Gonzalez, E., Messi, M. L., & Delbono, O. (2000). Contractile properties of single intact mouse extensor digitorum longus (EDL), flexor digitorum brevis (FDB) and soleus muscle fibers. *Journal of Membrane Biology*, 178, 175–183.

Gonzalez, E., Messi, M. L., Zheng, Z., & Delbono, O. (2003). IGF-1 prevents age-related decrease in specific-force and intracellular Ca2+ in single intact muscle fibres from transgenic mice. *Journal of Physiology*, 552, 833–844.

Grimby, G., & Saltin, B. (1983). The ageing muscle. *Clinical Physiology*, 3, 209–218.

Gutmann, E., & Hanzlikova, V. (1972). Age changes in the neuromuscular system. *Scientechnica, Bristol*, 1–168.

Gutmann, E., & Carlson, B. M. (1976). Regeneration and transplantation of muscles in old rats and between young and old rats. *Life Sciences*, 18, 109–114.

Hatakenaka, M., Ueda, M., Ishigami, K., Otsuka, M., & Masuda, K. (2001). Effects of aging on muscle T2 relaxation time. *Investigative Radiology*, 36, 692–698.

Hepple, R. T., Ross, K. D., & Rempfer, A. B. (2004). Fiber atrophy and hypertrophy in skeletal muscles of middle-aged Fischer 344′ brown Norway F1-hybrid rats. *Journal of Gerontology*, 59A, B108–B117.

Holloszy, J. O., & Khort, W. M. (1995). Exercise. In E. J. Masoro (Ed.), *Handbook of physiology of aging* (pp. 636–666). Oxford: Oxford University Press.

Holloszy, J. O., Chen, M., Cartee, G. D., & Young, J. C. (1991). Skeletal muscle atrophy in old rats: differential changes in the three fiber types. *Mechanisms of Ageing and Development*, 60, 199–213.

Hook, P., Li, X., Sleep, J., Hughes, S., & Larsson, L. (1999). *In vitro* motility speed of slow myosin extract from single soleus fibres from young and old rats. *Journal of Physiology*, 520, 463–471.

Hughes, V. A., Frontera, W. R., Wood, M., Evans, W. J., Dallal, G. E., Roubenoff, R., Fiatarone-Singh, M. A. (2001). Longitudinal muscle strength changes in older adults: influence of muscle mass, physical activity, and health. *Journal of Gerontology*, 56A, B209–B217.

Jacob, J. M., & Robbins, N. (1990). Differential effects of age on neuromuscular transmission in partially denervated mouse muscle. *Journal of Neuroscience*, 10, 1522–1529.

Janssen, I., Heymsfield, S. B., Wang, Z., & Ross, R. (2000). Skeletal muscle mass and distribution in 468 men and women aged 18–88 yr. *Journal of Applied Physiology*, 89, 81–88.

Kanda, K., & Hashizume, K. (1989). Changes in properties of medial gastrocnemius motor units in aging rats. *Journal of Neurophysiology*, 61, 737–746.

Larsson, L., & Edstrom, L. (1986). Effects of age on enzyme-histochemical fibre spectra and contractile properties of fast- and slow-twitch skeletal muscles in the rat. *Journal of the Neurological Sciences*, 76, 69–89.

Larsson, L., Li, X., & Frontera, W. R. (1997). Effects of aging on shortening velocity and myosin isoform composition in single human skeletal muscle cells. *American Journal of Physiology*, 272, C638–C649.

Lexell, J., Taylor, C., & Sjostrom, M. (1988). What is the cause of the ageing atrophy? Total number, size and proportion of different fiber types studies in whole vastus lateralis muscle from 15- to 83-year-old men. *Journal of Neurological Sciences*, 84, 275–294.

Li, X., & Larsson, L. (1996). Maximum shortening velocity and myosin isoforms in single muscle fibers from young and old rats. *American Journal of Physiology*, 270, C352–C360.

Lynch, N. A., Metter, E. J., Lindle, R. S., Fozard, J. L., Tobin, J. D., Roy, T. A., Fleg, J. L., & Hurley, B. F. (1999). Muscle quality. I. Age-associated differences between arm and leg muscle groups. *Journal of Applied Physiology*, 86, 188–194.

Mardini, I. A., McCarter, R. J. M., Neal, G. D., Wiederhold, M. L., & Compton, C. E. (1987). Contractile properties of laryngeal muscles in young and old baboons. *American Journal of Otolaryngology*, 8, 85–90.

McCarter, R. J. M. (1990). Age-related changes in skeletal muscle function. *Aging*, 2, 27–38.

McCarter, R. J. M., & McGee, J. (1987). Influence of nutrition and aging on the composition and function of rat skeletal muscle. *Journal of Gerontology*, 42, B432–B441.

McCarter, R. J. M., & Kelly, N. G. (1993). Cellular basis of aging in skeletal muscle. In Perry, M. H., Morley, J. E., & Coe, R. M. (Eds.), *Aging, musculoskeletal disorders* (pp. 45–67). New York: Springer.

Metter, E. J., Lynch, N., Conwit, R., Lindle, R., Tobin, J., & Hurley, B. (1999). *Journal of Gerontology*, 54A, B207–B218.

Musaro, A., Giacinti, C., Bonbellino, G., Dobrowolny, G., Pelosi, L., Cairns, L., Ottolengi, S., Cossu, G., Bernardi, G., Battistini, L., Molinaro, M., & Rosenthal, N. (2004). Stem cell-mediated muscle regeneration is enhanced by local isoform of insulin-like growth factor 1. *Proceedings of the National Academy of Sciences of the USA*, 101, 1206–1210.

Norton, M., Verstegeden, A., Maxwell, L. C., & McCarter, R. J. M. (2001). Constancy of masseter muscle structure and function with age in F344 rats. *Archives of Oral Biology*, 46, 139–146.

Olfert, I. M., Balouch, J., & Mathieu-Costello, O. (2004). Oxygen consumption during maximal exercise in Fischer 344X Brown Norway F1 hybrid rats. *Journal of Gerontology*, 59, M801–M808.

Overend, T., Cunningham, D., Dramer, J., Lefcoe, M., & Paterson, D. (1992). Knee extensor and knee flexor strength: cross-sectional area ratios in young and elderly men. *Journal of Gerontology*, 47, M204–M210.

Payne, A. P., Dodd, S. L., & Leeuwenburgh, C. (2003). Life-long calorie restriction in Fischer 344 rats attenuates age-related loss in skeletal muscle-specific force and reduces extracellular space. *Journal of Applied Physiology*, 95, 2554–2562.

Pette, D. (1980). *Plasticity of muscle*. Berlin: DeGruyter Press.

Phillips, S. K., Bruce, S. A., & Woledge, R. C. (1991). In mice, the muscle weakness due to age is absent during stretching. *Journal of Physiology*, 437, 63–70.

Phillips, S. K., Wiseman, R. W., Woledge, R. C., & Kushmerick, M. J. (1993). Neither changes in phosphorus metabolite levels nor myosin isoforms can explain the weakness in aged mouse muscle. *Journal of Physiology*, 463, 157–167.

Purslow, P. P. (1989). Strain-induced reorientation of an intramuscular connective tissue network: implications for passive muscle elasticity. *Journal of Biomechanics*, 22, 21–31.

Rantanen, T., Guralnik, J., Foley, D., Masaki, K., Leveile, S., Curb, J. D., & White, L. (1999). Midlife hand grip strength as a predictor of old age disability. *Journal of the American Medical Association*, 281, 558–560.

Reddan, W. G. (1980). Respiratory system and aging. In E. L. Smith & R. C. Serfass (Eds.), *Exercise and aging: the scientific basis* (pp. 89–107). Hillside, NJ: Enslow Publishers.

Renganathan, M., Messi, M. L., & Delbono, O. (1997). Dihydropyridine receptor-ryanodine receptor uncoupling in aged skeletal muscle. *Journal of Membrane Biology*, 157, 247–253.

Renganathan, M., Messi, M. L., & Delbono, O. (1998). Overexpression of IGF-1 exclusively in skeletal muscle prevents age-related decline in the number of dihydropyridine receptors. *Journal of Biological Chemistry*, 273, 28845–28851.

Rogers, M. A., & Evans, W. J. (1993). Changes in skeletal muscle with aging: effects of exercise training. *Exercise Sports Science Review*, 23, 65–102.

Rosenheimer, J. S., & Smith, D. O. (1985). Differential changes in the end-plate architecture of functionally diverse muscles during aging. *Journal of Neurophysiology*, 53, 1567–1581.

Roubenoff, R. (2003). Sarcopenia: effects on body composition and function. *Journal of Gerontology*, 58A, B1012–B1017.

Ryan, M., Butler-Browne, G., Erzen, I., Mouly, V., Thornell, L. E., Wernig, A., & Ohlendieck, K. (2003). Persistent expression of the alpha 1 S-dihydropyridine receptor in aged human skeletal muscle: implications for the excitation-contraction uncoupling hypothesis of sarcopenia. *International Journal of Molecular Medicine*, 11, 425–434.

Stålberg, R., & Fawcett, P. R, W. (1982). Macro EMG in healthy subjects of different ages. *Journal of Neurological Psychiatry*, 45, 870–878.

Tesch, P. A., Thorsson, A., & Kaiser, P. (1984). Muscle capillary supply and fiber type characteristics in weight and power lifters. *Journal of Applied Physiology*, 56, 35–38.

Thompson, L. V., & Brown, M. (1999). Age-related changes in contractile properties of single skeletal fibers from the soleus muscle. *Journal of Applied Physiology*, 86, 881–886.

Tomlinson, B. E., & Irving, D. (1977). The numbers of limb motor neurons in the human lumbosacral cord throughout life. *Journal of Neurological Science*, 34, 213–219.

Turturro, A., Witt, W., Lewis, S., Hass, B., Lipman, R., & Hart, R. (1999). Growth curves and survival characteristics of the animals used in the Biomarkers of Aging Program. *Journal of Gerontology*, 54, B492–B501.

Urbanchek, M. G., Picken, E. B., Kalliainen, L. K., & Kuzon, W. M. (2001). Specific force deficit in skeletal muscles of old rats is partially explained by the existence of denervated muscle fibers. *Journal of Gerontology*, 65A, B191–B197.

Walters, T. J., Sweeney, H. L., & Farrar, R. P. (1990). Aging does not affect contractile properties of Type IIB FDL muscle in Fischer 344 rats. *American Journal of Physiology*, 258, C1031–C1035.

Wang, K., McCarter, R., Wright, J. Beverly, J., & Ramirez-Mitchell, R. (1991). Regulation of skeletal muscle stiffness and elasticity by titin isoforms: a test of the segmental extension model of resting tension. *Proceedings of the National Academy of Sciences of the USA*, 88, 7101–7105.

Wang, Z-M., Messi, M. L., & Delbono, O. (2000). L-type Ca^{2+} channel charge movement and intracellular Ca^{2+} in skeletal muscle fibers from aging mice. *Biophysical Journal*, 78, 1947–1954.

Wang, Z-M., Messi, M. L., & Delbono, O. (2002). Sustained overexpression of IGF-1 prevents age-dependent decrease in charge movement and intracellular calcium in mouse skeletal muscle. *Biophysical Journal*, 82, 1338–1344.

Ward, W. F. (2000). The relentless effects of the aging process on protein turnover. *Biogerontology*, 1, 195–199.

Wineinger, M. A., Sharman, R. B., Stevenson, T. R., Carlsen, R. C., & McDonald, R. B. (1995). Peripheral nerve and muscle function in the aging Fischer 344/brown-Norway rat. *Growth, Development and Aging*, 59, 107–119.

Yamada, H. (1970). The locomotor system. In F. G. Evans (Ed.), *Strength of biological materials* (pp. 93–97). Baltimore: Williams and Wilkins.

Yu, B. P., Masoro, E. J., Bertrand, H. A., & Lynd, F. T. (1982). Lifespan study of SPF Fischer 344 male rats fed ad libitum or restricted diets: longevity, growth, lean body mass and disease. *Journal of Gerontology*, 37, 130–141.

Yu, F., Degens, H., Li, X., & Larssons, L. (1998). Effects of thyroid hormone, gender and age on contractility and myosin composition in single rat soleus fibres. *Pflugers Archives*, 437, 21–30.

Chapter 18

Aging, Body Fat, and Carbohydrate Metabolism

Marielisa Rincon, Radhika Muzumdar, and Nir Barzilai

I. Introduction

Aging is characterized by a decline in metabolic and cellular functions, with cells and organs gradually losing their capacity to work effectively and to respond successfully to injury (Anantharaju et al., 2002; Henry, 2000). Age also seems to endorse the development of obesity, alterations in body fat distribution, and insulin resistance (Enzi et al., 1986; Fraze et al., 1987). Easy access to food and sedentary lifestyle have doubled the prevalence of obesity in Western and westernizing countries over the past decade, with an estimated 315 million obese people worldwide (Caterson & Gill, 2002). Given these numbers, it is not surprising that the elderly are becoming heavier than in the past, with the additional burden of higher morbidity and mortality compared to younger individuals (Elia, 2001). Despite the increase in average life expectancy and advances in medical science in the past century, obesity and diabetes mellitus are taking a toll on humanity (National Task Force on the Prevention and Treatment of

Obesity, 2000). This will most likely be reflected in the rapidly growing population over age 65, with more individuals arriving to this age already dealing with major medical problems and decreasing their likelihood of an enjoyable old age.

This chapter reviews the effect of old age on body fat distribution and on carbohydrate metabolism, especially insulin secretion and insulin action.

II. Carbohydrate Metabolism and Body Composition in Aging

Aging is associated with increased insulin resistance and risk for diabetes (Chang & Halter, 2003). As stated by the Third National Health and Nutrition Examination Survey (NHANES III) conducted during 1988–1994 by the National Center for Health Statistics of the Centers for Disease Control and Prevention, the prevalence of diabetes based on American Diabetes Association criteria rises from 1 to 2 percent at ages 20 to 39 years to 18 to 20 percent at ages 60 to 74 years

(Harris *et al.*, 1998). When these rates were applied to U.S. population projections for 1997, the number of people 20 years of age and older who have diagnosed diabetes (fasting plasma glucose 126 mg/dl or above) and undiagnosed diabetes were estimated to be 10.2 million and 5.4 million, respectively. Moreover, the prevalence of impaired fasting glucose (fasting plasma glucose 110 to 126 mg/dl, which indicates a higher risk for diabetes) increased from age 20 to 39 years to age 60 to 74 years (Harris *et al.*, 1998).

The preceding statistics are not surprising considering the dramatic explosion of obesity. Approximately 64.5 percent of adult Americans are overweight or obese, with a 4.7 percent prevalence of extreme obesity (Body mass index ≥ 40) for the years 1999 to 2000 (Flegal *et al.*, 2002). This epidemic of obesity has an associated increase in morbidity and mortality (Allison *et al.*, 1999), mainly from atherosclerotic diseases (G. M. Reaven, 1988), cancer (Calle *et al.*, 1999), and diabetes mellitus (Kissebah, 1996). These risks decreased by 20 percent with weight reduction alone (Williamson *et al.*, 2000).

A. Body Composition in Aging

One of the most important factors that leads to insulin resistance in aging is the increase in fat mass (FM), especially visceral fat (VF). FM typically augments between the third and seventh decades of life (Andres *et al.*, 1985). The elderly are likely to have normal body weight but increase in waist circumference, indicating abdominal obesity. There is also progressive loss of muscle mass starting around age 30 (Elia, 2001). This change in lean body mass and fat distribution, with a predominant fat depot inside the abdominal cavity or visceral fat (VF), is clearly associated with insulin resistance (Bjorntrop, 1990, 1991; Kissebah, 1991, 1996), diabetes mellitus, and cardiovascular disease (Larson, 1992). Longitudinal

studies in humans have demonstrated a higher risk of developing impaired glucose tolerance (Carr *et al.*, 2004), type 2 diabetes (Boyko *et al.*, 2000; Hayashi *et al.*, 2003), and coronary heart disease (Fujimoto *et al.*, 1999; Lamarche *et al.*, 1998; St-Pierre *et al.*, 2002) in subjects with visceral adiposity. Decrease in VF by weight loss is associated with increases in insulin sensitivity (Boyko *et al.*, 2000; Hayashi *et al.*, 2003), favorable lipid profile (high HDL and low triglycerides) (Brochu *et al.*, 2003) and blood pressure (Brochu *et al.*, 2003; Kanai *et al.*, 1996), underscoring the physiologic significance of this depot. Similar disproportionate increase in VF with age (Ross & Bras, 1975) is also demonstrated in rodent models. In fact, rodent models have played a crucial role in the understanding of the complex relationship between aging, obesity, especially increased VF, and age-related diseases. They offer the unique advantage of dietary, drug, or surgical interventions to a homogenous group and subsequent outcome analysis specific to the manipulations (Barzilai & Gabriely, 2001), although the applicability of the conclusions derived from animal studies to the human paradigm should be considered cautiously (Barzilai & Gabriely, 2002).

Numerous human studies have shown that higher levels of moderate physical activity are associated with decreased risk of several age related diseases (Lee *et al.*, 1997), which ultimately could increase longevity. In addition, elderly people who routinely exercise are more likely to perceive themselves as healthy (Loland, 2004). Exercise has also been associated with decreased FM in the elderly (Mitchell *et al.*, 2003). Just as in humans, lifestyle plays a major role in body composition of rodents. Rodents in the wild are lean and maintain a high level of physical activity in their continuous search for food. In contrast, rodents in the lab tend to gain weight and FM due to restricted moving space and easy access to food. If provided with mechanically driven running wheels, they tend to exercise consistently as long as food is restricted (Russell *et al.*, 1987). The voluntary wheel-running decreases dramatically with aging (Poehlman *et al.*, 2001). Though exercise improves average longevity in rats (Holloszy, 1992, 1993), it is not clear how much of the life-prolonging effects of exercise are due to changes in body composition versus those due to the relative caloric restriction that occurs in rodents because they do not increase their intake to compensate for their energy expenditure (Poehlman *et al.*, 2001).

Dietary restriction in humans usually has more effect in body composition than does exercise training, but it is still rather unclear if any of these interventions prolong life span (Poehlman *et al.*, 2001). The role of caloric restriction (CR) in life extension and protection from age-related diseases has been demonstrated in many diverse species, such as rodents (rats, mice, hamsters) and nonmammalians (fish, flies, and water fleas) (Masoro, 2000). Although survival results of CR in long-lived nonhuman primates such as rhesus monkeys are not reported and studies are still ongoing, initial results indicate remarkable similarities with rodent studies in changes in body composition, development, reproduction, metabolism, and onset of age-related diseases (Mattison *et al.*, 2003). The reproduction of these results in humans could be difficult because there is no clear agreement as to what CR means in a human diet.

Restricting the food intake of laboratory rodents improves carbohydrate metabolism and extends their life dramatically. CR in rodents refers to a dietary regimen that is nutritious but with only ~60 percent of the usual caloric intake for the studied animals (Gabriely & Barzilai, 2001). The beneficial effects of CR on longevity have been explained by decreased fat mass, improved insulin sen-

sitivity (Masoro, 1999), reduction of oxidative stress (Sohal & Weindruch, 1996), and "hormesis," or the beneficial action(s) of a low-intensity stressor such as CR (Masoro, 1996).

ob/ob mice have been used to dissect whether food intake or adiposity is the critical component that retards the aging process in CR. *ob/ob* mice are leptin-deficient, which causes hyperglycemia, hyperinsulinemia, reduced energy expenditure, and early-onset morbid obesity, among other detrimental features (Coleman, 1978; Friedman & Halaas, 1998). Maximum longevity of the *ob/ob* food-restricted mice was extended by 46 percent, and they lived longer than *ad libitum*-fed animals despite maintaining relatively high body fat. Harrison and colleagues conclude that reduced food consumption, not reduced adiposity, was responsible for extending the longevity of these genetically obese mice (1984).

Apart from sedentary lifestyle, the decline in gonadal steroids (Barnett *et al.*, 2001; Munzer *et al.*, 2001), increase in cortisol production (Anderson *et al*, 2001), decline in GH axis (de Boer *et al.*, 1996; Hansen *et al.*, 1995), and age-dependent decrease of the GH/cortisol ratio (Nass & Thorner, 2002) have all been associated with increased accumulation of VF. A landmark randomized, double-blind, placebo-controlled study in healthy, ambulatory, community-dwelling U.S. women and men aged 65 to 88 years demonstrated that growth hormone (GH) increased lean body mass and decreased FM (Corpas *et al.*, 1993). However, the use of GH is limited because of its side-effects, which include insulin resistance, edema, and carpal-tunnel syndrome (Corpas *et al.*, 1993). Old rats demonstrate higher leptin levels but still continue to gain weight, demonstrating resistance to the effect of leptin. This resistance persists despite caloric restriction, suggesting that old age *per se*, independent of age-associated obesity, leads to leptin resistance (Gabriely et al., 2002b). The role of leptin in body composition and metabolism is demonstrated in many animal models that lack either leptin (ob/ob) or demonstrate defects in leptin signaling. db/db mice are leptin-resistant because of a leptin receptor mutation. They are morbidly obese, with many other problems, such as insulin resistance and diabetes (Chua et al., 1996; Coleman, 1978). Obese Zucker rats have mutations in the extracellular domain of the leptin receptor and exhibit hyperphagia, morbid obesity, impaired glucose tolerance, dyslipidemia, and other endocrinopathies. The fa/fa mutation in these rats reduces the expression of the leptin receptor on the cell surface, with decreased leptin binding and diminished signal transduction. A colony isolated from the Zucker rats, the Zucker Diabetic Fatty rats, become diabetic after about 8 weeks of high-fat diet (Chua et al., 1996; Yamashita et al., 1997). There are other important pathways that are also responsible for redistribution of body fat. Activation of peroxisome proliferator-activated receptor-γ (PPAR-γ, a nuclear receptor selectively expressed in VF compared to SC fat) by pharmacological agents like thioglitazones can also decrease visceral adipose tissue while total FM remains unchanged (Miyazaki et al., 2002).

B. Effect of Body Fat on Insulin Action

Physiologically, insulin regulates glycogenolysis and gluconeogenesis in the liver, to control hepatic glucose production. It promotes peripheral glucose uptake and glycogen synthesis in the muscle and triglyceride synthesis in the adipose tissues. Genetic models with tissue-specific knockout of insulin receptor have helped understand the critical role of various tissues, and especially the role of FM in life span (Blüher et al., 2003).

Fat-specific knockout of insulin receptor (FIRKO) appears to be beneficial and results in an increased life span. These animals were generated by crossing insulin receptor (IR) gene (lox/+) in which exon 4 of the IR is flanked by loxP sites, with IR (lox/+) mice that also express the Cre recombinase under the control of the adipose-specific fatty acid binding protein promoter/enhancer. This technique leads to the deletion of exon 4 of the IR gene only in fat tissue, with normal expression in the rest of the body (Blüher et al., 2002; Brüning et al., 1998). FIRKO mice have normal growth from birth to 8 weeks of age, followed after 3 months of age with 15 to 25 percent lower body weights and 50 to 75 percent reduction in body fat despite normal or increased food intake. They are healthy and are protected from age-related metabolic disturbances. The FIRKO mice have an 18 percent increase in mean life span compared to controls, with a maximum life-span extension of up to ~5 months (Blüher et al., 2003). FIRKO mice had a later onset of age-related mortality as seen in survival analysis. This group (Blüher et al., 2002) previously reported that the FIRKO mice have a loss of the normal relationship between plasma leptin and body weight, have changes in adipocytes, have lower triglycerides, and are protected against obesity and obesity-related glucose intolerance. The mechanisms for FIRKO mice longevity are not yet clear; still Blüher and colleagues (2003) concluded that it is their leanness and not food restriction that is responsible for their survival advantage. The authors also propose that pathways already associated with life-span regulation in nematodes and flies—such as free-radical damage (due to decreased fat mass) or, most likely, the selective loss of insulin signaling in fat tissue only (universal IR mutations are associated with insulin resistance, diabetes, and obesity)—could have a role in the longevity of FIRKO mice. Some critics of the conclusion that the life span of FIRKO mice is dependent on decreased fat mass alone rather than CR have suggested that the study designed by Bluher and colleagues (2003) does not provide enough evidence to conclude this because the group did not study CR in the animals (Masoro, 2003), especially considering that the elimination of the IR in the adipose tissue could potentially have an unknown role in longevity.

Other mouse models in which the IR has been knocked out do not achieve the same life-span extension as the FIRKO mice but have been successful in demonstrating insulin action in different tissues. Liver-specific IR knockout (LIRKO) mice demonstrate dramatic insulin resistance, severe glucose intolerance, unregulated hepatic glucose production, marked hyperinsulinemia, and decreased insulin clearance (Michael et al., 2000). Muscle-specific IR knockout (MIRKO) mice are protected against insulin resistance and diabetes under physiological conditions, despite a marked increase in FM and dyslipidemia. The epididymal fat (VF) of MIRKO mice is sensitized to insulin action with increased glucose utilization during euglycemic-hyperinsulinemic clamp. Furthermore, MIRKO adipocytes are able to maintain a favorable profile of fat-derived peptides. This model seems to confirm the crucial role of VF in the maintenance of insulin sensitivity (Cariou et al., 2004) and, perhaps, in longevity.

The brain-specific IR knockout (NIRKO) mice provide evidence that insulin may play a role in regulation of body weight at a central level (Baskin et al., 1999). Brüning and colleagues (2000) showed that female NIRKO mice exhibited a consistent 10 to 15 percent increase in body weight compared with controls. In addition, both male and female NIRKO mice demonstrated increased FM with an approximately two-fold increase in perigonadal white adipose tissue (VF) in females and a 1.5-fold increase in males.

Old-age-related increase in FM and VF is associated with hepatic and peripheral insulin resistance (Ferrannini et al., 1996; Peiris et al., 1988). Age-related increase in FM determines the age-related decline in peripheral insulin sensitivity (Bjorntrop, 1991; Folsom et al., 2000) and the occurrence of type 2 diabetes mellitus (Larson, 1992), coronary artery disease (Prineas et al., 1993), stroke (Larson, 1992), and death (Folsom et al., 1993). Use of the CR model supports the notion that FM plays an important role in determining hepatic and peripheral insulin resistance, as CR effectively reverses insulin resistance to the level of young rats (see Figure 18.1) (Barzilai et al., 1998; Gupta et al., 2000a).

Bjorntrop (1990) hypothesized that VF results in insulin resistance via a "portal" effect of free fatty acids (FFA) and glycerol released from increased omental fat. However, the observed relationship between increased FM and hepatic and peripheral insulin resistance may be caused by other endocrine and metabolic functions of VF, such as fat-derived peptides (FDPs) (Das et al., 2004). Adipose cells synthesize and secrete several metabolically active factors, such as leptin, tumor necrosis factor α (TNF-α) (Hofmann et al., 1994), resistin (Steppan et al., 2001), and ACRP30 (Combs et al., 2001). These factors circulate in plasma

YOUNG   **OLD**   **OLD - CR**

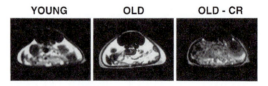

Figure 18.1. MRI scans of the abdomen in young, old, and CR rats. Marked reduction in VF can be visually appreciated in the MRI of typical Male Sprague-Dawley rats at ages 4 months (young) and 18 months (old) in cross-sectional cuts above the level of the pelvis. The white color depicts fat tissue. The old AL-fed rat has significantly more fat tissue (visceral and subcutaneous) compared to the young animal. In contrast, in old CR animals there was a marked reduction in both visceral and subcutaneous fat stores (Das et al., 2004).

and are active at distant tissues and organs. Many of the FDPs are differentially regulated (Atzmon et al., 2002), with an increased expression of many harmful FDPs from the VF, and may account for the differences in the metabolic functions between the two fat depots. Some of these factors are responsible for the development of insulin resistance (Wang et al., 1999). TNF-α (Gabriely & Barzilai, 2001; Hofmann et al., 1994), resistin (Steppan et al., 2001), and Acrp30 (Combs et al., 2001) genes are expressed in significantly higher amounts in VF compared to SC fat. Adiponectin (Barzilai & Gupta, 1999; Gabriely & Barzilai, 2001) increases insulin sensitivity. TNF-a mediates insulin resistance by decreasing insulin receptor tyrosine phosphorylation, insulin receptor substrate-1 phosphorylation, and downregulating the mRNA for GLUT-4 (insulin responsive glucose transporter). The markedly increased resistin expression in the VF of young rats and old diabetic rats (Steppan et al., 2001) suggests a potential role for this peptide in VF-mediated insulin resistance in rats; however, its role in humans is not clear. Resistin expression is decreased by insulin sensitizer rosiglitazone (Barzilai & Gupta, 1999; Steppan et al., 2001).

Surgically generated rat models in which different fat pads are removed (VF, subcutaneous fat, or both) allow further characterization of the significance of each fat depot. These surgical models have provided insight into the role of VF on insulin resistance and glucose intolerance in aging (Gabriely et al., 2002a). The specific role of VF in insulin resistance is highlighted in the model in which VF was surgically removed. Selective surgical removal of VF alters the natural history of glucose intolerance and diabetes of Zucker rats. Although CR results in a proportional decrease in all VF depots, the surgical intervention decreased specifically the epididymal and perinephric fat. This model suggests that

decreased VF could largely account for the beneficial metabolic effects of chronic CR. However, the relative contribution of the reduction in mass of mesenteric, epididymal, and perinephric fat depots in mediating CR effects was not quantified (Gabriely et al., 2002a). VF seems to play a causative role in peripheral and hepatic insulin resistance of aging. Gabriely and colleagues (2002a) showed that the ability of insulin to suppress endogenous glucose production (EGP) was significantly improved by removal of VF in rats. Still, there is the question of how VF induces insulin resistance. Although FFA was suggested as the mediator of hepatic insulin resistance through the increase in portal vein FFA level (Barzilai et al., 1999a), the models previously described had unchanged levels of venous and portal FFA levels. In addition, the perinephric and epididymal fat pads are drained by venous route, questioning whether portal FFA levels are involved in VF-induced insulin resistance. One possible explanation is that fat-derived peptides modulate insulin action, and by removal of VF, the role of these peptides decreases significantly (Gabriely & Barzilai, 2001).

Thus, aging-associated insulin resistance is determined to a large extent by the changes in body composition. Increase in fat mass and visceral fat significantly impairs insulin action. Exercise and caloric restriction exert beneficial effects, in part by favorable changes in body composition.

C. Changes on Insulin Secretion in Aging

Many studies on insulin function during aging suggest that there are defects in insulin secretion, action, and clearance (Chang & Halter, 2003). As in the younger age group, decreased physical activity and increased adiposity impair insulin sensitivity in the elderly, which is initially compensated by an increase in insulin secretion (Halter, 1995). However, the appearance of impaired glucose tolerance and type 2 diabetes suggests that adequate insulin secretion cannot be maintained over a period of time. Thus, relative insulin secretory defects in the presence of insulin resistance may contribute to the increased incidence of age-related glucose intolerance and diabetes (Muzumdar et al., 2004).

Oral glucose tolerance tests (GTTs) have been used to assess insulin response in aging; however, as the relative role of insulin resistance, ß-cell function, and gastrointestinal and neural factors cannot be deduced from these studies, they do not provide clear evidence that aging per se decreases insulin secretion (Chang & Halter, 2003; Gumbiner et al., 1989). Age-related decrease in insulin response has been demonstrated with intravenous GTT, suggesting impaired ß-cell function (Chen et al., 1985; Kahn et al., 1990). A clinical study utilizing a mixed meal and an intravenous injection of glucose demonstrated that age-related diminution in insulin secretion contributes to the glucose intolerance in the elderly (Basu et al., 2003). Although some studies have shown impairment in ß-cell function with aging (Fritsche et al., 2002), others have shown no differences in insulin secretion between young and old subjects (Bourey et al., 1993; Elahi et al., 1993).

Impaired insulin sensitivity is usually associated with a compensatory increase in insulin secretion (Chang & Halter, 2003) under basal and certain stimulated conditions. The newly proposed term *glucose allostasis* describes the slightly higher glucose levels, albeit within the normal range, in insulin-resistant states that continue to drive ß-cells to produce higher levels of insulin (Stumvoll et al., 2003). With aging, there is a decline in insulin action, and this has been demonstrated under euglycemic-hyperinsuline-

mic clamp conditions (DeFronzo, 1979). This decrease in insulin sensitivity is associated with a compensatory increase in insulin secretion. The ability to maintain insulin secretion, commensurate with the degree of insulin resistance, is maintained during a short physiologic stimulation; however, a more prolonged stimulation led to a decrease in insulin secretion (Muzumdar et al., 2004) in aging animals. In aging animals, a decline in insulin secretion can be demonstrated not in years but in just a few hours of stimulation, either by increasing the duration of the clamp or by increasing the glucose stimuli (Cases et al., 2001; Muzumdar et al., 2003; Zawich et al., 1990). Because insulin clearance may be decreased in aging (Fink et al., 1985; Minaker et al., 1982), lower insulin levels seen in old rats may underestimate the degree of the defect in insulin secretion. This is because there could be a falsely higher level of insulin in circulation than what is truly being secreted by the pancreas. In addition, parallel changes in C-peptide suggest a defect in insulin secretion. In light of a functional decrease in insulin secretion with aging, it is rather interesting that islet number, islet size, and secretory granules are actually increased in old Sprague-Dawley rats compared with young animals (Adelman, 1989; E. Reaven et al., 1983). Despite the increased size of the islets, release of insulin in response to glucose is decreased in old age *in vitro* (E. P. Reaven et al., 1979,1981, 1987; C. Reaven et al., 1983). This functional defect is demonstrable in both sexes and across strains of rats and is independent of body weight, although the pancreas of old males has more islet tissue coupled with more impaired secretion (E. P. Reaven et al., 1987). An impaired stimulation-secretion coupling has been demonstrated in the ß-cells of aging rats in response to glucose and arginine (Inoue et al., 1997).

A hyperbolic relationship between insulin action and insulin secretion has been demonstrated in many studies in humans through the use of a variety of techniques (Kahn *et al.*, 1993). Weyer and colleagues (1999) have shown that Pima Indians with increasing insulin resistance, when compensated, move on the hyperbolic curve, increasing insulin secretion capacity with time. Studies have also shown that subjects who eventually developed type 2 diabetes with time had declines in insulin secretion and moved "off the curve" (Weyer *et al.*, 1999). Inherent defects in insulin secretion with aging, when superimposed on increased insulin requirements, may contribute to the higher risk for abnormal glucose tolerance in old age. This is corroborated by a study in elderly humans using mixed-meal challenge and intravenous glucose infusion that showed a decrease in both insulin secretion and insulin action with aging, suggesting that the effect on insulin secretion is independent of the effects on insulin action (Basu *et al.*, 2003).

Interestingly, the defect in insulin secretion in old age appears to be specific to glucose. Additional stimulation with FFAs seems to be necessary to elicit a higher insulin response. FFAs are potent insulin secretagogues and augment insulin release only in the presence of glucose (Beysen *et al.*, 2002; Chalkley *et al.*, 1998), and this effect may be mediated through an increase in cytoplasmic long-chain acyl CoA (Deeney *et al.*, 2000; Prentki *et al.*, 1997).

Therefore, aging is associated with not only impaired insulin action, but also impaired insulin secretion, which contributes to the increased risk of insulin resistance, type 2 diabetes, and metabolic syndrome.

III. Conclusions

Alterations of fat distribution and carbohydrate metabolism seem to be a sine qua non feature of aging. These changes of metabolism are unfavorable, with an old age haunted by obesity, insulin resistance, diabetes mellitus, hyperlipidemia and other diseases. Changes in the amount and distribution of fat trigger an array of metabolic disturbances that ultimately alter insulin action, with terrible consequences. Animal models have provided insight into this chain of events. Further studies will be necessary to clearly identify the molecular mechanisms behind these metabolic changes and to eventually apply the new knowledge toward a healthy and enjoyable long life in humans.

References

Adelman, R. C. (1989). Secretion of insulin during aging. *Journal of the American Geriatric Society*, 37, 983–990.

Allison, D. B., Fontaine, K. R., Manson, J. E., Stevens, J., & VanItallie, T. B. (1999). Annual deaths attributable to obesity in the United States. *Journal of the American Medical Association*, 282, 1530–1538.

Anantharaju, A., Feller, A., & Chedid, A. (2002). Aging liver. *Gerontology*, 48, 343–353.

Anderson, L. A., McTernan, P. G., Barnett, A. H., & Kumar, S. (2001). The effects of androgens and estrogens on preadipocyte proliferation in human adipose tissue: influence of gender and site. *Journal of Clinical Endocrinology and Metabolism*, 86(10), 5045–5051.

Andres, R., Bierman, E. L., & Hazzard, W. R. (1985). *Principles of geriatric medicine.* New York: McGraw-Hill.

Atzmon, G., Yang, X. M., Muzumdar, R., Ma, X. H., Gabriely, I., & Barzilai, N. (2002). Differential gene expression between visceral and subcutaneous fat depot. *Hormone and Metabolic Research*, 34, 622–628.

Barnett, J. B., Woods, M. N., Rosner, B., McCormack, C., Longcope, C., Houser, R. F. Jr., & Gorbach, S. L. (2001). Sex hormone levels in premenopausal African-American women with upper and lower body fat phenotypes. *Nutrition and Cancer*, 41(1–2), 47–56.

Barzilai, N., & Gabriely, I. (2001). The role of fat depletion in the biological benefits of caloric restriction. *Journal of Nutrition*, 131, 903S–906S.

Barzilai, N., & Gabriely, I. (2002). Effect of age on the emergence of insulin resistance. In B. Hansen & E. Shafrir (Eds.), *Insulin resistance and insulin resistance syndrome* (1st ed., pp. 337–348). New York: Taylor & Francis.

Barzilai, N., & Gupta, G. (1999). Revisiting the role of fat mass in the life extension induced by caloric restriction. Journals of Gerontology *Series A Biological Sciences and Medical Sciences*, 54(3), B89–B96.

Barzilai, N., Banerjee, S., Hawkins, M., Chen, W., & Rossetti, L. (1998). Caloric restriction reverses hepatic insulin resistance in aging rats by decreasing visceral fat. *Journal of Clinical Investigation*, 101, 1353–1361.

Barzilai, N., She, L., Liu, L., Wang, J., Hu, M., Vuguin, P., & Rossetti, L. (1999). Decreased visceral adiposity account for leptin effect on hepatic but not peripheral insulin action. *American Journal of Physiology*, 277, E291–E298.

Barzilai, N., Wang, J., Massilon, D., Vuguin, P., Hawkins, M., & Rossetti, L. (1997). Leptin selectively decreases visceral adiposity and enhances insulin action. *Journal of Clinical Investigation*, 100, 3105–3110.

Basu, R., Breda, E., Oberg, A. L., Powell, C. C., Dalla Man, C., Basu, A., Vittone, J. L., Klee, G. G., Arora, P., Jensen, M. D., Toffolo, G., Cobelli, C., & Rizza, A. (2003). Mechanisms of age-associated deterioration in glucose tolerance: contribution of alterations in insulin secretion, action, and clearance. *Diabetes*, 52, 1738–1748.

Beysen, C., Karpe, F., Fielding, B. A., Clark, A., Levy, C., & Frayn, K. N. (2002). Interaction between specific fatty acids, GLP-1 and insulin secretion in humans. *Diabetologia*, 45, 1533–1541.

Bjorbaek, C., & Kahn B. B. (2004). Leptin signaling in the central nervous system and the periphery. *Recent Progress in Hormone Research*, 59, 305–331.

Bjorntrop, P. (1990). Portal adipose tissue as a generator of risk factors for cardiovascular disease and diabetes. *Arteriosclerosis*, 10, 493–496.

Bjorntrop, P. (1991). Metabolic implications of body fat distribution. *Diabetes Care*, 14, 1132–1143.

Blüher, M., Kahn, B., & Kahn, R. (2003). Extended longevity in mice lacking the insulin receptor in adipose tissue. *Science*, 299, 572–574.

Blüher, M., Michael, M. D., Peroni, O. D., Ueki, K., Carter, N., Kahn, B., & Kahn, R. (2002). Adipose tissue selective insulin receptor knockout protects against obesity and obesity-related glucose intolerance. *Developmental Cell*, 3, 25–38.

Bourey, R. E., Kohrt, W. M., Kirwan, J. P., Staten, M. A., King, D. S., & Holloszy, J. O. (1993). Relationship between glucose tolerance and glucose-stimulated insulin response in 65-year olds. *Journal of Gerontology*, 48, M122–M127.

Boyko, E. J., Fujimoto, W. Y., Leonetti, D. L., & Newell-Morris, L. (2000). Visceral adiposity and risk of type 2 diabetes: a prospective study among Japanese Americans. *Diabetes Care*, 23, 465–471.

Brochu, M., Tchernof, A., Turner, A. N., Ades, P. A., & Poehlman, E. T. (2003). Is there a threshold of visceral fat loss that improves the metabolic profile in obese postmenopausal women? *Metabolism*, 52, 599–604.

Brüning, J. C., Gautam, D., Burks, D. J., Gillette, J., Schubert, M., Orban, P. C., Klein, R., Krone, W., Muller-Wieland, D., & Kahn, C. R. (2000). Role of brain insulin receptor in control of body weight and reproduction. *Science*, 289, 2122–2125.

Brüning, J. C., Michael, M. D., Winnay, J. N., Hayashi, T., Hörsch, D., Accili, D., Goodyear, L. J., & Kahn, R. (1998). A muscle-specific insulin receptor knockout exhibits features of the metabolic syndrome of NIDDM without altering glucose tolerance. *Molecular Cell*, 3, 559–569.

Calle, E. E., Thun, M. J., Petrelli, J. M., Rodriguez, C., & Heath, C. W. Jr. (1999). Body-mass index and mortality in a prospective cohort of US adults. *New England Journal of Medicine*, 341, 1097–1105.

Carr, D. B., Utzschneider, K. M., Hull, R. L., Kodama, K., Retzlaff, B. M., Brunzell, J. D., Shofer, J. B., Fish, B. E., Knopp, R. H., & Kahn, S. E. (2004). Intra-abdominal fat is a major determinant of the National Cholesterol Education Program Adult Treatment Panel III criteria for the metabolic syndrome. *Diabetes*, 53, 2087–2094.

Cases, J. A., Gabriely, I., Ma, X. H., Yang, X. M., Michaeli, T., Fleischer, N., Rossetti, L.,

& Barzilai, N. (2001). Physiologic increase in plasma leptin markedly inhibits insulin secretion *in vivo*. *Diabetes*, 50, 348–352.

Caterson, I. D., & Gill, T. P. (2002). Obesity: epidemiology and possible prevention. *Best Practice & Research Clinical Endocrinology & Metabolism*, 16(4), 595–610.

Chalkley, S. M., Kraegen, E. W., Furler, S. M., Campbell, L. V., & Chisholm, D. J. (1998). NEFA elevation during a hyperglycemic clamp enhances insulin secretion. *Diabetic Medicine*, 15, 327–333.

Chang, A. M., & Halter, J. B. (2003). Aging and insulin secretion. *American Journal of Physiology-Endocrinology and Metabolism*, 284, E7–E12.

Chen, M., Bergman, R. N., Pacini, G., & Porte, D. (1985). Pathogenesis of age-related glucose intolerance in man: Insulin resistance and decreased beta cell function. *Journal of Clinical Endocrinology and Metabolism*, 60, 13–20.

Chua, S. C., Chung, W. K., Wu-Peng, X. S., Zhang, Y., Liu, S. M., Tartaglia, L., & Leibel, R. L. (1996). Phenotypes of mouse diabetes and rat fatty due to mutations in the OB (leptin) receptor. *Science*, 271, 994–996.

Chumlea, W. C., Rhyne, R. L., Garry, P. G., & Hunt, W. C. (1989). Changes in anthropometric indices of body composition with age in a healthy elderly population. *American Journal of Human Biology*, 1, 457–462.

Coleman, D. L. (1978). Obese and diabetes: two mutant genes causing diabetes-obesity syndromes in mice. *Diabetologia*, 14, 141–148.

Combs, T. P., Berg, A. H., Obici, S., Scherer, P. E., & Rossetti, L. (2001) Endogenous glucose production is inhibited by the adipose-derived protein Acrp30. *Journal of Clinical Investigation*, 108, 1875–1881.

Considine, R. V., Sinha, M. K., Heiman, A., Kriauciunas, T. W., Stephens, M. R., Nyce, J. P., Ohannesian, C. C., Marco, L. J., McKee, T., Bauer, T. L., & Caro, J. F. (1996). Serum immunoreactive-leptin concentrations in normal-weight and obese humans. *New England Journal of Medicine*, 334, 292–295.

Corpas, E., Harman, S. M., & Blackman, M. R. (1993). Human growth hormone and human aging. *Endocrine Reviews*, 14, 20–39.

Das, M., Gabriely, I., & Barzilai, N. (2004). Caloric restriction, body fat and aging in experimental models. *Obesity Reviews*, 5(1), 13–19.

de Boer, H., Blok, G. J., Voerman, B., Derriks, P., & van der Veen, E. (1996). Changes in subcutaneous and visceral fat mass during growth hormone replacement therapy in adult men. *International Journal of Obesity Related Metabolic Disorders*, 20(6), 580–587.

Deeney, J. T., Gromada, J., Hoy, M., Olsen, H. L., Rhodes, C. J., Prentki, M., Bergren, P. O., & Corkey, B. E. (2000). Acute stimulation with long chain acyl-coA enhances exocytosis in insulin-secreting cells (HIT T-15 and NMRI beta-cells). *Journal of Biological Chemistry*, 275, 9363–9368.

DeFronzo, R. A. (1979). Glucose intolerance and aging: evidence for tissue insensitivity to insulin. *Diabetes*, 28, 1095–1101.

Elahi, D., Muller, D. C., McAloon-Dyke, M., Tobin, J. D., & Andres, R. (1993). The effect of age on insulin response and glucose utilization during four hyperglycemic plateaus. *Experimental Gerontology*, 28, 393–409.

Elia, M. (2001). Obesity in the elderly. *Obesity Research*, 9 (Suppl. 4), 244S–248S.

Enzi, G., Gasparo, M., Binodetti, P. R., Fiore, D., Semisa, M., & Zurlo, F. (1986). Subcutaneous and visceral fat distribution according to sex, age and overweight, evaluated by computed tomography. *American Journal of Clinical Nutrition*, 44, 739–746.

Ferrannini, E., Vichi, S., Beck-Nielsen, H., Laakso, M., Paolisso, G., & Smith, U. (1996). Insulin action and age. *Diabetes*, 45, 947–953.

Fink, R. I., Revers, R. R., Kolterman, O. G., & Olefsky, J. M. (1985). The metabolic clearance of insulin and the feedback inhibition of insulin secretion are altered with aging. *Diabetes*, 34, 275–280.

Flegal, K. M., Carroll, M. D., Ogden, C. L., & Johnson, C. L. (2002). Prevalence and trends in obesity among US adults, 1999–2000. *Journal of the American Medical Association*, 288, 1723–1727.

Folsom, A. R., Kushi, L. H., Anderson, K. E., Mink, P. J., Olson, J. E., Hong, C. P., Sellers, T. A., Lazovich, D., & Prineas, R. J. (2000). Associations of general and abdominal obesity with multiple health outcomes in older women: the Iowa Women's Health Study. *Archives of Internal Medicine*, 160, 2117–2128.

Folsom, A. R., Sellers, T. A., Hong, C. P., Cerhan, J. R., & Potter, J. D. (1993). Body fat distribution and 5-year risk of death in older women. *Journal of the American Medical Association*, 269, 483–487.

Fraze, E., Chlou, M., Chen, Y., & Reaven, G. M. (1987). Age related changes in postprandial plasma glucose, insulin, and FFA concentrations in non-diabetic individuals. *Journal of the American Geriatric Society*, 35, 212–218.

Friedman, J. M., & Halaas, J. L. (1998). Leptin and the regulation of body weight in mammals. *Nature*, 395, 763–770.

Fritsche, A., Madaus, A., Stefan, N., Tschritter, O., Maerker, E., Teigeler, A., Haring, H., & Stumvol, M. (2002). Relationships among age, proinsulin conversion, and ß-cell function in nondiabetic humans. *Diabetes*, 51 (Suppl. 1), S234–S239.

Fujimoto, W. Y., Bergstrom, R. W., Boyko, E. J., Chen, K. W., Leonetti, D. L., Newell-Morris, L., Shofer, J. B., & Wahl, P. W. (1999). Visceral adiposity and incident coronary heart disease in Japanese-American men. The 10-year follow-up results of the Seattle Japanese-American Community Diabetes Study. *Diabetes Care*, 22, 1808–1812.

Gabriely, I., & Barzilai, N. (2001). The role of fat cell derived peptides in age-related metabolic alterations. *Mechanisms of Ageing and Development*, 122, 1565–1576.

Gabriely, I., Ma, X. H., Yang, X. M., Atzmon, G., Rajala, M. W., Berg, A. H., Scherer, P., Rossetti, L., & Barzilai, N. (2002a). Removal of visceral fat prevents insulin resistance and glucose intolerance of aging: an adipokine-mediated process? *Diabetes*, 51, 2951–2958.

Gabriely, I., Ma, X. H., Yang, X. M., Rossetti, L., & Barzilai, N. (2002b). Leptin resistance during aging is independent of fat mass. *Diabetes*, 51(4), 1016–1021.

Gumbiner, B., Polonsky, K. S., Beltz, W. F., Wallave, P., Bretchel, G., & Fink, R. I. (1989). Effects of aging on insulin secretion. *Diabetes*, 38, 1549–1556.

Gupta, G., Cases, J. A., She, L., Ma, X. H., Yang, X. M., Hu, M., Wu, J., Rossetti, L., & Barzilai, N. (2000a). Ability of insulin to modulate hepatic glucose production in aging rats is impaired by fat accumulation. *American Journal of Physiology-Endocrinology and Metabolism*, 278, E985–E991.

Gupta, G., She, L., Ma, X. H., Yang, X. M., Hu, M., Cases, J. A., Vuguin, P., Rossetti, L., & Barzilai, N. (2000b). Aging does not contribute to the decline in insulin action on storage of muscle glycogen in rats. *American Journal of Physiology. Regulatory Integrative Comparative Physiology*, 278, R111–R117.

Halter, J. B. (1995). Carbohydrate metabolism. In J. Masoro (Ed.), *Handbook of physiology: aging* (pp. 119–145). Bethesda, MD: American Physiology Society.

Hansen, T. B., Vahl, N., Jorgensen, J. O., Christiansen, J. S., & Hagen, C. (1995). Whole body and regional soft tissue changes in growth hormone deficient adults after one year of growth hormone treatment: a double-blind, randomized, placebo-controlled study. *Clinical Endocrinology (Oxf)*, 43(6), 689–696.

Harris, M. I., Flegal, K. M., Cowie, C. C., Eberhardt, M. S., Goldstein, D. E., Little, R. R., Wiedmeyer, H. M., & Byrd-Holt, D. D. (1998). Prevalence of diabetes, impaired fasting glucose, and impaired glucose tolerance in U.S. adults. The Third National Health and Nutrition Examination Survey, 1988–1994. *Diabetes Care*, 21(4), 475–476.

Harrison, D. E., Archer, J. R., & Astle, C. M. (1984). Effects of food restriction on aging: separation of food intake and adiposity. *Proceedings of the National Academy of Sciences of the USA*, 81(6), 1835–1838.

Hayashi, T., Boyko, E. J., Leonetti, D. L., McNeely, M. J., Newell-Morris, L., Kahn, S. E., & Fujimoto, W. Y. (2003). Visceral adiposity and the risk of impaired glucose tolerance: a prospective study among Japanese Americans. *Diabetes Care*, 26, 650–655.

Henry, C. J. (2000). Mechanisms of changes in basal metabolism during ageing. *European Journal of Clinical Nutrition*, 54 (Suppl. 3), S77–S91.

Hofmann, C., Lorenz, K., Braithwaite, S. S., Colca, J. R., Palazuk, B. J., & Hotamisliqil, G. S. (1994). Altered gene expression for tumor necrosis factor-alpha and its receptors during drug and dietary modulation of insulin resistance. *Endocrinology*, 134, 264–270.

Holloszy, J. O. (1992). Exercise and food restriction in rats. *Journal of Nutrition*, 122, 774–777.

Holloszy, J. O. (1993). Exercise increases average longevity of female rats despite increased food intake and no growth retardation. *Journal of Gerontology*, 48, B97–B100.

Inoue, K., Norgren, S., Luthman, H., Moller, C., & Grill, V. (1997). B cells of aging rats: impaired stimulus-secretion coupling but normal susceptibility to adverse effects of a diabetic state. *Metabolism*, 46, 242–246.

Kahn, S. E., Larson, V .J., Beard, J. C., Cain, K. C., & Abrass, I. B. (1990). Effect of exercise on insulin action, glucose tolerance and insulin secretion in aging. *American Journal of Physiology*, 258, E937–E943.

Kahn, S. E., Prigeo, R. L., McCulloch, D. K., Boyko, E. J., Bergman, R. N., Schwartz, M. W., Neifing, J. L., Ward, W. K., Beard, J. C., Palmer, J. P., & Porte, D. Jr. (1993). Quantification of the relationship between insulin sensitivity and ß-cell function in human subjects. Evidence for a hyperbolic function. *Diabetes*, 42, 1663–1672.

Kanai, H., Tokunaga, K., Fujioka, S., Yamashita, S., Kameda-Takemura, K. K., & Matsuzawa, Y. (1996). Decrease in intra-abdominal visceral fat may reduce blood pressure in obese hypertensive women. *Hypertension*, 27, 125–129.

Kershaw, E. E., & Flier, J. S. (2004). Adipose tissue as an endocrine organ. *Journal of Clinical Endocrinology & Metabolism*, 89(6), 2548–2556.

Kissebah, A. H. (1991). Insulin resistance in visceral obesity. *International Journal of Obesity*, 15, 109–115.

Kissebah, A. H. (1996). Intra-abdominal fat: it is a major factor in developing diabetes and coronary artery disease? *Diabetes Research and Clinical Practice*, (Suppl.), 25–30.

Lamarche, B., Lemieux, S., Dagenais, G. R., & Despres, J. P. (1998). Visceral obesity and the risk of ischaemic heart disease: insights from the Quebec Cardiovascular Study. *Growth Hormone & IGF Research*, 8 (Suppl. B), 1–8.

Larson, B. (1992). Regional obesity as a health hazard in men-prospective studies. *Acta Medica*, 723, 45–51.

Lawrence, J. C. Jr., Colvin, J., Cartee, G. D., & Holloszy, J. O. (1989). Effects of aging and exercise on insulin action in rat adipocytes are correlated with changes in fat cell volume. *Journal of Gerontology*, 44(4), B88–B92.

Lee, I. M., Paffenbarger, R. S. Jr., & Hennekens, C. H. (1997). Physical activity, physical fitness and longevity. *Aging (Milano)*, 9(1–2), 2–11.

Loland, N. W. (2004). Exercise, health, and aging. *Journal of Aging and Physical Activity*, 12(2), 170–184.

Ma, X. H., Muzumdar, R., Yang, X. M., Gabriely, I., Berger, R., & Barzilai, N. (2002). Aging is associated with resistance to effects of Leptin on fat distribution and insulin action. *Journal of Gerontology: Biological Science*, 57, B225–B231.

Masoro, E. J. (1996). Possible mechanisms underlying the antiaging actions of caloric restriction. *Toxicologic Pathology*, 24, 738–741.

Masoro, E. J. (2000). Caloric restriction and aging: an update. *Experimental Gerontology*, 35(3), 299–305.

Masoro, E. J. (2003). A forum for commentaries on recent publications. FIRKO mouse report: important new model but questionable interpretation. *Journals of Gerontology Series A: Biological Sciences and Medical Sciences*, 58, B871–B872.

Masoro, E. J., & Austad, S. N. (1996). The evolution of the antiaging action of dietary restriction: a hypothesis. *Journals of Gerontology: Series A Biological Science and Medical Sciences*, 51A, B387–B391.

Mattison, J. A., Lane, M. A., Roth, G. S., & Ingram, D. K. (2003). Calorie restriction in rhesus monkeys. *Experimental Gerontology*, 38(1–2), 35–46.

McCay, C., Crowell, M., & Maynard, L. (1935). The effect of retarded growth upon the length of life and upon ultimate size. *Journal of Nutrition*, 10, 63–79.

Michael, M. D., Kulkarni R. N., Postic, C., Previs, S. F., Shulman, G. I., Magnuson, M. A., & Kahn, C. R. (2000). Loss of insulin signaling in hepatocytes leads to severe insulin resistance and progressive hepatic dysfunction. *Molecular Cell*, 6(1), 87–97.

Minaker, K. J., Rowe, J. W., Tonino, R., & Plotta, J. A. (1982). Influence of age on clearance of insulin in man. *Diabetes*, 31, 851–855.

Mitchell, D., Haan, M. N., Steinberg, F. M., & Visser, M. (2003). Body composition in the elderly: the influence of nutritional factors and physical activity. *Journal of Nutrition, Health and Aging*, 7(3), 130–139.

Miyazaki, Y., Mahankali, A., Matsuda, M., Mahankali, S., Hardies, J., Cusi, K., Mandarino, L. J., & DeFronzo, R. A. (2002). Effect of pioglitazone on abdominal fat distribution and insulin sensitivity in type 2 diabetic patients. *Journal of Clinical Endocrinology and Metabolism*, 87(6), 2784–2791.

Munzer, T., Harman, S. M., Hees, P., Shapiro, E., Christmas, C., Bellantoni, M. F., Stevens, T. E., O'Connor, K. G., Pabst, K. M., St. Clair, C., Sorkin, J. D., & Blackman, M. R. (2001). Effects of GH and/or sex steroid administration on abdominal subcutaneous and visceral fat in healthy aged women and men. *Journal of Clinical Endocrinology and Metabolism*, 86(8), 3604–3610.

Muzumdar, R., Ma, X., Atzmon, G., Vuguin, P., Yang, X., & Barzilai, N. (2004). Decrease in glucose-stimulated insulin secretion with aging is independent of insulin action. *Diabetes*, 53(2), 441–446.

Muzumdar, R., Ma, X., Yang, X., Atzmon, G., Bernstein, J., Karkanias, G., & Barzilai, N. (2003). Physiologic effect of leptin on insulin secretion is mediated mainly through central mechanisms. *FASEB Journal*, J17, 1130–1132.

Nass, R., & Thorner, M. O. (2002). Impact of the GH-cortisol ratio on the age-dependent changes in body composition. *Growth Hormone & IGF Research*, 12, 147–161.

National Task Force on the Prevention and Treatment of Obesity. (2000). Overweight, obesity, and health risk. *Archives of Internal Medicine*, 160, 898–904.

Novelli, M., Pocai, A., Skalicky, M., Viidik, A., Bergamini, E., & Masiello, P. (2004). Effects of life-long exercise on circulating free fatty acids and muscle triglyceride content in ageing rats. *Experimental Gerontology*, 39, 1333–1340.

O'Rahilly, S., Yeo, G. S., & Farooqi, I. S. (2004). Melanocortin receptors weigh in. *Nature Medicine*, 10, 351–352.

Peiris, A. N., Struve, M. F., Mueller, R. A., Lee, M. B., & Kissebah, A. H. (1988). Glucose metabolism in obesity: influence of body fat distribution. *Journal of Clinical Endocrinology and Metabolism*, 67, 760–767.

Poehlman, E. T., Turturro, A., Bodkin, N., Cefalu, W., Heymsfield, S., Holloszy, J., & Kemnitz, J. (2001). Caloric restriction mimetics: physical activity and body composition changes. *Journals of Gerontology: Series A*, 56A, 45–54.

Prentki, M., Tornheim, K., & Corkey, B. (1997). Signal transduction mechanisms in nutrient-induced insulin secretion. *Diabetologia*, 40, S32–S41.

Prineas, R. J., Folsom, A. R., & Kaye, S. A. (1993). Central adiposity and increased risk of coronary artery disease mortality in older women. *Annals of Epidemiology*, 3, 35–41.

Rasmussen, M. H., Frystyk, J., Andersen, T., Breum, L., Christiansen, J. S., & Hilsted, J. (1994). The impact of obesity, fat distribution, and energy restriction on insulin-like growth factor-1 (IGF-1), IGF-binding protein-3, insulin, and growth hormone. *Metabolism*, 43(3), 315–319.

Reaven, C., Curry, D., Moore, J., & Reaven, G. (1983). Effects of age and environment factors on insulin release from perifused pancreas of the rats. *Journal of Clinical Investigation*, 71, 345–350.

Reaven, E., Wright, D., Solomon, R., Ho, H., & Reaven, G. M. (1983). Effect of age and diet on insulin secretion and insulin action in the rat. *Diabetes*, 32, 175–180.

Reaven, E. P., & Reaven, G. M.(1981). Structure and function changes in the endocrine pancreas of aging rats with reference to the modulating effects of exercise and caloric restriction. *Journal of Clinical Investigation*, 68, 75–84.

Reaven, E. P., Curry, D. L., & Reaven, G. M. (1987). Effect of age and sex on rat endocrine pancreas. *Diabetes*, 36, 1397–1400.

Reaven, E. P., Gold, G., & Reaven, G. M. (1979) Effect of age on glucose stimulated insulin release by the beta cell of the rat. *Journal of Clinical Investigation*, 64, 591–599.

Reaven, G. M. (1988). Role of insulin resistance in human disease (Banting lecture). *Diabetes*, 37, 1595–1607.

Ross, M., & Bras, G. (1975). Food preference and length of life. *Science*, 190, 165–167.

Rowe, J. W., Minaker, K. L., Plotta, J. A., & Flier, J. S. (1993). Characterization of the insulin resistance in aging. *Journal of Clinical Investigation*, 71, 1523–1535.

Russell, J. C., Epling, W. F., Pierce, D., Amy, R. M., & Boer, D. P. (1987). Induction of voluntary prolonged running by rats. *Journal of Applied Physiology*, 63, 2549–2553.

Sohal, R. S., & Weindruch, R. (1996). Oxidative stress, caloric restriction, and aging. *Science*, 273, 59–63.

Steppan, C. M., Bailey, S. T., Bhat, S., Brown, E. J., Banerjee, R. R. Wright, C. M., Patel, H. R., Ahima, R. S., & Lazar, M. A. (2001). The hormone resistin links obesity to diabetes. *Nature*, 409, 307–312.

St-Pierre, J., Lemieux, I., Vohl, M. C., Perron, P., Tremblay, G., Despres, J. P., Gaudet, D. (2002). Contribution of abdominal obesity and hypertriglyceridemia to impaired fasting glucose and coronary artery disease. *American Journal of Cardiology*, 90, 15–18.

Stumvoll, M., Tataranni, P. A., Stefan, N., Vozarova, B., & Bogardus, C. (2003). Glucose allostasis. *Diabetes*, 52, 903–909.

Tschöp, M., & Heiman, M. L. (2001). Rodent obesity models: an overview. Experimental and Clinical Endocrinology and Diabetes, 109, 307–319.

Wang, J., Liu, R., Liu, L., Chowdhury, R., Barzilai, N., Tan, J., & Rossetti, L. (1999). The effect of leptin on Lep expression is tissue-specific and nutritionally regulated. *Nature Medicine*, 5, 895–899.

Weyer, C., Bogardus, C., Mott, D. M., & Pratey, R. E. (1999). The natural history of insulin secretory dysfunction and insulin resistance in the pathogenesis of type 2 diabetes mellitus. *Journal of Clinical Investigation*, 104, 787–794.

Williamson, D. F., Thompson, J. T., Thun, M., Flanders, D., Pamuk, E., & Byers, E. (2000). Intentional weight loss and mortality among overweight individuals with diabetes. *Diabetes Care*, 23, 1499–1504.

Yamashita, T., Murakami, T., Iida, M., Kuwajima, M., & Shima, K. (1997). Leptin receptor of Zucker fatty rat performs reduced signal transduction. *Diabetes*, 46, 1077–1080.

Zawich, W. S., Zawich, K. C., Shulman, G. I., & Rossetti, L. (1990). Chronic *in vivo* hyperglycemia impairs phosphoinositide hydrolysis and insulin release in isolated perfused rat islets. *Endocrinology*, 126, 253–260.

Chapter 19

Growth and Aging: Why Do Big Dogs Die Young?

Richard A. Miller and Steven N. Austad

I. Introduction

Much of the published literature on aging has emerged from a research strategy in which young and old individuals are compared in some way. Fifty years ago, the comparison involved physiological properties, such as responses to immunization or to a glucose challenge, or neural conduction speed, or glomerular filtration rates. Over the next few decades, the comparisons began to involve enzyme levels, then mRNA levels one or two at a time, and then more recently mRNA levels evaluated wholesale. We now have at our disposal a vast literature documenting the effects of aging on cell, tissue, and system function in many kinds of animals.

This chapter focuses on a different research design, one that compares young individuals to try to see what distinguishes animals, within a species, that age at different rates. In particular, we will review evidence for or against the hypothesis that slow growth rates in early life produce, or are at least associ-

ated with, delayed aging and extended longevity.

II. Body Size and Aging in Dogs

The strongest evidence in favor of the idea linking early life growth rate and aging comes from analysis of size and mean life span among dog breeds. Figure 19.1A presents a data set accumulated by Norman Wolf and his colleagues (Li *et al.*, 1996). The life-span data were derived from Purdue University's Veterinary Medical Data Base, which compiles information on dogs treated at 20 American and two Canadian veterinary schools. This data set included information on age of death for 97 to >2,100 individuals in each of 17 stocks (=breeds), but only in "binned" format—that is, with age recorded only as within the intervals 4 to 7 years, 7 to 10 years, 10 to 15 years, and >15 years. Admittedly, this data set has its weaknesses. For instance, the collapsing of data from the longest-lived animals may underestimate the range of longevity

Handbook of the Biology of Aging, Sixth Edition

difference among stocks and does not allow analysis of maximum survival, often taken to be an important indicator of general aging rate. In addition, mortality statistics based on animals presented for care at specialized veterinary hospitals may not be fully representative of the larger population of pet dogs in American households or in other environments. Weight values were taken as the median of the range reported by the American Kennel Club as standard for each breed.

The squared correlation coefficient $R^2 = 0.56$ indicates that more than half of the life-span variation among breeds is explained by the factors—virtually all genetic—that modulate interbreed differences in body weight. The direction of causation here is unambiguous: dog breeders often select strongly for differences in body size to produce dogs with desired physical characteristics, rather than selecting for differences in life expectancy *per se*. Thus, the data suggest that the differences in life span among the dog breeds are unintended consequences of selective breeding for altered body size. Because body size represents the cumulative effects of growth

in utero, and in the postnatal and juvenile periods, the implication is that the timing of late-life illnesses, and thus life expectancy, can be dramatically altered by genes that affect early life growth processes. A second report (Patronek et al., 1997) included information from the same source about body weights and longevity of mixed-breed dogs. These data are shown in Figure 19.1B and show that there is a strong correlation between adult body weight and life span among dogs of mixed breed as well.

Another, independent analysis made use of data on 3,126 dogs developed through a questionnaire sent to British dog owners (Michell, 1999). Median survival was 12 years (with a mean value of 11 years), substantially higher than the ages seen in the Veterinary Medical Data Base (Li et al., 1996; Patronek et al., 1997), presumably reflecting a bias in selection of dogs that come to the attention of academic veterinary hospitals. In the British survey, 8 percent of the dogs lived longer than 15 years, and the longest-lived animal is said to have reached 22 years. The proportion of dogs dying of cancer ranged from 35 percent to

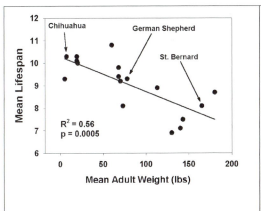 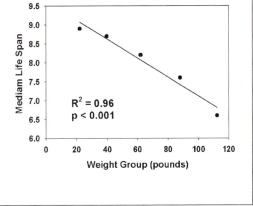

Figure 19.1 (A) Each symbol shows adult weight and life span for a different breed of dog. Three of the breeds are labeled with arrows. Data from Li and colleagues (1996). (B) Relationship between median life span and weight class for mixed-breed dogs, from Patronek and colleagues (1997). Weights are calculated as the midpoint of each of four intervals; dogs in the >100-pound class were assumed to have a median weight of 112 pounds.

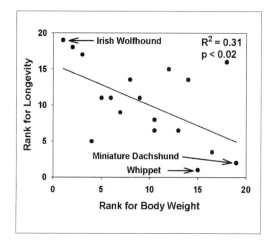

Figure 19.2 Small body size associated with longer life span among 19 breeds of dogs; data from each symbol represents data from a different breed.

50 percent, depending on sex and neutering status, with heart disease, kidney disease, and liver disease each accounting for 10 percent to 35 percent of the deaths to which a cause could be attributed. Figure 19.2 shows the relationship between rank of body weight and rank of longevity among 19 of the most common purebred breeds, using data derived from Michell (1999); the regression $R^2 = 0.31$ is significant at $p < 0.02$. Data from the British study also showed that within pairs of closely related breeds, such as springer versus cocker spaniels, miniature poodles versus standard poodles, whippets versus greyhounds, and miniature versus standard dachshunds, the smaller breed was typically longer lived, with one exception (equivalent longevity in standard versus miniature schnauzers). Thus, the association of small body size and longer life span is supported by two independent sets of data on purebred dogs as well as by the analysis of mixed-breed dogs (Patronek et al., 1997). The authors found no evidence for a relationship between breed life span and any cardiovascular parameter, such as heart rate or systolic or diastolic pressure.

The differences in longevity among dog breeds of different sizes seemingly

reflects not just survival *per se* but also real differences in aging rate in that multiple degenerative conditions and diseases appear earlier in larger breeds compared to smaller ones. Indeed, the age at which clinical veterinarians consider dogs to require "geriatric" care ranges from 6 to 9 years in giant breeds to 9 to 13 years in smaller breeds (Hoskins & McCurnin, 1997). As one example of the general trend for aging to track with body size, a large study of canine cataract found that among the six most common breeds examined, ranging in body mass from 6 kg to more than 30 kg, breed longevity (as measured in Michell, 1999) explained 55 percent of the variance in C_{50}, the age at which half the study population had developed detectable cataracts (Williams et al., 2004). Analysis of cataract risk in humans has also revealed increased risk in taller individuals (Schaumberg et al., 2000).

Generally speaking, large dogs differ from small dogs in growth and reproductive parameters as well as in aging rate. For instance, tiny breeds such as Boston Terriers or Chihuahuas may experience their first estrus as early as 5 months, although 6 to 7 months is more typical, whereas a giant breed such as an Irish Wolfhound may be 2 years old before first estrus. Age of puberty also varies by breed among male dogs, with small breeds generally reaching puberty earlier than large breeds (Johnston et al., 2001). It is also well documented that large breeds arrive at their adult body weight somewhat later than small breeds, such that a 7-kg Miniature Schnauzer will reach half of its adult body weight at 14 weeks of age and 99 percent of its adult body weight by 41 weeks, compared with a 67-kg English Mastiff that reaches those same growth points at 23 and 65 weeks, respectively (Hawthorne et al., 2004). In addition, large dog breeds are more fecund than small dogs. Litter size, which ranges between means of about 2 and 10, is highly correlated with dam body size ($r^2 = 0.89$) (Robinson, 1973). Neonate size also depends on dam size. Newborns of giant breeds can weigh six times as much as those of miniature breeds.

It is worth noting that the association between small body size and longer life span is contrary to the prediction of models that attribute long life span to lower metabolic rates. Smaller breeds of dogs, with relatively high area/volume ratios, must expend greater energy in maintaining body temperature and are thus expected to have higher than average metabolic demands, and indeed a comparison (Speakman *et al.*, 2003) among three breeds found 60 percent higher energy expenditure per kg lean body mass in the small, long-lived breed (Papillion) compared to the larger, short-lived breed (Great Dane).

There is relatively little information available about the mechanisms by which dog breeds differ in body size. Early work by Eigenmann showed a strong correlation between adult levels of circulating IGF-I and adult body size (see Figure 19.3). Even in a comparison among three closely related breeds (standard, miniature, and toy poodles) differences in body size were correlated with

variations in insulin-like growth factor-1 (IGF-I) levels in adult dogs, although these breeds did not differ in basal or stimulated growth hormone (GH) levels (Eigenmann *et al.*, 1984a). As for early life growth, a study of nursing puppies found that both growth rate and serum IGF-I levels were higher in Great Dane (giant breed) pups than in Beagles (medium-sized breed), and that IGF-I levels were 75 percent higher in the colostrums of the former breed compared with the latter (White *et al.*, 1999).

Somewhat confusingly, a later study (Favier *et al.*, 2001), which also compared beagles and Great Danes, focused on the post-weaning growth period from 6 to 24 weeks of age and found that these juvenile dogs of the two breeds did not differ in serum IGF-I or IGF-II levels at any age between 8 to 24 weeks, but that elevated levels of GH were characteristic of Great Danes. Furthermore, GH levels were elevated above average adult levels only up to 7 weeks of age in beagles, but were elevated above adult levels for at least 20 weeks in the Great Dane. It is not clear how to reconcile the apparent absence of IGF-I differences in this study with the major differences both in GH levels and in body weight gain trajectory, although the authors suggest that GH itself, rather than IGF-I or IGF-II, may be a primary regulator of growth in this breed.

III. Weight and Longevity in Mice

A. Selective Breeding for Body Weight

Several recent studies have addressed the question of whether the association between small body size and higher life expectancies in dogs represents a species-specific idiosyncrasy, or whether similar associations can be noted in mice. The first approach compared stocks of mice bred for differences in early life growth rate. Atchley and colleagues had produced 15 stocks of mice starting from

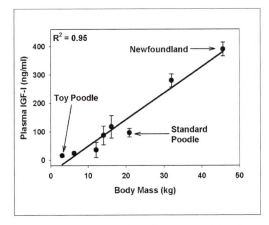

Figure 19.3 Relationship between adult body mass and plasma IGF-I levels in eight dog breeds. ($R^2 = 0.95$). Data from (Eigenmann *et al.*, 1984b; Eigenmann *et al.*, 1984c; Eigenmann *et al.*, 1988)

a single large population of genetically heterogeneous ICR mice. Three of the stocks were selected for slow rate of weight gain from birth to 10 days of age, and three others were selected for slow growth rate from 28 to 56 days; each of these six selection protocols produce mice that are relatively small as young adults. Six lines were selected in the opposite direction—that is, for rapid gain in body weight between 0 to 10 or between 28 to 56 days of age. In each case a "restricted selection index" was used, in which choice of parents for the next generation requires both differential weight gain over the chosen age interval as well as normal weight gain over the other age interval. In addition to these 12 selected stocks, three control stocks were produced in parallel, in which parents were selected at random without respect to weight gain trajectories.

Figure 19.4A shows the association between longevity and mean weight for each of the 15 stocks, regardless of cause of death. Stocks with the highest weight at 6 months tended to have shorter mean life span than mice in stocks that were smaller as young adults (Miller *et al.*, 2000a). Similar results were seen using data on weight measured at 91 days of age, or using peak body weight for each stock. Weight at 6 months was also a good predictor of maximal longevity ($R^2 = 0.54$, p $= 0.002$) among these 15 stocks. These

data thus suggest that genetic differences in body weight as early as 3 months of age are associated with dramatic differences in mean and maximal longevity not only in dogs, but also in mice.

In four of the stocks, neoplasia accounted for >80 percent of the deaths, and in five of the stocks, non-neoplastic deaths accounted for half or more of the deaths. Figure 19.4B shows that body weight at 6 months is a significant predictor of longevity when only deaths due to neoplasia are considered. Figure 19.4C still shows a negative relationship between weight and longevity for mice dying of non-neoplastic conditions, but here the effect does not reach statistical significance (p = 0.07).

These results are consistent with results of earlier studies evaluating the relationship between body size and longevity in mouse stocks generated by selective breeding. In one such study, a mouse stock selected for rapid early life weight gain was found to have a mean longevity 57 percent that of control stocks (Eklund & Bradford, 1977). A second group also found that a mouse stock selected for small body size over multiple generations was longer lived than a stock selected for unusually large body size (Roberts, 1961), although in a separate experiments mice selected for either large or small body size proved to be longer-lived than controls.

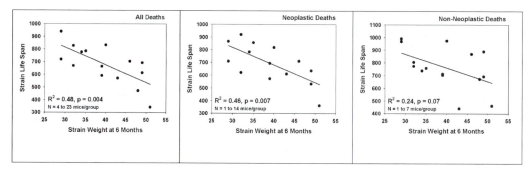

Figure 19.4 Mean life span versus mean adult weight for 15 stocks of mice selected for differences in early life growth trajectories. (A) All causes of death. (B) Deaths from neoplastic disease. (C) Deaths from non-neoplastic disease. Data from Miller and colleagues (2000a).

B. Correlation Between Weight and Life Span Among Genetically Heterogeneous Mice

A second approach (Miller *et al.*, 2002c) made use of a large group of genetically heterogeneous mice bred as the progeny of (BALB/cJ × C57BL/6J)F1 females and (C3H/HeJ × DBA/2J)F1 males; mice bred in this way are referred to UM-HET3 mice. A four-way cross of this kind, generated from four inbred mouse stocks, produces a set of test mice each of which is genetically unique but related as a full sib to each other mouse in the group. An analysis of 598 mice found that weight at 2 months was a significant predictor of life span among UM-HET3 mice; the association was significant at p < 0.01 and was found to be significant both for male and for female animals. The correlation between weight and longevity was significant for each age between 2 and 24 months, with the strongest correlation seen for mice examined at 5 months of age. Maximum weight attained by the mouse was not as good a predictor as weight at 2 to 5 months of age, and did not reach significance (p = 0.06) in the regression analysis. A similar regression analysis was performed on an independent set of 195 UM-HET3 mice for which weight at 6 months was available, and in this population as well, body weight was a significant predictor (p = 0.005) of life expectancy (Miller *et al.*, 2002c).

C. Mutations that Modulate GH and/or IGF-I Levels and Body Size

Data on mice bearing mutations in genes that modulate IGF-I production or response to IGF-I are also relevant to the question of how early growth trajectories might modulate the pace of aging and late life disease risk. Table 19.1 collects data on longevity in five such mutants. Two of the mouse lines, the Ames and Snell dwarf mice, have defects in embryonic pituitary development that

Table 19.1
Long-Lived Mouse Mutants with Altered GH/IGF-I Pathways

Experimental Model	Weight, % of Control	Control Life Span	Mutant Life Span	Life Span Difference	Background Stock	References
Prop1[df/df] (Ames dwarf)	~33%	721	1141	58%	Ames control stock	Brown-Borg *et al.*, 1996
Pit1[dwl/dw] (Snell dwarf)	25%	832	1178	42%	(DW × C3H)F1; similar effect in DW/J stock	Flurkey *et al.*, 2001
Ghrhr[lit/lit] (little)	60%	861	1082	26%	C57BL/6J	Flurkey *et al.*, 2001
GHR-KO (homozygous growth hormone receptor KO)	39%	789	954	21%	C57BL/6	Coschigano *et al.*, 2003
GHR-KO	ND	708	919	30%	Ola-BALB	Coschigano *et al.*, 2003
IGF-IR[+/−]	93%	577	718	24%	129/Sv	Holzenberger *et al.*, 2003

Notes: Weight is given as percent of control weight at 3 to 6 months of age. Life span refers to mean life span. For studies in which weight or life span is reported separately for each gender, the values presented are the average for males and females. Life-span difference is reported as a percentage of the control life span.

severely reduce production of growth hormone (GH), thyroid stimulating hormone (TSH), and prolactin. Because GH is the key regulator of hepatic production of IGF-I, these mice also have very low IGF-I levels throughout life. The body weight of young adult mice is reduced to 25 percent to 33 percent of that seen in controls, and mean life span is increased by 42 percent to 58 percent beyond that achieved by control mice, with maximum longevity extended to a similar extent (Brown-Borg et al., 1996; Flurkey et al., 2001). The "little" mouse mutant, which lacks the ability to produce GH-releasing hormone receptor, also exhibits lower levels of GH production. As young adults they are about 67 percent the size of control mice and have a 26 percent increase in mean life span (Flurkey et al., 2001). The GH-receptor mutant produced by Kopchick and his colleagues is defective not in GH production, but in response to GH, and thus IGF-I levels are about 20 percent of normal throughout life (Coschigano et al., 2003). These IGF-I-deficient mice show a life-span extension between 21 percent and 30 percent (comparing average control to average mutant life span across sexes), depending on the background stock used. Last, mice heterozygous for a loss-of-function allele of the IGF-I receptor show a 24 percent life span extension (averaged across sexes), although in this stock weight of young adults is only 7 percent below that of controls. Interpretation of the data on the IGF-I receptor mutant is complicated by the short life span of the control mice (mean survival was only 18 months), ambiguities about the infectious status of the colony (which was not specific pathogen-free) and its potential impact on survival, and the apparent sex-specificity of the effect, which was significant in females but not in males.

These five models differ greatly in their level of GH but share defects in the level of IGF-I signals, either because IGF-I is low or because the IGF-I receptor is itself diminished. Taken together, they make a strong case that diminished IGF-I effects can lead to delayed aging and life-span increase on multiple backgrounds in mice. In several of the models, evidence is accumulating to document that the effects on longevity represent merely one consequence of a generalized slowing down of the aging process per se. Thus, Snell dwarf mice, for example, show declines in the rate of joint pathology (Silberberg, 1972), collagen cross-linking (Flurkey et al., 2001), T-cell subset changes (Flurkey et al., 2001), as well as cataracts and glomerular disease (Vergara, Smith-Wheelock, Harper, Sigler, & Miller, 2004). Ames dwarf mice show a diminished incidence of neoplastic disease (Ikeno et al., 2003) and a slower age-dependent loss of locomotor activity and cognitive function (Kinney et al., 2001b), and GHR-KO mutants also retain cognitive function in old age (Kinney et al., 2001a).

It is noteworthy that mutants that combine low IGF-I levels with hypothyroidism—that is, the Snell and Ames dwarfs—seem to achieve more life-span extension than mutants that have primary effects on the GH/IGF-I pathway alone. Although mutant mice with primary defects in thyroid hormone levels are not notably long-lived (Flurkey & Harrison, 1990), it is quite plausible that the combination of hypothyroidism and low IGF-I responses in the Snell and Ames mutants may have a more potent influence than alterations of IGF-I responses by themselves. Genetic stocks in which key hormones, such as IGF-I and thyroxine, can be adjusted at will at specific stages of development and adult life are not yet available, but they will ultimately provide a better picture of the ways in which hormonal levels influence growth and modulate aging. To provide an initial foray into this arena, we have evaluated

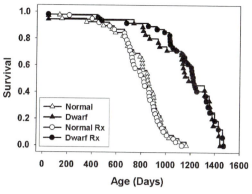

Figure 19.5 Snell dwarf mice treated with GH and T4 injections survive as long as saline-treated dwarf mice. Each symbol represents one mouse. Circles: mice received 55 injections of GH and T4 between age 4 and 15 weeks. Triangles: mice received saline injections as control. Reference: Vergara and colleagues, 2004.

longevity in Snell dwarf mice whose body weight was increased by about 50 percent through a program of GH and thyroxine injections between 4 and 15 weeks of age. Mice treated in this way were found to be as long-lived and as slow to develop cataracts and glomerular disease as Snell dwarf mice given saline injections instead of hormones. Figure 19.5 presents survival curves for treated and untreated normal and dwarf mice from this set of experiments. A more detailed account of this experiment is now in press (Vergara, Smith-Wheelock, Harper, Sigler, & Miller, 2004).

D. Wild-Derived Stocks

Nearly all of the mouse stocks commonly used for laboratory research have been molded by strong selective pressures for adaptation to vivarium husbandry and breeding conditions. Conversion of wild-trapped progenitor populations to laboratory stocks places a premium on alleles that promote rapid sexual maturation and large litter size; pressure for large litter size also imposes pressure for large body size needed to bear and nurse large numbers of pups.

Constant food availability and absence of competition for food and mating opportunities also place a premium on promiscuity and diminish the need to time reproductive effort based on sporadic access to food supplies. We hypothesized that intense selection for laboratory conditions might discard natural alleles that limit body size and growth rate, and which, by hypothesis, might also modulate aging. To test this idea, we captured wild mice from three locations (Idaho = Id, and the Pacific islands of Majuro = Ma and Pohnpei = Po), and created specific-pathogen-free laboratory stocks in such a way as to minimize loss of genetic heterogeneity. In good accord with the initial hypothesis, mice of all three stocks were found (Miller et al., 2000b) to be much smaller throughout adult life than a comparably heterogeneous control stock ("DC" for diversity control) developed by intercrosses from four standard laboratory inbred stocks (C57BL/6J, BALB/cJ, C3H/HeJ, and DBA/ 2J). The wild-derived stocks also had much smaller litter sizes (five pups/litter compared to 10 pups for the DC stocks.) The Id and Ma stocks were found (Miller et al., 2002b) to have shorter bodies and tail lengths than DC mice, and to have a slower pace of (at least) female reproductive maturation; Po mice were not tested for these traits. A life-span experiment then showed (Miller et al., 2002b) that Id mice had significantly longer life span than DC mice and had a larger "maximum" life span estimated by the age at death of the longest-lived 10 percent of the population. These data support the idea that genes promoting small body size and/or slow maturation might also promote longer life span, although it should be noted that the Po mice, although as small as Ma and Id mice, were not longer-lived than laboratory-derived DC mice. A replicate experiment (Miller et al., unpublished) has also shown longer life spans in independent populations of Id and Ma mice compared to a separate group of DC mice.

To what extent might the extended longevity of the Id (and, to a lesser extent, Ma) mice represent the effects of IGF-I, either in the developmental period or throughout adult life? IGF-I levels in serum, measured at 6 months of age, are significantly lower in Id mice than in DC mice (302 versus 591ng/ml, $p < 0.001$); levels in Ma mice are intermediate (464 ng/ml), although significantly lower than in DC. IGF-I levels were also measured in a segregating F2 population produced by breeding (Id $\times$ C57BL/6)F_1 mice, and in this population, low IGF-I levels at 6 months of age were predictors of longer life spans (J. M. Harper and R. A. Miller, in preparation). Low IGF-I was also associated with longer life span in a segregating (Ma $\times$ C57BL/6J)F_2 population. Data on IGF-I levels at ages prior to 6 months are not yet available, however, and it is not clear how the trajectory of IGF-I levels, and other endocrine circuits, might modulate growth rate, maturation rate, and longevity in these and related populations.

com/usuarios/j/jmgfall/engfaq.htm; www.ansi.okstate.edu/breeds/horses/ falabella), and the Gotland pony (www.gotlands.org/about_gotlands.htm).

Veterinarians specializing in the care of geriatric horses report that smaller breeds account for the majority of their patients aged 30 years or older (Brosnahan & Paradis, 2003). Of the 549 evaluations of equids over age 20 seen at a specialty clinic in a 10-year period, only 85 were for patients more than 30 years of age; pony breeds accounted for 48 percent of those seen at ages >30, although ponies made up only 13 percent of the total group of 549 visits ($p < 0.001$). Careful life-table data that could document differences in mortality risk profiles of standard size and miniature varieties of horse would be helpful to determine whether short stature is indeed associated with longevity in this species as well. Some, but not all, breeds of small horse and pony have been shown to have relatively low levels of IGF-I in serum (Malinowski et al., 1996); additional data on longevity of these breeds could help to sort out the relationships among size, IGF-I, and life span in mammals.

IV. Anecdotal Size-Longevity Reports on Horses

Information on longevity and stature in other mammalian species is sparse. There are many anecdotal reports, from experienced breeders and veterinarians, alleging that miniature breeds of horses tend to be remarkably long-lived with remarkably well-preserved health and vigor compared to full size horses, including claims for the Icelandic pony (www.allabouthorses.com/site/breeds/ icelandic.html;www.icelandichorses.ca/ horses.htm;www.angelfire.com/ca4/rock-ranch), the American miniature horse (www.guidehorse.com/ faq_horses.htm), the Falabella horse (http://webs. satlink.

V. Height and Longevity in Humans

Analysis of the relationships among growth trajectory, body size, and life span in human populations is complicated by interplay between biological and nonbiological factors. Both height and weight are modulated by genetic ancestry; differences in availability of food in utero, in postnatal development, and in adult life; differences in preferences for and availability of foods varying in fat content and micronutrients; and in social preferences for specific body shapes. Life span—a poor but necessary surrogate for the rate of aging—is similarly influenced by exposure to varying risks of death from infection and trauma, and varying exposure to carcinogens, exercise, and modern medical treatments, as well as underlying biological factors. The concern here is that correlated environmental factors, such as access to both high-protein diets and superior medical care, might increase height and life span in such a way as to obscure the postulated biological links between slow growth, small stature, and delayed or decelerated aging.

Samaras and his colleagues have assembled and summarized a variety of analyses in which small stature is associated with longer life span in small convenience samples—that is, samples chosen because they are easily accessible rather than through randomization from a well-defined reference population (Samaras & Elrick, 1999; Samaras & Storms, 1992; Samaras et al., 2003). Simple regression of age at death against adult height was used to document association between short stature and longer life span among men listed in Webster's American Biographies (R = −0.26, p < 0.005), among men listed in Current Biography Yearbook (R = −0.23, p < 0.005), among American

presidents, among 3,200 deceased professional baseball players, among men followed at a Veteran's hospital, among Harvard athletes, and among French men and women dying in the mid-1800s. The slopes of the regression lines, stated as years of life lost per additional centimeter of height, are surprisingly consistent: 0.35 years/cm for baseball players, 0.41 for persons listed in the Webster's biographical dictionary, 0.47 for patients treated at the VA medical center, 0.59 among French men and 0.43 among French women, with other examples given in the references cited. Two such examples are illustrated in Figure 19.6. Anecdotal regression studies of this kind have well-known flaws, including a failure to consider effects of potential confounders and population admixture, uncertainties in estimates calculated from small population samples, and a tendency to note significant relationships but to under-report negative or insignificant associations. In addition, it is unclear in many of these studies whether the height values were obtained at a consistent age (for example at the age of peak height). Because height declines with age,

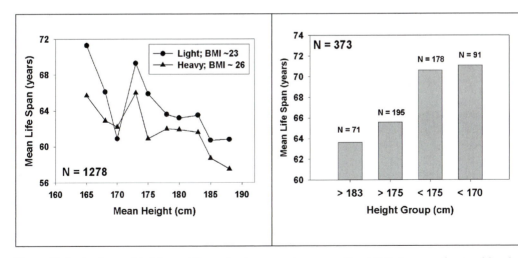

Figure 19.6 Analyses of height and longevity in convenience samples. (A) Data on professional baseball players, stratified by height decile; data are presented separately for those with relatively high or low body mass index. (B) Life span for height-based subsets of patients treated at a U.S. Veterans Administration Hospital. These and several similar data sets are presented in Samaras and Storms (1992).

height values obtained at or near death might show an artifactual association between short stature and increased age at death. Despite these technical concerns, the large size of the effects noted and the consistency of the findings among so many disparate convenience samples does provide some support for the idea that factors promoting increased height may also increase late-life mortality risks, at least in some modern American and European population groups.

Population-based prospective studies provide more convincing tests of such ideas, and here the data suggest that the relationship between height and life expectancy in humans may vary depending on cause of death, with short stature associated with protection against many forms of neoplastic disease but not against cardiovascular diseases or smoking-related neoplasias. One of the most comprehensive of such analyses (Davey et al., 2000) evaluated over 15,000 Scottish men and women, recruited at the ages of 45 to 63 between 1972 and 1976; 5,985 of these subjects had died by the time of analysis in the late 1990s. Although tall people had lower risks of all-cause mortality and lower mortality risks from coronary artery disease, stroke, and respiratory disease, the risks of death from colorectal, prostate, and hematopoietic cancers showed the opposite effect, with short stature associated with lower mortality risk.

Similarly, a study (Albanes et al., 1988) of over 12,000 participants in the U.S. National Health and Nutrition Examination Survey revealed a 40 to 60 percent increase in cancer incidence rates in taller people compared to those in the lowest quartile for height, after adjustment for race, income, and smoking status among men. A similar, significant, though weaker association was noted among women for both breast and colorectal cancer. A study of over 22,000 male American physicians with a 12-year follow-up period found a significant association between short stature and low incidence of malignancy after adjustment for age, smoking and alcohol use, exercise, and body mass index (Hebert et al., 1993). A study of 570,000 Norwegian women documented increased risk of breast cancer, at all ages, among the tallest individuals (Tretli, 1989). Tall height was also associated with increased risk of breast cancer in a study of over 400,000 American post-menopausal women (Petrelli et al., 2002), and with risk of esophageal cancer (though not stomach cancer) among 1.1 million Norwegian men and women (Tretli & Robsahm, 1999). An analysis comparing mortality risks by height among counties of England and Wales found that residents of counties with high mean heights tended to have lower all-cause mortality and lower risks of ischemic heart disease but higher mortality risks for breast, prostate, and ovarian cancer (Barker et al., 1990). Taken together, these papers point toward a consensus that short stature may be associated with protection against many forms of late-life neoplastic disease in humans, with perhaps the opposite association for cardiovascular disease. It should also be noted that studies of the relationship of height to risks of cardiovascular mortality in humans have not always reached the conclusion that short stature is associated with increased risk. Such studies are greatly complicated by the difficulties of adjusting for known and unknown confounder variables in admixtures of ethnic groups differing in genetic stocks, early and midlife food intake, exposure to environmental risk and protective factors, and so on. Cardiovascular illness is typically rare, for example, in societies that avoid Western diets rich in fats, salts, and refined sugars, and it would be informative to re-evaluate the relationship of growth trajectories and adult height to longevity and non-neoplastic diseases in such populations.

It seems plausible that high levels of IGF-I in middle-aged and older adults may increase their risk of cancer directly. *In vitro*, for example, IGF-I promotes survival of many cell types, including mammary epithelial cell lines (Rosfjord, 1999), and promotes production by colon cancer cells of VEGF, a key factor in tumor neovascularization (Akagi *et al.*, 1998). Prospective studies have shown that men with high levels of serum IGF-I have elevated risks of developing prostate and colon cancer (Chan *et al.*, 1998; Harman *et al.*, 2000; Ma *et al.*, 1999). These and similar studies are consistent with the data showing higher cancer risks in tall people, but they do not show whether these associations reflect an effect of IGF-I on cancer in late life or instead reflect an effect of early life hormone exposure on late-life tumor risk.

VI. Nutritional Manipulations that Modulate Longevity and Body Size

Life span of rodents can be extended by at least two classes of nutritional manipulations, those that diminish total caloric intake (Weindruch & Sohal, 1997; Weindruch & Walford, 1988) and those that restrict the levels of essential amino acids, such as methionine (Orentreich *et al.*, 1993; Richie *et al.*, 1994; Zimmerman *et al.*, 2003) or tryptophan (Segall & Timiras, 1976; Segall *et al.*, 1978). Both of these methods also lead to small body size, although whether they do so through distinct or overlapping metabolic pathways is still open to discussion. Effects of nutritional status on body weight and life span may also underlie a decades-long secular trend towards larger body size and shorter life spans among F344 rats used as controls for a series of studies at the National Center for Toxicologic Research (Turturro *et al.*, 1997; Turturro *et al.*, 1998). Although the basis

for the long-term trend toward higher body weight in these inbred rats is not known, these authors have speculated that unintentional changes in diet or husbandry conditions have contributed both to more rapid weight gain and to the dramatic decline in mean life span over the course of their series of investigations.

The calorie restriction story is presented in detail elsewhere in this handbook but has several implications worth stressing in respect to connections between body size and life span. To begin with, low levels of IGF-I are characteristic of calorically restricted (CR) mice, at least at early stages after imposition of the restricted diet (Breese *et al.*, 1991; Dunn *et al.*, 1997; Oster *et al.*, 1995), and reduction of amino acid intake can also depress serum IGF-I levels and hepatic production of IGF-I (Miller, Buehner, Chang, Harper, Sigler, & Smith-Wheelock, 2005; Straus, 1994; Underwood *et al.*, 1994).

Thus, small size and low IGF-I levels accompany extended life span in both dietary regimes as in the dwarf mouse stocks. There are, however, important differences between the genetic models currently available and the nutritional regimes that have been studied. For one thing, caloric restriction leads to a substantial reduction in adipose tissue mass, but dwarf mice have normal or above normal adiposity (Flurkey *et al.*, 2001). Second, the spectrum of gene expression differences between dwarf and control mice overlaps only to a limited degree the changes noted to distinguish young adult CR and control-diet mice (Miller *et al.*, 2002a; Tsuchiya *et al.*, 2004). Third, there is strong evidence that CR diets modulate the slope of the mortality risk curve, at least in rats (Holehan & Merry, 1986; Pletcher *et al.*, 2000), in contrast to the accumulating evidence that dwarf mutations may alter the age at which deaths are first noted rather than the rate of increase in mortality rate *per se* (Bartke *et al.*, 2001; Flurkey *et al.*, 2001).

It has long been apparent that CR diets can produce major increases in life span even when they are initiated at ages past the point at which rodents approach full adult stature, and furthermore that CR limited to the first six months of life is relatively ineffective (Yu et al., 1985). It now appears likely that, at least in some mouse stocks, imposition of a CR diet as late as ages 12 to 19 months can diminish subsequent mortality risks (Dhahbi et al., 2004; Pugh et al., 1999; Weindruch & Walford, 1982), even though the manipulation is started well after the age at which body size and weight are at full adult levels. It will be of interest to see to what extent mid-life initiation of CR delays, or even perhaps reverses, age-dependent changes in specific cell and tissue types, but the life span data make a *prima facie* case that the pathways through which CR improves health and postpones illness are not effective merely in the juvenile or early adult stages of the life span.

VII. Relation of Size to Longevity Among Different Species

The data presented above present a strong case that small body size is associated with longer life span in mice and dogs, and among people who die of many forms of neoplastic disease. This association at first appears paradoxical in view of the well-known association between body size and longevity among mammalian species, among which mice and rats have notably shorter lives than dogs, bears, and humans. Austad and Fischer (1991) have evaluated an extensive collection of data on size and life span among mammals and birds, and presented a more nuanced view and alternate explanations of the matter. Their discussion points out that the relationship between body size and life span is distinctly nonlinear, and shows no

evidence for association among mammals whose adult body weight is below approximately 1 kg. Further, they note that the relationship between body size and longevity is distinctly different between mammals that fly or glide and those that cannot: nonflying mammalian species tend to be much less long-lived than flying or gliding animals of the same body weight. Birds, too, are in general much longer-lived than nonflying mammalian species of the same weight, despite the metabolic demands, high blood-glucose levels, high body temperature, and high fuel utilization rates typical of flying bird species. These authors present the perspective that associations between large body size and longer life span among mammalian species principally reflect co-evolutionary pressures that promote anti-aging mechanisms among species large enough (or, in the case of bats and birds, agile enough) to avoid predation risk. In this model, small, predation-prone species can increase Darwinian fitness by rapid maturation and rapid production of large litters. In contrast, larger species, for which predation is less likely, may improve fitness by delaying aging effects long enough to permit production of multiple, smaller broods and to devote time to protection of young during their relatively long period of high-risk maturation. Such models postulate that the long life span of many larger mammalian species reflect co-evolved changes in size, growth rate, timing of maturation, and delay of aging and disease processes to optimize fitness to low-risk evolutionary niches. Such a model is consistent with the observation that the size/longevity association disappears among small mammals, for whom predation risk may be poorly linked to body size, and with the observation that predator-avoidance tactics such as flying or gliding, underground or cave habitat, or development of protective armor or spines may lead to evolution of anti-aging mechanisms even without the protection afforded by large body size.

A detailed discussion of the relationship between ecological niche and life history parameters is beyond the scope of this chapter. The differences between inter-species and intra-species comparisons, however, are worth careful consideration. The association of long life with large size among species does not call into question the strong evidence for the opposite relationship among mice or among dogs, but it certainly does call into question the naïve assumption that the developmental or hormonal factors that underlie the longevity of small dogs and small mice, and the cancer resistance of short people, also contribute to the anti-aging mechanisms that protect members of larger species with slower rates of development and maturation.

Before discussing connections between stature and longevity within and among species it should be noted that the mechanisms that modulate differences among species in growth rate and ultimate body size are not even remotely understood. Studies of worms and flies (Tatar et al., 2003) show that the family of insulin-related hormones, among which IGF-I plays a major role in mammalian growth, has evolutionarily deep connections to both size and longevity determination, and that reduced activity is often associated with both small size and longer life span. Studies in the genetically malleable invertebrate models (Murphy et al., 2003) are gradually revealing how these hormonally controlled pathways lead to improved resistance of multiple cell types to stress and hence to slower organismal aging, although it remains uncertain to what extent the details of these connections in worms and flies will lead to discoveries of analogous connections in mammals.

Evolutionary mechanisms within species differ in important ways from those that lead to changes among species. Classically (Mayr, 1989), each species can be considered as a pool of co-adapted gene complexes separated from other such pools and molded by natural selection to exhibit life histories appropriate for their environment (McKinnon et al., 2004). Species have thus traditionally been defined by the near absence of gene flow between them compared with extensive gene flow within them. Variation within a species is therefore variation on a limited theme, constrained in scope by the physiology and cell biology dictated by the species gene pool.

The overwhelming majority of alleles, protein activities, receptor affinities, signal transduction sensitivities, and other protein–protein interactions are expected to be similar even among diverse genotypes within a species, and these activities and interactions will be appropriately integrated to achieve the reproductive pattern natural selection favors. Alleles that modulate growth and/or life span within a species must do so within this set of species-specific constraints. In this context, it is striking that variations in body size, based at least to some extent on the IGF-I pathway, can lead to alterations in life span in dogs, mice, and probably horses, suggesting that ties between developmental levels of growth factors, and eventual risks of late-life diseases, either predate the mammalian radiation or are particularly likely to evolve through convergent mechanisms.

By contrast, once gene pools become isolated from one another due to ecological or geographic shifts, they will be subject to both adaptive and stochastic divergence from one another, limited by the necessity to maintain functional integration throughout development and adult life. Even closely related species such as mice and rats or humans and chimpanzees have undergone multiple genomic rearrangements relative to one another, some found in coding regions

(Frazer *et al.*, 2003; Zhao *et al.*, 2004) but others in regions that may modulate gene expression in specific cell types or at particular developmental stages. Evolutionary changes in the timing by which hormones, receptors, and other developmental coordinators are turned on or off in specific tissues may have major effects on key life history outcomes, including growth and aging, even if they do not greatly alter concentrations of these factors in the serum in adult life.

The extent of divergence of anti-aging protective mechanisms among species can be very striking. For example, if the malignant transformation of any single cell can kill a mouse or human, and a human consists of 2,000 times as many cells as a mouse, then human cells would need to be 2,000 times more resistant to malignant transformation than mouse cells, even if humans only lived a mouse-like 2 to 3 years. Because humans live roughly 30 times as long as mice, their cells must be roughly 60,000 times less vulnerable to malignant transformations than mouse cells (Miller, 1991). Development of large, long-lived species such as humans (or, in the extreme case, whales) thus requires construction of anti-neoplastic defenses that operate to reduce the risk of lethal neoplastic transformation by four to five orders of magnitude. The nature of these defenses is not yet well understood. There is modest support for the idea that larger, longer-lived species have reduced cellular vulnerability to extrinsic stress. For instance, Grube and Burkle (1992) found DNA repair correlated with species life span in peripheral white blood cells of 13 mammalian species. In addition, Kapahi and colleagues (1999) found that cultured fibroblast resistance to five sources of lethal stress was directly correlated with maximum life span of eight mammalian species ranging in size from hamsters to cows and in longevity from 4 to 100 years. Also, it has been recently shown that primary fibroblasts from mice and humans differ in their sensitivity to the damage caused by exposure to 20 percent oxygen during *in vitro* culture, with human cells less likely to be harmed than cells from mice (Parinello *et al.*, 2003), although cells from both species appear able to deal with oxygen levels (3 percent) similar to those typically encountered within tissues of intact mammals.

To be effective, evolutionary changes that block cancer must also lead to, or else be accompanied by, postponed vulnerability to changes in joints, muscles, immune defenses, hearing and sight, and neurological function that would limit life span even were cancer postponed indefinitely. Data from studies of dietary restriction and single gene mutations in mice, and on breed comparisons in dogs and horses, show that indeed it is possible for relatively simple interventions to retard both neoplastic and non-neoplastic aspects of mammalian aging; whether these processes are related to those that produce major differences among species in aging rate is a key unanswered question in biological gerontology.

VIII. General Discussion: Why Do Big Dogs Die Young, and Is It Worth Figuring This Out?

The evidence summarized above makes a strong case that genetic factors regulating body size influence aging rate and life expectancy in dogs and mice. The evidence includes studies comparing populations derived by selective breeding in both species, as well as analyses of mortality risks in genetically heterogeneous mice and mixed-breed dogs. Inadvertent selection for large body size during laboratory adaptation of wild-trapped mice is also accompanied by pressures toward more rapid reproductive maturation and diminished life span, although it is not known whether the genetic loci that contribute to the differences between wild-caught and laboratory-adapted stocks are related to the loci responsible for size/longevity associations among dog breeds, Atchley's growth-selected mouse stocks, and genetically heterogeneous stocks derived solely from laboratory mouse strains. Single gene mutants that interrupt IGF-I-dependent growth pathways also lead to dramatic increases in life span and delay or deceleration of multiple age-dependent changes.

Diets deficient in calories or in specific essential amino acids also lead to small size and to increased longevity as well as to diminished early life IGF-I levels, although it is still far from clear to what extent the beneficial effects of these diets involve mechanisms that play a role in the genetic systems that associate small size with longevity. The differences in the shape of the mortality risk curves seen in CR and in mutant dwarf models (Bartke *et al.*, 2001; Flurkey *et al.*, 2001), differences in the profile of altered gene expression, and the ability of restricted diets to extend longevity even when instituted at ages after attainment of full adult stature hint that the connections between size and longevity may be unrelated to, or only partially overlapping with, the pathways by which genetic polymorphisms regulate both size and life span. The observation that modulation of insulin sensitivity in adipose tissue can extend mouse life span (Bluher *et al.*, 2003), together with experiments implicating specific adipose depots as modulators of longevity and disease risk (Das *et al.*, 2004; Rincon *et al.*, 2004), suggest that modulation of adipose-derived hormones might also play a role in the anti-aging effects of CR diets, again in contrast to the dwarf mutants and selective breeding systems.

Leaving aside the nutritional intervention protocols, what then accounts for the longevity of small dogs and mice, and by extension perhaps the cancer resistance of short people? An initial hypothesis might be to look at physical factors through which small body size might in itself protect against late-life disease. Such factors might include differences in number of target cells exposed to neoplastic transformation, variations in heat loss mediated by surface area/ volume ratio, or changes in ratios in size among organs that do or do not scale in proportion to overall stature, including branching ratios and size-scaling patterns of vascular networks (West *et al.*, 1999). There are now multiple reasons for viewing this class of theories as unlikely. For one thing, the direction of the size/longevity regression is positive among mammals above 1kg, neutral among mammals less than 1kg, and negative within species such as mice and dogs. Secondly, Table 19.1 does not show any clear relationship between body-weight differences and life-span extension among the various single gene mutants. Life-span extension in the IGF-I receptor mutant, for example, is similar to that seen in the GHR-KO model, although the former are nearly as large as control mice and the latter are only 39 percent as large as controls. Similarly, our data on hormone-injected dwarf mice (see Figure 19.5) show that injections of GH and thyroxine (T4) into young adult Snell dwarf mice, although sufficient to increase body weight by 50 percent, do not diminish the long life span seen in this stock.

We believe it likely that the relationship between small body size and slow aging in the genetic models represents the effect of underlying factors, still to be identified, that influence both weight gain trajectory and, later, life span and late life diseases. From this perspective, body weight (or length) is merely a surrogate index, an indirect monitor of one or more developmental processes that alter both growth and aging. Body weight is influenced by multiple factors, including body dimensions (such as long bone growth) and the relative growth of multiple organs, notably including various adipose deposits. Background genetic differences, litter size and maternal nutritional status, intrauterine sex ratio, fat content of the postnatal diet, housing density, exposure to infectious agents, and food palatability, for example, may all influence body weight and length through paths that may be irrelevant to, or tangential to, the common factors that we postulate to link weight to aging. Furthermore, age at death is itself a crude and indirect surrogate for the pace of aging. The life span of any individual is influenced not only by aging but by risk factors, genetic and non-genetic, that may have differential effects on specific lethal diseases. Thus, for example, genetic factors that promote thymic lymphoma or lupus-like autoimmune syndromes have strong effects on life expectancy that are not mediated by a general modulation of the pace of age-dependent change in multiple systems. Given the indirect linkages between aging and longevity, and between body weight and the multiple developmental pathways that influence it, the very high correlations between size and life span seen in the selective breeding experiments appear all the more remarkable.

The scientific challenge, then, is to determine the mechanisms—hormonal, developmental, or cellular—that account for and in fact lead to the dramatic and consistent differences in life expectancy among small and large breeds and races within a given species. These mechanisms, a priori, need not be the same in each case; it is plausible, for example, that the small size of miniature dachshunds might be due to poor cellular responses to IGF-I, the small size of miniature mouse lines due to alterations in stem-cell commitment to proliferation,

and the small size of cancer-resistant people due to a mixture of multiple cellular, hormonal, and nutritional factors. The most promising current idea, however, focuses on the IGF-I pathway as a possible common denominator linking many of these phenomena. IGF-I signals are known to be diminished in each of the five long-lived mutants listed in Table 19.1, as well as the few miniature dog breeds that have been evaluated hormonally to date (but see Favier et al., 2001, for a contrary view). IGF-I levels are lower in wild-derived mice than in the shorter-lived laboratory-adapted stocks, and low IGF-I levels predict life span in segregating crosses between wild and laboratory mouse lines. Early life IGF-I levels are low in calorically restricted and methionine-restricted mice as well. It is not known, however, to what extent alterations in IGF-I levels or responses contribute to the size differences in other breeds of dogs, among the Atchley size-selected stocks, or in segregating populations of mice and people.

How, then, might differences among individuals in IGF-I levels, IGF-I responses, or parallel pathways triggered by other growth-related hormones influence age-sensitive change, including the increase with age in risks of diseases, disabilities, and death? Experiments in invertebrates, and recently in mice, suggest that changes in cellular resistance to stress may be a key link. Studies in worms and flies, reviewed elsewhere in this handbook, have shown that mutations identified by their ability to extend life span are often found to render the animal resistant to multiple forms of stress, including oxidants, heat, and heavy metals (Lithgow, 2000); many of these mutations cause downregulation of a pathway triggered by a worm analogue of the mammalian insulin or IGF-I receptor. Fibroblast cell lines from mutant mice whose long life span is due to declines in IGF-I or IGF-I receptor levels are also found to be resistant to multiple forms of cytotoxic stress, including ultraviolet light, heat, peroxide, paraquat, and the heavy metal cadmium (Holzenberger *et al.*, 2003; Murakami *et al.*, 2003). It is thus tempting to imagine an evolutionarily conserved pathway that evolved to allow adjustment of developmental processes to resource availability. In worms and flies, such a pathway might, if triggered by resource-poor circumstances, induce a set of organismic and cellular changes that protect the animal, and cells within it, from a wide range of lethal insults. In mammals, the same molecular apparatus might play a role at multiple stages, *in utero*, in postnatal life, and after attainment of full adult size, to adjust cellular properties in response to multiple signals, some of them influenced by genetic polymorphisms and others responsive to nutritional factors. Much more remains to be learned about the cell types responsive to these postulated endocrine factors, the specific developmental stages at which cells are susceptible to their influences, and the ways in which alterations in cellular stress resistance might contribute to the anti-aging defenses both in long-lived individuals and, perhaps, to individuals in long-lived species.

IX. Conclusions

One of the most promising avenues to improved understanding of the mechanisms that time the aging process relies on comparisons of animals that resemble each other closely but age at different rates. Many lines of evidence, from pituitary mutants, selective breeding in mice and dogs, correlation analysis in genetically polymorphic populations, and studies of calorie- or amino-acid restricted rodents, all suggest that the pace of aging may be regulated by hormonal pathways that also control growth and body size. This chapter marshals the current evidence and suggests new avenues

for dissection of the cellular pathways that might link early life and midlife growth hormone pathways to postponement of late-life illnesses in mammals.

Acknowledgements

Preparation of this review, and some of the original research reported, was supported by NIH grants AG13711, AG08808, and AG11687.

References

Akagi, Y., Liu, W., Zebrowski, B., Xie, K., & Ellis, L. M. (1998). Regulation of vascular endothelial growth factor expression in human colon cancer by insulin-like growth factor-I. *Cancer Research*, 58, 4008–4014.

Albanes, D., Jones, D.Y., Schatzkin, A., Micozzi, M.S., & Taylor, P. R. (1988). Adult stature and risk of cancer. *Cancer Research*, 48, 1658–1662.

Austad, S. N, & Fischer, K. E. (1991). Mammalian aging, metabolism, and ecology: evidence from the bats and marsupials. *Journal of Gerontology Biological Sciences*, 46, B47–B53.

Barker, D. J. P, Osmond, C., & Golding, J. (1990). Height and mortality in the counties of England and Wales. *Annals of Human Biology*, 17, 1–6.

Bartke, A., Wright, J. C., Mattison, J. A., Ingram, D. K., Miller, R. A., & Roth, G. S. (2001). Extending the lifespan of long-lived mice. *Nature*, 414, 412.

Bluher, M., Kahn, B. B., & Kahn, C. R. (2003). Extended longevity in mice lacking the insulin receptor in adipose tissue. *Science*, 299, 572–574.

Breese, C. R., Ingram, R. L., & Sonntag, W. E. (1991). Influence of age and long-term dietary restriction on plasma insulin-like growth factor-1 (IGF-I), IGF-I gene expression, and IGF-I binding proteins. *Journal of Gerontology Biological Sciences*, 46, B180–B187.

Brosnahan, M. M, & Paradis, M. R. (2003). Demographic and clinical characteristics of geriatric horses: 467 cases (1989–1999). *Journal of the American Veterinary Medical Association*, 223, 93–98.

Brown-Borg, H. M., Borg, K. E., Meliska, C. J., & Bartke, A. (1996). Dwarf mice and the ageing process. *Nature*, 384, 33.

Chan, J. M, Stampfer, M. J, Giovannucci, E., Gann, P. H., Ma, J., Wilkinson, P., Hennekens, C. H., & Pollak, M. (1998). Plasma insulin-like growth factor-I and prostate cancer risk: a prospective study. *Science*, 279, 563–566.

Coschigano, K. T., Holland, A. N., Riders, M. E., List, E. O., Flyvbjerg, A., & Kopchick, J.J. (2003). Deletion, but not antagonism, of the mouse growth hormone receptor results in severely decreased body weights, insulin, and insulin-like growth factor I levels and increased life span. *Endocrinology*, 144, 3799–3810.

Das, M., Gabriely, I., & Barzilai, N. (2004). Caloric restriction, body fat and ageing in experimental models. *Obesity Reviews*, 5, 13–19.

Davey, S. G., Hart, C., Upton, M., Hole, D., Gillis, C., Watt, G., & Hawthorne, V. (2000). Height and risk of death among men and women: aetiological implications of associations with cardiorespiratory disease and cancer mortality. *Journal of Epidemiology & Community Health*, 54, 97–103.

Dhahbi, J. M., Kim, H. J., Mote, P. L., Beaver, R. J., & Spindler, S. R. (2004). Temporal linkage between the phenotypic and genomic responses to caloric restriction. *Proceedings of the National Academy of Sciences of the USA*, 101, 5524–5529.

Dunn, S. E., Kari, F. W., French, J., Leininger, J. R., Travlos, G., Wilson, R., & Barrett, J. C. (1997). Dietary restriction reduces insulin-like growth factor I levels, which modulates apoptosis, cell proliferation, and tumor progression in p53-deficient mice. *Cancer Research*, 57, 4667–4672.

Eigenmann, J. E., Amador, A., & Patterson, D. F. (1988). Insulin-like growth factor I levels in proportionate dogs, chondrodystrophic dogs and in giant dogs. *Acta Endocrinologica*, 118, 105–108.

Eigenmann, J. E., Patterson, D. F., & Froesch, E. R. (1984a). Body size parallels insulin-like growth factor I levels but not growth hormone secretory capacity. *Acta Endocrinologica*, 106, 448–453.

Eigenmann, J. E., Patterson, D. F., Zapf, J., & Froesch, E. R. (1984b). Insulin-like growth

factor I in the dog: a study in different dog breeds and in dogs with growth hormone elevation. *Acta Endocrinologica*, 105, 294–301.

Eigenmann, J. E., Zanesco, S., Arnold, U., & Froesch, E. R. (1984). Growth hormone and insulin-like growth factor I in German shepherd dwarf dogs. *Acta Endocrinologica*, 105, 289–293.

Eklund, J., & Bradford, G. E. (1977). Longevity and lifetime body weight in mice selected for rapid growth. *Nature*, 265, 48–49.

Favier, R. P., Mol, J. A., Kooistra, H. S., & Rijnberk, A. (2001). Large body size in the dog is associated with transient GH excess at a young age. *Journal of Endocrinology*, 170, 479–484.

Flurkey, K., & Harrison, D. E. (1990). Use of genetic models to investigate the hypophyseal regulation of senescence. In D. E. Harrison (Ed.), *Genetic effects on aging II* (pp. 437–456). Caldwell, NJ: Telford Press.

Flurkey, K., Papaconstantinou, J., Miller, R. A., & Harrison, D. E. (2001) Lifespan extension and delayed immune and collagen aging in mutant mice with defects in growth hormone production. *Proceedings of the National Academy of Sciences of the USA*, 98, 6736–6741.

Frazer, K. A., Chen, X., Hinds, D. A., & Krshna Pant, P. B., Patil, N., Cox, D. R. (2003). Genomic DNA insertions and deletions occur frequently between humans and nonhuman primates. *Genome Res.*, 13, 341–346.

Grube, K., & Burkle, A. (1992). Poly (ADP-ribose) polymerase activity in mononuclear leukocytes of 13 mammalian species. *Proceedings of the National Academy of Sciences of the USA*, 89, 11759–11763.

Harman, S. M., Metter, E. J., Blackman, M. R., Landis, P. K., & Carter, H. B. (2000) Serum levels of insulin-like growth factor I (IGF-I), IGF-II, IGF-binding protein-3, and prostate-specific antigen as predictors of clinical prostate cancer. *Journal of Clinical Endocrinology and Metabolism*, 85, 4258–4265.

Hawthorne, A. J., Booles, D., Nugent, P. A., Gettinby, G., & Wilkinson, J. (2004). Body-weight changes during growth in puppies of different breeds. *Journal of Nutrition*, 134, 2027S–2030S.

Hebert, P. R., Rich-Edwards, J. W., Manson, J. E., Ridker, P. M., Cook, N. R., O'Connor, G. T., Buring J. E., & Hennekens C. H. (1993). Height and incidence of cardiovascular disease in male physicians. *Circulation*, 88, 1437–1443.

Holehan, A. M., & Merry, B. J. (1986). The experimental manipulation of ageing by diet. *Biological Reviews of the Cambridge Philosophical Society*, 61, 329–368.

Holzenberger, M., Dupont, J., Ducos, B., Leneuve, P., Geloen, A., Even, P. C., Cervera, P., & Le Bouc, Y. (2003). IGF-I receptor regulates lifespan and resistance to oxidative stress in mice. *Nature*, 421, 182–187.

Hoskins, J. D., & McCurnin, D. M. (1997). Geriatric care in the late 1990s. *Veterinary Clinics of North America-Small Animal Practice*, 27, 1273–1284.

Ikeno, Y., Bronson, R. T., Hubbard, G. B., Lee, S., & Bartke, A. (2003). Delayed occurrence of fatal neoplastic diseases in Ames dwarf mice: correlation to extended longevity. *Journals of Gerontology Series A: Biological Sciences & Medical Sciences*, 58, 291–296.

Johnston, S. D., Root Kustritz, M. V., & Olson, P. N. S. (2001). *Canine and feline theriogenology*. Philadelphia, PA: W. B. Saunders.

Kapahi, P., Boulton, M. E., Kirkwood, T. B. L., (1999). Positive correlation between mammalian life span and cellular resistance to stress. *Free Rad. Bio. Med.*, 26, 495–500.

Kinney, B. A., Coschigano, K. T., Kopchick, J. J., Steger, R. W., & Bartke, A. (2001a). Evidence that age-induced decline in memory retention is delayed in growth hormone resistant GH-R-KO (Laron) mice. *Physiology and Behavior*, 72, 653–660.

Kinney, B. A., Meliska, C. J., Steger, R. W., & Bartke, A. (2001b). Evidence that Ames dwarf mice age differently from their normal siblings in behavioral and learning and memory parameters. *Hormones and Behavior*, 39, 277–284.

Li, Y., Deeb, B., Pendergrass, W., & Wolf, N. (1996). Cellular proliferative capacity and life span in small and large dogs. *Journals of Gerontology Series A Biological Sciences and Medical Sciences*, 51, B403–B408.

Lithgow, G. J. (2000). Stress response and aging in *Caenorhabditis elegans*. *Results & Problems in Cell Differentiation*, 29, 131–148.

Ma, J., Pollak, M. N., Giovannucci, E., Chan, J. M., Tao, Y., Hennekens, C. H., & Stampfer, M. J. (1999). Prospective study of colorectal cancer risk in men and plasma levels of insulin-like growth factor (IGF)-I and IGF-binding protein-3. *Journal of the National Cancer Institute*, 91, 620–625.

Malinowski, K., Christensen, R. A., Hafs, H. D., & Scanes, C. G. (1996). Age and breed differences in thyroid hormones, insulin-like growth factor (IGF)-I and IGF binding proteins in female horses. *Journal of Animal Science*, 74, 1936–1942.

Mayr, E. (1989). Principles of Systematic Zoology. New York: McGraw-Hill.

McKinnon, J. S., Morl, S., Blackman, B. K., David, L., Kingsley, D. M., Jamieson, L., Chou, J., & Schluter, D. (2004). Evidence for ecology's role in speciation. *Nature*, 429, 294–298.

Michell, A. R. (1999). Longevity of British breeds of dog and its relationships with sex, size, cardiovascular variables and disease. *Veterinary Record*, 145, 625–629.

Miller, R. A. (1991). Gerontology as oncology: research on aging as the key to the understanding of cancer. *Cancer*, 68, 2486–2501.

Miller, R. A., Buehner, G., Chang, Y., Harper, J. M., Sigler, R., & Smith-Wheelock, M. (2005). Methionine-deficient diet extends mouse life span, slows immune and lens aging, alters glucose, T4, IGF-I and insulin levels, and increases hepatocyte MIF levels and stress resistance. *Aging Cell*, 4, 199–125.

Miller, R. A., Chang, Y., Galecki, A. T., Al-Regaiey, K., Kopchick, J. J., & Bartke, A. (2002a). Gene expression patterns in calorically restricted mice: partial overlap with long-lived mutant mice. *Molecular Endocrinology*, 16, 2657–2666.

Miller, R. A., Chrisp, C., & Atchley, W. R. (2000a). Differential longevity in mouse stocks selected for early life growth trajectory. *Journals of Gerontology Biological Sciences*, 55A, B455–B461.

Miller, R. A., Dysko, R., Chrisp, C., Seguin, R., Linsalata, L., Buehner, G., Harper, J. M., & Austad, S. (2000b). Mouse (*Mus musculus*) stocks derived from tropical islands: new models for genetic analysis of life history traits. *Journal of Zoology*, 250, 95–104.

Miller, R. A., Harper, J. M., Dysko, R. C., Durkee, S. J., & Austad, S. N. (2002b). Longer life spans and delayed maturation in wild-derived mice. *Experimental Biology and Medicine*, 227, 500–508.

Miller, R. A., Harper, J. M., Galecki, A., & Burke, D. T. (2002c). Big mice die young: early-life body weight predicts longevity in genetically heterogeneous mice. *Aging Cell*, 1, 22–29.

Murakami, S., Salmon, A., & Miller, R. A. (2003). Multiplex stress resistance in cells from long-lived dwarf mice. *FASEB Journal*, 17, 1565–1566.

Murphy, C. T., McCarroll, S. A., Bargmann, C. I., Fraser, A., Kamath, R. S., Ahringer, J., Li, H., & Kenyon, C. (2003). Genes that act downstream of DAF-16 to influence the lifespan of *Caenorhabditis elegans*. *Nature*, 424, 277–283.

Orentreich, N., Matias, J. R., DeFelice, A., & Zimmerman, J. A. (1993). Low methionine ingestion by rats extends life span. *Journal of Nutrition*, 123, 269–274.

Oster, M. H., Fielder, P. J., Levin, N., & Cronin, M. J. (1995). Adaptation of the growth hormone and insulin-like growth factor-I axis to chronic and severe calorie or protein malnutrition. *Journal of Clinical Investigation*, 95, 2258–2265.

Parinello, S., Samper, E., Krtolica, A., Goldstein, J., Melov, S., Campisi, J. (2003). Oxygen sensitivity severely limits the replicative lifespan of murine fibroblasts. *Nat. Cell Biol.*, 5, 741–747.

Patronek, G. J., Waters, D. J., & Glickman, L. T. (1997). Comparative longevity of pet dogs and humans: implications for gerontology research. *Journals of Gerontology Series A: Biological Sciences and Medical Sciences*, 52, B171–B178.

Petrelli, J. M., Calle, E. E., Rodriguez, C., & Thun, M. J. (2002). Body mass index, height, and postmenopausal breast cancer mortality in a prospective cohort of US women. *Cancer Causes and Control*, 13, 325–332.

Pletcher, S. D., Khazaeli, A. A., & Curtsinger, J. W. (2000). Why do life spans differ? Partitioning mean longevity differences in terms of age-specific mortality parameters. *Journals of Gerontology Series A: Biological Sciences and Medical Sciences*, 55, B381–B389.

Pugh, T. D., Oberley, T. D., & Weindruch, R. (1999). Dietary intervention at middle age: caloric restriction but not dehydroepiandrosterone sulfate increases lifespan and lifetime cancer incidence in mice. *Cancer Research*, 59, 1642–1648.

Richie, J. P. Jr., Leutzinger, Y., Parthasarathy, S., Malloy, V., Orentreich, N., & Zimmerman, J. A. (1994). Methionine restriction increases blood glutathione and longevity in F344 rats. *FASEB Journal*, 8, 1302–1307.

Rincon, M., Muzumdar, R., Atzmon, G., & Barzilai, N. (2004). The paradox of the insulin/IGF-I signaling pathway in longevity. *Mechanisms of Ageing and Development*, 125, 397–403.

Roberts, R. C. (1961). The lifetime growth and reproduction of selected strains of mice. *Heredity*, 16, 369–381.

Robinson, R. (1973). Relationship between litter size and weight of dam in the dog. *Veterinary Record*, 92, 221–223.

Rosfjord, E. C., & Dickson, R. B. (1999). Growth factors, apoptosis, and survival of mammary epithelial cells. *Journal of Mammary Gland Biology & Neoplasia*, 4, 229–237.

Samaras, T. T., & Elrick, H. (1999). Height, body size and longevity. *Acta Medica Okayama*, 53, 149–169.

Samaras, T. T., Elrick, H., & Storms, L. H. (2003). Is height related to longevity? *Life Sciences*, 72, 1781–1802.

Samaras, T. T., & Storms, L. H. (1992). Impact of height and weight on life span. *Bulletin of the World Health Organization*, 70, 259–267.

Schaumberg, D. A., Glynn, R. J., Christen, W. G., Hankinson, S. E., & Hennekens, C. H. (2000). Relations of body fat distribution and height with cataract in men. *American Journal of Clinical Nutrition*, 72, 1495–1502.

Segall, P. E., & Timiras, P. S. (1976). Patho-physiologic findings after chronic tryptophan deficiency in rats: a model for delayed growth and aging. *Mechanisms of Ageing and Development*, 5, 109–124.

Segall, P. E., Ooka, H., Rose, K., & Timiras, P. S. (1978). Neural and endocrine development after chronic tryptophan deficiency in rats: I. Brain monoamine and pituitary responses. *Mechanism of Ageing and Development*, 7, 1–17.

Silberberg, R. (1972). Articular aging and osteoarthritis in dwarf mice. *Pathology and Microbiology*, 38, 417–430.

Speakman, J. R., van Acker, A., & Harper, E. J. (2003). Age-related changes in the metabolism and body composition of three dog breeds and their relationship to life expectancy. *Aging Cell*, 2, 265–275.

Straus, D. S. (1994). Nutritional regulation of hormones and growth factors that control mammalian growth. *FASEB Journal*, 8, 6–12.

Tartar, M., Bartke, A., & Antebi, A. (2003). The endocrine regulation of aging by insulin-like signals. *Science*, 299, 1346–1351.

Tretli, S. (1989). Height and weight in relation to breast cancer morbidity and mortality. A prospective study of 570,000 women in Norway. *International Journal of Cancer*, 44, 23–30.

Tretli, S., & Robsahm, T. E. (1999). Height, weight and cancer of the oesophagus and stomach: a follow-up study in Norway. *European Journal of Cancer Prevention*, 8, 115–122.

Tsuchiya, T., Dhahbi, J. M., Cui, X., Mote, P. L., Bartke, A., & Spindler, S. R. (2004). Additive regulation of hepatic gene expression by dwarfism and caloric restriction. *Physiological Genomics*, 17, 307–315.

Turturro, A., Hass, B., Hart, R. W., & Allaben, W. T. (1998). Body weight impact on spontaneous diseases in chronic bioassays. *International Journal of Toxicology*, 17 (Suppl. 2), 79–99.

Turturro, A., Leakey, J., Allaben, W. T., & Hart, R. W. (1997). Fat (and thin) rats distort results. *Nature*, 389, 326.

Underwood, L. E., Thissen, J. P., Lemozy, S., Ketelslegers, J. M., & Clemmons, D. R. (1994). Hormonal and nutritional regulation of IGF-I and its binding proteins. *Hormone Research*, 42, 145–151.

Vergara, M., Smith-Wheelock, M., Harper, J. M., Sigler, R., & Miller, R. A. (2004). Hormone-treated Snell dwarf mice regain fertility but remain long-lived and disease resistant. *Journal of Gerontology: Biological Sciences*, 59, 1244–1250.

Weindruch, R., & Sohal, R. S. (1997). Seminars in medicine of the Beth Israel Deaconess Medical Center. Caloric intake and aging. *New England Journal of Medicine*, 337, 986–994.

Weindruch, R., & Walford, R. L. (1982). Dietary restriction in mice beginning at 1 year of age: effect on life span and spontaneous cancer incidence. *Science*, 215, 1415–1418.

Weindruch, R., & Walford, R. L. (1988). *The retardation of aging and disease by dietary restriction*. Springfield, IL: Charles C Thomas.

West, G. B., Brown, J. H., & Enquist, B. J. (1999). The fourth dimension of life: fractal geometry and allometric scaling of organisms. *Science*, 284, 1677–1679.

White, M. E., Hathaway, M. R., Dayton, W. R., Henderson, T., & Lepine, A. J. (1999). Comparison of insulin-like growth factor-I concentration in mammary secretions and serum of small- and giant-breed dogs. *American Journal of Veterinary Research*, 60, 1088–1091.

Williams, D. L., Heath, M. F., & Wallis, C. (2004) Prevalence of canine cataract: preliminary results of a cross-sectional study. *Veterinary Ophthalmology*, 7, 29–35.

Yu, B. P., Masoro, E. J., & McMahan, C. A. (1985). Nutritional influences on aging of Fischer 344 rats: I. Physical, metabolic, and longevity characteristics. *Journal of Gerontology*, 40, 657–670.

Zhao, S., Shetty, J., Hou, L., Delcher, A., Zhu, B., Osoegawa, K., deJong, P., Nierman, W. C., Strausberg, Fraser, C. M. (2004). Human, mouse, and rate genome large-scale rearrangements: stability versus speciation. *Genome Res.*, 14, 1851–1860.

Zimmerman, J. A., Malloy, V., Krajcik, R., & Orentreich, N. (2003). Nutritional control of aging. *Experimental Gerontology*, 38, 47–52.

Chapter 20

Growth Hormone, Insulin-Like Growth Factor-1, and the Biology of Aging

Christy S. Carter and William E. Sonntag

I. Introduction

The functional decline in tissues and organs that are the hallmarks of aging were recognized by the earliest scientists and writers. However, it was not until the advent of techniques in the 1970s to accurately measure circulating hormones that the age-related decline in anabolic hormones was finally documented and its contribution to the biological changes of aging proposed. Since that time, the role of growth hormone and its anabolic mediator, insulin-like growth factor-1 (IGF-1) in the development of the aging phenotype, onset of age-related pathology, and regulation of life span has been under intense investigation. However, despite numerous studies on this topic, the biological effects of these hormones and their contribution to aging remain highly controversial. Studies in both humans and animals clearly indicate a progressive decrease in growth hormone and IGF-1 with age. Replacement of growth hormone reverses the age-related decline in IGF-1 and subsequently the decline in lean body mass,

bone density, skin thickness, immune function, learning and memory, myocardial function, as well as the increase in adiposity that are part of aging. The results of these numerous studies evolved into the concept that the aged phenotype results from a deficiency in anabolic hormones of which a deficiency of growth hormone and, subsequently, IGF-1 have a particularly important role.

The remarkable progress in understanding the genetics of life span in invertebrate models, primarily through mutagenesis techniques, has permitted the identification of specific genes and signaling pathways that modulate longevity. For example, disruption of signaling in the *daf-2* pathway (including mutations in the *daf-2* or *age-1* genes) in *C. elegans* extends life span up to 100 percent (Johnson, 1990; Kenyon *et al.*, 1993). Heteroallelic mutation of *InR* extends female life span in *D. melanogaster* by 85 percent (Clancy *et al.*, 2001). Similarly, mutation of *C. cerevisiae Sch9*, which encodes a protein kinase involved in glucose-dependent signaling that is homologous to that encoded by mammalian *Akt*, can double replicative life span (Fabrizio *et al.*, 2001). Because these invertebrate genes exhibit substantial homology to the insulin/IGF-1 receptor and signaling pathways in other species, the possibility exists that genetic modification to the insulin/IGF-1 signaling cascade may represent a common pathway for regulating life span (see Figure 20.1).

The similarities among the signaling pathways for insulin/IGF-1 in invertebrates and mammals raised the possibility that genetic modifications to this pathway may extend life span in mammals. This conclusion appeared to be supported by studies in Ames and Snell dwarf mice (resulting from *Pit1* or *Prop1* mutations that produce deficiencies in growth hormone, thyroid-stimulating hormone, and

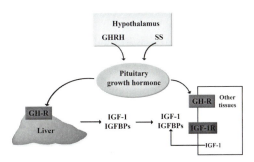

Figure 20.1 Growth hormone, produced in the anterior pituitary, is modulated by two hypothalamic hormones, growth hormone-releasing hormone (GHRH), which stimulates both the synthesis and secretion of growth hormone, and somatostatin (SS), which inhibits growth hormone release in response to GHRH. Growth hormone also feeds back to inhibit GHRH secretion and probably has a direct inhibitory effect on secretion from the somatotroph (growth hormone–producing cells). Basal concentrations of growth hormone in blood are very low. In mammals, growth hormone is secreted in pulsatile bursts from the anterior pituitary gland, a pattern that is necessary to achieve full biological activity. Although 90 percent of circulating IGF-1 is synthesized and secreted by the liver, many types of cells, including some found in the brain and vasculature, are capable of IGF-1 production. Reprinted from *Trends in Genetics*, Volume 18, No. 6, 2002, pp. 295–301, with permission from Elsevier.

prolactin) as well as in transgenic mice with a knockout of the growth hormone receptor (GHR/BP-KO) that reduces IGF-1 levels. All these strains demonstrated markedly increased life span (Brown-Borg *et al.*, 1996; Flurkey *et al.*, 2001; Hauck *et al.*, 2001). Although the specific mechanisms continue to be debated, an opposing point of view—that growth hormone and IGF-1 accelerate aging—became well established in the literature.

These two disparate concepts—that growth hormone and IGF-1 ameliorate impairments of biological aging and that growth hormone and IGF-1 accelerate aging—are at the center of the current controversy and the focus of this chapter. Here, we review the endocrine pathway and mechanisms of action of growth hormone and IGF-1, detail the effects of growth hormone and/or IGF-1 replacement on the aging phenotype, and review the various models that, in our opinion, have given rise to some aspects of these controversies. Finally, we propose an integrated view of the actions of growth hormone and IGF-1 and suggest that the dynamic changes in these hormones throughout the life span have evolutionary significance.

II. Biological Actions of Growth Hormone

Bovine growth hormone was first isolated from the pituitary gland by Li and colleagues (1945) and was subsequently shown to stimulate fatty acid mobilization; amino acid uptake; DNA, RNA, and protein synthesis; and have a role in cell division and tissue hypertrophy. Although the importance of growth hormone in regulating body growth was established soon after these initial studies, current research in the regulation and effects of growth hormone began with the development of sensitive assays that accurately measure hormone levels in the circulation. These studies led to the discovery that growth hormone is secreted into the blood in pulsatile bursts from the anterior pituitary gland, a pattern necessary to achieve full biological activity. In humans, the majority of secretion occurs at night in association with slow-wave sleep (Born et al., 1988). Although similar pulses are observed in rodents, high-amplitude secretory pulses occur every 3.5 hours in males (Tannenbaum & Martin, 1976) and hourly in females (see Figure 20.2).

It was later discovered that the regulation of these pulses involved at least two hormones released by the hypothalamus: growth hormone-releasing hormone (GHRH), which increases growth hormone release (Ling et al., 1984; Rivier et al., 1982) and somatostatin, which inhibits its release (Brazeau et al., 1973). The dynamic interactions between these hormones are responsible for high-amplitude, pulsatile growth hormone secretion. It is generally believed that somatostatin tone is dominant during trough periods and that growth hormone is released in response to secretion of GHRH and suppression of somatostatin (Tannenbaum & Ling, 1984).

Both growth hormone and IGF-1 inhibit growth hormone release in a typical endocrine feedback relationship either directly at the level of the pituitary or by stimulating somatostatin and/or inhibiting GHRH release (Berelowitz et al., 1981). Although the precise function of this ultradian pattern remains unknown, the pulsatile nature of growth hormone release has been confirmed in every species examined to date and is necessary for full biological potency of the hormone.

Growth hormone binds with high affinity to its receptor, found in tissues throughout the body, and activation of this receptor stimulates the synthesis and secretion of IGF-1 (Le Roith et al., 2001). This receptor belongs to the cytokine family of receptors and its activation facilitates the association of intracellular components of the receptor with JAK2 into a complex with subsequent phosphorylation of both proteins (Argetsinger et al., 1993; Campbell et al., 1992; Gronowski et al., 1995; Sotiropoulos et al., 1994; also see review by Roupas & Herington, 1994). Several other intracellular proteins are subsequently phosphorylated, including mitogen-activated protein kinase (MAP

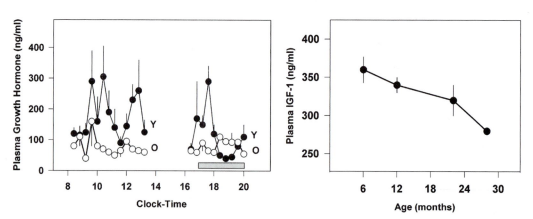

Figure 20.2 Age-related changes in the growth hormone/IGF-1 axis. (A) Growth hormone secretory pulses in young (6-month-old) (blue symbols) and old (20-month-old) (red symbols) Sprague-Dawley rats. Serial samples of blood were removed at 20-minute intervals from conscious, freely moving animals and analyzed by radioimmunoassay. The green bar represents the dark phase of the light/dark cycle. (B) Age-related changes in plasma IGF-1. Data represents mean ± sem. Reprinted from *Trends in Genetics*, Volume 18, No. 6, 2002, pp. 295–301, with permission from Elsevier.

kinase), S6 kinase, and STAT proteins (signal transducer and activator of transcription). The result of growth hormone receptor activation is an increase in *c-fos*, *c-jun*, serine phosphatase inhibitor-1, and IGF-1 gene expression and secretion (Bichell *et al.*, 1992).

Although 90 percent of circulating IGF-1 is synthesized and secreted by the liver, many types of cells, including those found in the brain and vasculature, are capable of IGF-1 production (Lopez-

Fernandez *et al.*, 1996; Yamamoto & Murphy, 1995), although it is unclear whether these sources contribute to circulating levels of IGF-1. As with hepatic IGF-1 that is secreted into the bloodstream and constitutes the endocrine IGF-1 pathway, the local or paracrine sources of IGF-1 are also regulated by growth hormone. The processing of IGF-1 mRNA by these tissues produces several transcripts that are homologous to pro-insulin, and the resulting protein, IGF-1,

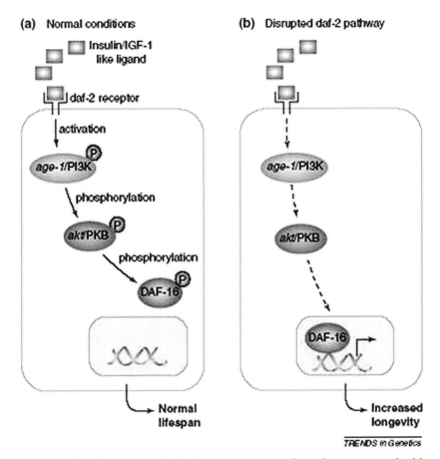

TRENDS in Genetics

Figure 20.3 *C. elegans* daf-2 pathway. (A) Under permissive growth conditions, an insulin-like substrate binds the *daf-2*-encoded receptor, initiating a cascade of events, including activation of the *age-1* encoded homolog of mammalian phosphoinositide-3-OH kinase (PI3K). PI3K activates the *Akt*-encoded protein kinase B (PKB), which phosphorylates the *daf-16* transcription factor, preventing its translocation to the nucleus. (B) Disruption of the *daf-2* pathway (including mutations in *daf-2*, *age-1*, or *Akt* genes) prohibits the phosphorylation of the *daf-16* transcription factor, permitting its translocation to the nucleus. The role of *daf-16* in transcription is believed to extend life. Reprinted from *Trends in Genetics*, Volume 18, No. 6, 2002, pp. 295–301, with permission from Elsevier.

is primarily responsible for the anabolic actions of growth hormone through regulation of cellular DNA, RNA, and protein synthesis (Cohick & Clemmons, 1993). Blood and tissue levels as well as activity of the peptide are regulated by at least six IGF-1 binding proteins (IGFBPs) that are capable of facilitating or inhibiting IGF activity (Cohick & Clemmons, 1993). Although it was initially proposed that all of the actions of growth hormone were mediated through IGF-1, data from several studies (Daughaday, 1989; Isaksson et al., 1988) support direct roles for growth hormone in the regulation of lipolysis and insulin sensitivity that are independent of IGF-1.

III. Aging and the Growth Hormone Axis

More than 25 years ago, it was reported that elderly individuals experience a decline in the ability to secrete growth hormone in response to several stimuli, including insulin-induced hypoglycemia and arginine administration (Laron et al., 1970). Subsequent studies revealed a loss of the nocturnal surges of growth hormone (Carlson et al., 1972; Finkelstein et al., 1972) and a decrease in plasma IGF-1 that paralleled the decline in growth hormone pulse (Johanson & Blizzard, 1981; Rudman et al., 1981). These early studies in humans have been extended to rodents (Sonntag et al., 1980), and currently, the decline in high-amplitude growth hormone secretion and plasma IGF-1 concentrations are some of the most robust and well-characterized endocrine alterations that occur with age.

Shortly after the documentation of decreases in growth hormone secretion in humans, studies confirmed an age-related decline in the amplitude of growth hormone pulses in rodents (Sonntag et al., 1980) that led to the decline in plasma IGF-1 (Florini et al.,

1981). These studies progressed to an investigation of the hypothalamic and pituitary mechanisms responsible for the deficiency in growth hormone secretion. A decline in in vivo pituitary response to GHRH with age was reported in both animals and humans (Ceda et al., 1986; Shibasaki et al., 1984; Sonntag et al., 1985); however, studies attempting to detail the specific deficits within the pituitary gland were controversial. The latter findings ultimately were attributed to either differential responses of older animals to the pharmacological agents used to suppress endogenous growth hormone pulses during in vivo testing (Sonntag & Boyd, 1988; Sonntag et al., 1983) or technical limitations in culturing anterior pituitary cells from older animals (Spik & Sonntag, 1989).

Research efforts were eventually directed to an analysis of hypothalamic release and inhibiting hormones based on studies indicating that (1) acute administration of somatostatin antiserum in vivo increased growth hormone release identically in both young and old animals (Sonntag et al., 1981); (2) passive immunization with somatostatin antiserum reversed the in vivo deficiency in pituitary response to GHRH (Sonntag & Gough, 1988); and (3) stimulation of hypothalamic synaptosomes from old animals in a superfusion system released greater amounts of somatostatin than those of young animals (Sonntag et al., 1986). Increased somatostatin concentrations also have been reported in pituitary extracts from older animals, again suggesting increased release of this peptide from hypothalamic neurons (Sonntag et al., 1986). These results provided evidence that increased somatostatin tone is an important factor in the decline in growth hormone pulses with age. Furthermore, these conclusions were supported by research studies in humans, where administration of cholinergic agonists or arginine, considered to preferentially inhibit somatostatin release (Penalva *et al.*, 1989), were capable of increasing growth hormone secretion in older individuals (Ghigo *et al.*, 1990).

Although the previously mentioned studies did not address the synthesis and release of GHRH, related studies indicated that a decline in this hormone is another contributing factor in the decrease in growth hormone secretion with age. In a series of experiments, investigators demonstrated that GHRH mRNA decreased with age (DeGennaro *et al.*, 1989) and that the feedback relationship between growth hormone and hypothalamic neurons is impaired (DeGennaro Colonna *et al.*, 1993). In this latter study, growth hormone administration in older animals increased GHRH mRNA and decreased somatostatin mRNA, but GHRH neurons remained non-responsive to GHRH. Thus, the data suggest that decreases in growth hormone secretion with age result from alterations within the hypothalamus involving regulation of both GHRH and somatostatin.

Although a decline in the amplitude of growth hormone pulses is an important determinant of the decrease in plasma IGF-1, growth hormone-induced IGF-1 secretion also is diminished in elderly individuals and suggests that resistance to the actions of growth hormone may be an additional contributing factor in the low plasma IGF-1 concentrations (Lieberman *et al.*, 1994). In rodents, a two-fold increase in hepatic growth hormone receptors has been observed with age, but this fails to compensate for the reduction in growth hormone secretion (Takahashi & Meites, 1987; Xu *et al.*, 1995). A more detailed investigation revealed that the K_D and apparent size of the growth hormone receptor were not altered, whereas the capacity of growth hormone to induce IGF-1 gene expression and secretion was 40 to 50 percent less in old than in young animals. These results demonstrated that impairment in growth hormone receptor signal transduction is

another contributing factor in the decline in IGF-1 in both animals and man.

The reduced response to growth hormone appears to be the consequence of deficiencies in intracellular signaling mechanisms. Studies by Xu and colleagues (1995) reported that phosphorylation of JAK2 and the growth hormone receptor complex were suppressed in aged rodents in response to growth hormone, and these decreases were accompanied by a decline in MAP kinase activity. More recent studies demonstrated that growth hormone–induced STAT3 activation and nuclear translocation are also decreased with age (Xu & Sonntag, 1996). Although these studies did not address the etiology of the decrease in JAK2 activity, they clearly indicated that diminished growth hormone receptor signal transduction is a contributing factor in the functional alterations in tissues with age.

Because the specific deficits in growth hormone signal transduction in aged animals appear to be an early event in receptor signaling, it was postulated that production of splice variants that are resistant to phosphorylation or a decrease in turnover of the growth hormone receptor, perhaps resulting from oxidative damage, contribute to the signaling deficits with age. However, data from our laboratory demonstrated that growth hormone receptor turnover *in vivo* increases with age, and no obvious changes in receptor mRNA structure were evident when analyzed by RT-PCR. Mechanisms that may potentially contribute to the decline in growth hormone receptor signaling include point mutations, post-translational modifications in receptor protein, and enhanced phosphotyrosine phosphatase activity. Although the specific mechanisms for the decline in growth hormone signal transduction remain poorly understood, the deficiency in growth hormone signal transduction together with concomitant decreases in growth hormone secretion appear to be major factors involved in the decline in plasma IGF-1 with age.

IV. Studies of Growth Hormone/IGF-1 Replacement

Classical endocrine studies to determine the consequences of hormone deficiency require replacement of highly purified hormone under physiological conditions. In the case of growth hormone and IGF-1, the physiological significance of the age-related decline in these hormones was assessed by administration of growth hormone to either aged animals or humans. Consistent with the concept that aging is a catabolic process, age-related decreases in skeletal muscle mass, bone mass, immune function, and skin thickness were shown to be ameliorated by growth hormone administration. More recently, memory deficits as well as age-associated rarefaction of cerebrovasculature and cardiac microvasculature were found to be reversed by growth hormone and/or IGF-1 therapy (Khan et al., 2001; Lembo et al., 1996; Sonntag et al., 1999; Thornton et al., 2000). The positive results of these studies provided evidence that the decrease in these hormones contributes to some of the biochemical and physiological impairments of aging.

Despite the fact that growth hormone and IGF-1 supplementation have been shown to reverse the age-related decline in several specific measures of tissue function, technical limitations related to the restoration of endogenous, diurnal growth hormone pulses have hindered progress in this area. These issues have been compounded by the limited availability of rat growth hormone for long-term replacement studies. In fact, there have been only two studies in which the effects of growth hormone on life span were assessed for periods longer than four months. Unfortunately, both studies

used human growth hormone, which is both antigenic and prolactogenic in rodents, potentially confounding the experimental results. Nevertheless, these authors reported either no detrimental effect of growth hormone administration on life span when initiated at 18 months of age in rats (Kalu et al., 1998) or an increase in life span when administered to mice beginning at 17 months of age (Khansari & Gustad, 1991).

The impaired secretion of growth hormone and the subsequent decline in IGF-1 appear to influence the maintenance and viability of multiple organ systems as well as subsequent functional and behavioral outcomes. However, there are often deleterious effects associated with growth hormone replacement therapy in the elderly, including edema, arthralgias, carpal tunnel, muscle pain and bloating, thereby questioning whether growth hormone supplementation is recommended for use in the elderly before more longer-term randomized controlled trials are conducted (Harman & Blackman, 2003).The following sections briefly review the impact of loss of growth hormone/IGF-1 on specific physiological systems.

A. Cognitive Function

There are numerous reports addressing a possible relationship between serum IGF-1 levels and human cognitive function. Others have observed statistically significant associations between both perceptual-motor performance and information processing speed and IGF-1 levels in a sample of 25 subjects 65 to 76 years of age (Aleman et al., 1999). The same subject group demonstrated a significant association between serum IGF-1 and fluid intelligence, a cognitive measure that is sensitive to aging (Aleman et al., 2001). In a two-year prospective study involving 186 participants between 55 and 80 years of age, high total serum

IGF-1 concentrations and high IGF-1/ IGFBP-3 ratios were significantly correlated with decreased age-adjusted cognitive decline determined by scores on the 30-point MMSE (Kalmijn et al., 2000). In 19 healthy centenarians, a significant correlation was reported between IGF-1/IGFBP-3 molar ratios, which have been postulated to reflect the amount of biologically available IGF-1, and MMSE scores (Juul et al., 1995; Paolisso et al., 1997). Rollero and colleagues (1998) documented a direct correlation between serum IGF-1 concentrations and MMSE scores in 22 subjects between 65 and 86 years of age (Rollero et al., 1998). Morley and colleagues (1997) reported a significant correlation between IGF-1/growth hormone ratio and both visual and auditory learning in men 20 to 84 years of age (Morley et al., 1997). In a three-year longitudinal study of cognitive decline in 1,318 subjects 65 to 88 years of age, Dik and colleagues (2003) observed an association between low serum levels of IGF-1 and deficits in information processing speed (Dik et al., 2003). However, Papadakis and colleagues (1995) reported no association between serum IGF-1 levels and age-adjusted cognitive status in 104 healthy older men, and others observed no correlation between IGF-1 levels and attention, fluid intelligence, or memory (Aleman et al., 2000).

While these correlational observations have offered valuable information related to connections between the growth hormone/IGF-1 axis and human cognitive function, intervention studies offer a more realistic picture of the therapeutic potential of growth hormone or IGF-1 replacement. However, very few such investigations have been performed to date. A report in women over 60 years of age, given one-year IGF-1 treatment, sufficient to increase plasma IGF-1 to that found in younger subjects, had no effect on memory in name-face and word-list recall tasks (Friedlander et al., 2001).

Nevertheless, six-month growth hormone treatment in men of mean age 75 resulted in significant improvements on the Trails B test compared to those receiving placebo (Papadakis et al., 1996). Dissention among investigators regarding the success of growth hormone and IGF-1 replacement for the attenuation of age-related cognitive impairment in humans necessitates additional studies. In fact, other factors that influence levels of IGF-1, such as level of physical activity, comorbidities, and body composition, may also influence cognitive competency. Therefore, more closely controlled studies will be necessary in order to clarify these findings.

Studies in rodents are more promising. Although information on the direct effects of growth hormone on neuronal function are limited, convincing evidence exists that IGF-1 has an important role in regulating numerous aspects of brain function, in general, and neuronal function specifically (Noguchi et al., 1987; Shemer et al., 1987; Werther et al., 1990). IGF-1 has been reported to stabilize tubulin mRNA (Fernyhough et al., 1989), stimulate DNA and RNA synthesis in brain (Han et al., 1988; Lenoir & Honegger, 1983; Shemer et al., 1987; Torres-Aleman et al., 1989) and neurite formation (Recio-Pinto & Ishii, 1984; Recio-Pinto et al., 1984; Toran-Allerand et al., 1988), enhance oligodendrocyte proliferation (McMorris & Dubois-Dalcq, 1988; McMorris et al., 1986; van der Pal et al., 1988), and increase survival of neurons and glia in culture (Recio-Pinto et al., 1986). In vivo, increases in neurogenesis, survival of differentiating neurons, and increased synaptic complexity have been reported (Lichtenwalner et al., 2000). Recent evidence suggests that IGF-1 participates in the regulation of intracellular calcium and increases the expression of the proto-oncogene c-fos (Ghahary et al., 1998; Renganathan et al., 1997), paired pulse facilitation (Ramsey, Weiner,

Moore, Carter & Sonntag 2004), and AMPA receptor activity (Ramsey, Ariwodola, et al., 2004). Although there are large volumes of data supporting an active role for IGF-1 in brain function, there are fewer in vivo studies of IGF-1 replacement, in part because of the lack of appropriate animal models and simple, reliable techniques to regulate IGF-1 levels in brain.

Although plasma growth hormone and IGF-1 clearly have a role in brain function, the specific sources of IGF-1 that influence the brain are less clear. The majority of evidence suggests that growth hormone does not readily cross the blood-brain barrier, although it is known that hypophysectomy (which decreases both growth hormone and plasma IGF-1) decreases IGF-1 mRNA in brain, and concentrations can be restored by growth hormone administration (Hynes et al., 1987). Recently published studies suggest that administration of growth hormone raises brain IGF-1 levels (Lopez-Fernandez et al., 1996), and peripheral injections of IGF-1 have been shown to protect neurons from cell death after ischemic injury (Pulford et al., 1997). Recent evidence supports the conclusion that plasma IGF-1 is actively transported through the blood-brain barrier (Reinhardt & Bondy, 1994), but the specific transport mechanism for this process is poorly understood. Because IGF-1 is also produced in endothelial and smooth muscle cells (Delafontaine, Lou, & Alexander, 1991; Delafontaine, Bernstein, & Alexander, 1991; Engelmann et al., 1989), the possibility exists that both plasma IGF-1 and vascular-derived IGF-1 (possibly under the regulation of growth hormone and/or IGF-1) are important sources of IGF-1 in the brain.

IGF-1 is an important neurotrophic factor that decreases with age. As with earlier studies of growth hormone replacement to assess the impact of growth hormone deficiency on the aging phenotype, intracerebroventricular IGF-1 replacement has been shown to reverse the age-related decline in learning and memory as well as several biochemical measures linked to cognitive ability. Studies using the Morris Water Maze revealed that icv administration of IGF-1 for 28 days to old animals increased both working and reference memory (Bennett et al., 1997). In addition, prevention of the age-related decline in growth hormone pulse amplitude and plasma IGF-1 by daily injections of [D-Ala^2]GHRH for 18 months ameliorated the age-related decline in reference memory. In this latter study, performance of old animals treated with [D-Ala^2]GHRH to raise growth hormone and IGF-1 levels was indistinguishable from that of young animals on the reference memory task . The improved performance in older animals appears to be associated with increased hippocampal glucose metabolism and NMDA receptor density (specifically NMDAR2a-c) (Bennett et al., 1997), an effect that can be mimicked by peripheral injections of growth hormone (Nyberg, 1997). Similarly, recent studies indicate that peripheral growth hormone administration for four to six months reverses age-related impairments in paired-pulse facilitation suggesting improved hippocampal GABAergic function (Ramsey et al., 2004). Finally, growth hormone replacement was able to ameliorate the age-related rise in oxidative stress in hippocampus assessed as GSH/GSSH ratios. Since NMDA receptors (specifically NMDA R2A and R2B) have been strongly implicated in the process of memory acquisition (Altman & Quartermain, 1983; Dubrovina & Il'iuchenok, 1990; Gasbarri et al., 1993; Shaywitz & Pearson, 1978; Smith et al., 1973), it was proposed that the behavioral improvement noted in response to IGF-1 is based, in part, on the regulation of excitatory neurotransmitter systems. However, the diverse actions of growth hormone and IGF-1 on the aging brain suggest that these hormones may regulate an underlying process critical for brain aging. Such processes may include regulation of blood flow, metabolism (see below), oxidative stress, or a combination of these factors.

B. Cerebral Microvascular Density and Blood Flow

Decreases in cerebral blood flow with age have been reported in rodents, non-human primates, and humans and have the potential to be an important contributing factor in brain aging (Amano et al., 1982; Bell & Ball, 1990; Goldman et al., 1987; Jucker et al., 1990; Kety, 1956; Melamed et al., 1980; Shaw et al., 1984). Although the etiology of the age-related decrease in blood flow has not been determined, contributing factors may be increases in vascular resistance (most likely resulting from an age-related increase in arteriolar vessel segment length between branches) or a decrease in arteriolar density (Cook et al., 1992). In other vascular beds (e.g. skeletal muscle), Hutchins and colleagues (1982, 1996) reported a decline in the total number of arterioles, in the rat, between 3 and 30 weeks of age. These results suggest that a reduction in arteriolar density is a primary factor in the decrease in blood flow to skeletal muscle. A similar hypothesis (Rosenblum & Kontos, 1974) (reduction in arteriolar density) was proposed to account for the decrease in cerebral blood flow with age. Subsequent analysis of arteriolar density on the cortical surface demonstrated an age-related rarefaction of arteries, arteriolar-to-arteriolar anastomoses, and venules. Because vasculature on the surface of brain is generally representative of vasculature in other brain regions, it was suggested that the decrease in the number of arterioles may be the critical factor in the decline in brain blood flow with age.

The maintenance of arteriolar density is a complex process involving a number of growth factors. Both growth hormone and IGF-1 have an important regulatory role in blood vessel growth and repair (Delafontaine, 1995; Delafontaine, Bernstein, & Alexander, 1991; Folkow et al., 1988; Gould et al., 1995). For example, blood vessels have receptors for growth hormone and IGF-1, and several studies indicate that immunoreactive IGF-1 within vessels increases during periods of vessel growth and repair (Hansson et al., 1987; Hansson et al., 1989). Furthermore, IGF-1 has been shown to potentiate the actions of several vascular growth factors, including VEGF, bFGF, and PDGF (Sato et al., 1993). Both growth hormone and IGF-1 stimulate endothelial cell proliferation, tube formation, and angiogenesis in a number of tissues. Growth hormone, for example, has been shown to stimulate angiogenesis in chorioallantoic membranes of the chick embryo (Gould et al., 1995), whereas IGF-1 has been reported to stimulate the growth of endothelial cells in the retina (Grant et al., 1993) and the proliferation of omental microvessel endothelial cells (Sato et al., 1993). Similarly, IGF-1 increases angiogenesis and migration of endothelial cells in both rat aortic rings and bovine carotid artery cells. Tube formation in endothelial cells derived from the carotid artery also has been reported in response to IGF-1 (Nakao-Hayashi et al., 1992; Nicosia et al., 1994). In addition to the apparent ability of IGF-1 to stimulate vascular growth independently, several investigators report that the actions of other growth factors, including tissue plasminogen activator (tPA) and hepatocyte growth factor, are facilitated by IGF-1 (Sato et al., 1993). These studies support the hypothesis that growth hormone and IGF-1 regulate vascular growth *in vitro*, and our recent data are consistent with the conclusion that a decline in the secretion of these hormones contribute to age-associated vascular deficiencies.

The effects of growth hormone replacement on vascular changes within the aging brain were assessed by administration of growth hormone to older animals over a 30-day period. As expected, vehicle-treated young and old animals exhibited no changes in vascular density during this period; however, a substantial increase in vascular growth in older animals treated with growth hormone was observed (Sonntag et al., 1997). Although the vascular growth observed in these animals represented only small arterioles, the results provide compelling evidence that growth hormone (and/or IGF-1) participate in the regulation of vascular growth, and the age-related reduction in these hormones contribute to the decline in cerebrovascular density.

C. Cardiovascular System

The concepts that growth hormone has effects on the cardiovascular system and may reverse age-related changes in cardiovascular function are based on both in vivo and in vitro studies. Cardiac myocytes contain receptors for growth hormone (Adamafio et al., 1991; Haro et al., 1999; Mathews et al., 1989) and cultured myocytes are responsive to growth hormone administration (Adamafio et al., 1991). Growth hormone has been shown to regulate cardiac growth in vivo (including myocyte growth) (Kupfer & Rubin, 1992), to increase left ventricular function, and to regulate left ventricular remodeling and contractile processes in pigs with congestive heart failure (CHF) (Houck et al., 1999). Two studies have suggested that IGFR stimulation results in activation of the β-adrenergic receptor (Karoor et al., 1998; Lembo et al., 1996) and may partially reverse the age-related decline in β-adrenergic activity. Therefore, the current data support the concept that growth hormone, either directly or through IGF-1, has potent effects on the heart and has

the capacity to improve myocardial function in aged animals or in response to specific diseases that affect the cardiovascular system.

Administration of growth hormone to rodents in physiological doses ameliorates many age-related changes in the cardiovascular system. The age-related rarefaction of myocardial vessels (Khan et al., 2001) is partially reversed by administration of bovine growth hormone (similar to the reversal observed in brain) (Sonntag et al., 1997). It is of interest that in this latter study, the effects of growth hormone on microvascular density were limited to specific regions of the heart, and it was suggested that predisposing pathology (fibrosis) may limit or prevent the angiogenic actions of growth hormone. Nevertheless, growth hormone administration to aged rats also increased coronary blood flow (Sonntag et al., 1997) and cardiac myofilament contractility (Wannenburg et al., 2001). Thus, physiological doses of growth hormone are able to reverse some of the changes in cardiovascular structure and function with age, supporting the conclusion that age-related decreases in growth hormone have the potential to contribute to impairments in cardiovascular function observed in aged animals.

Several investigators have examined the differential and synergistic cardiac effects of growth hormone and IGF-1. Cittadini and colleagues (1996), for example, administered recombinant human growth hormone, recombinant human IGF-1, or a combination of both hormones to 3-month-old Sprague-Dawley rats. Echocardiography revealed that combination therapy with growth hormone and IGF-1 did not have synergistic effects on myocardial growth or function. However, cardiac output and stroke volume were increased in response to IGF-1 and/or in response to the combination of growth hormone and IGF-1 compared to controls and animals treated with growth hormone alone. Another study examined the *in vitro* effects of growth hormone and IGF-1 on intracellular calcium (Stromer *et al.*, 1996). No acute effects of growth hormone were found on cardiac function, although IGF-1 caused an increase in isovolumic developed pressure without a change in intracellular $Ca2^+$ concentration. Further studies of isolated ferret papillary muscles demonstrated that the effects of IGF-1 on contractility could be blocked by wortmannin, an inhibitor of PI-3 (phosphatidylinositol-3 kinase), an intracellular kinase stimulated by IGF-1 receptor activation (Cittadini *et al.*, 1998). These results suggest that IGF-1 is able to increase cardiac contractility *in vitro* by altering myofilament calcium sensitivity rather than through increasing intracellular calcium. Studies utilizing combination therapy with growth hormone and IGF-1 suggest that some of the effects of growth hormone on the heart are mediated through IGF-1 and that, in addition, both hormones exert independent and interacting effects on cardiac structure and function.

Growth hormone administration has been considered as a possible treatment for heart failure (Frustaci *et al.*, 1992) and has been shown to improve left ventricular contractility in rats with experimental heart failure and cardiomyopathy. In response to left coronary artery ligation (Yang *et al.*, 1995), growth hormone administration increased stroke volume and decreased mean arterial pressure through a decrease in systemic vascular resistance. Left ventricular (LV) contractility, as measured by LV dP/dt, was also improved by growth hormone. With the exception of an increase in body weight and a decrease in mean arterial pressure, growth hormone administration did not have a significant effect in control animals. A recent study by Ryoke and colleagues (1999) examined the effects of growth hormone administration on LV dysfunction in cardiomyopathic hamsters. This strain

becomes cardiomyopathic due to an autosomal recessive mutation of the gene for d-sarcoglycan, part of the dystrophin complex (Nigro *et al.*, 1997; Sakamoto *et al.*, 1997). LV contractility improved with growth hormone treatment, but to a greater degree in the younger versus older animals. LV wall stress at end systole was reduced by growth hormone administration in 4-month-old animals, whereas wall stress increased at end diastole in response to growth hormone in 10-month-old animals. Therefore, the conclusion was made that growth hormone administration has beneficial effects on LV contractility and wall stress, but the response is blunted with age.

Studies in humans have also suggested that growth hormone deficiency can result in cardiomyopathy. A positive correlation between mean nocturnal growth hormone plasma levels and ejection fraction was demonstrated in 12 patients with cardiomyopathy (Giustina *et al.*, 1996). In a single case report of a patient with hypopituitarism, dilated cardiomyopathy was partially reversible with growth hormone administration (Frustaci *et al.*, 1992), and growth hormone withdrawal resulted in recurrent thinning of the myocardial wall and a decrease in LV ejection fraction. Others have demonstrated that growth hormone replacement improved cardiac function in patients with ischemic cardiomyopathy (Genth-Zotz *et al.*, 1999). Interestingly, growth hormone was administered at a relatively low dose—half the dose shown to be effective in growth hormone deficient cardiomyocytes (Frustaci *et al.*, 1992). Exercise capacity, cardiac output, and myocardial wall thickness increased, whereas end systolic and diastolic volume indices decreased. However, there was no increase in LV ejection fraction. The effects were maintained for three months and diminished after withdrawal of growth hormone therapy. It is unknown whether these effects were mediated by increased IGF-1 levels or changes in myocardial structure.

D. Body Composition and Physical Performance

During the adult life span, human males average a 12 kg loss in lean mass and an increase in fat mass. In women, the ratio is more in favor of fat mass gain (15 kg) with a much smaller loss of lean mass (5 kg). The age-related loss of muscle mass, or sarcopenia, has been correlated with a loss of function and disability (Roubenoff & Rall, 1993). Rudman and colleagues (1990) described this association in a population of community-dwelling men over 60 years old. Individuals were randomized to receive growth hormone replacement or no treatment for six months. Individuals receiving GH supplementation had increases in IGF-1 levels along with an increase in lean body mass and a decrease in adipose-tissue mass. They also reported an increase in average lumbar vertebral bone density and skin thickness. More recently, Harman and Blackman (2003) described the effects of growth hormone alone or in combination with sex hormone replacement therapy. In a cohort of healthy, ambulatory, community-dwelling men and women between 65 and 88 years of age, 26 weeks of treatment resulted in increases in lean and decreases in fat mass; however, only males receiving combined therapy of growth hormone and testosterone show an increase in total body strength. In contrast, Friedlander and colleagues (2001) demonstrated no effect of 12 months of IGF-1 administration in a population of post-menopausal women over 60 years of age on any measure of body composition.

Only one randomized study to date has used functional status after GH replacement as an outcome. Papadakis and colleagues (1995) randomized a group of men over the age of 69 to either six months of hormone replacement therapy or no treatment. They found an increase in lean body mass accompanied by a decrease in fat mass. There were no changes in muscle strength as measured by grip strength, endurance, or knee flexion. Nor were there changes in measures of physical performance as measured by requiring the subjects to write a prescribed sentence, transfer kidney beans using a teaspoon, place a heavy book on a shelf, remove a jacket, pick up a penny from the floor, turn 360 degrees, walk a 50-foot walking test course, and climb stairs to determine speed and the number of flights climbed before the development of fatigue. They concluded that although there were increases in lean body mass, it would only be possible to observe benefits related to physical function at pharmacological rather than the physiological doses used in the study. However, a number of side effects (lower extremity edema and diffuse arthralgias, among others) were observed even at this low physiological dose; therefore, the practicality of increasing growth hormone levels further is questionable.

Rodents undergo shifts in body composition similar to humans (e.g., increased fat and decreased lean mass with an eventually loss of fat mass late in life as well). These results have been described by Wolden-Hanson and colleagues in a cross-sectional analysis of male brown Norway rats aged 3, 8, 17, and 29 months. Body weight, lean mass, and absolute and percentage fat increased with age, whereas percentage of lean mass decreased (Wolden-Hanson et al., 1999). In contrast others have shown that, in Fisher 344 rats, lean body mass does not progressively decline with increasing age, but rather the decline occurred only after the onset of the terminal disease process. Fat mass increases up to about 70 percent survival but declines thereafter (Bertrand et al., 1980; Yu et al., 1982).

Our lab and others have shown that many age-related deficits of muscle mass (Cartee *et al.*, 1996) and function, as well as the increase in fat body mass accumulation, are attenuated with growth hormone replacement. Senescent animals (24 to 30 months of age) receiving bovine growth hormone replacement from 24 to 30 months of age demonstrated a modest but significant increase in grip strength compared to controls (unpublished data, Carter *et al.*). Furthermore, in mice over-expressing IGF-1 in skeletal muscle, the age-related loss of specific force, a measurement of quality of muscle that compares the ratio of muscle mass to muscle force, is attenuated (Delbono, 2000).

The body of knowledge concerning hormone replacement therapy in the elderly is still controversial, although experimental studies in rodents appear to support a beneficial role. The effects are generally small in magnitude, and the increases in muscle strength are inconsistent. Using pharmacological doses of these hormones might very well increase the benefit of replacement therapy, but the side effects and increased risk for serious disease have, to date, limited enthusiasm for replacement therapy.

E. Immune Function

Growth hormone replacement in a variety of models of growth hormone deficiency including both aging (French *et al.*, 2002; Goya *et al.*, 1992; Goff *et al.*, 1987; Knyszynski *et al.*, 1992) and dwarf models (Murphy *et al.*, 1992), demonstrate clear effects on immune function. A decline in growth hormone correlates with a progressive atrophy of the thymus gland and thymocyte progenitors derived from bone marrow. IGF-1 acts, in part, by increasing the migration and colonization of these bone marrow–derived precursors to the thymus. Growth hormone replacement *in vivo* to aged rats is associated with reversal of age-related hypocellularity

of hematopoietic cells and the increased accumulation of adipocytes in bone marrow (French *et al.*, 2002). Growth hormone administration also restores thymic morphology, increases thymic lymphoid and bone marrow myeloid cells, and reduces adipocyte accumulation. This effect was extended to spleen, liver, and adrenal gland.

In contrast, others have characterized immune function in Ames and Snell dwarf murine models (Flurkey *et al.*, 2001). Aging in normal animals results in an increase in the proportion of CD4 and CD8 cells that express the CD44 surface marker, typical of a memory cell. These dwarf models display delay aging of T cell surface markers and responder T cell frequencies that is correlated with increased survival. However, these authors also recognize that work with these dwarf models does not identify growth hormone specifically as the agent responsible for these aging effects due to their multiple endocrine deficiencies.

F. Cell Proliferation and Tissue Pathology

Several *in vitro* studies suggest that IGF-1 is an important mitogenic factor. For example, serum (which contains high quantities of IGF-1) is necessary for cell survival and antibodies against IGF-1 are able to inhibit the ability of 5 percent serum to stimulate DNA synthesis in Balb/c-3T3 cells (Russell *et al.*, 1984). In addition, Balb/c-3T3 cells transfected with IGF-1 and type 1 IGF receptors grow in serum-free media (Pietrzkowski *et al.*, 1992) and antagonists to the IGF receptor inhibit cellular growth (Pietrzkowski *et al.*, 1992). Other growth factors, including platelet-derived growth factor (PDGF) and epidermal growth factor (EGF) (Pietrzkowski *et al.*, 1992), also increase cellular IGF-1 synthesis, and it has been proposed that their effects may be mediated in whole, or in part, through the IGF-1 system. Similar stimulatory effects of IGF-1 on cellular growth also have been reported *in vivo* (Desai *et al.*, 1999) and form the basis for the concept that IGF-1 is potentially pathogenic.

Many human cancers and transformed cell lines produce IGF-1 or its receptor (see review by Werner & LeRoith, 1996), and overexpression of the type 1 IGF receptor in 3T3 fibroblasts leads to the formation of tumors in nude mice (Kaleko *et al.*, 1990). Finally, passive immunization with antibodies against the type 1 IGF receptor inhibits the pro-liferation of numerous cell types and cancers (El Badry *et al.*, 1989; Furlanetto *et al.*, 1994; Gansler *et al.*, 1989; Kappel *et al.*, 1994; Lahm *et al.*, 1994; Peyrat & Bonneterre, 1992; Raile *et al.*, 1994). As expected, transgenic rodents expressing very high levels of human GH (and sub-sequently high levels of plasma IGF-1) exhibit an increase in spontaneous mam-mary tumors (Steger *et al.*, 1993).

Numerous studies indicate a positive correlation between plasma IGF-1 and caloric intake, with a 40 percent reduc-tion in caloric intake associated with a corresponding 40 to 50 percent decline in circulating IGF-1 levels. Since caloric restriction (CR; 40 percent reduction in caloric intake compared to *ad libitum*-fed animals) is the most robust intervention known to delay aging and age-related pathology and increase life span, it has been postulated that part of the beneficial actions of CR may be mediated through a reduction in IGF-1 levels. Interactions between the effects of CR on pathology and levels of IGF-1 are originally based on studies by Dunn and colleagues in p53 mice. These inves-tigators demonstrated that calorically restricted animals with low levels of IGF-1 are resistant to *p*-cristine-induced bladder cancer; replacement of IGF-1 restored the incidence of bladder cancer to that of *ad libitum*-fed controls (Dunn *et al.*, 1997).

Although no specific studies of the effects of growth hormone and IGF-1 on age-related pathology are available, other studies demonstrate that reduced levels of IGF-1 protect against chemical-induced carcinogenesis. Using growth hormone–deficient dwarf models or transgenic animals with low IGF-1 levels, results indicate that low levels of IGF-1 protect against 7,12-dimethylbenz[a]anthracene (DMBA)-induced mammary carcinogene-sis and GI metastasis (LeRoith *et al.*, 1993; Ramsey *et al.*, 2002), and in one study replacement of growth hormone produced a dose-related rise in tumor incidence in response to DMBA. Similar relationships between IGF-1 and cancer have been proposed in humans because elevated IGF-1 levels are a risk factor for breast cancer (Brunner *et al.*, 1992; Lee *et al.*, 1994; Osborne *et al.*, 1990; Torrisi *et al.*, 1993), lung cancer (Ankrapp & Bevan, 1993; Kaiser *et al.*, 1993; Rotsch *et al.*, 1992; Shigematsu *et al.*, 1990). and prostate cancer (Wang & Wong, 1998). The mechanisms through which plasma GH and IGF-1 influence age-related pathologies and life span and the specific stage in the life span when these effects are manifest remain unanswered.

The importance of GH and IGF-1 in preventing apoptosis or programmed cell death also has been recognized for some time. IGF-1 inhibits apoptosis in a number of systems (Dunn *et al.*, 1997; Lee-Kwon *et al.*, 1998), and this effect of IGF-1 contributes to the generation of age-related pathologies (Gobe *et al.*, 1999; Yu & Berkel, 1999;). Part of the basis for this view is that transgenic animals over-expressing bcl-2 (an intracellular protein that inhibits apoptosis) exhibit pathogenic changes in a number of tissues (Baker *et al.*, 1999; Van Molle *et al.*, 1999). Furthermore, suppression of apoptosis has been reported to increase oxidative stress and tumorigenesis *in vitro* while several antitumor agents act by stimulat-ing apoptosis (Magnetto *et al.*, 1999).

Most recently, suppression of apoptosis has been reported to enhance both oxidative DNA damage and mutagenesis and has been proposed as a potential mechanism of carcinogenesis (Kuo *et al.*, 1999).

V. Growth Hormone, IGF-1, and Life Span

Technical difficulties in manipulating growth hormone and IGF-1 over the life span of the animal have been a significant impediment in advancing our understanding of the effects of these hormones on aging and life span. The ideal model for investigating the effects of growth hormone/IGF-1 on aging would undoubtedly demonstrate a specific and limited alteration in these hormones. Unfortunately, the diverse action of these and other hormones as well as the interdependence that exists between endocrine systems are such that a major alteration in one hormone induces compensation by others. Therefore, an analysis of the specific effects of growth hormone and IGF-1 require a limited reduction or rise in hormone levels, whereas more dramatic alterations in hormone levels require extreme caution with interpretation. Despite these limitations, several models of chronic growth hormone/IGF-1 deficiency and overexpression have been used to investigate the effects of these hormones on the biological processes that contribute to aging. Several of these animal models that affect the growth hormone/IGF-1 axis are described below. As noted, every model has strengths and weaknesses, but conclusions related to effects on biological aging and life span require a clear understanding of both the endocrine, pathological, and biological manifestations of the model. Although life-span studies have been completed on several of these models,

others have only recently been developed, and therefore studies are likely in progress.

A. Growth Hormone or IGF-1 Overexpression

Mice that overexpress growth hormone were some of the earliest transgenic animals (Palmiter *et al.*, 1983) and have been used to indirectly support the argument that growth hormone deficiency increases life span (Brown-Borg *et al.*, 1996). These animals carry either a human or bovine growth hormone gene driven by a metallothionine or phosphoenolpyruvate promoter and, as one might expect, exhibit a drastic reduction in life span. Three groups of transgenic mice were subsequently engineered with varying levels of growth hormone overexpression (MThGH—high GH; PCKbGH—medium GH; MTbGH—low GH), resulting in an inverse relationship between growth hormone expression and life span. The reduction in life span observed with high expression of growth hormone is generally attributed to increased pathologies, primarily renal lesions, hepatic alterations, and a high frequency of hepatocellular tumors, including adenoma and carcinoma (Steger *et al.*, 1993). Furthermore, it has been proposed that the reduced life span in models of growth hormone overexpression supports the hypothesis that physiological levels of growth hormone accelerate aging (Brown-Borg *et al.*, 1996). However, growth hormone levels in the overexpression model are 1,000 to 10,000 times greater than those found under physiological conditions, a concern that makes the increased pathologies in this model of limited relevance to the investigation of the actions of growth hormone and IGF-1 under normal physiological conditions.

In a more directed approach, investigators have created transgenics that overexpress growth hormone or IGF-1 in specific tissues. For example, overexpression of human IGF-1 exclusively in skeletal muscle of transgenic mice (Coleman *et al.*, 1995) increases muscle mass and prevents the age-related decline in the number of dihydropyridine receptors that are necessary for excitation–contraction uncoupling (Renganathan *et al.*, 1998). Furthermore, selective IGF-1 overexpression in brain increases synaptic density (Dentremont *et al.*, 1999; O'Kusky *et al.*, 2000), although their effect on the age-related decrease in cortical synapse density has not been investigated. Obviously, tissue-specific models of IGF-1 overexpression or underexpression are useful for the investigation of functional parameters that change with age; nevertheless, their applicability to analysis of the underlying mechanisms of aging has not been resolved.

B. *Prop1* and *Pit1* Mutants

The Ames dwarf mouse has a mutation at the prophet of *Pit1* or *Prop1* locus, resulting in deficiencies in growth hormone, prolactin, and thyroid-stimulating hormone (Sornson *et al.*, 1996). Ames dwarves demonstrate markedly

increased longevity (see Figure 20.4) (Brown-Borg *et al.*, 1996); however, a wide range of physiological alterations in these animals is present, suggesting that the underlying mechanisms for the increased longevity are complex. Phenotypically, these animals differ from the wildtype in a number of ways, including (1) lower body temperature, (2) increased levels of enzymes responsible for the removal of reactive oxygen species (catalase and Cu/Zn superoxide dimutase), (3) increased insulin sensitivity, and (4) smaller body size (Bartke *et al.*, 1998). Although investigators generally attribute the increased life span of Ames dwarves exclusively to growth hormone/IGF-1 deficiency, multiple factors in this model (other than growth hormone/IGF-1) have the potential to influence life span. For example, hypothyroidism alone has been reported to extend longevity (Ooka *et al.*, 1983), and the reduction in basal glucose levels found in these animals leads to a reduction in insulin concentrations that mayexert independent effects on longevity. Smaller body size alters cardiovascular parameters and energy requirements, and these factors may

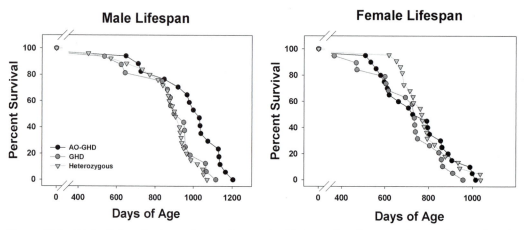

Figure 20.4 (A) Snell dwarf mice and normal controls. (B) Ames dwarf mice and normal controls. The graphs show proportion of animals remaining alive within the group. Reprinted from *Experimental Gerontology*, Volume 36, Issue 1, 2001, p. 3, with permission from Elsevier.

influence oxidative stress, independent of growth hormone or IGF-1 deficiency. Finally, increased levels of glucocorticoids found in Ames dwarves further complicate the task of determining whether increases in life span are mediated specifically by changes in the growth hormone/IGF-1 axis.

Snell dwarf mice, first described in 1929 (Snell, 1929), are homozygous for a mutation at the Pituitary-1 or *Pit1* locus, which is similar to the Ames mutation (Li *et al.*, 1990). These animals exhibit an absence of pituitary cells secreting growth hormone (somatotrophs), prolactin (lactotrophs), and thyroid-stimulating hormone (thyrotrophs). Phenotypically, they are normal at birth but grow slowly and achieve only one-third the body weight of normal animals. Silberberg was the first to propose the idea that that deficiency in growth hormone and IGF-1 may slow the functional deterioration of tissues often associated with aging. In a series of experiments (Silberberg, 1972, 1973), she suggested that protection from bone aging and osteoarthritis observed in Snell dwarf mice was due to their GH deficiency. Most recently, Flurkey and colleagues have shown that Snell dwarves demonstrate increased longevity (see Figure 20.4) and exhibit a delay in the age-related increase in collagen synthesis as well as delayed impairments in immune function (Flurkey *et al.*, 2001).

C. Ghrhr−/Ghrhr− Little Mice

The Ghrhr−/Ghrhr− or *lit/lit* mouse exhibits a mutation in the growth hormone releasing hormone (GHRH) receptor (Godfrey *et al.*, 1993). Mice homozygous for this mutation are defective in their response to GHRH, have lower circulating levels of growth hormone and IGF-1, and are approximately two-thirds the weight of their wildtype littermates. Flurkey and colleagues (2001) reported an approxi-

mately 20 to 25 percent increase in life span, which they speculated may have resulted from the low-fat (4 percent) diet, since earlier preliminary life span studies in the same strain of mice on higher-fat diets were inconclusive (Flurkey *et al.*, 2002). The animals also exhibit alterations in glucose, insulin, and glucocorticoids that complicate interpretations related to the biological effects of a primary effect of growth hormone/IGF-1 deficiency.

D. Growth Hormone Receptor Knockout

The growth hormone (GH) receptor/binding protein knockout (GHR/BP-KO) mouse, first described in 1997, has a disruption in the GHR/BP gene that codes for both the growth hormone receptor and the truncated form of the receptor that acts as a circulating growth hormone binding protein (Baumann, 1990). Therefore, growth hormone levels are increased, whereas plasma IGF-1 is reduced by 90 percent (Coschigano *et al.*, 2000). Studies examining longevity in this strain have shown that mice homozygous for the mutated allele have a 50 percent reduction in body size and greater longevity compared with their heterozygous and wildtype counterparts (Hauck *et al.*, 2001).

A recent study by Hauck and Bartke (2000) argues that the GHR/BP-KO model is phenotypically and physiologically similar to the Ames and Snell dwarves but without the complications of multiple hormone deficiency. Furthermore, they conclude that results from this model provide definitive support for the conclusion that growth hormone/ IGF-1 deficiency increases life span. Nevertheless, a reduction in thyroid hormones and core body temperature are evident, and basal levels of glucose and insulin are decreased in females and male GHR/BP-KO mice. Basal corticosterone levels are significantly higher in both sexes, as is the case

Table 20.1

Primary and secondary alterations in mammalian models of growth hormone deficiency

Model	Mutation	GH	IGF-1	TSH	PRL	CORT	Basal Glucose/Insulin	GTT	Body Temp	Body Size	Adult-onset	Lifespan
Snell mouse	pit-1	↓	↓	↓	↓	–	↓	?	↓	↓	no	↑
Ames mouse	prop^{-1}	↓	↓	↓	↓	–	↓	?	↓	↓	no	↑
GHR/BP KO mouse	GHR$^{-/-}$	–	↓	↑	–	?	↑	?	↓	↓	no	↑
Ghrhr^{Lit} mouse	GHRHR$^{-/-}$	↓	↓	?	?	?	↓	?	?	↓	no	↑
IGFR$^{+/-}$ mouse	IGFR$^{+/-}$	?	↓	?	?	?	–	1	?	↓	no	↑$^{(f)}$
LID mouse	Hepatic IGF-1	↑	↓	?	?	?	↑	2	?	↓	no	→
Tg/–	GH antisense	–	↓	?	?	?	↓	?	?	↓	no	↑
GHA	GH antagonist	–	↓	?	?	?	–	?	?	↓	no	–
dw/dw rat (AO-GHD)	Unknown GH deficiency	↓	↓	–	–	–	–	–	–	↓	yes	↑$^{(m)}$

GH-growth hormone; GHR/BP- growth hormone receptor binding protein; GHR- growth hormone receptor; IGF-1-insulin-like growth factor-1; PRL-prolactin; Cort-corticosterone; TSH-thyroid stimulating hormone; 1- insulin levels during GTT not reported (in males), glucose hypersecretion; 2- Insulin hypersecretion – normal glucose levels; (m)- males; (f)-females; ? - unknown at this time.

in male Ames dwarfs (Borg *et al.*, 1995). Therefore, despite a primary deficiency in IGF-1, this model exhibits many of the same complexities evident in the Ames and Snell dwarves (see Table 1).

E. IGF-1 Knockout

Multiple primary endocrine deficiencies evident in the Ames and Snell dwarves and secondary endocrine deficiencies present in the GHR/BP-KO mice confound analyses of results related to the specific actions of growth hormone on biological aging and life span. However, it has been suggested that a more targeted disruption of growth hormone/ IGF-1 signaling pathways in mammals may eliminate some of these confounding variables. Transgenic IGF-1 knockout mice resulting from homologous recombination have been generated by Beck and colleagues (1995). Unfortunately, this mutation is lethal in a large percentage of animals, resulting in severe growth retardation and deficiencies in development of bone, muscle, and reproductive organ systems in the remainder of the population (Liu *et al.*, 2000). Although the animals are viable at birth, mortality rates range from 32 to 95 percent (depending on strain), and death is generally attributed to respiratory difficulties or severe muscle dystrophy. Both males and females are infertile as a result of impairments of gonadal steroidogenesis and other organs, including the kidney, heart, liver, and brain, are enlarged.

In an attempt to improve the postnatal survival of these animals, Liu and colleagues used the *Cre/loxP* system to create transgenic mice with variable IGF-1 expression (Liu *et al.*, 1998). Relative to wildtype controls, the resulting homozygous animals are smaller at birth, grow at a slower rate, and have severely reduced levels of IGF-1. This is in contrast to animals with only one recombinant allele, which grow only marginally slower than the wildtype, achieve nearly normal size (81 to 85 percent weight of wildtype), exhibit reduced levels of IGF-1, and are fertile.

In another model of IGF-1 deficiency, a 75 percent reduction in circulating levels of plasma IGF-1 is achieved by specific deletion of the gene encoding hepatic IGF-1(Li *et al.*, 1990). IGF-1 gene expression in other tissues, including heart, brain, kidney, and fat, is not altered in this model. These animals grow to normal size, are fertile, and it appears that high levels of growth hormone (due to absence of negative feedback at the pituitary gland) increase paracrine or tissue IGF-1 levels, compensating for the lower plasma levels of IGF-1.

Interestingly, a transgenic animal with a *loxP*-IGF-1 exon 4 has recently been developed, and mating of these animals with mice carrying the *Cre recombinase* gene will permit for the first time the deletion of IGF-1 at a specific age. The application of this model to the study of the effects of growth hormone and IGF-1 on aging will undoubtedly advance our understanding of the role of growth hormone and IGF-1 in the regulation of aging and life span.

F. IGF-1 Receptor Knockout

Another model of IGF deficiency in mice results from inactivation of the IGF-1R gene by homologous recombination using *Cre-loxP* technology (Holzenberger *et al.*, 2003). Heterozygous knockout mice (Igf1r$^{+/-}$), with a 50 percent reduction in IGF-1 receptors were assessed since null mutants were not viable. Male and female Igf1r$^{+/-}$ mice survive 16 percent and 33 percent longer, respectively, than their wildtype littermates; however, only the difference in females is significant. Furthermore, the Igf1r$^{+/-}$ mice do not develop dwarfism, dysregulation of energy metabolism, or a reduction in physical activity, fertility, or food intake. Plasma IGF-1 levels are elevated in both male and females, perhaps due to autoregulatory feedback mechanisms that are activated in the presence of low levels of receptor. Fasting glucose and non-fasting insulin did not differ significantly between groups. However, glucose tolerance testing indicates insulin deficiency in males and slightly decreased glucose response in females.

In the same study, the investigators explored the relationship between oxidative stress and IGF receptor status. Male and female $Igf1r^{+/-}$ mice receiving intraperitoneal injections of an oxidant, paraquat survived longer than wildtype controls, and these effects were particularly salient in the females. *In vitro* studies also confirm these results in that $Igf1r^{+/-}$ mice display greater resistance to H_2O_2 induced oxidative stress. The authors conclude that the IGF-1 receptor may be a central regulator of mammalian life span, perhaps mediated via its effects on oxidative stress pathways.

G. Growth Hormone Deficiency

The *dw/dw* rat is a specific model of limited growth hormone/IGF-1 deficiency. This animal has a deficiency of the transcription factor necessary for somatotroph development in the pituitary resulting in a decrease in growth hormone secretion (Tierney & Robinson, 2002). One advantage of this animal is that the modest decreases in plasma IGF-1 do not induce differences in basal plasma T_4, corticosterone, glucose, insulin, or insulin/glucose ratios (Carter *et al.*, 2002; Sonntag *et al.*, 1999). The animals are a normal size at birth and first demonstrate indications of growth hormone/IGF-1 deficiency at 26 to 28 days of age when high-amplitude growth hormone pulses are necessary to stimulate the rise in IGF-1. Porcine growth hormone (90 percent homologous to the structure of rat growth hormone) or vehicle is injected to mimic the peripubertal rise in growth hormone, resulting in IGF-1 levels and body weights that are equivalent to normal animals. After 10 weeks of growth hormone

treatment to ensure pancreatic islet development, animals either continue on growth hormone treatment (GH Replete) or are switched to vehicle, creating a model of adult-onset growth hormone deficiency (AO-GHD). Animals are compared to dwarf littermates that only received vehicle (Growth hormone deficient— GHD) or heterozygous-normal animals. The reduction in plasma IGF-1 in the growth hormone–deficient dwarf animal is approximately 40 percent. In this model, no differences in mean or maximal life span are evident between GHD animals and their heterozygous siblings. Surprisingly, replacement of growth hormone to dwarf animals for 10 weeks (AO-GHD animals) results in a 12.7 percent increase in mean and maximal life span. The increase in life span in males is associated with a reduction in age-associated pathology— suggesting that modification of age-related pathology is an important underlying mechanism for effects on life span (Sonntag *et al.*, in press).

H. Comments on Dwarf and Transgenic Animal Studies

The results of many dwarf and transgenic animal studies have been interpreted to suggest that growth hormone/IGF-1 deficiency has a primary action on biological aging and slows a "biological clock" (Bartke *et al.*, 2001), an effect dissociable from a simple reduction in age-related pathology proposed by others. In support of this perspective, it has been argued that robust changes associated with biological aging are ameliorated in models of growth hormone/IGF-1 deficiency (Flurkey *et al.*, 2001). The availability of mutant and transgenic animals undoubtedly has advanced our understanding of biological aging by demonstrating that alterations in endocrine systems have the potential to regulate life span. However, there exist two basic concerns with these interpretations. First, there are no established markers of biological aging that could be used to conclude that the "rate of aging" is delayed. Alterations in immune function and collagen cross-linking are of interest but cannot, at present, be used as a surrogate marker for "biological aging." Second, part of the issue with interpretation of results derives from the issue of whether the decrease in growth hormone and IGF-1 exert a primary effect on aging or whether alterations in these hormones produce downstream effects that are then manifest as alterations in life span. The difference between primary and secondary effects of growth hormone and IGF-1 is not simply a semantic issue because this information guides the development of future research in the field. Finally, pathology undoubtedly exerts a key influence on life span. Previous studies indicate that animals expressing a growth hormone receptor antagonist exhibit no increase in life span, and the increase in life span in the growth hormone receptor knockout appears to be both strain- and gender-dependent. For example, in the C57BL/6J background, no differences in life span are evident between GHR$^{-/-}$ animals compared to controls at 50 percent mortality (although modest effects were detectable at different ages), whereas the effects of the mutation on life span appeared to be more robust in females and in both males and females of the Ola-Balb/cJ background (Coschigano et al., 2003). Thus, as previously noted, the underlying pathology of the parent strain may be a critical factor in life span.

The concept that pathology has a critical role in determination of life span is, of course, not a novel idea. However, there are few studies that routinely assess end-of-life pathology with life span. In the model of adult-onset growth hormone deficiency described previously (Sonntag et al., 2005), in contrast to males, no increase in life span of either GHD or AO-GHD animals was observed compared to heterozygous females. Analysis of end-of-life pathology revealed the presence of large, prolactin-secreting pituitary tumors in all groups regardless of treatment, which undoubtedly was the primary factor in death in all groups. In fact, there appeared to be early deaths from pituitary tumors in GHD and AO-GHD females (beginning around 400 to 500 days of age in GHD and AO-GHD animals and 600 days in heterozygous females), but this effect did not reach statistical significance. Despite this potential acceleration of pituitary pathology, growth hormone and IGF-1 deficiency appeared to reduce the number of palpable mammary tumors in both AO-GHD and GHD animals by approximately 50 percent. These latter results are consistent with the absence of DMBA-induced mammary cancer in GHD animals and the dose-related rise in DMBA-induced mammary cancer in response to growth hormone administration previously reported for this strain (Ramsey et al., 2002). Thus, the presence of "plasma IGF-1 dependent" and "plasma IGF-1 independent" pathologies that are present in the dw/dw model are certain to have an impact on life span. Without specific knowledge of end-of-life pathology of the parent strain and alterations in pathology induced in the mutant, the effects of interventions designed to assess life span are compromised.

Finally, the conclusion that the effects of an intervention on aging and life span are mediated primarily by a reduction in growth hormone and/or IGF-1 when the intervention modifies, either directly or indirectly, multiple systems must be carefully considered. However, the specific mechanisms that regulate life span in relatively nonspecific models of growth hormone/IGF-1 deficiency (e.g., Ames, Snell, GHRKO mice) and more specific models (models of adult-onset GH deficiency in dw/dw rats) have not been resolved. Nevertheless, without solid evidence to the contrary, one must consider that these effects are mediated primarily by modifying/reducing age-specific pathology.

VI. Pleiotropic Effects of Growth Hormone and IGF-1

Despite repeated evidence that growth hormone replacement in older animals improves function, the dichotomy between the beneficial and deleterious effects of growth hormone has received little attention. The outcome of the many studies of life span in transgenic and mutant strains have been interpreted to suggest that it may be possible to achieve "cost-free aging" through a modest reduction in activity of the growth hormone/IGF-1 axis (e.g., increased life span at no expense to the health or well-being of the organism). It is difficult to consider, however, that the profound rise in growth hormone and IGF-1 levels during the peripubertal period that occurs in virtually all mammals does not impart a physiological and evolutionary advantage to the organism. There is, and has been, sufficient laboratory, clinical, and empirical data to conclude that the rise in growth hormone and IGF-1 immediately before puberty is important to optimize reproductive fecundity and increase the growth and perhaps even the survival of offspring. However, the effects of growth hormone and IGF-1 go well beyond optimization of reproduction function. During the peripubertal period these hormones ensure the maturation of sufficient pancreatic islets, which may help to protect against diabetes (Chen *et al.*, 2004) and stimulate the development of sufficient bone mass and cartilage to delay or prevent osteoporosis (Veldhuis *et al.*, 2005). One major concern is that by inducing major alterations in the growth hormone and IGF-1 axis, organ and system development is affected,

thereby compromising interpretation of the specific effects of these hormones. Furthermore, animals, especially humans, rarely live their life under environmentally controlled conditions with little stress and an abundant supply of food. The presence of anabolic hormones such as growth hormone and IGF-1 may ultimately be necessary to support tissue development, maintenance, and repair—ensuring survival and hence reproductive fitness.

There has been substantial controversy surrounding the question of whether growth hormone and/or IGF-1 contribute to the development of the aged phenotype, whether administration of these hormones to the elderly is warranted, and whether the actions of these hormones on the aging phenotype have evolutionary significance. Growth hormone and IGF-1 are important for reproductive success early in life, for developing an adequate tissue architecture to delay degenerative changes that contribute to disability (e.g., loss of cartilage, vascular degeneration), and to provide optimal tissue function throughout life (e.g., maintenance of cognitive function). However, the levels of growth hormone and IGF-1 found in normal animals throughout the life span contribute to the development of both neoplastic and non-neoplastic disease. The paradoxical and pleiotropic actions of these hormones are consistent with a model in which expression of specific genes influence biological aging through both beneficial and deleterious effects on the organism at different stages of the life span—antagonistic pleiotropy (Rose & Charlesworth, 1980). In reference to growth hormone and IGF-1, effects on reproductive success may result in selection for high levels of these hormones in early adulthood; however, there is little or no evolutionary pressure to suppress expression of these hormones because the pathological actions are not manifest until after reproductive senescence. Thus, the reduction in age-associated neoplastic disease, nephropathy, pathological burden, and increased life span possible through a specific reduction in growth hormone/IGF-1 levels is obtained at the risk of increased functional impairments and degenerative disease with age.

VII. Conclusion

After 20 years of research, there is no consensus for biomarkers of aging. However, over the same time frame, the changes in growth hormone and IGF-1 levels are among the most robust and well documented to date. In all instances, what is clear is that these hormones contribute to the biological fitness of organisms and that replacement results in positive results for many aspects of physiological and behavioral functioning. What is not clear is whether replacement in older individuals contributes to the risk of age-related disease. This is the question for the next 20 years.

Models of growth hormone deficiency have contributed intriguing evidence related to the regulation of life span. If one defines aging using life span alone, then age-related reductions in growth hormone and IGF-1 most likely increase life span and therefore delay aging in mice and rats. However, if one uses functional measures (physical function, cognitive function, and/or cardiovascular function), then the reductions in these hormones may (or may not) accelerate aging. Do growth hormone and IGF-1 accelerate or retard aging? This is the conundrum that defines the current issues in the field.

The issues raised with the dwarf animal model raise broader questions for the field of gerontology. How do we define aging and determine whether an intervention modifies aging? Life-span studies appear to be the most readily accepted "gold standard," yet most of the current studies are published with little or no end-of-life pathology, and the numbers of animals associated with these studies range from as few as six to greater than 30 per group. Interventions may have a positive benefit for aging (e.g., delay in functional deterioration of tissue or a decrease in a specific pathology) without affecting life span. Without supporting functional and pathological data, it is difficult to interpret whether an intervention is successful. Furthermore, interpretation of results when the control group exhibits a relatively short mean life span and the intervention increases mean life span to more "acceptable" levels needs to be carefully evaluated. Should all animals in life-span studies be housed under specific pathogen–free conditions? To date, there are many life-span studies conducted in nonspecific pathogen–free facilities, raising additional concerns about cause of death. Do growth hormone and IGF-1 accelerate or retard aging? This issue will only be resolved when we broaden our understanding of several endpoints that are relevant for aging rather than concentrating on life span alone and become aware of the diverse actions of hormones that are critical to the organism throughout the life span.

Acknowledgements

The authors would like to thank Ms. Rhonda Ingram, Ms. Colleen Bennett, Mr. Randy Gooch, and Ms. Tracy Moore for their excellent technical assistance. The authors would also like to thank Drs. Melinda Ramsey, Amir Khan, Judy Brunso-Bechtold, and David Riddle for their valuable discussions regarding the content of the chapter. Finally, the authors would like to thank Dr. Kevin Flurkey for his expert review of this chapter. The following grants from the National Institute on Aging supported this work: P01AG011370–08A10002 and P30AG021332.

References

Adamafio, N. A., Towns, R. J., & Kostyo, J. L.
(1991). Growth hormone receptors and
action in BC3H-1 myocytes. *Growth
Regulation*, 1, 17–22.

Aleman, A., de Vries, W. R., de Haan,
E. H., Verhaar, H. J., Samson, M. M., &
Koppeschaar, H. P. (2000). Age-sensitive
cognitive function, growth hormone
and insulin-like growth factor 1
plasma levels in healthy older men.
Neuropsychobiology, 41, 73–78.

Aleman, A., de Vries, W. R., Koppeschaar, H.
P., Osman-Dualeh, M., Verhaar, H. J.,
Samson, M. M. Bol, E., de Haan, E. H. (2001).
Relationship between circulating levels of
sex hormones and insulin-like growth
factor-1 and fluid intelligence in older men.
Experimental Aging Research, 27, 283–291.

Aleman, A., Verhaar, H. J., De Haan, E. H.,
De Vries, W. R., Samson, M. M., Drent, M. L.,
Van der Veen, E. A., Koppeschaar, H. P.
(1999). Insulin-like growth factor-I and
cognitive function in healthy older men.
*Journal of Clinical Endocrinology
and Metabolism*, 84, 471–475.

Altman, H. J., & Quartermain, D. (1983).
Facilitation of memory retrieval by
centrally administered catecholamine
stimulating agents. *Behavioural Brain
Research*, 7, 51–63.

Amano, T., Meyer, J. S., Okabe, T., Shaw, T.,
& Mortel, K. F. (1982). Stable xenon CT
cerebral blood flow measurements
computed by a single compartment—
double integration model in normal aging
and dementia. *Journal of Computer
Assisted Tomography*, 6, 923–932.

Ankrapp, D. P., & Bevan, D. R. (1993).
Insulin-like growth factor-I and human
lung fibroblast-derived insulin-like
growth factor-I stimulate the proliferation
of human lung carcinoma cells in vitro.
Cancer Research, 53, 3399–3404.

Argetsinger, L. S., Campbell, G. S., Yang, X.,
Witthuhn, B. A., Silvennoinen, O., Ihle, J. N.,
Carter-Su, C. (1993). Identification of JAK2
as a growth hormone receptor-associated
tyrosine kinase. *Cell*, 74, 237–244.

Baker, N. L., Carlo, R., V, Bernard, O.,
D'Ercole, A. J., & Werther, G. A. (1999).
Interactions between bcl-2 and the
IGF system control apoptosis in the

developing mouse brain. *Brain
Research-Developmental Brain
Research*, 118, 109–118.

Bartke, A., Brown-Borg, H. M., Bode, A. M.,
Carlson, J., Hunter, W. S., & Bronson, R. T.
(1998). Does growth hormone prevent or
accelerate aging? *Experimental
Gerontology*, 33, 675–687.

Bartke, A., Brown-Borg, H., Mattison, J.,
Kinney, B., Hauck, S., & Wright, C. (2001).
Prolonged longevity of hypopituitary dwarf
mice. *Experimental Gerontology*, 36,
21–28.

Baumann, G. (1990). Growth hormone
binding proteins and various forms of
growth hormone: implications for
measurements. *Acta Paediatrica
Scandinavica*, 370 (Suppl.), 72–80.

Beck, K. D., Powell-Braxton, L., Widmer, H. R.,
Valverde, J., & Hefti, F. (1995). Igf1 gene
disruption results in reduced brain size, CNS
hypomyelination, and loss of hippocampal
granule and striatal parvalbumin-containing
neurons. *Neuron*, 14, 717–730.

Bell, M. A., & Ball, M. J. (1990). Neuritic
plaques and vessels of visual cortex in aging
and Alzheimer's dementia. *Neurobiology of
Aging*, 11, 359–370.

Bennett, S. A., Xu, X., Lynch, C. D., &
Sonntag, W. E. (1997). Insulin-like growth
factor-1 (IGF-1) regulates NMDAR1 in the
hippocampus of aged animals. *Society for
Neuroscience Abstracts*, 23, 349.

Berelowitz, M., Szabo, M., Frohman, L. A.,
Firestone, S., Chu, L., & Hintz, R. L. (1981).
Somatomedin-C mediates growth hormone
negative feedback by effects on both the
hypothalamus and the pituitary. *Science*,
212, 1279–1281.

Bertrand, H. A., Lynd, F. T., Masoro, E. J., &
Yu, B. P. (1980). Changes in adipose mass
and cellularity through the adult life of rats
fed ad libitum or a life-prolonging restricted
diet. *Journal of Gerontology*, 35, 827–835.

Bichell, D. P., Kikuchi, K., & Rotwein, P.
(1992). Growth hormone rapidly activates
insulin-like growth factor I gene
transcription *in vivo*. *Molecular
Endocrinology*, 6, 1899–1908.

Borg, K. E., Brown-Borg, H. M., & Bartke, A.
(1995). Assessment of the primary adrenal
cortical and pancreatic hormone basal levels
in relation to plasma glucose and age in the
unstressed Ames dwarf mouse. *Proceedings*

of the Society for Experimental Biology and Medicine. Society for Experimental Biology and Medicine, 210, 126–133.

Born, J., Muth, S., & Fehm, H. L. (1988). The significance of sleep onset and slow wave sleep for nocturnal release of growth hormone (GH) and cortisol. Psychoneuroendocrinology, 13, 233–243.

Brazeau, P., Vale, W., Burgus, R., Ling, N., Butcher, M., Rivier, J., Guillemin, R. (1973). Hypothalamic polypeptide that inhibits the secretion of immunoreactive pituitary growth hormone. Science, 179, 77–79.

Brown-Borg, H. M., Borg, K. E., Meliska, C. J., & Bartke, A. (1996). Dwarf mice and the ageing process. Nature, 384, 33.

Brunner, N., Moser, C., Clarke, R., & Cullen, K. (1992). IGF-I and IGF-II expression in human breast cancer xenografts: relationship to hormone independence. Breast Cancer Research and Treatment, 22, 39–45.

Campbell, G. S., Pang, L., Miyasaka, T., Saltiel, A. R., & Carter-Su, C. (1992). Stimulation by growth hormone of MAP kinase activity in 3T3-F442A fibroblasts. Journal of Biological Chemistry, 267, 6074–6080.

Carlson, H. E., Gillin, J. C., Gorden, P., & Snyder, F. (1972). Absence of sleep-related growth hormone peaks in aged normal subjects and in acromegaly. Journal of Clinical Endocrinology and Metabolism, 34, 1102–1105.

Cartee, G. D., Bohn, E. E., Gibson, B. T., & Farrar, R. P. (1996). Growth hormone supplementation increases skeletal muscle mass of old male Fischer 344/brown Norway rats. The Journals of Gerontology Series A, Biological Sciences and Medical Sciences, 51, B214–B219.

Carter, C. S., Ramsey, M. M., Ingram, R. L., Cashion, A. B., Cefalu, W. T., Wang, Z. Q., Sonntag, W. E. (2002). Models of growth hormone and IGF-1 deficiency: applications to studies of aging processes and life-span determination. Journals of Gerontology Series A, Biological Sciences and Medical Sciences, 57, B177–B188.

Ceda, G. P., Valenti, G., Butturini, U., & Hoffman, A. R. (1986). Diminished pituitary responsiveness to growth hormone-releasing factor in aging male rats. Endocrinology, 118, 2109–2114.

Chen, W., Salojin, K. V., Mi, Q. S., Grattan, M., Meagher, T. C., Zucker, P., Delovitch, T. L. (2004). Insulin-like growth factor (IGF)-I/IGF-binding protein-3 complex: therapeutic efficacy and mechanism of protection against type 1 diabetes. Endocrinology, 145(2), 627–38.

Cittadini, A., Ishiguro, Y., Stromer, H., Spindler, M., Moses, A. C., Clark, R., Douglas, P. S., Ingwall, J. S., Morgan, J. P. (1998). Insulin-like growth factor-1 but not growth hormone augments mammalian myocardial contractility by sensitizing the myofilament to Ca2+ through a wortmannin-sensitive pathway: studies in rat and ferret isolated muscles. Circulation Research, 83, 50–59.

Cittadini, A., Stromer, H., Katz, S. E., Clark, R., Moses, A. C., Morgan, J. P., Douglas, P. S. (1996). Differential cardiac effects of growth hormone and insulin-like growth factor-1 in the rat. A combined in vivo and in vitro evaluation. Circulation, 93, 800–809.

Clancy, D. J., Gems, D., Harshman, L. G., Oldham, S., Stocker, H., Hafen, E., Leevers, S. J., Partridge, L. (2001). Extension of life-span by loss of CHICO, a Drosophila insulin receptor substrate protein. Science, 292, 104–106.

Cohick, W. S., & Clemmons, D. R. (1993). The insulin-like growth factors. Annual Review of Physiology, 55, 131–153.

Coleman, M. E., DeMayo, F., Yin, K. C., Lee, H. M., Geske, R., Montgomery, C., Schwartz, R. J. (1995). Myogenic vector expression of insulin-like growth factor I stimulates muscle cell differentiation and myofiber hypertrophy in transgenic mice. Journal of Biological Chemistry, 270, 12109–12116.

Cook, J. J., Wailgum, T. D., Vasthare, U. S., Mayrovitz, H. N., & Tuma, R. F. (1992). Age-related alterations in the arterial microvasculature of skeletal muscle. Journal of Gerontology, 47, B83–B88.

Coschigano, K. T., Clemmons, D., Bellush, L. L., & Kopchick, J. J. (2000). Assessment of growth parameters and life span of GHR/BP gene-disrupted mice. Endocrinology, 141, 2608–2613.

Coschigano, K. T., Holland, A. N., Riders, M. E., List, E. O., Flyvbjerg, A., & Kopchick, J. J.

(2003). Deletion, but not antagonism, of the mouse growth hormone receptor results in severely decreased body weights, insulin, and insulin-like growth factor I levels and increased life span. *Endocrinology, 144,* 3799–3810.

Daughaday, W. H. (1989). A personal history of the origin of the somatomedin hypothesis and recent challenges to its validity. *Perspectives in Biology and Medicine, 32,* 194–211.

DeGennaro Colonna, V., Fidone, F., Cocchi, D., & Muller, E. E. (1993). Feedback effects of growth hormone on growth hormone-releasing hormone and somatostatin are not evident in aged rats. *Neurobiology of Aging, 14,* 503–507.

DeGennaro Colonna, V., Zoli, M., Cocchi, D., Maggi, A., Marrama, P., Agnati, L. F., Muller, E. E. (1989). Reduced growth hormone releasing factor (GHRF)-like immunoreactivity and GHRF gene expression in the hypothalamus of aged rats. *Peptides, 10,* 705–708.

Delafontaine, P. (1995). Insulin-like growth factor I and its binding proteins in the cardiovascular system. *Cardiovascular Research, 30,* 825–834.

Delafontaine, P., Bernstein, K. E., & Alexander, R. W. (1991). Insulin-like growth factor I gene expression in vascular cells. *Hypertension, 17,* 693–699.

Delafontaine, P., Lou, H., & Alexander, R. W. (1991). Regulation of insulin-like growth factor I messenger RNA levels in vascular smooth muscle cells. *Hypertension, 18,* 742–747.

Delbono, O. (2000). Regulation of excitation contraction coupling by insulin-like growth factor-1 in aging skeletal muscle. *Journal of Nutrition Health and Aging, 4,* 162–164.

Dentremont, K. D., Ye, P., D'Ercole, A. J., & O'Kusky, J. R. (1999). Increased insulin-like growth factor-I (IGF-I) expression during early postnatal development differentially increases neuron number and growth in medullary nuclei of the mouse. *Brain Research. Developmental Brain Research, 114,* 135–141.

Desai, D. M., Adams, G. A., Wang, X., Alfrey, E. J., Sibley, R. K., & Dafoe, D. C. (1999). The influence of combined trophic factors on the success of fetal

pancreas grafts. *Transplantation, 68,* 491–496.

Dik, M. G., Pluijm, S. M., Jonker, C., Deeg, D. J., Lomecky, M. Z., & Lips, P. (2003). Insulin-like growth factor I (IGF-I) and cognitive decline in older persons. *Neurobiology of Aging, 24,* 573–581.

Dubrovina, N. I., & Il'iuchenok, R. I. (1990). The role of the dopaminergic system and GABA-benzodiaze. *Fiziologicheskii Zhurnal, 36,* 3–8.

Dunn, S. E., Kari, F. W., French, J., Leininger, J. R., Travlos, G., Wilson, R., Barrett, J. C. (1997). Dietary restriction reduces insulin-like growth factor I levels, which modulates apoptosis, cell proliferation, and tumor progression in p53-deficient mice. *Cancer Research, 57,* 4667–4672.

El Badry, O. M., Romanus, J. A., Helman, L. J., Cooper, M. J., Rechler, M. M., & Israel, M. A. (1989). Autonomous growth of a human neuroblastoma cell line is mediated by insulin-like growth factor II. *Journal of Clinical Investigation, 84,* 829–839.

Engelmann, G. L., Boehm, K. D., Haskell, J. F., Khairallah, P. A., & Ilan, J. (1989). Insulin-like growth factors and neonatal cardiomyocyte development: ventricular gene expression and membrane receptor variations in normotensive and hypertensive rats. *Molecular and Cellular Endocrinology, 63,* 1–14.

Fabrizio, P., Pozza, F., Pletcher, S. D., Gendron, C. M., & Longo, V. D. (2001). Regulation of longevity and stress resistance by Sch9 in yeast. *Science, 292,* 288–290.

Fernyhough, P., Mill, J. F., Roberts, J. L., & Ishii, D. N. (1989). Stabilization of tubulin mRNAs by insulin and insulin-like growth factor I during neurite formation. *Brain Research Molecular Brain Research, 6,* 109–120.

Finkelstein, J. W., Roffwarg, H. P., Boyar, R. M., Kream, J., & Hellman, L. (1972). Age-related change in the twenty-four-hour spontaneous secretion of growth hormone. *Journal of Clinical Endocrinology and Metabolism, 35,* 665–670.

Florini, J. R., Harned, J. A., Richman, R. A., & Weiss, J. P. (1981). Effect of rat age on serum levels of growth hormone and somatomedins. *Mechanisms of Ageing and Development*, 15, 165–176.

Flurkey, K., Papaconstantinou, J., Miller, R. A., & Harrison, D. E. (2001). Lifespan extension and delayed immune and collagen aging in mutant mice with defects in growth hormone production. *Proceedings of the National Academy of Sciences of the USA*, 98, 6736–6741.

Flurkey, K., Papaconstantinou, J., Harrison, D. E. (2002). The Snell dwarf mutation Pit1 (dw) can increase life span in mice. *Mechanisms of Ageing and Development*, 123, 121–30.

Folkow, B., Isaksson, O. P., Karlstrom, G., Lever, A. F., & Nordlander, M. (1988). The importance of hypophyseal hormones for structural cardiovascular adaptation in hypertension. *Journal of Hypertension*, 6 (Suppl.), S166–S169.

French, R. A., Broussard, S. R., Meier, W. A., Minshall, C., Arkins, S., Zachary, J. F., Dantzer, R., Kelley, K. W. (2002). Age-associated loss of bone marrow hematopoietic cells is reversed by GH and accompanies thymic reconstitution. *Endocrinology*, 143, 690–699.

Friedlander, A. L., Butterfield, G. E., Moynihan, S., Grillo, J., Pollack, M., Holloway, L., Friedman, L., Yesavage, J., Matthias, D., Lee, S., Marcus, R., Hoffman, A. R. (2001). One year of insulin-like growth factor I treatment does not affect bone density, body composition, or psychological measures in postmenopausal women. *Journal of Clinical Endocrinology and Metabolism*, 86, 1496–1503.

Frustaci, A., Perrone, G. A., Gentiloni, N., & Russo, M. A. (1992). Reversible dilated cardiomyopathy due to growth hormone deficiency. *American Journal of Clinical Pathology*, 97, 503–511.

Furlanetto, R. W., Harwell, S. E., & Frick, K. K. (1994). Insulin-like growth factor-I induces cyclin-D1 expression in MG63 human osteosarcoma cells *in vitro*. *Molecular Endocrinology*, 8, 510–517.

Gansler, T., Furlanetto, R., Gramling, T. S., Robinson, K. A., Blocker, N., Buse, M. G., Sens, D. A., Garvin, A. J. (1989). Antibody to type I insulinlike growth factor receptor inhibits growth of Wilms' tumor in culture and in athymic mice. *American Journal of Pathology*, 135, 961–966.

Gasbarri, A., Introini-Collison, I. B., Packard, M. G., Pacitti, C., & McGaugh, J. L. (1993). Interaction of cholinergic-dopaminergic systems in the regulation of memory storage in aversively motivated learning tasks. *Brain Research*, 627, 72–78.

Genth-Zotz, S., Zotz, R., Geil, S., Voigtlander, T., Meyer, J., & Darius, H. (1999). Recombinant growth hormone therapy in patients with ischemic cardiomyopathy: effects on hemodynamics, left ventricular function, and cardiopulmonary exercise capacity. *Circulation*, 99, 18–21.

Ghahary, A., Shen, Q., Shen, Y. J., Scott, P. G., & Tredget, E. E. (1998). Induction of transforming growth factor beta 1 by insulin-like growth factor-1 in dermal fibroblasts. *Journal of Cellular Physiology*, 174, 301–309.

Ghigo, E., Goffi, S., Nicolosi, M., Arvat, E., Valente, F., Mazza, E., Ghigo, M. C., Camanni, F. (1990). Growth hormone (GH) responsiveness to combined administration of arginine and GH-releasing hormone does not vary with age in man. *Journal of Clinical Endocrinology and Metabolism*, 71, 1481–1485.

Giustina, A., Lorusso, R., Borghetti, V., Bugari, G., Misitano, V., & Alfieri, O. (1996). Impaired spontaneous growth hormone secretion in severe dialated cardiomyopathy. *American Heart Journal*, 131, 620–622.

Gobe, G., Zhang, X. J., Cuttle, L., Pat, B., Willgoss, D., Hancock, J., Barnard, R., Endre, R. B. (1999). Bcl-2 genes and growth factors in the pathology of ischaemic acute renal failure. *Immunology and Cell Biology*, 77, 279–286.

Godfrey, P., Rahal, J. O., Beamer, W. G., Copeland, N. G., Jenkins, N. A., & Mayo, K. E. (1993). GHRH receptor of little mice contains a missense mutation in the extracellular domain that disrupts receptor function. *Nature Genetics*, 4, 227–232.

Goff, B. L., Roth, J. A., Arp, L. H., & Incefy, G. S. (1987). Growth hormone treatment stimulates thymulin production in aged dogs. *Clinical and Experimental Immunology*, 68, 580–587.

Goldman, H., Berman, R. F., Gershon, S., Murphy, S. L., & Altman, H. J. (1987).

Correlation of behavioral and cerebrovascular functions in the aging rat. *Neurobiology of Aging*, 8, 409–416.

Gould, J., Aramburo, C., Capdevielle, M., & Scanes, C. G. (1995). Angiogenic activity of anterior pituitary tissue and growth hormone on the chick embryo chorio-allantoic membrane: a novel action of GH. *Life Sciences*, 56, 587–594.

Goya, R. G., Gagnerault, M. C., De Moraes, M. C., Savino, W., & Dardenne, M. (1992). *In vivo* effects of growth hormone on thymus function in aging mice. *Brain, Behavior, and Immunity*, 6, 341–354.

Grant, M. B., Mames, R. N., Fitzgerald, C., Ellis, E. A., Caballero, S., Chegini, N. (1993). Insulin-like growth factor I as an angiogenic agent. *In vivo* and *in vitro* studies. *Annals of the New York Academy of Sciences*, 692, 230–242.

Gronowski, A. M., Zhong, Z., Wen, Z., Thomas, M. J., Darnell, J. E. Jr., & Rotwein, P. (1995). *In vivo* growth hormone treatment rapidly stimulates the tyrosine phosphorylation and activation of Stat3. *Molecular Endocrinology*, 9, 171–177.

Han, V. K., Lauder, J. M., & D'Ercole, A. J. (1988). Rat astroglial somatomedin/insulin-like growth factor binding proteins: characterization and evidence of biologic function. *Journal of Neuroscience*, 8, 3135–3143.

Hansson, H. A., Brandsten, C., Lossing, C., & Petruson, K. (1989). Transient expression of insulin-like growth factor I immunoreactivity by vascular cells during angiogenesis. *Experimental and Molecular Pathology*, 50, 125–138.

Hansson, H. A., Jennische, E., & Skottner, A. (1987). Regenerating endothelial cells express insulin-like growth factor-I immunoreactivity after arterial injury. *Cell and Tissue Research*, 250, 499–505.

Harman, S. M., & Blackman, M. R. (2003). The effects of growth hormone and sex steroid on lean body mass, fat mass, muscle strength, cardiovascular endurance and adverse events in healthy elderly women and men. *Hormone Research*, 60, 121–124.

Haro, L. S., Bustamante, J., Hernandez, P., Flores, R., Aguilar, R., Lopez-Guajardo, C., Martinez, A. O. (1999). Biochemistry and pharmacology of rabbit cardiac growth hormone (GH) receptors. *Molecular and Cellular Endocrinology*, 152, 179–187.

Hauck, S. J., & Bartke, A. (2000). Effects of growth hormone on hypothalamic catalase and Cu/Zn superoxide dismutase. *Free Radical Biology & Medicine*, 28, 970–978.

Hauck, S. J., Hunter, W. S., Danilovich, N., Kopchick, J. J., & Bartke, A. (2001). Reduced levels of thyroid hormones, insulin, and glucose, and lower body core temperature in the growth hormone receptor/binding protein knockout mouse. *Experimental Biology and Medicine*, 226, 552–558.

Holzenberger, M., Dupont, J., Ducos, B., Leneuve, P., Geloen, A., Even, P. C., Cervera, P., Le Bouc, Y. (2003). IGF-1 receptor regulates lifespan and resistance to oxidative stress in mice. *Nature*, 421, 182–187.

Houck, W. V., Pan, L. C., Kribbs, S. B., Clair, M. J., McDaniel, G. M., Krombach, R. S., Merritt, W. M., Price, C., Iannini, J. P., Mukherjee, R., Spinale, F. G. (1999). Effects of growth hormone supplementation on left ventricular morphology and myocyte function with the development of congestive heart failure. *Circulation*, 100, 2003–2009.

Hutchins, P. M., Dusseau J. W., Marr M. C., & Greenough, W. T. (1982). The role of arteriolar structural changes in hypertension. *Microvascular Aspects of Spontaneous Hypertension*, 10, 41–53.

Hutchins, P. M., Lynch, C. D., Cooney, P. T., & Curseen, K. A. (1996). The microcirculation in experimental hypertension and aging. *Cardiovascular Research*, 32, 772–780.

Hynes, M. A., Van Wyk, J. J., Brooks, P. J., D'Ercole, A. J., Jansen, M., & Lund, P. K. (1987). Growth hormone dependence of somatomedin-C/insulin-like growth factor-I and insulin-like growth factor-II messenger ribonucleic acids. *Molecular Endocrinology*, 1, 233–242.

Isaksson, O. G., Lindahl, A., Nilsson, A., & Isgaard, J. (1988). Action of growth hormone: current views. *Acta paediatrica Scandinavica.Supplement*, 343, 12–18.

Johanson, A. J., & Blizzard, R. M. (1981). Low somatomedin-C levels in older men rise in response to growth hormone administration. *Johns Hopkins Medical Journal*, 149, 115–117.

Johnson, T. E. (1990). Increased life-span of age-1 mutants in *Caenorhabditis elegans* and lower Gompertz rate of aging. *Science*, 249, 908–912.

Jucker, M., Battig, K., & Meier-Ruge, W. (1990). Effects of aging and vincamine derivatives on pericapillary microenvironment: stereological characterization of the cerebral capillary network. *Neurobiology of Aging*, 11, 39–46.

Juul, A., Dalgaard, P., Blum, W. F., Bang, P., Hall, K., Michaelsen, K. F., Muller, J., Skakkebaek, N. E. (1995). Serum levels of insulin-like growth factor (IGF)-binding protein-3 (IGFBP-3) in healthy infants, children, and adolescents: the relation to IGF-I, IGF-II, IGFBP-1, IGFBP-2, age, sex, body mass index, and pubertal maturation. *Journal of Clinical Endocrinology and Metabolism*, 80, 2534–2542.

Kaiser, U., Schardt, C., Brandscheidt, D., Wollmer, E., & Havemann, K. (1993). Expression of insulin-like growth factor receptors I and II in normal human lung and in lung cancer. *Journal of Cancer Research and Clinical Oncology*, 119, 665–668.

Kaleko, M., Rutter, W. J., & Miller, A. D. (1990). Overexpression of the human insulinlike growth factor I receptor promotes ligand-dependent neoplastic transformation. *Molecular and Cellular Biology*, 10, 464–473.

Kalmijn, S., Janssen, J. A., Pols, H. A., Lamberts, S. W., & Breteler, M. M. (2000). A prospective study on circulating insulin-like growth factor I (IGF-I), IGF-binding proteins, and cognitive function in the elderly. *Journal of Clinical Endocrinology and Metabolism*, 85, 4551–4555.

Kalu, D. N., Orhii, P. B., Chen, C., Lee, D. Y., Hubbard, G. B., Lee, S., Olatunji-Bello, Y. (1998). Aged-rodent models of long-term growth hormone therapy: lack of deleterious effect on longevity. *Journals of Gerontology Series A, Biological Sciences and Medical Sciences*, 53, B452–B463.

Kappel, C. C., Velez-Yanguas, M. C., Hirschfeld, S., & Helman, L. J. (1994). Human osteosarcoma cell lines are dependent on insulin-like growth factor I for in vitro growth. *Cancer Research*, 54, 2803–2807.

Karoor, V., Wang, L., Wang, H. Y., & Malbon, C. C. (1998). Insulin stimulates sequestration of beta-adrenergic receptors and enhanced association of beta-adrenergic receptors with Grb2 via tyrosine 350. *Journal of Biological Chemistry*, 273, 33035–33041.

Kenyon, C., Chang, J., Gensch, E., Rudner, A., & Tabtiang, R. (1993). A *C. elegans* mutant that lives twice as long as wild type. *Nature*, 366, 461–464.

Kety, S. S. (1956). Human cerebral blood flow and oxygen consumption as related to aging. *Research Publications: Association for Research in Nervous and Mental Disease*, 35, 31–45.

Khan, A. S., Lynch, C. D., Sane, D. C., Willingham, M. C., & Sonntag, W. E. (2001). Growth hormone increases regional coronary blood flow and capillary density in aged rats. *Journals of Gerontology Series A, Biological Sciences and Medical Sciences*, 56, B364–B371.

Khansari, D. N., & Gustad, T. (1991). Effects of long-term, low-dose growth hormone therapy on immune function and life expectancy of mice. *Mechanisms of Ageing and Development*, 57, 87–100.

Knyszynski, A., Adler-Kunin, S., & Globerson, A. (1992). Effects of growth hormone on thymocyte development from progenitor cells in the bone marrow. *Brain, Behavior, and Immunity*, 6, 327–340.

Kuo, M. L., Shiah, S. G., Wang, C. J., & Chuang, S. E. (1999). Suppression of apoptosis by Bcl-2 to enhance benzene metabolites-induced oxidative DNA damage and mutagenesis: a possible mechanism of carcinogenesis. *Molecular Pharmacology*, 55, 894–901.

Kupfer, J. M., & Rubin, S. A. (1992). Differential regulation of insulin-like growth factor I by growth hormone and thyroid hormone in the heart of juvenile hypophysectomized rats. *Journal of Molecular and Cellular Cardiology*, 24, 631–639.

Lahm, H., Amstad, P., Wyniger, J., Yilmaz, A., Fischer, J. R., Schreyer, M., Givel, J. C. (1994). Blockade of the insulin-like growth-factor-I receptor inhibits growth of human colorectal cancer cells: evidence of a functional IGF-II-mediated autocrine loop. *International Journal of Cancer*, 58, 452–459.

Laron, Z., Doron, M., & Arnikan, B. (1970). Plasma growth hormone in men and women over 70 years of age. *Medicine, Sports, Physical Activity and Aging*, 4, 126–129.

Le Roith, D., Bondy, C., Yakar, S., Liu, J. L., & Butler, A. (2001). The somatomedin hypothesis: 2001. *Endocrine Reviews*, 22, 53–74.

Lee, A. V., Darbre, P., & King, R. J. (1994). Processing of insulin-like growth factor-II (IGF-II) by human breast cancer cells. *Molecular and Cellular Endocrinology*, 99, 211–220.

Lee-Kwon, W., Park, D., & Bernier, M. (1998). Nucleotide excision repair is not required for the antiapoptotic function of insulin-like growth factor 1. *Experimental Cell Research*, 241, 458–466.

Lembo, G., Rockman, H. A., Hunter, J. J., Steinmetz, H., Koch, W. J., Ma, L., Prinz, M. P., Ross, J. Jr., Chien, K. R., Powell-Braxton, L. (1996). Elevated blood pressure and enhanced myocardial contractility in mice with severe IGF-1 deficiency. *Journal of Clinical Investigation*, 98, 2648–2655.

Lenoir, D., & Honegger, P. (1983). Insulin-like growth factor I (IGF I) stimulates DNA synthesis in fetal rat brain cell cultures. *Brain Research*, 283, 205–213.

LeRoith, D., Adamo, M. L., Shemer, J., Lanau, F., Shen-Orr, Z., Yaron, A., Roberts, C. T. Jr., Clemmons, D. R., Sheikh, M. S., Shao, Z. M. (1993). Retinoic acid inhibits growth of breast cancer cell lines: the role of insulin-like growth factor binding proteins. *Growth Regulation*, 3, 78–80.

Li, C. H., Evans, H. M., & Simpson, M. E. (1945). Isolation and properties of the anterior pituitary hypophyseal growth hormone. *Journal of Biological Chemistry*, 159, 353–356.

Li, S., Crenshaw, E. B. III, Rawson, E. J., Simmons, D. M., Swanson, L. W., & Rosenfeld, M. G. (1990). Dwarf locus mutants lacking three pituitary cell types result from mutations in the POU-domain gene pit-1. *Nature*, 347, 528–533.

Lichtenwalner, R. J., Forbes, M. E., Bennett, S. A., Lynch, C. D., Sonntag, W., & Rifai, N. (2000). IGF-1 increases cell survival and the size of the dentate gyrus in aged rats. *30th Annual Meeting of the Society for Neuroscience*.

Lieberman, S. A., Mitchell, A. M., Marcus, R., Hintz, R. L., & Hoffman, A. R. (1994). The insulin-like growth factor I generation test: resistance to growth hormone with aging and estrogen replacement therapy. *Hormone and Metabolic Research*, 26, 229–233.

Ling, N., Esch, F., Bohlen, P., Brazeau, P., Wehrenberg, W. B., & Guillemin, R. (1984). Isolation, primary structure, and synthesis of human hypothalamic somatocrinin: growth hormone-releasing factor. *Proceedings of the National Academy of Sciences of the USA*, 81, 4302–4306.

Liu, J. L., Grinberg, A., Westphal, H., Sauer, B., Accili, D., Karas, M., LeRoith, D. (1998). Insulin-like growth factor-I affects perinatal lethality and postnatal development in a gene dosage-dependent manner: manipulation using the Cre/loxP system in transgenic mice. *Molecular Endocrinology*, 12, 1452–1462.

Liu, J. L., Yakar, S., & LeRoith, D. (2000). Conditional knockout of mouse insulin-like growth factor-1 gene using the Cre/loxP system. *Proceedings of the Society for Experimental Biology and Medicine*, 223, 344–351.

Lopez-Fernandez, J., Sanchez-Franco, F., Velasco, B., Tolon, R. M., Pazos, F., & Cacicedo, L. (1996). Growth hormone induces somatostatin and insulin-like growth factor I gene expression in the cerebral hemispheres of aging rats. *Endocrinology*, 137, 4384–4391.

Magnetto, S., Boissier, S., Delmas, P. D., & Clezardin, P. (1999). Additive antitumor activities of taxoids in combination with the bisphosphonate ibandronate against invasion and adhesion of human breast carcinoma cells to bone. *International Journal of Cancer*, 83, 263–269.

Mathews, L. S., Enberg, B., & Norstedt, G. (1989). Regulation of rat growth hormone receptor gene expression. *Journal of Biological Chemistry*, 264, 9905–9910.

McMorris, F. A., & Dubois-Dalcq, M. (1988). Insulin-like growth factor I promotes cell proliferation and oligodendroglial commitment in rat glial progenitor cells developing in vitro. *Journal of Neuroscience Research*, 21, 199–209.

McMorris, F. A., Smith, T. M., DeSalvo, S., & Furlanetto, R. W. (1986). Insulin-like growth factor I/somatomedin C: a potent inducer of oligodendrocyte development. *Proceedings of the National Academy of Sciences of the USA*, 83, 822–826.

Melamed, E., Lavy, S., Bentin, S., Cooper, G., & Rinot, Y. (1980). Reduction in regional cerebral blood flow during normal aging in man. *Stroke*, 11, 31–35.

Morley, J. E., Kaiser, F., Raum, W. J., Perry, H. M., 3rd, Flood, J. F., Jensen, J., Sillver, A. J., Roberts, E. (1997). Potentially predictive and manipulable blood serum correlates of aging in the healthy human male: progressive decreases in bioavailable testosterone, dehydroepiandrosterone sulfate, and the ratio of insulin-like growth factor 1 to growth hormone. *Proceedings of the National Academy of Sciences of the USA*, 94, 7537–7542.

Murphy, W. J., Durum, S. K., Anver, M. R., & Longo, D. L. (1992). Immunologic and hematologic effects of neuroendocrine hormones. Studies on DW/J dwarf mice. *Journal of Immunology*, 148, 3799–3805.

Nakao-Hayashi, J., Ito, H., Kanayasu, T., Morita, I., & Murota, S. (1992). Stimulatory effects of insulin and insulin-like growth factor I on migration and tube formation by vascular endothelial cells. *Atherosclerosis*, 92, 141–149.

Nicosia, R. F., Nicosia, S. V., & Smith, M. (1994). Vascular endothelial growth factor, platelet-derived growth factor, and insulin-like growth factor-1 promote rat aortic angiogenesis in vitro. *American Journal of Pathology*, 145, 1023–1029.

Nigro, V., Okazaki, Y., Belsito, A., Piluso, G., Matsuda, Y., Politano, L., Nigro, G., Ventura, C., Abbondanza, C., Molinari, A. M., Acampora, D., Nishimura, M., Hayashizaki, Y., Puca, G. A. (1997). Identification of the Syrian hamster cardiomyopathy gene. *Human Molecular Genetics*, 6, 601–607.

Noguchi, T., Kurata, L. M., & Sugisaki, T. (1987). Presence of a somatomedin-C-immunoreactive substance in the central nervous system: immunohistochemical mapping studies. *Neuroendocrinology*, 46, 277–282.

Nyberg, F. (1997). Aging effects on growth hormone receptor binding in the brain. *Experimental Gerontology*, 32, 521–528.

O'Kusky, J. R., Ye, P., & D'Ercole, A. J. (2000). Insulin-like growth factor-I promotes neurogenesis and synaptogenesis in the hippocampal dentate gyrus during postnatal development. *Journal of Neuroscience*, 20, 8435–8442.

Ooka, H., Fujita, S., & Yoshimoto, E. (1983). Pituitary-thyroid activity and longevity in neonatally thyroxine-treated rats. *Mechanisms of Ageing and Development*, 22, 113–120.

Osborne, C. K., Clemmons, D. R., & Arteaga, C. L. (1990). Regulation of breast cancer growth by insulin-like growth factors. *Journal of Steroid Biochemistry and Molecular Biology*, 37, 805–809.

Palmiter, R. D., Norstedt, G., Gelinas, R. E., Hammer, R. E., & Brinster, R. L. (1983). Metallothionein-human GH fusion genes stimulate growth of mice. *Science*, 222, 809–814.

Paolisso, G., Ammendola, S., Del Buono, A., Gambardella, A., Riondino, M., Tagliamonte, M. R., Rizzo, M. R. Carella, C., Varricchio, M. (1997). Serum levels of insulin-like growth factor-I (IGF-I) and IGF-binding protein-3 in healthy centenarians: relationship with plasma leptin and lipid concentrations, insulin action, and cognitive function. *Journal of Clinical Endocrinology and Metabolism*, 82, 2204–2209.

Papadakis, M. A., Grady, D., Black, D., Tierney, M. J., Gooding, G. A., Schambelan, M., Grunfeld, C. (1996). Growth hormone replacement in healthy older men improves body composition but not functional ability. *Annals of Internal Medicine*, 124, 708–716.

Papadakis, M. A., Grady, D., Tierney, M. J., Black, D., Wells, L., & Grunfeld, C. (1995). Insulin-like growth factor 1 and functional status in healthy older men. *Journal of the American Geriatrics Society*, 43, 1350–1355.

Penalva, A., Burguera, B., Casabiell, X., Tresguerres, J. A., Dieguez, C., & Casanueva, F. F. (1989). Activation of cholinergic neurotransmission by pyridostigmine reverses the inhibitory effect of hyperglycemia on growth hormone (GH) releasing hormone-induced GH secretion in man: does acute hyperglycemia act through hypothalamic release of somatostatin? *Neuroendocrinology*, 49, 551–554.

Peyrat, J. P., & Bonneterre, J. (1992). Type 1 IGF receptor in human breast diseases. *Breast Cancer Research and Treatment*, 22, 59–67.

Pietrzkowski, Z., Wernicke, D., Porcu, P., Jameson, B. A., & Baserga, R. (1992). Inhibition of cellular proliferation by peptide analogues of insulin-like growth factor 1. *Cancer Research*, 52, 6447–6451.

Pulford, B. E., Whalen, L. R., & Ishii, D. N. (1997). Subcutaneous IGF administration spares loss of the limb withdrawal reflex in 6-OHDA lesioned rats. *Society for Neuroscience Abstracts*, 23, 1705.

Raile, K., Hoflich, A., Kessler, U., Yang, Y., Pfuender, M., Blum, W. F., Kolb, H., Schwarz, H. P., Kiess, W. (1994). Human osteosarcoma (U-2 OS) cells express both insulin-like growth factor-I (IGF-I) receptors and insulin-like growth factor-II/mannose-6-phosphate (IGF-II/M6P) receptors and synthesize IGF-II: autocrine growth stimulation by IGF-II via the IGF-I receptor. *Journal of Cellular Physiology*, 159, 531–541.

Ramsey, M., Ariwodola, O., Sonntag, W., & Weiner, J. (2004). Functional characterization of Des-IGF-1 action at excitatory synapses in the CA1 region of the rat hippocampus. *(In preparation)*

Ramsey, M. M., Ingram, R. L., Cashion, A. B., Ng, A. H., Cline, J. M., Parlow, A. F., Sonntag, W. E. (2002). Growth hormone-deficient dwarf animals are resistant to dimethylbenzanthracine (DMBA)-induced mammary carcinogenesis. *Endocrinology*, 143, 4139–4142.

Ramsey, M., Weiner, J., Moore, T., Carter, C., & Sonntag, W. (2004). Growth hormone treatment attenuates age-related deficits in short-term plasticity and spatial learning. *Neuroscience*, 129, 119–127.

Recio-Pinto, E., & Ishii, D. N. (1984). Effects of insulin, insulin-like growth factor-II and nerve growth factor on neurite outgrowth in cultured human neuroblastoma cells. *Brain Research*, 302, 323–334.

Recio-Pinto, E., Lang, F. F., & Ishii, D. N. (1984). Insulin and insulin-like growth factor II permit nerve growth factor binding and the neurite formation response in cultured human neuroblastoma cells. *Proceedings of the National Academy of Sciences of the USA*, 81, 2562–2566.

Recio-Pinto, E., Rechler, M. M., & Ishii, D. N. (1986). Effects of insulin, insulin-like growth factor-II, and nerve growth factor on neurite formation and survival in cultured sympathetic and sensory neurons. *Journal of Neuroscience*, 6, 1211–1219.

Reinhardt, R. R., & Bondy, C. A. (1994). Insulin-like growth factors cross the blood-brain barrier. *Endocrinology*, 135, 1753–1761.

Renganathan, M., Messi, M. L., & Delbono, O. (1998). Overexpression of IGF-1 exclusively in skeletal muscle prevents age-related decline in the number of dihydropyridine receptors. *Journal of Biological Chemistry*, 273, 28845–28851.

Renganathan, M., Sonntag, W. E., & Delbono, O. (1997). L-type Ca2+ channel-insulin-like growth factor-1 receptor signaling impairment in aging rat skeletal muscle. *Biochemical and Biophysical Research Communications*, 235, 784–789.

Rivier, J., Spiess, J., Thorner, M., & Vale, W. (1982). Characterization of a growth hormone-releasing factor from a human pancreatic islet tumour. *Nature*, 300, 276–278.

Rollero, A., Murialdo, G., Fonzi, S., Garrone, S., Gianelli, M. V., Gazzerro, E., Barreca, A., Polleri, A. (1998). Relationship between cognitive function, growth hormone and insulin-like growth factor I plasma levels in aged subjects. *Neuropsychobiology*, 38, 73–79.

Rose, M., & Charlesworth, B. (1980). A test of evolutionary theories of senescence. *Nature*, 287, 141–142.

Rosenblum, W. I., & Kontos, H. A. (1974). The importance and relevance of studies of the pial microcirculation. *Stroke*, 5, 425–428.

Rotsch, M., Maasberg, M., Erbil, C., Jaques, G., Worsch, U., & Havemann, K. (1992). Characterization of insulin-like growth factor I receptors and growth effects in human lung cancer cell lines. *Journal of Cancer Research and Clinical Oncology*, 118, 502–508.

Roubenoff, R., & Rall, L. C. (1993). Humoral mediation of changing body composition during aging and chronic inflammation. *Nutrition Reviews*, 51, 1–11.

Roupas, P., & Herington, A. C. (1994). Postreceptor signaling mechanisms for growth hormone. *Trends in Endocrinological Metabolism*, 5, 154–158.

Rudman, D., Feller, A. G., Nagraj, H. S., Gergans, G. A., Lalitha, P. Y., Goldberg, A. F., Schlenker, R. A., Cohn, L., Rudman, I. W., Mattson, D. E. (1990). Effects of human growth hormone in men over 60 years old. *New England Journal of Medicine*, 323, 1–6.

Rudman, D., Kutner, M. H., Rogers, C. M., Lubin, M. F., Fleming, G. A., & Bain, R. P. (1981). Impaired growth hormone secretion in the adult population: relation to age and adiposity. *Journal of Clinical Investigation*, 67, 1361–1369.

Russell, W. E., Van Wyk, J. J., & Pledger, W. J. (1984). Inhibition of the mitogenic effects of plasma by a monoclonal antibody to somatomedin C. *Proceedings of the National Academy of Sciences of the USA*, 81, 2389–2392.

Ryoke, T., Gu, Y., Mao, L., Hongo, M., Clark, R. G., Peterson, K. L., Ross, J. Jr. (1999). Progressive cardiac dysfunction and fibrosis in the cardiomyopathic hamster and effects of growth hormone and angiotensin-converting enzyme inhibition. *Circulation*, 100, 1734–1743.

Sakamoto, A., Ono, K., Abe, M., Jasmin, G., Eki, T., Murakami, Y., Masaki, T., Toyo-oka, T., Hanaoka, F. (1997). Both hypertrophic and dilated cardiomyopathies are caused by mutation of the same gene, delta-sarcoglycan, in hamster: an animal model of disrupted dystrophin-associated glycoprotein complex. *Proceedings of the National Academy of Sciences*, 94, 13873–13878.

Sato, Y., Okamura, K., Morimoto, A., Hamanaka, R., Hamaguchi, K., Shimada, T., Ono, M., Kohno, K., Sakata, T., Kuwano, M. (1993). Indispensable role of tissue-type plasminogen activator in growth factor-dependent tube formation of human microvascular endothelial cells in vitro. *Experimental Cell Research*, 204, 223–229.

Shaw, T. G., Mortel, K. F., Meyer, J. S., Rogers, R. L., Hardenberg, J., & Cutaia, M. M. (1984). Cerebral blood flow changes in benign aging and cerebrovascular disease. *Neurology*, 34, 855–862.

Shaywitz, B. A., & Pearson, D. A. (1978). Effect of phenobarbital on activity and learning in 6-hydroxydopamine treated rat pups. *Pharmacology, Biochemistry, and Behavior*, 9, 173–179.

Shemer, J., Raizada, M. K., Masters, B. A., Ota, A., & LeRoith, D. (1987). Insulin-like growth factor I receptors in neuronal and glial cells. Characterization and biological effects in primary culture. *Journal of Biological Chemistry*, 262, 7693–7699.

Shibasaki, T., Shizume, K., Masuda, A., Nakahara, M., Hizuka, N., Miyakawa, N., Takano, K., Demura, H., Wakabayashi, I., Ling, N. (1984). Age-related changes in plasma growth hormone response to growth hormone-releasing factor in man. *Journal of Clinical Endocrinology and Metabolism*, 58, 212–214.

Shigematsu, K., Kataoka, Y., Kamio, T., Kurihara, M., Niwa, M., & Tsuchiyama, H. (1990). Partial characterization of insulin-like growth factor I in primary human lung cancers using immunohistochemical and receptor autoradiographic techniques. *Cancer Research*, 50, 2481–2484.

Silberberg, R. (1972). Articular aging and osteoarthrosis in dwarf mice. *Pathologia et Microbiologia*, 38, 417–430.

Silberberg, R. (1973). Vertebral aging in hypopituitary dwarf mice. *Gerontologia*, 19, 281–294.

Smith, R. D., Cooper, B. R., & Breese, G. R. (1973). Growth and behavioral changes in developing rats treated intracisternally with 6-hydroxydopamine: evidence for involvement of brain dopamine. *Journal of Pharmacology and Experimental Therapeutics*, 185, 609–619.

Snell, G. D. (1929). Dwarf, a new Mendelian recessive character of the house mouse. *Proceedings of the National Academy of Sciences of the USA*, 15, 733–734.

Sonntag, W. E., & Boyd, R. L. (1988). Chronic ethanol feeding inhibits plasma levels of insulin-like growth factor-1. *Life Sciences*, 43, 1325–1330.

Sonntag, W. E., Carter, C. S., Ikeno, Y., Ekenstedt, K., Carlson, C. S., Loeser, R. F., Chakrabarty, S., Lee, S., Bennett, C., Ingram, R., Moore, T., Ramsey, M. (2005). Adult-onset growth hormone and insulin-like growth factor 1 deficiency reduces neoplastic disease, modifies age-related pathology, and increases life span. *Endocrinology*, 146(7), 2920–32.

Sonntag, W. E., Forman, L. J., Miki, N., Steger, R. W., Ramos, T., Arimura, A., Meites, J. (1981). Effects of CNS active drugs and somatostatin antiserum on growth hormone release in young and old male rats. *Neuroendocrinology*, 33, 73–78.

Sonntag, W. E., Gottschall, P. E., & Meites, J. (1986). Increased secretion of somatostatin-28 from hypothalamic neurons of aged rats *in vitro*. *Brain Research*, 380, 229–234.

Sonntag, W. E., & Gough, M. A. (1988). Growth hormone releasing hormone induced release of growth hormone in aging male rats: dependence on pharmacological manipulation and endogenous somatostatin release. *Neuroendocrinology*, 47, 482–488.

Sonntag, W. E., Hylka, V. W., & Meites, J. (1983). Impaired ability of old male rats to secrete growth hormone in vivo but not in vitro in response to hpGRF(1–44). *Endocrinology*, 113, 2305–2307.

Sonntag, W. E., Hylka, V. W., & Meites, J. (1985). Growth hormone restores protein synthesis in skeletal muscle of old male rats. *Journal of Gerontology*, 40, 689–694.

Sonntag, W. E., Lynch, C. D., Cefalu, W. T., Ingram, R. L., Bennett, S. A., Thornton, P. L., Khan, A. S. (1999). Pleiotropic effects of growth hormone and insulin-like growth factor (IGF)-1 on biological aging: inferences from moderate caloric-restricted animals. *Journals of Gerontology Series A, Biological Sciences and Medical Sciences*, 54, B521–B538.

Sonntag, W. E., Lynch, C. D., Cooney, P. T., & Hutchins, P. M. (1997). Decreases in cerebral microvasculature with age are associated with the decline in growth hormone and insulin-like growth factor 1. *Endocrinology*, 138, 3515–3520.

Sonntag, W. E., Steger, R. W., Forman, L. J., & Meites, J. (1980). Decreased pulsatile release of growth hormone in old male rats. *Endocrinology*, 107, 1875–1879.

Sornson, M. W., Wu, W., Dasen, J. S., Flynn, S. E., Norman, D. J., O'Connell, S. M., Gukovsky, I., Carriere, C., Ryan, A. K., Miller, A. P., Zuo, I., Gleiberman, A. S., Andersen, B., Beamer, W. G., Rosenfeld, M. G. (1996). Pituitary lineage determination by the Prophet of Pit-1 homeodomain factor defective in Ames dwarfism. *Nature*, 384, 327–333.

Sotiropoulos, A., Perrot-Applanat, M., Dinerstein, H., Pallier, A., Postel-Vinay, M. C., Finidori, J., Kelly, P. A. (1994). Distinct cytoplasmic regions of the growth hormone receptor are required for activation of JAK2, mitogen-activated protein kinase, and transcription. *Endocrinology*, 135, 1292–1298.

Spik, K., & Sonntag, W. E. (1989). Increased pituitary response to somatostatin in aging male rats: relationship to somatostatin receptor number and affinity. *Neuroendocrinology*, 50, 489–494.

Steger, R. W., Bartke, A., & Cecim, M. (1993). Premature ageing in transgenic mice expressing different growth hormone genes. *Journal of Reproduction and Fertility*, 46 (Suppl.), 61–75.

Stromer, H., Cittadini, A., Douglas, P. S., & Morgan, J. P. (1996). Exogenously administered growth hormone and insulin-like growth factor-I alter intracellular Ca^{2+} handling and enhance cardiac performance. *In vitro* evaluation in the isolated isovolumic buffer-perfused rat heart. *Circulation Research*, 79, 227–236.

Takahashi, S., & Meites, J. (1987). GH binding to liver in young and old female rats: relation to somatomedin-C secretion. *Proceedings of the Society for Experimental Biology and Medicine*, 186, 229–233.

Tannenbaum, G. S., & Ling, N. (1984). The interrelationship of growth hormone (GH)-releasing factor and somatostatin in generation of the ultradian rhythm of GH secretion. *Endocrinology*, 115, 1952–1957.

Tannenbaum, G. S., & Martin, J. B. (1976). Evidence for an endogenous ultradian rhythm governing growth hormone secretion in the rat. *Endocrinology*, 98, 562–570.

Thornton, P. L., Ingram, R. L., & Sonntag, W. E. (2000). Chronic [D-Ala2]-growth hormone-releasing hormone administration attenuates age-related deficits in spatial memory. *Journals of Gerontology Series A: Biological Sciences and Medical Sciences*, 55, B106–B112.

Tierney, T., & Robinson, I. C. (2002). Increased lactotrophs despite decreased somatotrophs in the dwarf (dw/dw) rat: a defect in the regulation of lactotroph/somatotroph cell fate? *Journal of Endocrinology*, 175, 435–446.

Toran-Allerand, C. D., Ellis, L., & Pfenninger, K. H. (1988). Estrogen and insulin synergism in neurite growth enhancement *in vitro*: mediation of steroid effects by interactions with growth factors? *Brain Research*, 469, 87–100.

Torres-Aleman, I., Naftolin, F., & Robbins, R. J. (1989). Growth promoting effects of IGF-I on fetal hypothalamic cell lines under serum-free culture conditions. *International Journal of Developmental Neuroscience*, 7, 195–202.

Torrisi, R., Pensa, F., Orengo, M. A., Catsafados, E., Ponzani, P., Boccardo, F., Costa, A., Decensi, A. (1993). The synthetic retinoid fenretinide lowers plasma insulin-like growth factor I levels in breast cancer patients. *Cancer Research*, 53, 4769–4771.

van der Pal, R. H., Koper, J. W., van Golde, L. M., & Lopes-Cardozo, M. (1988). Effects of insulin and insulin-like growth factor (IGF-I) on oligodendrocyte-enriched glial cultures. *Journal of Neuroscience Research*, 19, 483–490.

Van Molle, W., Denecker, G., Rodriguez, I., Brouckaert, P., Vandenabeele, P., & Libert, C. (1999). Activation of caspases in lethal experimental hepatitis and prevention by acute phase proteins. *Journal of Immunology*, 163, 5235–5241.

Veldhuis, J. D., Roemmich, J. N., Richmond, E. J., Rogol, A. D., Lovejoy, J. C., Sheffield-Moore, M., Mauras, N., Bowers, C. Y. (2005). Endocrine control of body composition in infancy, childhood, and puberty. *Endocrine Reviews*, 26(1), 114–46.

Wang, Y. Z., & Wong, Y. C. (1998). Sex hormone-induced prostatic carcinogenesis in the noble rat: the role of insulin-like growth factor-I (IGF-I) and vascular endothelial growth factor (VEGF) in the development of prostate cancer. *Prostate*, 35, 165–177.

Wannenburg, T., Khan, A. S., Sane, D. C., Willingham, M. C., Faucette, T., & Sonntag, W. E. (2001). Growth hormone reverses age-related cardiac myofilament dysfunction in rats. *American Journal of Physiology: Heart and Circulatory Physiology*, 281, H915–H922.

Werner, H., & LeRoith, D. (1996). The role of the insulin-like growth factor system in human cancer. *Advances in Cancer Research*, 68, 183–223.

Werther, G. A., Abate, M., Hogg, A., Cheesman, H., Oldfield, B., Hards, D., Hudson, P., Power, B., Freed, K., Herington, A. C. (1990). Localization of insulin-like growth factor-I mRNA in rat brain by in situ hybridization—relationship to IGF-I receptors. *Molecular Endocrinology*, 4, 773–778.

Wolden-Hanson, T., Marck, B. T., Smith, L., & Matsumoto, A. M. (1999). Cross-sectional and longitudinal analysis of age-associated changes in body composition of male Brown Norway rats: association of serum leptin levels with peripheral adiposity. *Journals of Gerontology Series A: Biological Sciences and Medical Sciences*, 54, B99–B107.

Xu, X., & Sonntag, W. E. (1996). Growth hormone-induced nuclear translocation of Stat-3 decreases with age: modulation by caloric restriction. *American Journal of Physiology*, 271, E903–E909.

Xu, X., Bennett, S. A., Ingram, R. L., & Sonntag, W. E. (1995). Decreases in growth hormone receptor signal transduction contribute to the decline in insulin-like growth factor I gene expression with age. *Endocrinology*, 136, 4551–4557.

Yamamoto, H., & Murphy, L. J. (1995). Enzymatic conversion of IGF-I to des(1–3)IGF-I in rat serum and tissues: a further potential site of growth hormone regulation of IGF-I action. *Journal of Endocrinology*, 146, 141–148.

Yang, R., Bunting, S., Gillett, N., Clark, R., & Jin, H. (1995). Growth hormone improves cardiac performance in experimental heart failure. *Circulation*, 92, 262–267.

Yu, B. P., Masoro, E. J., Murata, I., Bertrand, H. A., & Lynd, F. T. (1982). Life span study of SPF Fischer 344 male rats fed ad libitum or restricted diets: longevity, growth, lean body mass and disease. *Journal of Gerontology*, 37, 130–141.

Yu, H., & Berkel, H. (1999). Insulin-like growth factors and cancer. *Journal of the Louisiana State Medical Society*, 151, 218–223.

Chapter 21

Aging of the Female Reproductive System

Phyllis M. Wise

I. Introduction

This chapter reviews the changes that occur in the female reproductive system with age. For most physiological processes, male organisms are studied more frequently than females in any area of biology. Thus, it is unusual that in terms of reproductive aging, more attention has been paid to females than to males. This is probably because (1) menopause occurs relatively early during the aging process so may serve as a model system in which to study the biology of aging of other systems, and (2) in humans and Old World monkeys, female reproductive aging is clearly punctuated by an easily observed endpoint: the cessation of menstrual bleeding. Therefore, it is relatively easy to document changes before and after this endpoint and, when desirable, to normalize the timing of specific changes relative to this endpoint. In males, changes are more gradual, and functional decline is not marked by an easily measurable endpoint; thus, it has been more difficult to document when the reproductive axis declines and when these changes have functional repercussions.

Emphasis will be placed on changes that occur in humans and animal models. The majority of basic science studies that have been performed using animal models have been performed in rats and mice, although some work has been done in nonhuman primates. Therefore, the majority of the work that will be reviewed in this chapter is from studies performed with these species.

II. Menopause

Although there is considerable variation in the exact age of menopause, the majority of women go through menopause at approximately 51 years of age (Treloar, 1981; Treloar et al., 1967), and the timing of this change has remained essentially the same since medical records have been maintained. Menopause occurs around the time that the ovarian follicular reserve becomes exhausted, and, in fact, marked variation in the follicular

Handbook of the Biology of Aging, Sixth Edition

reserve correlates with variation in deterioration of regular menstrual cyclicity. Because these cells are not only the source of germ cells but also are the key cells that produce and synthesize ovarian steroids and peptide hormones, plasma levels of all of these hormones drop dramatically after menopause and remain low for the remainder of a woman's life. In particular, the ovarian steroids, estrogens and progestins, decrease dramatically and remain low unless a woman chooses to take hormone therapy. During the past decade, investigators have realized that ovarian steroids are not only reproductive hormones, but that they are hormones that play roles in a wide variety of nonreproductive functions as disparate as bone and mineral metabolism, memory and cognition, cardiovascular function, and the immune system. Thus, the end of reproductive life and the cessation of synthesis and secretion of estrogens, progestins, and peptide hormones have far-reaching implications for the health and quality of life of women. With the dramatic increase in the average life span of humans from approximately 50 years to over 80 years, which has occurred during the last 100 years, and the relatively unchanging age of menopause, the number and the proportion of women who are destined to spend over one-third of their lives in the postmenopausal state with unique gender-related medical and social challenges has become substantial. It should not be surprising then that an increasing number of clinical and basic science studies have focused on understanding fully the physiological changes that accompany menopause, the mechanisms that drive reproductive aging, and the impact of these changes on women's health.

A better understanding of reproductive changes will be important to gerontologists because the female reproductive system deteriorates early during the aging process, in the absence of pathological changes that often confound gerontological studies. Therefore, we hope that the understanding and concepts derived from our deepening understanding of menopause and the aging reproductive system may apply more generally to the process of the biology of aging of other systems.

It is interesting to note that nonhuman primates exhibit a similar transition to acyclicity; however, in general, it occurs at a much later stage of the life span, and many nonhuman primate species do not have a prolonged postmenopausal period (Bellino, 2000). In fact, in some nonhuman primate species, reproductive cyclicity does not completely cease in some individuals before they die. Whether this is a fundamental difference between humans and nonhuman primates or whether this is the result of inadequate knowledge as to how to optimally maintain these species in "laboratory" environments is not clear. If it is the latter, we would predict that by improving their diets or health care, the way we have been able to intervene in human populations during the past 100 years, we will be able to prolong their average life spans. It will be interesting to observe whether menopause will then occur closer to the middle of this more prolonged life span.

There has been an ongoing and lively debate as to whether rodents serve as a good model for human reproductive aging. In some sense, because rodents do not undergo a true menstrual cycle—that is, there in no sloughing of the uterine wall at the end of each cycle and the resultant vaginal bleeding—rodents cannot undergo a true "meno-pause." In addition, in rats and mice, there is no true luteal phase of the estrous cycle because the corpus luteum regresses rapidly after ovulation and progesterone is not secreted for a prolonged period of time. Arguments that rodents are not good models center primarily around two findings. First, in women, the loss of primordial follicles is log-linear during the initial stages of life and accelerates dramatically around the time women are 37 years old. This accelerated loss leads to the total absence of follicles when women are between 50 and 55 years old, when they are postmenopausal (Crowley *et al.*, 1985). In contrast, different strains and species of rodents exhibit striking variation in the rate of follicular loss. Although no studies have followed the rate of follicular loss across the entire life span, Faddy and colleagues (1987) showed that during the first 100 days of life, if anything, the rate of follicular loss decreases with age in mice. These data would suggest that, by the time rodents are reproductively senescent, the follicular pool may not be a limiting factor. Ovarian aging does play some role even in rodents since Gosden and colleagues (1983) showed a correlation between the size of the follicular reserve and entrance into irregular cyclicity. In addition, grafting young ovaries into mice about to become anovulatory extends their cycling life span (Felicio *et al.*, 1986). Second, in postmenopausal women, gonadotropins (hormones secreted from the anterior pituitary gland) concentrations in the circulation are elevated. It is thought that this is primarily in response to lowered estradiol secretion from the ovary because gonadotropin concentrations decrease in response to estrogen therapy. In contrast, gonadotropin concentrations remain relatively normal in old acyclic, repeatedly pseudopregnant rats. Thus, despite decreases in estradiol, gonadotropins do not appear to exhibit the dramatic increases observed in women. This suggests that decreased hypothalamic function leads to the post-reproductive state in rodents. The differences and similarities in reproductive aging between humans and rodent or nonhuman primate models are considered in detail later in this chapter.

III. Definitions

A. Terminology Used to Define Stages of Human Menopause

Investigators have used several terms to define different stages of the period of women's lives that surround the end of their reproductive life: perimenopause, climacteric, menopause, and postmenopause. *Perimenopause*, also called the *climacteric*, begins before menopause. This interval, which lasts approximately fours years, is the entire transition from the reproductive to the post-reproductive period of women's lives (Lobo, 1998; Prior, 1998). Symptoms such as hot flashes and irregular menstrual cycles may start to appear. By definition, perimenopause continues through the 12 months following the last menstrual period. Menopause is the permanent cessation of menstruation. Despite significant variation, menopause normally occurs spontaneously at approximately 51 years of age and is associated with the depletion of the ovarian follicular reserve. The term *surgical menopause* is defined as the cessation of menstrual cyclicity that results from the removal of a woman's ovaries when she would not normally undergo reproductive aging. Although both result in the cessation of menstrual cycles and the onset of infertility, the repercussions of natural menopause and surgical menopause may be different because the age of normal menopause is considerably greater than surgical menopause. Hence, changes in reproductive hormones in older women may result from interactions between chronological aging of the whole organism and aging of the reproductive system, whereas in younger women who are experiencing fewer age-related changes in other systems, the changes are likely to be related specifically to changes in the feed-forward and feed-back of the reproductive axis. Table 21.1 summarizes the definitions that are recommended by the World Health Organization.

Table 21.1
Definitions

Terminology	Definition
Menopause	Permanent cessation of menstruation associated with loss of ovarian follicular activity
Perimenopause or Climacteric	Period immediately prior to and at least one year after menopause, characterized by physiological and clinical features of altered ovarian function
Postmenopause	Period of life remaining after menopause
Premenopause	The reproductive period prior to menopause

B. "Menopause" in Species Other than Humans

Investigators once thought that menopause was restricted to human females. However, several papers (Gilardi *et al.*, 1997; Gould *et al.*, 1981; Graham *et al.*, 1979; Hodgen *et al.*, 1977) demonstrate that several species of nonhuman primates undergo a process very similar to that which women experience across menopause. However, these changes occur later in their average life span; therefore, the postmenopausal period is considerably shorter in these nonhuman primates species compared to women. At the present time, we do not know whether this is because menopause is truly delayed in nonhuman primates compared to humans or whether the nonhuman primate species that have been studied have not been maintained under optimal laboratory conditions and therefore their postmenopausal life span could be extended under different, more optimal environmental conditions. Currently, the populations of nonhuman primates that are available for study, which are maintained under controlled laboratory conditions, are small, and few studies have focused on aging. However, there are distinct advantages to using these species as models: longitudinal characterization from a population of animals that have been followed through their reproductive life span should be possible; intensive monitoring of hormonal changes through urinary samples is feasible; and records of reproductive history, in terms of numbers of pregnancies and live young, can be obtained. In addition, it is possible to perform longitudinal studies that are invasive and sometimes terminal in these species. Together, this means that use of these species in aging research will allow us to probe the underlying mechanisms that drive the menopausal transition. Such studies are expensive and labor-intensive; however, because an increasing number of nonhuman primate colonies have been maintained in captivity at several research centers, such studies will provide new data in the next several years.

Studies reveal several similarities in hormone profiles in older female rhesus monkeys and women during the transition from regular to irregular menstrual cycles. Variable inter-menstrual intervals and delay of ovulation interspersed with breakthrough uterine bleeding were found in perimenopausal rhesus monkeys (Gilardi *et al.*, 1997) and women in the fifth decade (Shideler *et al.*, 1989). However, it appears that not all of the hallmarks of human menopause punctuate the menopausal transition in the rhesus monkey. Importantly, in initial studies (Shideler *et al.*, 2001), the harbinger of impending reproductive decline, a selective rise in follicle stimulating hormone (FSH) concentrations in the absence of any change in luteinizing hormone (LH) levels, does not appear to occur in monkeys approaching menopause prior to overt changes in menstrual cycle length. In addition, rhesus monkeys do not exhibit frequent periods of high, unopposed estrogen in association with the transition to the menopausal state as has been observed in women (Gilardi *et al.*, 1997; Santoro *et al.*, 1996). Studies are ongoing to determine whether the baboon may be a better nonhuman primate model of human menopause; however, aging colonies of this species are even less available than rhesus monkeys. It is clear from these initial tantalizing results that considerably more work is required before we will know which of these other species can be used to model human menopause.

IV. Role of the Ovary in Reproductive Aging

A. Depletion and Aging of the Oocyte Reserve

A large body of evidence suggests that, in women, exhaustion of ovarian follicular reserve is the major factor that underlies the timing of perimenopause and menopause. Thus, ultimately, the permanent cessation of menstrual cyclicity can be largely attributed to changes within the ovaries. It appears that females are born with an enormous, but finite, postmitotic, nonrenewable endowment of follicles. This follicular reserve is set down during fetal development: germ cells undergo mitosis for a time while they are outside the ovary proper and migrate into the undifferentiated gonad. They then cease replicating, initiate meiosis, organize into primordial follicles, and most remain dormant for many months to years. Once mitosis stops, no new germ cells will ever be added to the original reserve. This basic tenet of mammalian ovarian biology has been challenged recently in a study performed in mice (Johnson *et al.*, 2004). However, the methods used in this paper make it

important to perform further experiments before a paradigm shift in our thinking is warranted. Within this follicular stockpile, a selected few will be recruited to undergo all of the steps that lead to the step of fertilization: growth, differentiation, and ovulation. The vast majority will re-awaken from the dormant pool and begin the path of growth and differentiation but will never undergo this entire process of development, differentiation, and maturation. Instead, they will undergo atresia through apoptic mechanisms of cell death before they are ever recruited to grow or at a step of the differentiation and maturation process (see Gougeon, 1996; Hirshfield, 1991 for reviews). Because atretic follicles cannot be replaced, the number of follicles continues an inexorable decline until relatively few, poorly responsive follicles remain at the time of menopause.

From fetal life through childhood into the reproductive years and ending at menopause, follicles reawaken and mature from primordial to secondary follicles. In postmenopausal women, the endowment of ovarian follicles is completely depleted (Block, 1952; Costoff & Mahesh, 1975;). In fact, Richardson and colleagues (1987) demonstrated that middle-aged women who had already begun menopausal transition and were exhibiting irregular menstrual cyclicity had 10 times fewer follicles in their ovaries than women who continued to cycle regularly. One of the most intriguing and provocative findings in the area of ovarian aging is that the rate of follicular loss is not log-linear (see Figure 21.1) (Gougeon *et al.*, 1994; Richardson *et al.*, 1987). Instead, the rate of follicular loss accelerates three- to six-fold when women are approximately 39 years of age. This change occurs at least 10 years prior to menopause and leads to complete depletion of the follicular endowment by the time women are in their fifties.

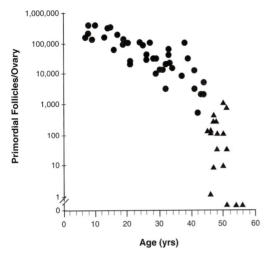

Figure 21.1 Age-related decrease in the total number of primordial follicles within both human ovaries from birth to menopause. As a result of recruitment, the number of follicles decreases in a log-linear fashion until approximately 37 years of age (circles), then the rate of decrease in the follicular pool accelerates (triangles) such that there are virtually no follicles left in the ovary at the time of menopause. From Richardson *et al.*, 1987; Copyright 1987, The Endocrine Society.

Gougeon and colleagues (1994) differentiated between the rate of disappearance of primordial non-growing follicles versus early growing follicles over the life span. Their results support the view that depletion of the pool of non-growing follicles is caused mainly by atresia of dormant primordial follicles in younger women, but mainly by the entrance of non-growing follicles into the growing pool in older women. If the rate of follicular loss did not change during this critical interval, the reserve of ovarian follicles would not be exhausted until women were between 70 and 80 years old. Thus, if the size of the follicular pool is the rate-limiting factor in female reproductive aging, the timing of reproductive senescence might not differ remarkably compared to the timing of decline of multiple other physiological systems. What leads to this accelerated loss of follicles during middle age? Unfortunately, few answers are available

because the mechanisms leading to atresia within the non-growing dormant pool of primordial follicles and the regulation of the re-entry of resting follicles into the growing pool and their initial stages of growth are largely unknown, even in young females. The very early stages of follicular development appear to be independent of hormonal influences, such as gonadotropin levels or patterns of secretion or intraovarian concentrations of steroids or ovarian peptides. However, the final stages of follicular development and differentiation depend on hormone concentrations and their patterns of secretion, and only if the proper amount, proper patterns of secretion, and proper sequence of hormonal events occur do primordial follicles fully mature and ovulate. Because the primary factor that determines the rate of exhaustion is the rate at which dormant follicles re-awaken and move into the growing pool, this parameter is the critical factor—but probably the most difficult—to study. Some believe that the number of follicles in the primordial endowment is itself the major factor that determines the rate at which follicles begin to grow. According to this theory, and when the follicular reserve goes below a "threshold," regulation is compromised (Krarup *et al.*, 1969). Several studies support this view. Unilateral ovariectomy of older rats, or more drastic ovarian resection, accelerated the loss of the remaining primordial follicles (Meredith & Butcher, 1985; Meredith *et al.*, 1992). Meredith and colleagues (1992) found that unilateral ovariectomy only affected the rate of loss of follicles in older rats. In contrast, no difference was observed in numbers of follicles remaining in the single ovary or their rate of depletion in younger rats. In addition, destruction of a portion of the follicular stockpile by prenatal treatment with busulfan (Hirshfield, 1994) or postnatal treatment with xenobiotics (Krarup *et al.*, 1969), which caused younger animals to have a follicular reserve that was more similar to middle-aged rats, also increased the rate at which the remaining primordial follicles moved into the growing pool. Taken together, these data suggest that a decrease in the number of primordial follicles results in an amplifying cascade that exacerbates the further loss of the follicular reserve.

Declining fertility and fecundity have been well documented prior to the exhaustion of the follicular pool (Santoro et al., 2003). Evidence suggests that the predominant effect of age on fertility is due to abnormalities present in the older oocyte; however, changing uterine receptivity and embryo-uterine crosstalk certainly contribute to the lower rates of fertility and fecundity. Oocytes from normal younger and older reproductive aged women, examined at the second metaphase of meiosis, exhibited distinct structural differences and chromosomal abnormalities (Angell, 1994; Battaglia et al., 1996; Battaglia et al., 1997). The most compelling evidence for an effect of the aging oocyte on female fertility comes from clinical studies of donor oocyte in in vitro fertilization programs. Pregnancy and delivery rates are much more strongly correlated with age of the donor than age of the recipient or the age of the sperm donor (Klein & Soules, 1998).

B. Age-Related Changes in Ovarian Hormone Secretion

For many years, it was thought that decreased estradiol concentrations heralded the onset of the perimenopausal transition and that changes in pituitary gonadotropin levels followed as a result of decreased negative feedback. In fact, we now know that middle-aged women exhibit changes in FSH and inhibin before any obvious change in estradiol occurs (Klein et al., 1996; Reame et al., 1996). In fact, older ovulatory women who continue to have menstrual cycles of normal length show preovulatory urinary estrogen levels that are elevated and rise earlier in the menstrual cycle than younger women (Santoro et al., 1996). Santoro and colleagues found that daily urinary steroid metabolites, estrone conjugates and pregnanediol glucuronide, were higher in premenopausal women 43 years old and older and compared these hormones to women between 19 and 38 years of age during both the follicular and luteal phase of the menstrual cycle (see Figure 21.2). Because FSH levels were also elevated in these women, the change in this hormone may have led to an earlier selection and development of the dominant follicle, which, in turn, could lead to relative increases in early follicular phase estradiol secretion (Klein et al., 1996). It is interesting that elevated estradiol during the early follicular phase rise (i.e., day 3 of the menstrual cycle) is an excellent predictor of a poor response to treatments for infertility (Licciardi et al., 1995). The pattern of age-related changes in estradiol in laboratory rats is strikingly similar to that reported in women: estradiol levels are essentially normal during the middle-age period of time when animals continue to cycle (Lu et al., 1985; Nass et al., 1984; Wise, 1982b;). Thus, in rats as in humans, it is not until the later stages of reproductive senescence that estradiol concentrations are clearly lower than those observed in young (Metcalf et al., 1981; Santoro et al., 1996).

One of the earliest detectable changes in ovarian hormone levels is a change in inhibin levels that are associated with a monotropic rise in FSH concentrations (Klein et al., 1996; MacNaughton et al., 1992) (see Figure 21.3). These data have led to the conclusion that the decrease in the number of primordial and early antral follicles remaining in the ovaries of older women leads to decreased inhibin B concentration. This small rise in the

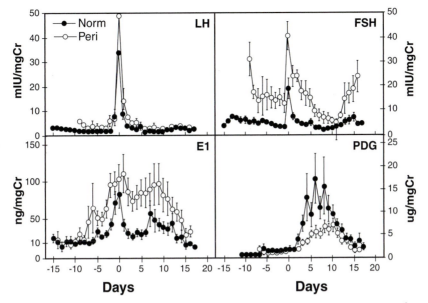

Figure 21.2 Daily urinary gonadotropin and sex steroid secretion patterns in perimenopausal women aged 43 compared to women between 19 and 38 years. Urinary FSH and estrone metabolites are significantly higher in perimenopausal women than in young controls. Data are standardized to day 0, the presumed day of ovulation and expressed as mean ± S.E. From Santoro *et al.*, 1996, Copyright 1996, The Endocrine Society.

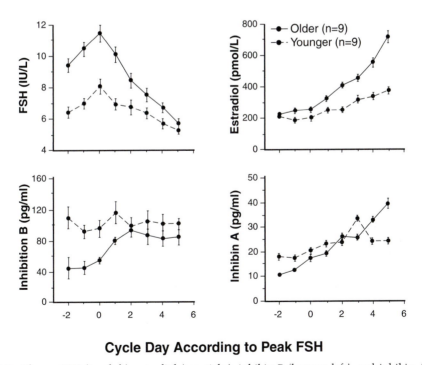

Cycle Day According to Peak FSH

Figure 21.3 Plasma FSH (top left), estradiol (top right), inhibin B (bottom left), and inhibin A (bottom right) in younger (dashed lines) and older (solid lines) women. In older women, FSH concentrations are higher and inhibin B concentrations are lower than in young women. From Klein *et al.*, 1996, Copyright 1996, The Endocrine Society.

concentrations of FSH, unaccompanied by a rise in LH, becomes evident in both women (Klein *et al.*, 1996; Sherman & Korenman, 1975) and laboratory rats (DePaolo & Chappel, 1986) before any overt changes in cycle length. It is not caused by any loss in bioactivity of the FSH molecule, as there is no difference observed in the bioactive:immunoactive FSH ratio between women in their early twenties compared to those in their early forties (Klein *et al.*, 1996). This sentinel change is considered a predictor of impending reproductive decline and the marker that irregularity in cycle length will soon occur. As reproductive aging progresses, LH levels also increase, and changes in the

pattern of LH secretion have been documented prior to the onset of perimenopause (Santoro *et al.*, 1996).

At later stages of the perimenopausal transition and postmenopausal period, multiple ovarian and pituitary hormones (Jaffe, 1999; Sherman *et al.*, 1976) exhibit changes in both concentrations and patterns of secretion. The detailed hormone profiles of Sherman and Korenman over the course of the perimenopausal period in individual women clearly establish that the pattern of ovarian steroid secretion that normally occurs over the course of a month is no longer predictable (see Figure 21.4). The highly

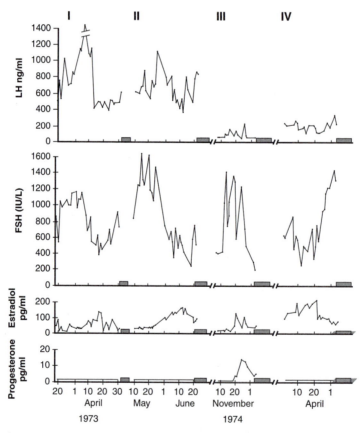

Figure 21.4 Daily concentration of serum luteinizing hormone (LH), follicle stimulating hormone (FSH), estradiol, and progesterone during four cycles in one 49-year-old subject during the menopausal transition. Hormone levels are arrayed by calendar date, and the hatched areas indicate menstruation. During menopausal transition, hormone patterns show discordant regulation relative to the normal menstrual hormone relationship: FSH concentrations are elevated and not inhibited by high estrogen levels, whereas LH levels are in the normal or low range. From Sherman *et al.*, 1976, Copyright 1976, The Endocrine Society.

erratic concentrations, patterns, and relationships among the hormones raises the real possibility that all aspects of the reproductive axis are no longer coordinated in the normal feed-forward and feed-back manner. During postmenopause, estrogens decrease dramatically, and androgens, including testosterone and weaker androgens, decrease to a lesser magnitude (Zumoff *et al.*, 1995). Blood samples drawn from the ovarian vein compared to peripheral concentrations show that the majority of circulating estrogens are derived from peripheral conversion rather than ovarian synthesis (Judd & Korenman, 1982).

V. Role of the Central Nervous System in Female Reproductive Aging

A. Changes in Hypothalamic Signaling Contribute to Reproductive Aging

An alternative perspective that has gained attention is that the brain is a critical partner in reproductive aging: it is a pacemaker in the sequence of events leading to reproductive senescence. Several lines of evidence that will be discussed below support this contention. However, it should be emphasized that ultimately, exhaustion of ovarian follicles limits the reproductive life span. The elegant studies of Nelson, Felicio, and their colleagues emphasize the complexities of the partnership of the central nervous system and the ovary. These studies, performed in mice, led the authors to the conclusion that the hypothalamo-pituitary axis plays a role in the transition from regular to irregular estrous cycles during middle age, but the ovary is the primary factor in timing the actual cessation of ovulatory cycles. Parallel studies have not been performed in rats or nonhuman primate models.

It was once thought that the exhaustion of ovarian follicles was the most important factor leading to the transition to age-related permanent infertility. More recently, we realize that reproductive senescence is more complex and that there are probably multiple pacemakers involved in this process. What is clear from a wealth of data accumulated over many years is that an exquisite temporal order of signaling among the major components of the reproductive axis (brain, anterior pituitary, and ovary) is required for the occurrence of regular reproductive cycles. Of equal importance, the ultradian (intervals of minutes to hours) and diurnal (intervals of 24 hours) patterns and the amplitude of the hormonal excursions influence the regularity of cycles, the terminal stages of ovarian follicular growth and differentiation, and the occurrence of ovulation. Precise synchronization of the orchestrated ultradian, circadian, and infradian (intervals greater than 24 hours) events is the signature of the intricate communication required for successful reproductive cyclicity. Thus, the synthesis and secretion of gonadotropin releasing hormone (GnRH) from neurons within the hypothalamus are regulated by a repertoire of neurotransmitters. Which one(s) are primary and which are permissive are still not completely understood or universally accepted by investigators. The secretory pattern of GnRH determines the level of LH and FSH gene expression, their synthesis, their secretory patterns, the ratio of LH to FSH released, and the density of GnRH receptors in the pituitary gland. In turn, the patterns of gonadotropin secretion determine the success or failure of the final stages of follicular growth, development, and differentiation, and, hence, the pattern of steroid secretion. Most studies would suggest that the hormonal milieu does not influence the re-entry of dormant primordial follicles into the growing pool and/or the initial stages of growth from primordial to primary or secondary follicles. However, controversy remains in this realm, and the final conclusions are not clear at the present time. The nature of steroid feedback— negative and positive—to the level of the anterior pituitary gland and hypothalamus is determined not only by the levels of steroid, but the duration of the elevation in steroid secretion and the ratio of estrogens/progestins and the temporal order of increases in these two steroids (see Knobil & Neill, 1994, for excellent chapter reviews of each of these topics).

Subtle changes in the temporal pattern and synchrony of neurochemical and neuroendocrine signals become detectable during middle age in both women (Matt et al., 1998) and laboratory animal models (Wise et al., 1997). They precede the cessation of reproductive cycles and may explain the accelerated loss of follicles that occurs during the perimenopausal period. The dynamics of specific neurotransmitters that regulate the secretion of GnRH changes with age (discussed below). However, the body of data suggests that it is more than any single neurotransmitter or neuropeptide that determines the role of the central nervous system in female reproductive aging. Multiple studies demonstrate that the temporal order and the pattern of multiple signals are altered during aging. These observations suggest that the dampening and desynchronization of the precisely orchestrated ultradian, circadian, and infradian neural signals lead to miscommunication between the brain and the pituitary-ovarian axis. In turn, an increasing desynchronization of neuroendocrine signals may contribute to the accelerated rate of follicular loss and the decreasing frequency of regular cycles that occurs during middle age.

Direct measurement of neurotransmitter dynamics (e.g., release, the density of receptors, uptake of neurotransmitters at post-synaptic sites, and re-uptake at pre-synaptic sites) over a prolonged period remains methodologically impossible in humans. Perhaps in the future, in vivo imaging methods will allow us to monitor these changes in real time. However, until now, virtually all of the work that forms the foundation of this research has been performed in laboratory animal models. Studies in young, middle-aged, and old animals have revealed that age-related changes are progressive and more exaggerated in older rats that had completed the transition to acyclicity. These changes are subtle: investigators who measured indices of neural function at any one time of day in aging animals are unlikely to detect significant differences among age groups. However, together, disruption of the synchrony and coordination of multiple neural signals that regulate the precise timing of GnRH release may ultimately lead to important changes in the ability of rats to maintain regular estrous cycles.

B. Pituitary Hormone Secretion as a Surrogate of Brain Aging

GnRH is the primary hypothalamic hormone that regulates both LH and FSH secretion. In turn, its synthesis and secretion is regulated by a panoply of neurotransmitters and by estradiol negative feedback. Unfortunately, GnRH is not detectable in peripheral plasma because high concentrations exist only in the hypophysial portal blood, into which it is secreted from terminal boutons in the median eminence of the hypothalamus. Therefore, pulsatile patterns of secretion of LH have been used as a surrogate and are thought to reflect changes in the pattern of secretion of GnRH (Levine & Duffy, 1988). Changes in pulse amplitude can result from changes at the hypothalamic and/or pituitary level, whereas changes in the inter-pulse interval and duration of pulses are thought to reflect more purely changes in the hypothalamic pulse generator and the accuracy with which it generates discrete, robust signals.

Changes in the patterns of pulsatile LH secretion have been detected in both perimenopausal women and middle-aged rats. In women, reports of changes in the pattern of pulsatility are contradictory. Matt and colleagues (1998) reported that in middle-aged women whose menstrual cycles remain the normal length, the frequency of LH pulses decreases and the width of the peak increases prior to any change in plasma estradiol. However, when the menstrual cycle length shortens, Reame and colleagues (1996) reported that LH pulse frequency was higher in older women. Similar changes have been reported in rodent models. Scarbrough and Wise (1990) monitored pulsatile LH release in ovariectomized young and middle-aged rats and found that the inter-pulse interval and average duration of individual pulses increased (see Figure 21.5). As in studies performed in women, these results from studies performed in rats strongly suggest that subtle changes in the integrity of the GnRH pulse generator occur early, prior to the transition from regular to irregular cycles, and may be a component of the cascade of events that contribute to reproductive aging.

C. GnRH Secretion During Aging

As we focus our attention on potential changes that occur at the level of the central nervous system, it is important to emphasize that virtually all of these studies have been performed in laboratory rodents. Very recently, Gore and colleagues (2004) have published work on changes in pulsatile GnRH secretion in the aging female Rhesus monkey. It is possible that not all of the factors that regulate GnRH secretion in rodents and nonhuman primates are identical to those that regulate secretion in humans. However, these species have been excellent experimental models and have provided important insights into the mechanisms and factors that regulate development of the reproductive system, puberty, and maintenance of regular cycles in the adult. We anticipate that the information gained from these species can be applied to humans and will provide an understanding that can be generalized to human reproductive aging.

Even in rodent models, it has been problematic to monitor GnRH activity and secretion. Only between 1,000 to 2,000 GnRH neurons exist in the brain, and they are widely and diffusely distributed through the septo-preoptico-infundibular pathway of rodents and the medial basal hypothalamus of humans (Silverman, 1994). Furthermore, because GnRH receptors are expressed in diverse regions of the brain that do not appear to be in anatomical locations that could influence pituitary gonadotropin secretion, it is thought that GnRH may have multiple functions, not all of which are directly related to gonadotropin secretion. We do not know whether anatomically distinct subpopulations of GnRH neurons are specifically dedicated to regulating LH and FSH, although recent data (Petersen *et al.*, 1993; Rance & Uswandi, 1996) suggest that they may exist. For all of these reasons, it has been extremely difficult to correlate GnRH activity patterns over time in individual animals under controlled experimental conditions, although a few investigators have successfully achieved this technically challenging feat in rats (e.g., Levine & Duffy, 1988; Levine & Ramirez, 1982; Rubin & Bridges, 1989) and monkeys (Terasawa, 1995). Other methods, including quantitation of

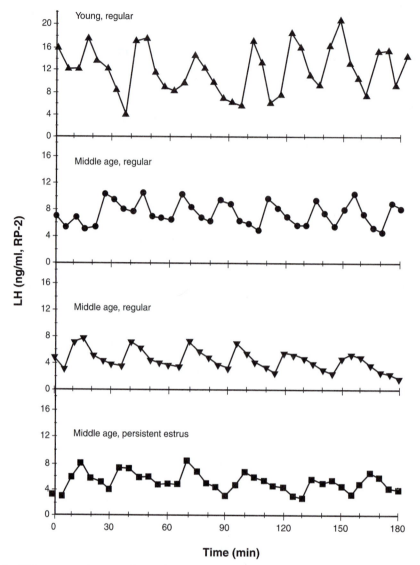

Figure 21.5 LH concentrations are shown from a representative young regularly cycling and middle-aged rats at various stages of reproductive senescence (regularly cycling, irregularly cycling, and acyclic persistent estrous). All rats were ovariectomized for four weeks prior to blood collection. Blood samples were collected at five-minute intervals for a three-hour period. From Scarbrough & Wise, 1990, Copyright 190; The Endocrine Society.

mRNA levels to assess gene expression and use of dual label immunocytochemistry to identify fos expression in GnRH neurons, an index of activation, have allowed us to monitor the activity of GnRH neurons in aging animals. Rubin and Bridges (1989) reported alterations in GnRH release from the mediobasal hypothalamus of steroid-primed middle-aged rats, as monitored by push-pull cannula methods. These functional changes become apparent prior to any detectable change in the number of immunoreactive GnRH neurons (Lloyd et al., 1994), in morphology or distribution of GnRH neurons of aging male rats (Witkin, 1987), or any age-related differences in the distribution of GnRH-immunoreactive forms expressed in GnRH neurons (Hoffman & Finch, 1986). Thus, functional changes in GnRH neurons appear to precede changes in the ability to maintain regular estrous cyclicity and appear to be a more sensitive measure of the status of GnRH neuronal activity than morphological criteria or alterations in the absolute concentrations of GnRH.

Equivalent studies are impossible in humans. To our knowledge, only two investigations that assessed GnRH have been performed in human females. Both monitored GnRH in postmenopausal women; no studies have assessed GnRH neuronal changes prior to or during the perimenopausal transition. The existing data are contradictory: Parker and Porter (1984) reported that radioimmunoassayable GnRH concentrations in the mediobasal hypothalamus were lower in postmenopausal women than in young. More recently, Rance and Uswandi (1996) found that GnRH mRNA levels in the tuberoinfundibular region were elevated in postmenopausal women. A possible interpretation of these seemingly contradictory findings is that, in the presence of low estrogen characteristic of the postmenopausal state, transcription of the GnRH gene increases, and release of the peptide is elevated to an even greater extent, such that steady-state mRNA levels are elevated but the stored pool of GnRH in the mediobasal hypothalamus is lower than in young women. Obviously much more needs to be done before we can clearly interpret these data or draw conclusions as to the factors that lead to such changes.

Observations that rhythmicity is altered have led investigators to question whether deterioration of a master pacemaker may explain the desynchronization of multiple neuroendocrine rhythms. The suprachiasmatic nucleus (SCN) of the hypothalamus is considered the master circadian pacemaker, or biological clock, in mammals (Moore-Ede et al., 1982; Turek & Van Cauter, 1994). These bilateral nuclei, which are located at the base of the brain dorsal to the optic chiasm, exhibit endogenous circadian rhythmicity: they continue to exhibit circadian electrophysiological activity and neuropeptide secretion patterns even when removed and maintained in vitro (Turek, 1985). Neurons from the SCN communicate extensively with each other, send efferents to many regions of the brain, and drive the timing of multiple outputs so that almost all physiological functions show a pervasive daily rhythm. For the female reproductive system to maintain regular cycles, the circadian system must be intact. This is most evident in laboratory animals that are maintained in controlled laboratory conditions (Everett & Sawyer, 1950; Legan & Karsch, 1975). However, even in humans where activity and light-dark and sleep-wake cycles are not rigorously controlled, reproductive functions exhibit a diurnal rhythmicity (Casper et al., 1988; Czeisler et al., 1990; Khoury et al., 1987; Testart et al., 1982). The biochemical mechanism by which time-of-day information is transmitted from the SCN to other regions of the brain is through several key neuropeptides. They are an integral part of the inputs or outputs of the clock. The SCN sends projections directly to GnRH neurons (Hoorneman & Buijs, 1982; van der Beek et al., 1993) and may communicate temporal information to the reproductive axis. Thus, deterioration in this neural pacemaker or the coupling to its outputs may initiate the gradual disintegration of the temporal organization of neurotransmitter rhythms that are critical for stable, precise, and regular cyclic GnRH secretion. In turn, this deterioration and desynchronization of multiple neuropeptides of the clock may initiate a cascade that leads to the transition to irregular cycles and ultimately contributes to acyclicity. Several lines of evidence suggest that aging results in a decline of this critical master pacemaker and that this leads to a desynchronization of multiple physiological rhythms, including ones that are required for cyclic gonadotropin secretion and follicular development and differentiation.

Numerous reports that multiple circadian rhythms are compromised in aging organisms support the concept that the clock itself or its coupling to an array of outputs may deteriorate with age: the period of rhythms decrease, the phase of many outputs of the clock advances, and the amplitude of multiple rhythms is attenuated with age (see Figure 21.6) (for review, see Brock, 1991; Richardson, 1990). In addition, temporal desynchronization of two or more rhythms, fragmentation of circadian rhythms, and altered responsiveness to stimuli that induce phase shifts are a common occurrence in older organisms. Thus, declining reproductive function may be only one of many physiological endpoints to suffer from the fragmentation of temporal organization of physiological functions.

There appears to be a difference between aging of the reproductive system in humans and rats in the secretory patterns of LH. In women, most reports suggest that the average plasma LH levels do not rise until later during the menopausal transition, despite alterations in FSH secretion. Korenman and colleagues (1978) monitored LH levels in individual women over several months during the perimenopausal transition. These studies show that LH levels are highly variable during this period and cannot be consistently explained by the changes in estradiol negative or positive feedback. No changes have been observed in the average concentrations of LH secreted during the preovulatory surge (Klein et al., 1996;

Korenman et al., 1978). In contrast, in rats, the preovulatory LH surge is both delayed and attenuated in middle-aged rats prior to overt changes in the length or regularity of the LH surge (Cooper et al., 1980; Nass et al., 1984; Wise, 1982a). Intriguingly, Nass and colleagues (1984) found that regularly cycling rats that were destined to become irregular cyclers exhibited delayed and attenuated LH release compared to those that would continue to cycle for at least the following six months.

D. Multiple Neurotransmitters that Regulate GnRH Change with Age

Changes in the pattern of GnRH expression and secretion may result from changes in one or more of the repertoire of neurotransmitters and neuropeptides that modulate neuronal activity. Investigators have examined monoamine activity, neurotransmitter receptor densities, and the gene expression of some of the neuropeptide neuromodulators of GnRH. It appears that during middle age, the diurnal rhythmicity in the activity of many neurotransmitters, the density of their receptors, and/or the level of gene expression is dampened or undetectable in hypothalamic regions involved in regulating the pattern of GnRH neuronal activity. Age-related changes have been detectable by the time animals were middle-aged, as they were entering the transition to irregular cycles. For example, changes in the pattern of proopiomelanocortin (POMC) gene expression can be used as an example of the many neurochemical events that exhibit changes in rhythmicity. In young rats, POMC gene expression exhibited a diurnal rhythm (see Figure 21.7). This rhythm was undetectable when rats were middle-aged or older. Similar age-related changes have been reported in many of the neuromodulators of GnRH release. Thus, it would appear that, during middle age,

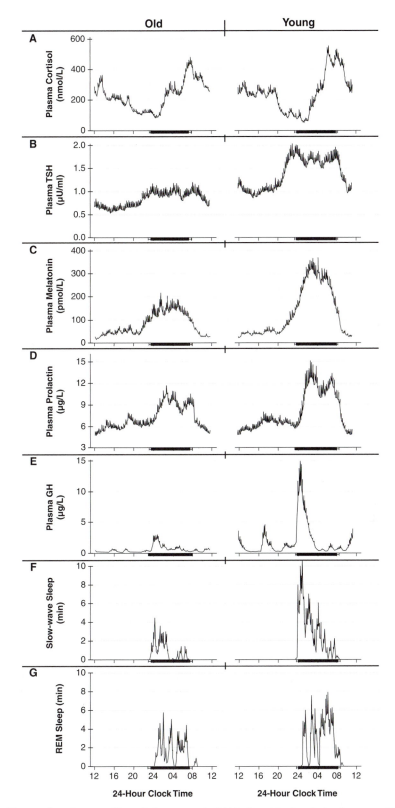

Figure 21.6 Twenty-four-hour profiles of plasma cortisol (A), thyroid-stimulating hormone TSH (B), melatonin (C), prolactin (D), and growth hormone (GH) (E) levels and distribution of slow wave (SW) (F), and rapid-eye movement (REM) (G) stages in old and young subjects. Distribution of sleep stages is expressed in minutes in each 15-minute interval between blood samplings spent in SW or REM stage. Mean ± S.E. black bars correspond to mean sleep period. From van Coevorden *et al.*, 1991, Copyright 1991, The American Physiological Society.

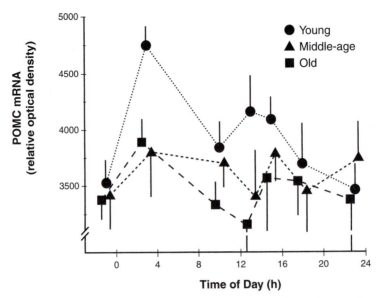

Figure 21.7 Proopiomelanocortin (POMC) mRNA concentrations in the arcuate nucleus of young (circles), middle-aged (triangles), and old (squares) rats. In young rats, POMC mRNA levels exhibit diurnal rhythmicity. This rhythm disappears by the time animals become middle-aged (mean ± S.E.). From Weiland *et al.*, 1992, Copyright 1992, The Endocrine Society.

the precise, synchronized, and interactive patterns of hypothalamic neurotransmitter and neuropeptide activity, which are critical to maintain a specific pattern of GnRH secretion, become less ordered. Similar changes may occur in humans and may be manifested by the occurrence of hot flushes, a hallmark of deterioration of the hypothalamic thermoregulatory centers. Some researchers propose that this deterioration in communication among the neurotransmitters that regulate GnRH secretion causes the initial changes in patterns of gonadotropin secretion and that these changes herald the imminent transition to the perimenopausal state.

VI. Conclusion

In summary, considerable evidence has accumulated that both the ovary and the brain exhibit changes during aging. The most recent studies show that multiple

events at different levels of the reproductive axis lead to reproductive decline. The roles of the brain and ovary may be different: the brain may be more involved in the initial deterioration in reproductive cycle regularity, whereas the ovarian follicular reserve may be the ultimate driver of the cessation in cyclicity. Our goals for the future are to better understand the repertoire of factors that interact to maintain regular reproductive cyclicity and how this dynamic balance changes with age. It will be important to determine which alterations are primary and cause decline in reproduction and which are secondary correlates of the primary changes.

References

Angell, R. (1994). Aneuploidy in older women. *Human Reproduction, 9,* 119–1201.

Battaglia, D., Goodwin, P., Klein, N., & Soules, M. (1996). Influence of maternal age on meiotic spindle assembly in oocytes from naturally cycling women. *Human Reproduction*, 11, 2217–2222.

Battaglia, D. E., Klein, N. A., & Soules, M. R. (1997). Changes in centrosomal domains during meiotic maturation in the human oocyte. *Molecular Human Reproduction*, 2, 845–851.

Bellino, F. L. (2000). Nonprimate animal models of menopause: workshop report. *Menopause*, 7, 14–24.

Block, E. (1952). Quantitative morphological investigations of the follicular system in women. Variations at different ages. *Acta Anatomica*, 14, 108–123.

Brock, M. A. (1991). Chronobiology and aging. *Journal of the American Geriatrics Society*, 39, 74–91.

Casper, R. F., Erskine, H. J., Armstrong, D. T., Brown, S. E., Daniel, S. A., Graves, G. R., & Yuzpe, A. A. (1988). *In vitro* fertilization: diurnal and seasonal variation in luteinizing hormone surge onset and pregnancy rates. *Fertility and Sterility*, 49, 644–648.

Cooper, R. L., Conn, P. M., & Walker, R. F. (1980). Characterization of the LH surge in middle-aged female rats. *Biology of Reproduction*, 23, 611–615.

Costoff, A., & Mahesh, V. B. (1975). Primordial follicles with normal oocytes in the ovaries of postmenopausal women. *Journal of the American Geriatrics Society*, 23, 193–196.

Crowley, W. F. Jr., Filicori, M., Spratt, D. I., & Santoro, N. F. (1985). The physiology of gonadotropin-releasing hormone (GnRH) secretion in men and women. *Recent Progress in Hormone Research*, 41, 473–531.

Czeisler, C. A., Rogacz, S., & Duffy, J. F. (1990). Reproductive function in women: circadian interaction. In F. Naftolin, J. N. Gutmann, A. H. DeCherney, & P. M. Sarrel (Eds.), *Ovarian secretions and cardiovascular and neurological function* (Serono Symposia Publications, Vol. 80, pp. 239–247). New York: Raven Press.

DePaolo, L. V., & Chappel, S. C. (1986). Alterations in the secretion and production of follicle-stimulating hormone precede age-related lengthening of estrous cycles in rats. *Endocrinology*, 118, 1127–1133.

Everett, J. W., & Sawyer, C. H. (1950). A 24-hour periodicity in the "LH-release

apparatus" of female rats, disclosed by barbiturate sedation. *Endocrinology*, 47, 198–218.

Faddy, M. J., Telfer, E., & Gosden, R. G. (1987). The kinetics of pre-antral follicle development in ovaries of CBA/Ca mice during the first 14 weeks of life. *Cell and Tissue Kinetics*, 20, 551–560.

Felicio, L. S., Nelson, J. F., & Finch, C. E. (1986). Prolongation and cessation of estrous cycles in aging C57BL/6J mice are differentially regulated events. *Biology of Reproduction*, 34, 849–858.

Gilardi, K. V., Shideler, S. E., Valverde, C. R., Roberts, J. A., & Lasley, B. L. (1997). Characterization of the onset of menopause in the rhesus macaque. *Biology of Reproduction*, 57, 335–340.

Gore, A. C., Windsor-Engnell, B. M., & Terasawa, E. (2004). Menopausal increases in pulsatile GnRH release in a non-human primate (*Macaca mulatta*). *Endocrinology*, 145, 4653–4659.

Gosden, R. G., Laing, S. C., Felicio, L. S., Nelson, J. F., & Finch, C. E. (1983). Imminent oocyte exhaustion and reduced follicular recruitment mark the transition to acyclicity in aging C57BL/6J mice. *Biology of Reproduction*, 28, 255–260.

Gougeon, A. (1996). Regulation of ovarian follicular development in primates: facts and hypotheses. *Endocrine Reviews*, 17, 121–155.

Gougeon, A., Ecochard, R., & Thalabard, J. C. (1994). Age-related changes of the population of human ovarian follicles: increase in the disappearance rate of non-growing and early-growing follicles in aging women. *Biology of Reproduction*, 50, 653–663.

Gould, K. G., Flint, M., & Graham, C. E. (1981). Chimpanzee reproductive senescence: a possible model for evolution of the menopause. *Maturitas*, 3, 157–166.

Graham, C. E., Kling, O. R., & Steiner, R. A. (1979). Reproductive senescence in female non-human primates. In D. M. Bowden (Ed.), *Aging in non-human primates* (pp. 183–202). New York: Van Nostrand Reinhold.

Hirshfield, A. N. (1991). Development of follicles in the mammalian ovary. *International Review of Cytology*, 124, 43–101.

Hirshfield, A. N. (1994). Relationship between the supply of primordial follicles and the onset of follicular growth in rats. *Biology of Reproduction*, 50, 421–428.

Hodgen, G. D., Goodman, A. L., O'Connor, A., & Johnson, D. K. (1977). Menopause in rhesus monkeys: model for study of disorders in the human climacteric. *American Journal of Obstetrics and Gynecology*, 127, 581–584.

Hoffman, G. E., & Finch, C. E. (1986). LHRH neurons in the female C57BL/6J mouse brain during reproductive aging: no loss up to middle age. *Neurobiology of Aging*, 7, 45–48.

Hoorneman, E. M. D., & Buijs, R. M. (1982). Vasopressin fiber pathways in the rat brain following suprachiasmatic nucleus lesioning. *Brain Research*, 243, 235–241.

Jaffe, R. B. (1999). Menopause and aging. In Yen, S. S. C. & Jaffe, R. B. (Ed.), *Reproductive endocrinology physiology, pathophysiology, and clinical management* (pp. 301–319). Philadelphia: W.B. Saunders.

Johnson, J., Canning, J., Kaneko, T., Pru, J. K., & Tilly, J. L. (2004). Germline stem cells and follicular renewal in the postnatal mammalian ovary. *Nature*, 428, 145–150.

Judd, H. L., & Korenman, S. G. (1982). Effects of aging on reproductive function in women. In S. G. Korenman (Ed.), *Endocrine aspects of aging* (pp. 163–197). New York: Elsevier Science Publishing Company.

Khoury, S. A., Reame, N. E., Kelch, R. P., & Marshall, J. C. (1987). Diurnal patterns of pulsatile luteinizing hormone secretion in hypothalamic amenorrhea: reproducibility and responses to opiate blockade and an alpha2-adrenergic agonist. *Journal of Clinical Endocrinology and Metabolism*, 64, 755–762.

Klein, N. A., & Soules, M. R. (1998). Endocrine changes of the perimenopause. *Clinical Obstetrics and Gynecology*, 41, 912–920.

Klein, N. A., Illingworth, P. J., Groome, N. P., McNeilly, A. S., Battaglia, D. E., & Soules, M. R. (1996). Decreased inhibin B secretion is associated with the monotropic FSH rise in older, ovulatory women: a study of serum and follicular fluid levels of dimeric inhibin A and B in spontaneous menstrual cycles. *Journal of Clinical Endocrinology and Metabolism*, 81, 2742–2745.

Knobil, E., & Neill, J. D. (1994). *The physiology of reproduction*, 2nd ed. New York: Raven Press.

Korenman, S. G., Sherman, B. M., & Korenman, J. C. (1978). Reproductive hormone function: the perimenopausal period and beyond. *Clinics in Endocrinology and Metabolism*, 7, 625–643.

Krarup, T., Pedersen, T., & Faber, M. (1969). Regulation of oocyte growth in the mouse ovary. *Nature*, 224, 187–188.

Legan, S. J., & Karsch, F. J. (1975). A daily signal for the LH surge in the rat. *Endocrinology*, 96, 57–62.

Levine, J. E., & Duffy, M. T. (1988). Simultaneous measurement of luteinizing hormone (LH)-releasing hormone, LH, and follicle-stimulating hormone release in intact and short-term castrate rats. *Endocrinology*, 122, 2211–2221.

Levine, J. E., & Ramirez, V. D. (1982). Luteinizing hormone-releasing hormone release during the rat estrous cycle and after ovariectomy, as estimated with push-pull cannulae. *Endocrinology*, 111, 1439–1448.

Licciardi, F., Liu, H., & Rosewaks, Z. (1995). Day 3 estradiol serum concentrations as prognosticators of ovarian stimulation response and pregnancy outcome in patients undergoing *in vitro* fertilization. *Fertility and Sterility*, 64, 991–994.

Lloyd, J. M., Hoffman, G. E., & Wise, P. M. (1994). Decline in immediate early gene expression in gonadotropin-releasing hormone neurons during proestrus in regularly cycling, middle-aged rats. *Endocrinology*, 134, 1800–1805.

Lobo, R. A. (1998). The perimenopause. *Clinical Obstetrics and Gynecology*, 41, 895–897.

Lu, J. K. H., Lapolt, P. S., Nass, T. E., Matt, D. W., & Judd, H. L. (1985). Relation of circulating estradiol and progesterone to gonadotropin secretion and estrous cyclicity in aging female rats. *Endocrinology*, 116, 1953–1959.

MacNaughton, J., Banah, M., McCloud, P., Hee, J., & Burger, H. (1992). Age related changes in follicle stimulating hormone, luteinizing hormone, oestradiol and immunoreactive inhibin in women of reproductive age. *Clinical Endocrinology*, 36, 339–345.

Matt, D. W., Kauma, S. W., Pincus, S. M., Veldhuis, J. D., & Evans, W. S. (1998). Characteristics of luteinizing hormone secretion in younger versus older premenopausal women. *American Journal of Obstetrics and Gynecology*, 178, 504–510.

Meredith, S., & Butcher, R. L. (1985). Role of decreased numbers of follicles on reproductive performance in young and aged rats. *Biology of Reproduction*, 32, 788–794.

Meredith, S., Dudenhoeffer, G., Butcher, R. L., Lerner, S. P., & Walls, T. (1992). Unilateral Ovariectomy increases loss of primordial follicles and is associated with increased metestrous concentration of follicle-stimulating hormone in old rats. *Biology of Reproduction*, 47, 162–168.

Metcalf, M. G., Donald, R. A., & Livesey, J. H. (1981). Pituitary-ovarian function in normal women during the menopausal transition. *Clinical Endocrinology*, 14, 245–255.

Moore-Ede, M. C., Sulzman, F. M., & Fuller, C. A. (1982). Characteristics of circadian clocks. In M. C. Moore-Ede, F. M. Sulzman, & C. A. Fuller (Eds.), *The clocks that time us* (pp. 30–112). Cambridge, MA: Harvard University Press.

Nass, T. E., Lapolt, P. S., Judd, H. L., & Lu, J. K. H. (1984). Alterations in ovarian steroid and gonadotrophin secretion preceding the cessation of regular oestrous cycles in ageing female rats. *Journal of Endocrinology*, 100, 43–50.

Parker, C. R. Jr., & Porter, J. C. (1984). Luteinizing hormone-releasing hormone and thyrotropin-releasing hormone in the hypothalamus of women: effects of age and reproductive status. *Journal of Clinical Endocrinology and Metabolism*, 58, 488–491.

Petersen, S. L., McCrone, S., Coy, D., Adelman, J. P., & Mahan, L. C. (1993). GABA$_A$ receptor subunit mRNAs in cells of the preoptic area: colocalization with LHRH mRNA using dual-label *in situ* hybridization histochemistry. *Endocrine Journal*, 1, 29–34.

Prior, J. C. (1998). Perimenopause: the complex endocrinology of the menopausal transition. *Endocrine Reviews*, 19, 397–428.

Rance, N. E., & Uswandi, S. V. (1996). Gonadotropin-releasing hormone gene expression is increased in the medial basal hypothalamus of postmenopausal women. *Journal of Clinical Endocrinology and Metabolism*, 81, 3540–3546.

Reame, N. E., Kelch, R. P., Beitins, I. Z., Yu, M.-Y., Zawacki, C. M., & Padmanabhan, V. (1996). Age effects on follicle-stimulating hormone and pulsatile luteinizing hormone secretion across the menstrual cycle of premenopausal women. *Journal of Clinical Endocrinology and Metabolism*, 81, 1512–1518.

Richardson, G. S. (1990). Circadian rhythms and aging. In E. L. Schneider & J. W Rowe (Eds.), *Handbook of the biology of aging* (pp. 275–305). New York: Academic Press.

Richardson, S. J., Senikas, V., & Nelson, J. F. (1987). Follicular depletion during the menopausal transition: evidence for accelerated loss and ultimate exhaustion. *Journal of Clinical Endocrinology and Metabolism*, 65, 1231–1237.

Rubin, B. S., & Bridges, R. S. (1989). Alterations in luteinizing hormone-releasing hormone release from the mediobasal hypothalamus of ovariectomized, steroid-primed middle-aged rats as measured by push-pull perfusion. *Neuroendocrinology*, 49, 225–232.

Santoro, N., Brown, J. R., Adel, T., & Skurnick, J. H. (1996). Characterization of reproductive hormonal dynamics in the perimenopause. *Journal of Clinical Endocrinology and Metabolism*, 81, 1495–1501.

Santoro, N., Isaac, B., Neal-Perry, G., Tovaghol, A., Weigel, L., Nussbaum, A., Thakur, S., Jinnai, H., Khosla, N., & Barad, D. (2003). Impaired folliculogenesis and ovulation in older reproductive aged women. *Journal of Clinical Endocrinology and Metabolism*, 88, 5502–5509.

Scarbrough, K., & Wise, P. M. (1990). Age-related changes in the pulsatile pattern of LH release precede the transition to estrous acyclicity and depend upon estrous cycle history. *Endocrinology*, 126, 884–890.

Sherman, B. M., & Korenman, S. G. (1975). Hormonal characteristics of the human menstrual cycle throughout reproductive life. *Journal of Clinical Investigation*, 55, 699–706.

Sherman, B. M., West, J. H., & Korenman, S. G. (1976). The menopausal transition: analysis of LH, FSH, estradiol, and progesterone concentrations during menstrual cycles of older women. *Journal of Clinical Endocrinology and Metabolism*, 42, 629–636.

Shideler, S. E., DeVane, G. W., Kalra, P. S., Benirschke, K., & Lasley, B. L. (1989). Ovarian-pituitary hormone interactions during the perimenopause. *Maturitas*, 11, 331–339.

Shideler, S. E., Gee, N. A., Chen, J., & Lasley, B. L. (2001). Estrogen and progesterone metabolites and follicle stimulating hormone in the aged macaque female. *Biology of Reproduction*, 65, 1718–1725.

Silverman, A.-J. (1994). The gonadotropin-releasing hormone (GnRH) neuronal systems: immunocytochemistry and *in situ* hybridization. In E. Knobil & J. Neill (Eds.), *The physiology of reproduction* (pp. 1683–1709). New York: Raven Press.

Terasawa, E. (1995). Control of luteinizing hormone-releasing hormone pulse generation in nonhuman primates. *Cellular and Molecular Neurobiology*, 15, 141–163.

Testart, J., Frydman, R., & Roger, M. (1982). Seasonal influence of diurnal rhythms in the onset of the plasma luteinizing hormone surge in women. *Journal of Clinical Endocrinology and Metabolism*, 55, 374–377.

Treloar, A. E. (1981). Menstrual activity and the pre-menopause. *Maturitas*, 3, 249–264.

Treloar, A. E., Boynton, R. E., Behn, B. G., & Brown, B. W. (1967). Variation of the human menstrual cycle through reproductive life. *International Journal of Fertility*, 12, 77–126.

Turek, F. W. (1985). Circadian neural rhythms in mammals. *Annual Review of Physiology*, 47, 49–64.

Turek, F. W., & Van Cauter, E. (1994). Rhythms in reproduction. In E. Knobil & J. Neill (Eds.), *The physiology of reproduction* (pp. 487–540). New York: Raven Press.

van Coevorden, A., Mockel, J., Laurent, E., Kerkhofs, M., L'Hermite-Baleriaux, M., Decoster, C., Neve, P., & Van Cauter, E. (1991). Neuroendocrine rhythms and sleep in aging men. *American Journal of Physiology*, 260, E651–E661.

van der Beek, E. M., Wiegant, V. M., van der Donk, H. A., van den Hurk, R., & Buijs, R. M. (1993). Lesions of the suprachiasmatic nucleus indicate the presence of a direct vasoactive intestinal polypeptide-containing projection to gonadotropin-releasing hormone neurons in the female rat. *Journal of Neuroendocrinology*, 5, 137–144.

Weiland, N. G., Scarbrough, K., & Wise, P. M. (1992). Aging abolishes the estradiol-induced suppression and diurnal rhythm of proopiomelanocortin gene expression in the arcuate nucleus. *Endocrinology*, 131, 2959–2964.

Wise, P. M. (1982a). Alterations in proestrous LH, FSH, and prolactin surges in middle-aged rats. *Proceedings of the Society for Experimental Biology and Medicine*, 169, 348–354.

Wise, P. M. (1982b). Alterations in the proestrous pattern of median eminence LHRH, serum LH, FSH, estradiol and progesterone concentrations in middle-aged rats. *Life Sciences*, 31, 165–173.

Wise, P. M., Kashon, M. L., Krajnak, K. M., Rosewell, K. L., Cai, A., Scarbrough, K., Harney, J. P., McShane, T., Lloyd, J., & Weiland, N. G. (1997). Aging of the female reproductive system: a window into brain aging. *Recent Progress in Hormone Research*, 52, 279–305.

Witkin, J. W. (1987). Aging changes in synaptology of luteinizing hormone-releasing hormone neurons in male rat preoptic area. *Neuroscience*, 22, 1003–1013.

Zumoff, B., Strain, G., Miller, L., & Rosner, W. (1995). Twenty-four hour mean plasma testosterone concentration declines with age in normal premenopausal women. *Journal of Clinical Endocrinology and Metabolism*, 80, 1429–1430.

Author Index

Numbers in italics refer to the pages on which the complete references are listed.

Subject Index